Springer Series in Biomaterials Science and Engineering

Volume 10

Series editor

Prof. Min Wang, Department of Mechanical Engineering
The University of Hong Kong, Pokfulam Road, Hong Kong
e-mail: memwang@hku.hk

Aims and Scope

The Springer Series in Biomaterials Science and Engineering addresses the manufacture, structure and properties, and applications of materials that are in contact with biological systems, temporarily or permanently. It deals with many aspects of modern biomaterials, from basic science to clinical applications, as well as host responses. It covers the whole spectrum of biomaterials—polymers, metals, glasses and ceramics, and composites/hybrids—and includes both biological materials (collagen, polysaccharides, biological apatites, etc.) and synthetic materials. The materials can be in different forms: single crystals, polycrystalline materials, particles, fibers/wires, coatings, non-porous materials, porous scaffolds, etc. New and developing areas of biomaterials, such as nano-biomaterials and diagnostic and therapeutic nanodevices, are also focuses in this series. Advanced analytical techniques that are applicable in R&D and theoretical methods and analyses for bio-materials are also important topics. Frontiers in nanomedicine, regenerative medicine and other rapidly advancing areas calling for great explorations are highly relevant.

The Springer Series in Biomaterials Science and Engineering aims to provide critical reviews of important subjects in the field, publish new discoveries and significant progresses that have been made in both biomaterials development and the advancement of principles, theories and designs, and report cutting-edge research and relevant technologies. The individual volumes in the series are thematic. The goal of each volume is to give readers a comprehensive overview of an area where new knowledge has been gained and insights made. Significant topics in the area are dealt with in good depth and future directions are predicted on the basis of current developments. As a collection, the series provides authoritative works to a wide audience in academia, the research community, and industry.

More information about this series at http://www.springer.com/series/10955

Jing Liu · Liting Yi

Liquid Metal Biomaterials

Principles and Applications

Springer

Jing Liu
Department of Biomedical Engineering
Tsinghua University
Beijing, China

Liting Yi
Technical Institute of Physics and Chemistry
Chinese Academy of Sciences
Beijing, China

ISSN 2195-0644 ISSN 2195-0652 (electronic)
Springer Series in Biomaterials Science and Engineering
ISBN 978-981-10-5606-2 ISBN 978-981-10-5607-9 (eBook)
https://doi.org/10.1007/978-981-10-5607-9

Library of Congress Control Number: 2018948625

This Springer imprint is published by the registered company Springer Nature Singapore Pte Ltd.
The registered company address is: 152 Beach Road, #21-01/04 Gateway East, Singapore 189721, Singapore

Preface

Conventional biomaterials like metals, polymers, composites, ceramics, and those naturally derived matters may encounter medical challenges sometimes. At around body temperature, most of such materials especially metals mainly stay at solid state and are often difficult to shape due to their high melting point. Meanwhile, although classical electrolyte solutions own perfect flexibility, their electrical conductivities appear rather low which evidently restricted their utilizations to compose medical devices. From an alternative, the newly emerging liquid metal materials, such as gallium, bismuth, or their alloy which could easily switch between liquid and solid state at around room temperature, are becoming powerful new generation functional materials and have increasingly displayed many unconventional properties superior than that of traditional biomaterials. This is because liquid metal simultaneously owns a great many capabilities like high fluidity, excellent electrical and thermal conductivities, good biocompatibility, outstanding radiopacity, controllable behaviors accompanied with reversible liquid–solid phase transition, easy manufacture, and low cost. Such unique versatile features as "One material, diverse capabilities" are rather unusual among many existing top materials. It is for this reason that liquid metals are reshaping modern sciences and technologies and have in fact demonstrated surprising virtues in tackling a wide variety of tough biomedical challenges which are hard to solve otherwise.

To push forward further researches and rapid applications along the above important frontier, this book is dedicated to draft a new biomedical category: the liquid metal biomaterials. The major advancements as achieved before will be summarized, and future directions worth of pursuing will be outlined. Representative applications enabled by liquid metal biomaterials from both therapeutic and diagnostic aspects will be reviewed. Particularly, endeavors will be made to interpret a group of representative typical trials which include but are not limited to: vascular embolization tumor therapy, targeted minimally invasive thermal ablation of tumor, reversible bone cement materials, flexible exoskeleton device, nerve reconnection and functional recovery, injectable 3D medical electronics, X-ray angiography, and skin electronics, etc. Related efforts of employing liquid metals to resolve modern biomedical issues were also discussed. Perspective for future development in liquid metal biomaterials area was given. It is clear that, with continuous technical progresses and fundamental discoveries made along this direction, the liquid metals are expected to offer more and more fantastic opportunities as a new class of biomaterials which are promising an exciting area in revolutionizing disease diagnostics, therapy, and the general health care.

The present book is an output of our lab's more than 10 years' continuous academic endeavors. Over the past few years, a group of our colleagues, postdoctoral research fellows, graduate students, and collaborators have made important contributions to mold this new area of liquid metal biomaterials. Without their persistence, patience, and creativity, presenting such a book with many brand new fundamentals or technical categories inside is almost impossible. At the end of finalizing this book, the authors would like to take this chance to express their sincere appreciations to those people who have offered their professional contribution: Prof. Qian Wang, Prof. Zhongshan Deng, Prof. Wei Rao, Dr. Yang Yu, Dr. Jie Zhang, Dr. Cangran Guo, Dr. Lei Sheng, Dr. Fujun Liu, Dr. Yueguang Deng, Ms. Xuelin Wang, Ms. Xuyang Sun, Ms. Han Gui, Mr. Rui Guo, Ms. Xi Zhao, Ms. Shuo Xu, Mr. Xudong Zhang, Mr. Sen Chen, and Ms. Yue Sun et al. Meanwhile, we also wish to thank the Springer editors Dr. Na Xu, Dr. Suganya Gnanamani for their invitation, encouragement and very helpful suggestions for us to initiate and complete the tough task in preparing this book. Last but not least, the senior author of this book would like to acknowledge the generous support from the Frontier Project of the Chinese Academy of Sciences, Special Foundation of President of the Chinese Academy of Sciences, the NSFC Key Project under Grant No. 91748206, and Tsinghua University Initiative Scientific Research Program. Thanks for all these valuable supports, the present book could now become a reality.

We humbly hope that this book could serve as start point for the academics and industrial society to quickly grasp the basics of the liquid metal biomaterials and thus better advance the area. We would very much welcome any critical comments and constructive suggestions from the readers for us to further enhance our book which would be incorporated into its future possible updated version.

Beijing, China
March 2018

Jing Liu
Liting Yi

Contents

Abstract

Conventional biomaterials like metals, polymers, composites, ceramics, and naturally derived matters may not work well when facing certain medical challenges. At around body temperature, most of such materials mainly stay at solid state and are often difficult to shape due to their high melting point. Meanwhile, although electrolyte solutions own excellent flexibility, their electrical conductivities appear rather low which limited their utilizations to compose medical devices. As an alternative, the room temperature liquid metal materials are quickly emerging as a new generation functional material which displayed many unconventional properties superior than traditional biomaterials. This book is dedicated to draft a new biomedical category termed as liquid metal biomaterials and illustrates the science and art therein. The major advancements as made before will be summarized, and future directions worth of pursuing will be outlined. Representative applications enabled by liquid metal biomaterials from both therapeutic and diagnostic aspects will be presented. Related efforts of employing liquid metals to resolve touch biomedical challenges will be discussed. This book would help readers grasp a basic understanding of the technical progresses and fundamental discoveries in the frontier of liquid metal biomaterials, and thus better investigate and utilize them to tackle various critical needs in the coming time.

Keywords Biomaterial · Liquid metal · Disease treatment · Health care
Medical electronics

Chapter 1
Introduction

Abstract This chapter introduces a new biomedical category of the liquid metal biomaterials which consists of the core theme of the present book. The major advancements as made before will be briefly summarized and future directions worth of pursuing will be outlined. Representative applications enabled by liquid metal biomaterials from both therapeutic and diagnostic aspects will be pointed out. Potential efforts of employing liquid metals to resolve modern biomedical issues will be discussed. Perspective for future development in liquid metal biomaterials area will be given.

Keywords Disease · Metallic biomaterial · Liquid metal · Physical property Manufacture

1.1 Background

Conventional biomaterials like metals, polymers, composites, ceramics and those naturally derived matters, may not work well when facing certain medical challenges. At around body temperature, most of such materials especially metals mainly stay at solid state and are often difficult to shape due to their high melting point. Meanwhile, although electrolyte solutions own good flexibility, their electrical conductivities appear rather low which often limited their utilizations to compose medical devices. As an alternative, the room temperature liquid metal materials, such as gallium, bismuth or their alloy are recently emerging as a new generation functional material which depicted many unconventional properties superior than traditional biomaterials. This is because liquid metal simultaneously owns multiple capabilities like high fluidity, excellent electrical and thermal conductivities, good biocompatibility, sufficient radiopacity, controllable behaviors accompanied with reversible liquid-solid phase transition, easy manufacture and low cost etc. Such outstanding versatile feature as "One material, diverse capabilities" is rather unique among many existing materials. It is clear that liquid metals are reshaping modern sciences and technologies and have shown rather promising

J. Liu and L. Yi, *Liquid Metal Biomaterials*,
Springer Series in Biomaterials Science and Engineering10,
https://doi.org/10.1007/978-981-10-5607-9_1

values in tackling a wide variety of tough biomedical challenges which are hard to solve otherwise. With continuous technical progresses and fundamental discoveries made along this direction, the liquid metals are expected to offer more and more outstanding merits as a new class of biomaterials which are promising a generalized strategy towards resolving many latest biomedical challenges. This chapter is dedicated to introduce a new biomedical category of the liquid metal biomaterials which consists of the core theme of the present book. The major advancements as made before will be briefly summarized and future directions worth of pursuing will be outlined. Representative applications enabled by liquid metal biomaterials from both therapeutic and diagnostic aspects will be pointed out. Potential efforts of employing liquid metals to resolve modern biomedical issues will be discussed. Perspective for future development in liquid metal biomaterials area will be given.

1.2 Conventional Biomaterials and Challenges Involved

For a long time, human beings have suffered from various diseases which can occur almost anywhere throughout the whole body [1]. Such disease may gradually develop in some serious cases even lead to pathological changes of important organs or tissues, such as heart, vessel, nerve, bone and muscle, inducing pain, physical disability, even death (Fig. 1.1). Although the world health care situation and medical technology have been improved significantly over the past few decades, the number of disability-adjusted life-years (DALYs) still remained increasing for most specific non-communicable diseases from 2005 to 2013 [2]. Without any doubt, there are tremendous demands on developing highly advanced medical technologies which can fulfill the urgent health care needs. To enhance the average life expectancy and improve the patients' living quality, clinicians, researches and engineers have been struggling to find various possible methodologies in diagnosis, therapy and monitoring to fight against these diseases.

Among the numerous endeavours ever made, biomaterials have played an imperative role in clinical practices even since ancient times [3–5]. The term biomaterials commonly encompass the materials involved in both intra-corporeal and extracorporeal utilization for medical practices. With the advancements of modern science and technology, a wide variety of materials have been developed in the area. So far, conventional biomaterials generally include metals, polymers, composites, ceramics and naturally derived matters (Fig. 1.2) [6]. With intrinsic merits, these materials take their particular functions from different aspects [7, 8]. For instance, metals have been widely used to replace and repair the damaged hard tissues [9, 10]. And, polymers have been investigated and prepared as artificial organs, such as artificial muscles [11] and vessels [12]. A huge population of patients have in fact benefited from such technical progresses. Nevertheless, there also exist a lot of challenges facing traditional biomaterials. For example, biomaterials derived from nature or human body such as allograft generally encounter limited sources and probably would induce rejection despite of their high cost.

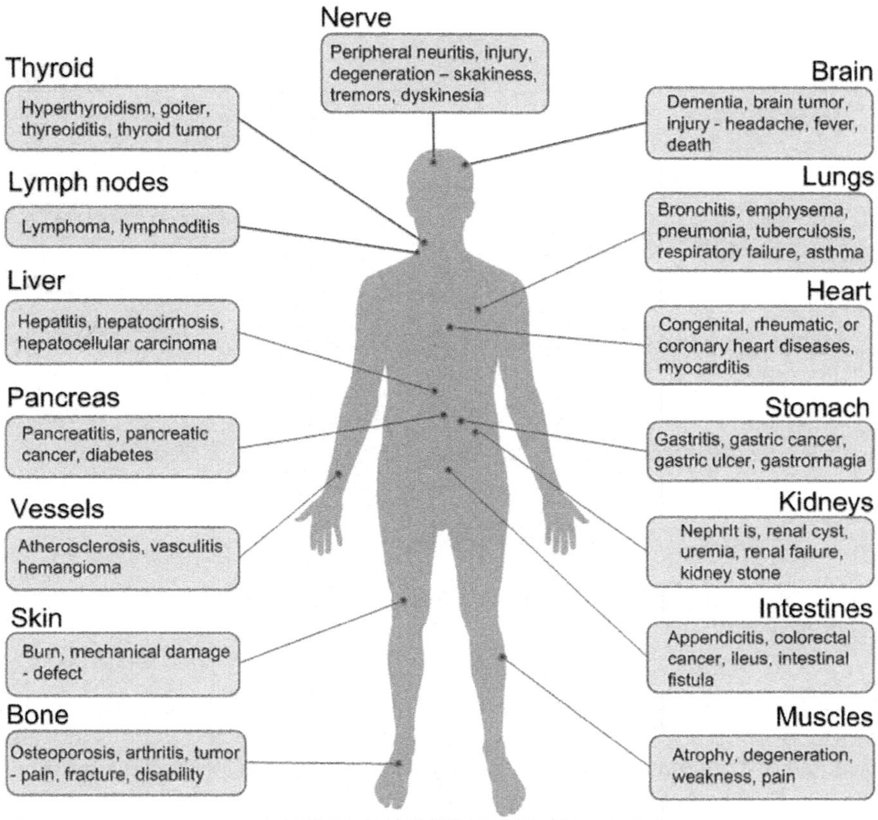

Fig. 1.1 Schematic of human anatomy and related diseases [1]. Picture reproduced with permission

Meanwhile, common metal biomaterials would exhibit high melting point which results in the difficulty in their conformal shaping at or near body temperature. Moreover, non-metallic materials have poor electrical or thermal conductivity and lack of radiopaque capability. In general, most of these biomaterials do not possess diverse functions and therefore could not make up the absence in a lot of practical situations. Taking a typical case for example, conventional materials are rigid which are hard to achieve free deformation according to the demands like micro robot swimming in vessels with varying size. Consequently, more smart biomaterials are urgently requested to fulfil various tough needs.

Recently, a group of metals with low melting point come into the eye of researchers and kept attracting increasing attentions. These materials own the interesting behaviours that could stay at liquid state at or near room temperature, such as gallium, mercury, caesium and eutectic alloys. It thus opens many possibilities of extending soft metal materials into diverse areas, naturally including biomedical sciences. However, because of the unavoidable toxicity and

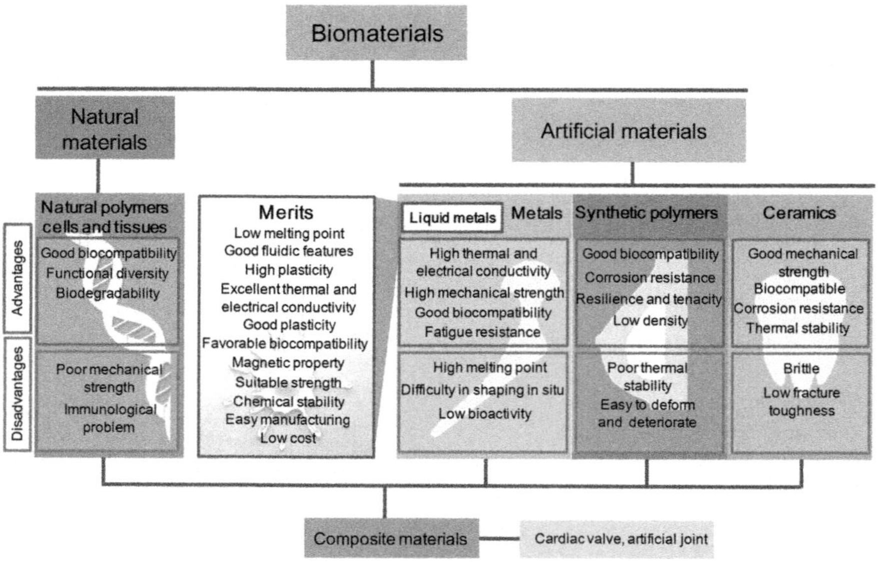

Fig. 1.2 Typical properties of general biomaterials and diverse capability of liquid metal [1]. Picture reproduced with permission

radioactivity issues, some of these metals like mercury, caesium and lead are hard to be widely utilized from practical aspects. Fortunately, more and more works also disclosed that gallium, bismuth or their alloys present outstanding merits for safety concern. Such materials have been normally used in industry fields over the past few decades [13–15]. Starting from their low melting point behaviour, other distinctive properties of liquid metal are also being revealed. It has been proven that the liquid metal not only owns excellent properties in electricity and thermal conductivity but also shows low viscosity, favourable fluidity, plasticity and biocompatibility etc. By virtue of these versatile advantages, the latest findings have uncovered a series of novel roles of liquid metal in biomedical area. Particularly, such technologies offer unconventional and effective solutions and in fact are showing big capacities in tackling a group of rather tough biomedical challenges which are hard to treat otherwise. With such outstanding multi-role material feature as “One material, diverse capabilities”, a new area of liquid metal biomaterials is incubating which will be very possible to reshape modern biomedical sciences and technologies. The following section is dedicated to draft the fundamental category of liquid metal biomaterials, with major scientific issues preliminarily outlined.

As a comparison with conventional metal biomaterials, we begin to briefly introduce the applications of rigid metal materials in biomedical area. Then we move to focus on the recent advances regarding the biomedical uses of special metal materials i.e. room-temperature liquid metal. Additionally, a series of typical methods employing the liquid metal to important needs spanning from disease therapy, diagnosis to monitoring etc. are described. Clearly, challenges always coexist with opportunities. Therefore, the difficulties may be encountered in developing future materials and technologies are also interpreted as a start point for the readers to prepare well for digesting the whole book.

1.3 Classical Metallic Biomaterials

Metallic materials have been developed as one significant biomaterial with a long history [16]. Up to now, the role of such materials in biomedical area has been almost unchanged that they are generally applied as implants to replace the damage or diseased hard tissues. To be suitable for use in vivo, metallic implants should own all or at least in special case one of the following key characteristics:

1. Adequate mechanical strength, including short-term performance (compressive strength, tensile strength and shear strength) and long-term behaviors (fatigue resistance), which should be similar to that of biological tissue to be replaced.
2. Appropriate corrosion resistance and chemical stability, allowing the substitute to work effectively.
3. Biocompatibility, which is to guarantee its safety to biological tissues.
4. Low cost, wide source and easy machining.

Currently, the common metallic biomaterials generally include gold, silver, stainless steel, Co–Cr alloys and Ti alloys etc. They are widely used in orthopedics applications such as dental restoration, knee and hip implant and fractured bone fixation for a long time with excellent success [17]. Metallic materials are superior to ceramics and polymeric materials due to their high mechanical strength. However, this merit also implied as a disadvantage that the strength of the metal implant is much higher than that of bone tissues (Table 1.1) [18–20], thus inducing the adverse effect of stress shielding. Moreover, corrosion is another problem for these metals as applied in physiological environment.

In general, corrosion is unfavorable factor for metal implant in vivo, but except that for magnesium material. By virtue of the degradability, magnesium and its alloys have been developed as temporary implants providing short-term structural

Table 1.1 Mechanical strength of bone tissue and typical metals

Materials	Tensile strength (MPa)	Elastic modulus (GPa)
Cancellous bone	1.5–38	0.01–1.57
Cortical bone	35 Trans. 283 Long.	5–23
Stainless steel	480–620	193–200
Titanium alloys	550–985	100–125
Cobalt alloys	450–960	195–230
Magnesium	185–232	73–117

Note Data from Refs. [18–20]

support and dissolving after the damage is cured, which avoids the second injury from removal of implant [21]. Such degradable materials have been applied for numerous clinical applications, such as cardiovascular stent, wound closing devices and musculoskeletal surgery [22]. Notably, biodegradable batteries mainly based on Mg were investigated as transient electronics, which are potential in assisting or monitoring a transient biological event [23]. Although magnesium is a safe element, there is limit concentration of every element for human body to tolerate. Thus, great efforts have been devoted to controlling the corrosion rate of Mg by using various methods such as purification, alloying, anodizing, and surface coating [24, 25]. Although these processing methods have gained certain success, the study of the precise controllability according to requirement is still a significant subject serving as a future opportunity for further optimizing the effects of Mg-based implants.

1.4 Basics About Liquid Metal

As mentioned above, liquid metal which can easily stay at liquid state at around room temperature is providing a wide variety of unique biomaterial merits that are hardly available in existing rigid metal materials. Before enabling such materials into biomedical practices, their basic characteristics should be briefly understood, which are necessary for assessing their feasibility in making biomaterials. In principle, biomaterials can generally be characterized through satisfying various specific requirements like application site, high stability, good biocompatibility and easy operation. Based on the previous studies, the properties relevant to liquid metal biomaterials will be preliminarily introduced in this chapter, including melting point, fluidic features, thermal and electrical properties, plasticity, chemical stability, magnetic property, mechanical performance, biocompatibility, manufacturing method and cost etc. This can serve as a start point for the discussion of the whole book.

1.5 Low Melting Point Properties of Liquid Metal

Table 1.2 comparatively lists the primary physical properties of water and several typical metals [26–30]. Thereinto, gallium has a low melting point of 29.8 °C. Owing to its supercooling character, such material remains liquid at room temperature. It is noteworthy that gallium-based binary and ternary alloys could possess even much lower melting temperature than gallium. For example, EGaIn alloy (eutectic gallium indium alloy) with a typical composition of Ga 80% and In 20% owns a melting point of 16 °C, and galinstan, which consists of 67% Ga, 20.5% In and 12.5% Sn, melts at a lower temperature of 10.5 °C. Though their melting point is higher than that of mercury (−38.87 °C), they have excellent fluidity as mercury does at body temperature.

Table 1.2 Physical properties of water and typical metals

	Melting point (°C)	Density (kg/m^3)	Thermal conductivity W/(m K)	Electrical conductivity (S/m)	Viscosity mPa s
Water	0	1000	0.6	$\leq 0.1 \times 10^{-3}$ (25 °C)	1.002 (20 °C)
Mercury	−38.87	13,546 (25 °C)	8.34 (25 °C)	1.04×10^6	1.526 (25 °C)
Ag	962	10,530 (20 °C)		6.3×10^7 (20 °C)	
Gallium	29.8	5907 (50 °C)	29.4 (50 °C)	2.2×10^6	1.2 (77 °C)
$GaIn_{20}$	16.0	6335	26.58 (20 °C)		
$Ga_{67}In_{20.5}Sn_{12.5}$	10.5	6360	16.5	3.1×10^6	
$Bi_{35}In_{48.6}Sn_{16}Zn_{0.4}$	58.3	7898	10.9 (25 °C)	7.3×10^6 (25 °C)	4.0 (74 °C)

Another group of alloy, the main ingredients of which generally include metallic elements bismuth (Bi), lead (Pb), tin (Sn), cadmium (Cd) and indium (In), is known as fusible alloy. With the increasing importance of green concept, toxic metals and the one causing environmental pollution should always be avoided to use. For this reason, Bi-based alloy has been selected and applied aiming to replace the lead alloy. Among the promising candidates, the melting point of BiInSnZn alloy can be regulated to 58.3 °C. Although this value is a little higher than that of gallium-based alloy, it is still much lower than most of the common metallic biomaterials, e.g. iron, aluminum, and titanium. Based on such moderate melting temperature, the liquid-solid phase transition of eutectic alloy is facile to be easily achieved under gentle condition.

1.6 Fluidic Features

Taking advantages of the low melting point, metals can stay at liquid phase at around the room temperature. As the most typical representative of liquid, water demonstrates prominent flow characteristics. Viscosity is one of the most important physical parameters in describing this behavior. The data in Table 1.2 shows that the viscosity of gallium is approximately low to that of water [29]. Additionally, the splashing dynamics has been compared between water and $GaIn_{24.5}$ alloy droplet (Fig. 1.3a) [31]. The phenomena of such two kinds of droplets impacting vertically on a pool composed of the same liquid were recorded using a high speed camera. Clearly, they both can form crown and display other similar impact behaviours during the splashing processes at the same moment. It is also found that the splashing phenomenon of liquid metal droplet is not so obvious when the oxide

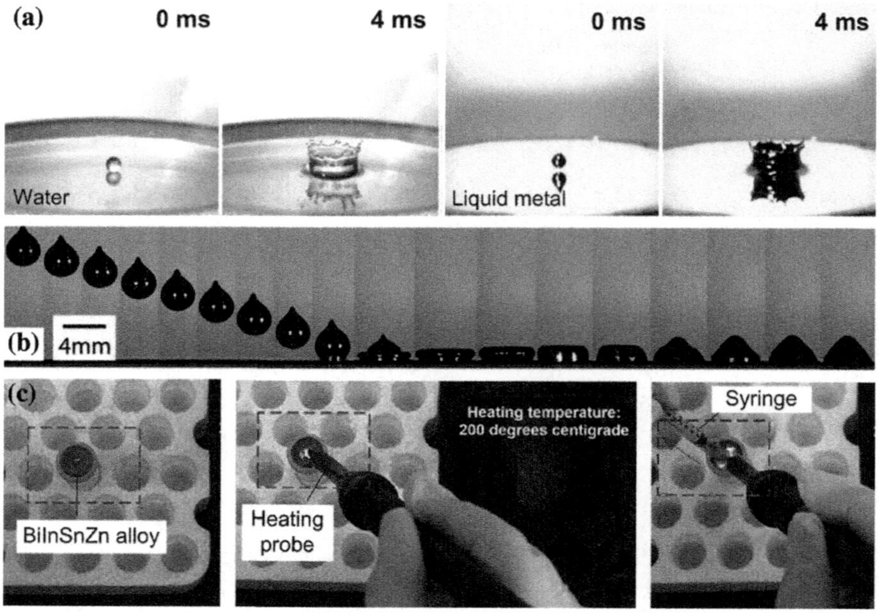

Fig. 1.3 The fluidic features of liquid metal. **a** Comparison of water and $GaIn_{24.5}$ droplets impacting their respective liquid pools during the splashing processes at the same moment (25 °C) [31]. **b** Photos of galinstan pendant droplet dropped on a silicon wafer surface [32]. **c** The flexible liquid-solid phase transition of BiInSnZn alloy. The melting alloy with good fluidity can be removed by syringe [30]. All pictures reproduced with permission

skin is formed on its surface [31, 32]. Figure 1.3b exhibits the impacting process of galinstan droplet on the silicon wafer [32]. As reflected in the photos, a crown-like rim has an obtuse contact angle at the impact and a more even conical shape is formed finally. The reason lies in that existing of the oxide skin maintains the shape and restrains the free flow of liquid metal. Consequently, the viscosity of gallium alloy can be controlled by the degree of oxidation. Similarly, the viscosity of melting BiInSnZn alloy is 4.0 mPa s [30]. Such material appears in solid phase at room temperature, thus, the flow features of this alloy are capable of being altered by the variations of temperature. For example, the solidified BiInSnZn alloy can be heated to melting and then sucked into syringe easily (Fig. 1.3c) [30]. All these evidences verify that the low-melting point metal owns excellent flow features.

1.7 Thermal Features

Such property is critical in thermally related biomedical practices including those situations where quick switch between liquid and solid state of the metallic materials is urgently needed. Originally, liquid metal is mainly used in chip cooling area.

Since the fluid is always employed for heat transport or energy delivery, the one with good thermal conductivity will play a significant role in current industry. Water is a kind of familiar liquid for circulating cooling. However, its thermal conductivity is 0.5 W/(m K) which is pretty small for transferring low grade heat [33]. The thermal conductivity of $GaIn_{20}$ is 26.58 W/(m K) at 20 °C. Compared with water and other inorganic/organic fluids, it is evident that liquid metal owns a much higher thermal conductivity. Consequently, the low-melting point metal with high heat transfer capacity has been investigated as excellent coolant and thermal interface material [27, 34]. And it is able to cool the computer chip with excellent efficiency [35]. With these dual capabilities, the liquid metal fluid has been introduced as soft microwave electrode in delivering energy for tumor ablation which meanwhile could transfer the heat to the outside to avoid over heating of the nearby tissues [36].

1.8 Electrical Features and Plasticity

Metal materials exhibit not only outstanding thermal behaviours but also excellent electrical conductivity. Silver (Ag) perhaps owns the highest electrical conductivity in the metal family which can reach 6.3×10^7 S/m. Such merit is embodied on the liquid metal as well. Electrolyte solutions are the most commonly applied conductive fluids in various micro-scale electronics [37, 38]. The conductivity of these solutions is only a few S/m, whereas that of gallium is 2.2×10^6 S/m. Compared with the electrolyte solutions, liquid metals clearly offer much higher conductivity with orders of magnitude less resistive loss in conducting electrical signals [32].

In addition, the liquid metal is a perfect flexible material that can be easily manipulated into any desired shape in various scales from microscopic to macroscopic [34]. Figure 1.4a, b shows that EGaIn alloy was frozen into geometries with certain thickness and depth [39]. In combination with the good conductivity, the functional components such as resistive strain sensing (Fig. 1.4c) can be fabricated utilizing EGaIn alloy through the patterned polydimethylsiloxane (PDMS) mould. Kramer et al. had ever produced GaIn circuits embedded elastomer devices with features smaller than 200 μm and edge-to-edge separations as small as 25 μm [40]. Interestingly, the liquid metal droplets in micro scale are able to be prepared via channelless approach. Yu et al. [41] found that injecting gallium material from a syringe with a dispersing needle to the water solution of surfactant sodium dodecyl sulfate (SDS) would generate tremendous tiny liquid metal droplets (Fig. 1.4d). As the plunger is pushed, a large number of liquid metal droplets are quickly fabricated. Through a statistical measurement of size distribution in Fig. 1.4e, the corresponding histogram displays that the diameter of the liquid metal droplets ranges from 200 to 400 μm (Fig. 1.4f). Furthermore, it can also be managed to produce the droplets with diameter smaller than 50 μm by means of regulating diameters of pinheads and jetting velocity. Through such method, the fabrication of metal droplets has advantages of low cost, high efficiency and simple operation, compared

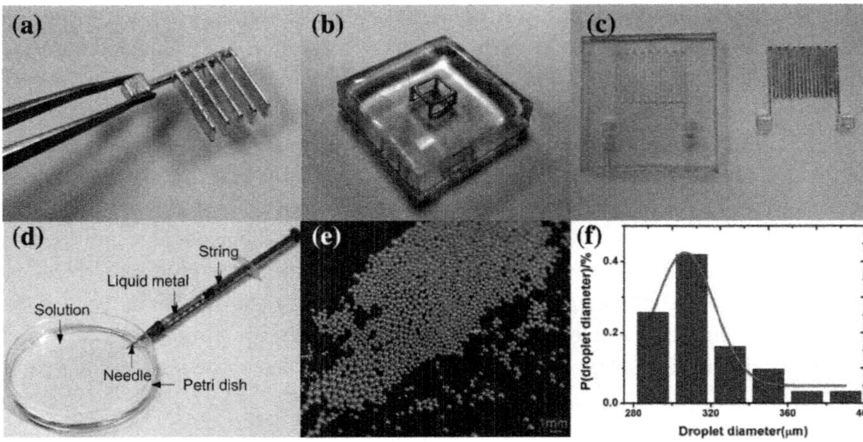

Fig. 1.4 The plasticity of liquid metal. **a** EGaIn can be molded into different structures through freezing in specially designed geometries. **b** The frozen EGaIn encapsulated in elastomer. **c** The frozen EGaIn made as serpentine wire segments which can be adopted for resistive strain sensing and easily removed from the patterned PDMS mold [39]. **d** Device for injectable liquid metal droplets fabrication. **e** Bottom view of liquid metal micro-droplets using microscope. **f** Histogram of droplet diameter distribution in the sample [41]. All pictures reproduced with permission

with the conventional method. Such tiny liquid metal droplets can be used in a wide variety of biomedical practices such as microfluidic system, nano carrier, MEMS devices and tumor therapy etc. [41].

1.9 Chemical Stability

As exposed in air with humidity, the liquid metal containing gallium is ease to be oxidized. It has been proven that Ga is predominantly oxidized compared to the other two elements for GaInSn alloy [42]. Such gallium oxide film covers on the surface of the liquid metal, which can be efficiently removed by acid or alkaline solution, such as HCl and NaOH solution [38]. As is well known, Al can react with NaOH solution, meanwhile releasing hydrogen. When this reaction system is added with liquid metal, interesting story happens. The present lab found that, if attaching Al flake to the EGaIn or Galinstan in electrolyte solution, the liquid metal would penetrate into aluminium and continuously keep running for a surprisingly long time like more than 1 h [43]. This unusual phenomenon would not occur on separate Al or liquid metal alone. It is because that the liquid metal destroys the oxide skin of Al surface, which deeply activates the reaction between Al and NaOH solution, accelerating the generation and release of H_2 bubbles [44]. Additionally, the galvanic cell is formed based on this reaction system, which induces beneficial bipolar electrochemical reaction for actuation. This basic effect based on integrating multiple metals together will contribute a lot to self-fuelled tiny motor or soft robot which can be found useful in developing future smart biomedical systems.

1.10 Magnetic Property

Generally, the compositions of low melting point metals and alloys do not involve the magnetic metallic elements. In other words, such materials themselves are non-magnetic. Nevertheless, the liquid metal behaves unmorally under magnetic field, and recent studies have revealed related phenomena, meanwhile, illustrating their mechanisms. Wang et al. set galinstan alloy between a pair of concentric ring electrodes in the NaOH solution on the permanent magnet [45]. In this situation, the liquid metal sphere can be induced to rotate centrifugally around the central electrode. The rotating speed increases with the voltage and is influenced by the concentration of NaOH solution. Unexpectedly, such speed will not slow down when the volume of liquid metal increases in some extent. On the contrary, the requirement of driving voltage is lower than that of smaller volume. Such magnetic field effect on liquid metal can be utilized to develop liquid metal motor in medical device and soft robot etc. Apart from that, magnetic field can restrict the motion of self-fuelled motor composed of $GaIn_{10}$ alloy and aluminium [46]. The liquid metal droplets with diameter less than 1 mm are found to be bounced off by magnetic trap effect from the boundary of magnet. These behaviours have been interpreted as that the strong magnetic field influences the electrical charges generated from the reaction between Al and GaIn alloy. On this basis, such mechanism can be employed to control the motion of liquid metal in definite direction. Moreover, it will be of great sense if the liquid metal material itself owns magnetic property, making the control more direct and flexible. Researchers have mixed carbon nano tubes together with liquid metal which significantly improves the thermal conductivity of liquid metal [47]. Similar to that, the magnetic component such as nickel nanoparticles can also be loaded into liquid metal for further improvements of its magnetic characteristics.

1.11 Mechanical Strength of Solidified Liquid Metal

For some metals, they own a little higher melting point than room temperature liquid metal, such as BiInSnZn alloy. Notably, these metals not only have good fluidity in liquid state, but also exhibit certain strong mechanical strength when they become solidified at the temperature below their melting point. Our group has tested the mechanical properties of BiInSnZn alloy in comparison with the commonly used hard biomaterial i.e. PMMA (polymethyl methacrylate) [30]. Under the same conditions based on international testing standard, the measured magnitudes of short term characteristics including compressive strength and bending stress of

BiInSnZn alloy were 37.6 ± 1.56 and 35.31 ± 1.09 MPa which are slightly smaller than those of PMMA. Except for these, BiInSnZn alloy owns larger or comparable bending modulus (6.41 ± 0.81 GPa), crack resistance (KQ = 4.85 ± 0.05 $MPam^{1/2}$) and fatigue property (number of cycles to failure = 109,373, 106,549, 78,594 and 76,892). Especially, this alloy material is able to withstand obvious deformations under certain stress without being broken, indicating its excellent ductile property. Comprehensively being measured on various mechanical performances, the solidified liquid metals have already been able to meet the strength requirements of non load-bearing position repair. To broaden the applications fields, modified methods can be implemented to further improve the mechanical strength of these metals. Moreover, there are still tremendous options of low-melting point alloys whose mechanical properties vary with the different constituents, waiting for people to test and learn more.

1.12 Biocompatibility

Liquid metals are becoming increasingly popular due to their unique properties. Although mercury is the most widely known material among various liquid metals, unfortunately, it has strong poison which restrains its further applications. Typical low-melting alloys with potential biomedical values are generally composed of Ga, In, Sn and Bi elements. In medical field, gallium compounds have gained importance in the past decades. For example, they play roles as anti-inflammatory, antimicrobial agents and immunosuppressive activity in animal models of human disease. Gallium and gallium nitrate can be used as diagnostic and therapeutic agents in cancer and disorders of calcium and bone metabolism [48]. In addition, tin has been made into container for food and drink with a long history. It is a kind of indispensable trace element for human body, with the safe limit value for fruit conserves being ca. 250–500 mg/kg, and for fruit juices 500–1000 mg/kg [49]. Considering another element, indium is the major component in electric engineering, and its occupational exposure limit was recommended to be 3 mg/L in serum by Japan Society [50]. In fact, galinstan alloy has been applied as dental filling biomaterials clinically, whose safety has been confirmed before [51, 52]. In industry, bismuth metal as a kind of green and clean material is utilized to replace the toxic lead. Bismuth compound based medicine i.e. pepto-bismol is rather common and easily available in the market. According to the clinical report, the limited value of bismuth blood level is 50 mg/ml [53].

Corrosion behaviours of BiInSnZn alloy in physiological condition have been simulated via immersion tests [30]. After 1, 2, 5, 9 and 14 days immersion at 37 °C, metallic elements released into the Hank's solution from such alloy were quantitatively analysed. As zinc is a kind of active metal, its release rate was slightly increased along with the time and its concentration was 0.8 ± 0.1 mg/mL after 14 days. In comparison, Bi, In, and Sn elements were barely detectable in physiological solution during two weeks' immersion. In addition, the cytotoxicity was evaluated by using this soaking solution to culture BALB/c 3T3 cells. The result demonstrates that composition in solution did not affect the cell viability. Further, the biocompatibility was proven via in vivo experiments as well. Alloy specimens were embedded subcutaneously in mice for 1, 7 and 14 days. It was found that the activities of mice and the histological staining of tissue directly contacting with the alloy were normal, indicating the good biocompatibility of BiInSnZn alloy in a relatively long period of time. Besides, there is another study on magnesium alloy containing bismuth as degradable bone implants [54]. The in vivo experiment shows that the implants did not affect the typical biochemical indexes and the pathological examinations of liver and kidney were normal without necrotic areas. Generally speaking, gallium and bismuth based low melting point alloys are quite safe for human body use which are advantages in replacement of highly toxic mercury [55].

1.13 Manufacturing Method

As is well known, electrical conductivity varies in response to the deformation of electrical wiring or sensors. On this basis, liquid metal especially gallium or its alloys can be manufactured into various shapes together with elastomers for multiple applications which has been proven to be a means of realizing flexible electronics, such as interconnects [56], stretchable radiofrequency antennas [57–60] and force sensors [61–63]. Currently, liquid alloys are generally patterned with needle-injection [39] or masked deposition [40, 64]. Our studies have demonstrated that the slightly oxidized alloy ink is able to be flexibly printed on nearly every kind of substrate materials [65–68]. Hence, the innovative printed patterns are developed and carried out by direct printing techniques such as syringe pumped dispensing needle [69], roller-ball pen [70], micro contact printing [71] and desktop printer (Fig. 1.5) [72]. Figure 1.5a displays the printing procedure of GaIn24.5 on coated paper under control of digitalized program. Various patterns of liquid metal, e.g. wires (Fig. 1.5a) and coil (Fig. 1.5b) can be printed easily by utilizing this method. Figure 1.5c, d shows the SEM photos of the liquid metal ink printed on the coated paper from front and side view respectively. The results exhibit that the adhesion between liquid metal and coated paper is close, thus the stability of the patterns printed are ensured. Meanwhile, another alloy, i.e. $Bi_{35}In_{48.6}Sn_{16}Zn_{0.4}$ with a little higher melting point has been demonstrated printable in forming multiple three dimensional structures by 3D printer (Fig. 1.5e, f) [73]. Figure 1.5g, h demonstrates the basic principle of the liquid phase 3D printing. The metallic droplet can join together to form a column under the control of printer with the process of melting and solidification. In such sense, easy going mechanization greatly improves the accuracy and efficiency and reduces the cost of manufacture based on low-melting metal.

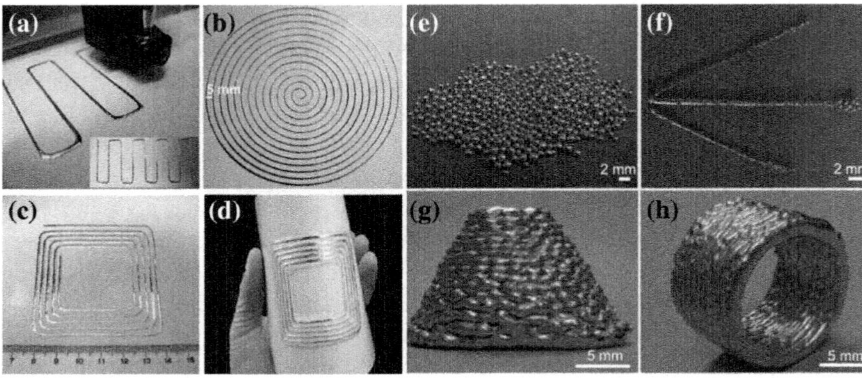

Fig. 1.5 Liquid metal printed typical conductive antennas or structures. **a** Physical diagram of $GaIn_{24.5}$ based liquid alloy directly printed on coated paper by a dispenser printer and optical images for conductive wires on coated paper. Optical images for printed inductance coil (**b**). SEM images of surface (**c**) and cross-section (**d**) of printed liquid metal RFID antenna on coated paper [72]. 3D structures made by liquid phase 3D printing method: **e** liquid metal balls; **f** frustum of a cone structure. **g**, **h** The droplet deposition process in ethanol cooling fluid (the droplet falling velocity is 5.65 mm/s) [73]. All pictures reproduced with permission

1.14 Cost Affairs

The cost of biomaterials is another important issue worthy of consideration before large scale practical application and popularization. According to the report from recent metallic market in China, the bulk price of typical materials is listed in Table 1.3. Despite the good properties, the extensive application of silver is restricted with its high cost when large amount is consumed. In Table 1.3, it is found that the price of silver is much higher than that of Ga, Bi, Sn and In. Although In is the most expensive among the compositions of low-melting alloy materials, the total price of alloy decreases due to reduced use of its content and the lower price of other components. Overall, the cost of the low-melting alloy is comparable to that of mercury which is acceptable.

Generally, low-melting metals offer various favorable attributes including low viscosity, good fluidity and plasticity, high thermal and electrical conductivity, easy printing, low toxicity and acceptable cost. The excellent outcome of such alloys makes them a better substitute for mercury. Most importantly, their characteristics are nearly all in accordance with the requirements of the biomaterials. More and more studies have verified their possibility to be used in many aspects of biomedicine.

Table 1.3 Price of typical metallic materials in China (in the year of 2015)

Bulk price (US$/kg)	Mercury	Silver	Gallium	Bismuth	Indium	Tin
	75	550	150	12	250	17

1.15 Conclusion

This book is the first ever trial on illustrating the science and art of liquid metal biomaterials. It is an output of our lab's more than 10 years' continuous academic endeavors. However, as a new area in the biomedical engineering, what presented in this book is only an initial draft with much inspiration for future. Our endeavors here will be mainly to interpret a group of representative typical advancements. To name a few of them, these include but will not limit to: vascular embolization tumor therapy, targeted minimally invasive thermal ablation of tumor, reversible bone cement materials, flexible exoskeleton device, nerve reconnection, injectable 3D medical electronics, X-ray angiography, wearable and skin electronics etc. Related efforts of employing liquid metals to resolve modern biomedical issues were discussed. Perspective for future development in liquid metal biomaterials area was given. With continuous technical progresses and fundamental discoveries made along this direction, the liquid metals are expected to offer more and more opportunities to develop new class of biomaterials which are promising a generalized strategy towards resolving biomedical challenges.

References

1. Yi L, Liu J (2017) Liquid metal biomaterials: a newly emerging area to tackle modern biomedical challenges. Int Mater Rev 62:415–440
2. Murray CJ, Barber RM, Foreman KJ, Ozgoren AA, Abd-Allah F, Abera SF et al (2015) Global, regional, and national disability-adjusted life years (DALYs) for 306 diseases and injuries and healthy life expectancy (HALE) for 188 countries, 1990-2013: quantifying the epidemiological transition. Lancet 386(10009):2145–2191
3. Hench LL, Polak JM (2002) Third-generation biomedical materials. Science 295(5557):1014–1017
4. Kohn J (2004) New approaches to biomaterials design. Nat Mater 3(11):745–747
5. Huebsch N, Mooney DJ (2009) Inspiration and application in the evolution of biomaterials. Nature 462(7272):426–432
6. Bhat S, Kumar A (2013) Biomaterials and bioengineering tomorrow's healthcare. Biomatter 3 (3):e24717
7. Dean MN, Swanson BO, Summers AP (2009) Biomaterials: properties, variation and evolution. Integr Comp Biol 49:15–20
8. Rezaie HR, Bakhtiari L, Öchsner A (2015) Application of biomaterials. Biomaterials and their applications. Springer
9. Webster TJ, Ejiofor JU (2004) Increased osteoblast adhesion on nanophase metals: Ti, Ti6Al4V, and CoCrMo. Biomaterials 25(19):4731–4739
10. Bencharit S, Byrd WC, Altarawneh S, Hosseini B, Leong A, Reside G et al (2014) Development and applications of porous tantalum trabecular metal-enhanced titanium dental implants. Clin Implant Dent Relat Res 16(6):817–826
11. Haines CS, Lima MD, Li N, Spinks GM, Foroughi J, Madden JD et al (2014) Artificial muscles from fishing line and sewing thread. Science 343(6173):868–872
12. Tamura K, Mizuno H, Okada K, Katoh H, Hitomi S, Teramatsu T et al (1985) Experimental application of polyvinyl alcohol-silica for small artificial vessels. Biomat Med Dev Artif Organs 13(3–4):133–152

13. Abbott F (1942) The use of fusible alloy in vapor diffusion pumps. Rev Sci Instrum 13(4):187
14. Brunetti B, Gozzi D, Iervolino M, Piacente V, Zanicchi G, Parodi N et al (2006) Bismuth activity in lead-free solder Bi-In-Sn alloys. Calphad 30(4):431–442
15. Moelans N, Kumar KH, Wollants P (2003) Thermodynamic optimization of the lead-free solder system Bi-In-Sn-Zn. J Alloy Compd 360(1):98–106
16. Crubzy E, Murail P, Girard L, Bernadou JP (1998) False teeth of the Roman world. Nature 391:29
17. Bahraminasab M, Hassan MR, Sahari BB (2010) Metallic biomaterials of knee and hip—a review. Trends Biomat Artif Organs 24(2):69–82
18. Poinern GEJ, Brundavanam S, Fawcett D (2012) Biomedical magnesium alloys: a review of material properties, surface modifications and potential as a biodegradable orthopaedic implant. Am J Biomed Eng 2(6):218–240
19. Staiger MP, Pietak AM, Huadmai J, Dias G (2006) Magnesium and its alloys as orthopedic biomaterials: a review. Biomaterials 27(9):1728–1734
20. Valiathan MS, Krishnan VK (1999) Biomaterials: an overview. Natl Med J India 12(6): 270–274
21. Zberg B, Uggowitzer PJ, Loffler JF (2009) MgZnCa glasses without clinically observable hydrogen evolution for biodegradable implants. Nat Mat 8:887–891
22. Lim GB (2013) Atherosclerosis: addition of niacin to optimal statin therapy does not affect plaque regression. Nat Rev Cardiol 10(10):554
23. Yin L, Huang X, Xu H, Zhang Y, Lam J, Cheng J, Rogers JA (2014) Materials, designs, and operational characteristics for fully biodegradable primary batteries. Adv Mater 26(23):3879–3884
24. Zheng YF, Gu XN, Witte F (2014) Biodegradable metals materials. Mat Sci Eng 77(2):1–34
25. Yun Y, Dong Z, Lee N, Liu Y, Xue D, Guo X, Kuhlamann J, Doepke A, Halsall HB, Sundaramurthy S et al (2009) Revolutionizing biodegradable metals. Mater Today 12(10):22–32
26. Wang L, Liu J (2014) Compatible hybrid 3D printing of metal and nonmetal inks for direct manufacture of end functional devices. Sci China Technol Sci 57(11):2089–2095
27. Zhang Q, Liu J (2013) Nano liquid metal as an emerging functional material in energy management, conversion and storage. Nano Energy 2(5):863–872
28. Liu T, Sen P, Kim CJC (2012) Characterization of nontoxic liquid-metal alloy galinstan for applications in microdevices. J Microelectromech Syst 21(2):443–450
29. Spells K (1936) The determination of the viscosity of liquid gallium over an extended range of temperature. Proc Phys Soc 48(2):299
30. Yi L, Jin C, Wang L, Liu J (2014) Liquid-solid phase transition alloy as reversible and rapid molding bone cement. Biomaterials 35(37):9789–9801
31. Li H, Mei S, Wang L, Gao Y, Liu J (2014) Splashing phenomena of room temperature liquid metal droplet striking on the pool of the same liquid under ambient air environment. Int J Heat Fluid Flow 47:1–8
32. Sivan V, Tang SY, O'Mullane AP, Petersen P, Eshtiaghi N, Kalantar-zadeh K et al (2013) Liquid metal marbles. Adv Func Mater 23(2):137
33. Li P, Liu J (2011) Harvesting low grade heat to generate electricity with thermosyphon effect of room temperature liquid metal. Appl Phys Lett 99(9):094106
34. Gao Y, Liu J (2012) Gallium-based thermal interface material with high compliance and wettability. Appl Phys A 107(3):701–708
35. Liu J, Zhou YX, Lv YG, Li T (2005) Liquid metal based miniaturized chip-cooling device driven by electromagnetic pump. In: ASME 2005 international mechanical engineering congress and exposition. American Society of Mechanical Engineers
36. Wang Q, Liu J (2013) Liquid metal based microwave delivery wire, fabrication and application. China Patent No. 201310259413.7, China
37. Kaltenbrunner M, Kettlgruber G, Siket C, Schwödiauer R, Bauer S (2010) Arrays of ultracompliant electrochemical dry gel cells for stretchable electronics. Adv Mater 22 (18):2065–2067

38. Li G, Parmar M, Lee DW (2015) An oxidized liquid metal-based microfluidic platform for tunable electronic device applications. Lab Chip 15(3):766–775
39. Fassler A, Majidi C (2013) 3D structures of liquid-phase GaIn alloy embedded in PDMS with freeze casting. Lab Chip 13(22):4442–4450
40. Kramer RK, Majidi C, Wood RJ (2013) Masked deposition of gallium-indium alloys for liquid-embedded elastomer conductors. Adv Func Mater 23(42):5292–5296
41. Yu Y, Wang Q, Yi L, Liu J (2014) Channelless fabrication for large-scale preparation of room temperature liquid metal droplets. Adv Eng Mater 16(2):255–262
42. Scharmann F, Cherkashinin G, Breternitz V, Knedlik C, Hartung G, Weber T et al (2010) Viscosity effect on GaInSn studied by XPS. Surf Interface Anal 36(8):981–985
43. Zhang J, Yao Y, Sheng L, Liu J (2015) Self-fueled biomimetic liquid metal mollusk. Adv Mater 27(16):2648–2655
44. Ilyukhina A, Ilyukhin A, Shkolnikov E (2012) Hydrogen generation from water by means of activated aluminum. Int J Hydrogen Energy 37(21):16382–16387
45. Wang L, Liu J (2015) Electromagnetic rotation of a liquid metal sphere or pool within a solution. Proc Royal Soc London 471(2178):20150177
46. Tan SC, Gui H, Yuan B, Liu J (2015) Magnetic trap effect to restrict motion of self-powered tiny liquid metal motors. Appl Phys Lett 107(7):071904
47. Ma KQ, Liu J (2007) Nano liquid-metal fluid as ultimate coolant. Phys Lett A 361(3): 252–256
48. Chitambar CR (2010) Medical applications and toxicities of gallium compounds. Int J Environ Res Public Health 7(5):2337–2361
49. Graf GG (2005) Tin, tin alloys, and tin compounds. Ullmann's Encyclopedia of Industrial Chemistry
50. Tanaka A, Hirata M, Kiyohara Y, Nakano M, Omae K, Shiratani M et al (2010) Review of pulmonary toxicity of indium compounds to animals and humans. Thin Solid Films 518 (11):2934–2936
51. Cadwallader LC (2003) Gallium safety in the laboratory. Idaho National Laboratory
52. Dunne S, Abraham R (2000) Restorative dentistry: dental post-operative sensitivity associated with a gallium-based restorative material. Br Dent J 189(6):310–313
53. Serfontein W, Mekel R (1979) Bismuth toxicity in man ii. review of bismuth blood and urine levels in patients after administration of therapeutic bismuth formulations in relation to the problem of bismuth toxicity in man. Res Commun Chem Pathol Pharmacol 26(2):391–411
54. Remennik S, Bartsch I, Willbold E, Witte F, Shechtman D (2011) New, fast corroding high ductility Mg-Bi-Ca and Mg-Bi-Si alloys, with no clinically observable gas formation in bone implants. Mater Sci Eng, B 176(20):1653–1659
55. Zhang Q, Zheng Y, Liu J (2012) Direct writing of electronics based on alloy and metal (DREAM) ink: a newly emerging area and its impact on energy, environment and health sciences. Front Energy 6(4):311–340
56. Kim HJ, Son C, Ziaie B (2008) A multiaxial stretchable interconnect using liquid-alloy-filled elastomeric microchannels. Appl Phys Lett 92(1):011904
57. Cheng S, Rydberg A, Hjort K, Wu Z (2009) Liquid metal stretchable unbalanced loop antenna. Appl Phys Lett 94(14):144103
58. Kubo M, Li X, Kim C, Hashimoto M, Wiley BJ, Ham D et al (2010) Stretchable microfluidic radiofrequency antennas. Adv Mater 22(25):2749–2752
59. Jeong SH, Hjort K, Wu Z (2014) Tape transfer printing of a liquid metal alloy for stretchable RF electronics. Sensors 14(9):16311–16321
60. Nawaz AA, Mao X, Stratton ZS, Huang TJ (2013) Unconventional microfluidics: expanding the discipline. Lab Chip 13(8):1457–1463
61. Jung T, Yang S (2015) Highly stable liquid metal-based pressure sensor integrated with a microfluidic channel. Sensors 15(5):11823–11835
62. Park YL, Majidi C, Kramer R, Bérard P, Wood RJ (2010) Hyperelastic pressure sensing with a liquid-embedded elastomer. J Micromech Microeng 20(12):125029

63. Wong RDP, Posner JD, Santos VJ (2012) Flexible microfluidic normal force sensor skin for tactile feedback. Sens Actuators, A 179:62–69
64. Shan W, Lu T, Majidi C (2013) Soft-matter composites with electrically tunable elastic rigidity. Smart Mater Struct 22(8):085005
65. Gao Y, Li H, Liu J (2012) Direct writing of flexible electronics through room temperature liquid metal ink. PLoS ONE 7(9):e45485
66. Li H, Yang Y, Liu J (2012) Printable tiny thermocouple by liquid metal gallium and its matching metal. Appl Phys Lett 101(7):073511
67. Mei S, Gao Y, Li H, Deng Z, Liu J (2013) Thermally induced porous structures in printed gallium coating to make transparent conductive film. Appl Phys Lett 102(4):041905
68. Zhang Q, Gao Y, Liu J (2014) Atomized spraying of liquid metal droplets on desired substrate surfaces as a generalized way for ubiquitous printed electronics. Appl Phys A 116(3):1091–1097
69. Boley JW, White EL, Chiu GTC, Kramer RK (2014) Direct writing of gallium-indium alloy for stretchable electronics. Adv Func Mater 24(23):3501–3507
70. Zheng Y, Zhang Q, Liu J (2013) Pervasive liquid metal based direct writing electronics with roller-ball pen. AIP Adv 3(11):112117
71. Tabatabai A, Fassler A, Usiak C, Majidi C (2013) Liquid-phase gallium-indium alloy electronics with microcontact printing. Langmuir 29(20):6194–6200
72. Zheng Y, He Z, Gao Y, Liu J (2013) Direct desktop printed-circuits-on-paper flexible electronics. Sci Rep 3:1786-1-7
73. Wang L, Liu J (2014) Liquid phase 3D printing for quickly manufacturing conductive metal objects with low melting point alloy ink. Sci China Technol Sci 57(9):1721–1728

Chapter 2
Unconventional Fluidic Properties of Liquid Metal

Abstract To promote deep understanding of liquid metal in future biomedical applications where hybrid even multiple phase fluids are often involved, this chapter illustrates the unconventional hydrodynamics from experiment, theory, and simulation aspects. Typical phenomena and basic working mechanisms are explained. Some representative simulation methods are incorporated to tackle the governing functions of the electrohydrodynamics. Further, prospects and challenges are raised, which is to offer a startup insight into the new physics of the hybrid fluid under applied fields.

Keywords Liquid metal · Fluidic property · Hybrid fluids · Unconventional flow

2.1 Background

Unlike former academic endeavors on a single fluid, liquid metals are found uniquely important when used along with other solution which is especially critical in many biomedical environments or application situations. In this sense, the hydrodynamic properties of liquid metal and allied fluids made of liquid metal/aqueous solution are elementary in the design and operation of various biomedical functional devices or systems involved. In terms of the general physical and chemical properties, such as density, thermal conductivity and electrical conductivity, the huge differences between the two fluidic phases of liquid metal and conventional fluid raise a big challenge for quantifying the hybrid flow behaviors [1]. Interesting enough, the liquid metal immersed in the solution would easily move and deform when administrated with external non-contact electromagnetic force, or even induced by redox reaction, which is entirely different from the cases of a single fluid or conventional contacting force. Owing to its remarkable capability in flow and deformation, liquid metal immersed in the solution is apt to deform on an extremely large scale, resulting in marked changes on its boundary and interface. However, until now, the working mechanisms of the movement and deformation of liquid metal in the allied solution environment still lack appropriate

J. Liu and L. Yi, *Liquid Metal Biomaterials*,
Springer Series in Biomaterials Science and Engineering10,
https://doi.org/10.1007/978-981-10-5607-9_2

models to describe such scientific issues via a set of well-established unified theories. To promote deep understanding of liquid metal in future biomedical applications where hybrid even multiple phase fluids are often involved, this chapter is dedicated to illustrate the unconventional hydrodynamics from experiment, theory, and simulation aspects. Typical phenomena and basic working mechanisms are explained. Some representative simulation methods are incorporated to tackle the governing functions of the electrohydrodynamics. Further, prospects and challenges are raised, which is to offer a startup insight into the new physics of the hybrid fluid under applied fields.

2.2 Hybrid Fluid Made of Liquid Metal and Allied Solution

As is well known, the hybrid fluid hydrodynamics can be applied to various industrial fields such as oil extraction [2, 3], electrostatic spraying [4], inkjet printing [5], and metal recycling [6]. The liquid metal drops immersed in immiscible solution under electric field will present intriguing phenomena such as movement [7–10], deformation [10], rotation [11], breakup [10, 12], oscillating [13], collision and coalescence [14, 15]. So far, precise description of the electrohydrodynamics of liquid metal drops still remains unclear, due to the mutual coupling of the electric field and the flow field.

The room temperature liquid metal (RTLM) is an attractive material option owing to its combination of advantages of metals such as high electrical conductivity, thermal conductivity and reflectivity, with the inherently dynamic nature of fluids [16]. Though mercury is the most well-known RTLM, its further applications are limited by the hyper toxicity involved. In contrast to mercury, gallium-based alloys have little toxicity and a low vapor pressure at a high temperature, on the order of 10^{-9} atm at 538 °C and nearly zero at room temperature [17]. Recently, it was gradually disclosed that liquid metal immersed in immiscible solutions under applied fields displays rather unconventional hydrodynamic characteristics, including planar locomotion [18], rotation [18], self-propelled [19], oscillation [20], climbing [21], breathing [22], deformation [16, 21], and surfing [23]. The potential of fluidic metallic liquid metal has been verified in a variety of very different fields such as chip cooling [24–26], heat dissipation [27, 28], energy harvest [29, 30], drug delivery [31], liquid pump [32, 33], soft robot manufacture [34], and printed electronics [35, 36], etc.

Distinctive from the classical hybrid fluid in nature such as oil/water hybrid fluid and debris flow, the liquid metal/aqueous solution hybrid flow is rather unique in the following aspects: (1) Liquid metal immersed in the solution can move and deform when exerted with non-contact electromagnetic force, or even the force induced by redox reaction, which is significantly different from the conventional contact force. (2) Owing to its excellent characteristics of flow and deformation, liquid metal is apt to deform on a large scale, resulting in marked changes on the boundary between the liquid metal and the solution. (3) Because of the strong disparity in density between liquid metal (5907 kg/m^3) [37] and water (1000 kg/m^3), liquid metal invariably sinks into the bottom of the container. The surface tension of liquid metal (700 mN/m) [38], another leading property in hybrid flow study, is almost ten times larger than that of water (72 mN/m, 25 °C) [39]. Besides, the electrical conductivity of liquid metal is 7 orders of magnitude higher than that of water. (4) Chemical reactions such as the transformation between gallium and its oxide have an important effect on the movement and deformation of the liquid metal. In light of the uniqueness of liquid metal/aqueous solution, the working mechanism of the movement and deformation of liquid metal is not yet clear enough, with no suitable theoretical model established to describe it with a set of unified equations.

In the following sections, we mainly illustrated the unconventional fluid mechanics of the movement and deformation of liquid metal in aqueous solutions.

2.3 Experimental Fluidic Behaviors of Liquid Metal

Liquid metal possesses proprieties of both liquid and metal. Apart from the ability to move and deform under the pressure field, many intriguing phenomena occur under electric field [18, 27, 40, 41], magnetic field [42, 43], and chemical field [19, 21, 44–46] as well.

2.3.1 Electric Field Actuated Liquid Metal Flow

It was observed that when the spherical liquid metal was exposed to the electric field after the electrodes were rearranged, self-rotation of the metal accompanied by two vortexes of water could occur (Fig. 2.1). Meanwhile, planar locomotion of the sphere was initiated as a result of the driving forces applied by the electric field. Both the self-rotation and the planar locomotion could be adopted to control the movement of liquid objects [18]. Such flexible capabilities are of important value for developing biomedical fluidic systems.

Figure 2.2 shows an electrohydrodynamic shooting phenomenon of liquid metal stream. Here, a low voltage direct current electric field would be strong enough to induce the ejection of liquid metal inside the capillary tube, which ultimately shoot into sodium hydroxide solution and form discrete droplets [47].

Tang et al. [33] demonstrated a system called the liquid metal enabled pump capable of driving liquid with modest electric field, abandoning traditional mechanical moving parts. This pump incorporates a droplet of liquid metal, which induces liquid flow at high flow rates, yet with exceptionally low power consumption by electrowetting/deelectrowetting at the metal surface. Figure 2.3

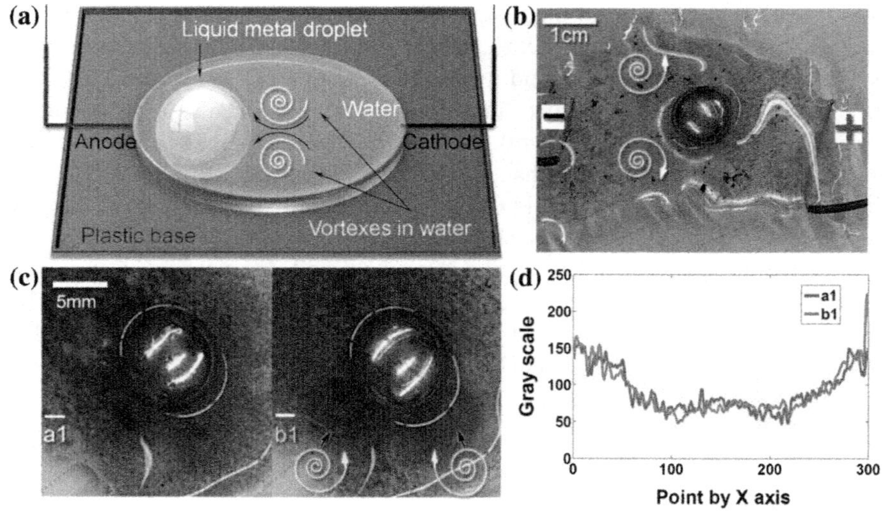

Fig. 2.1 Electric field induced rotation of a liquid metal sphere in electrolyte [18]. All pictures reproduced with permission

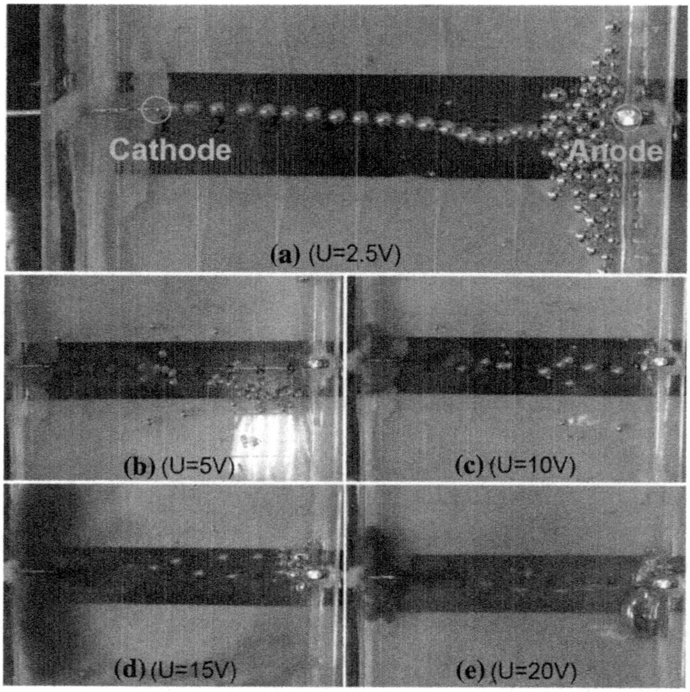

Fig. 2.2 An electrohydrodynamic shooting phenomenon of liquid metal stream. Sequential snapshots of liquid metal shooting in NaOH solution of 0.25 mol/L with different voltages [47]. Picture reproduced with permission

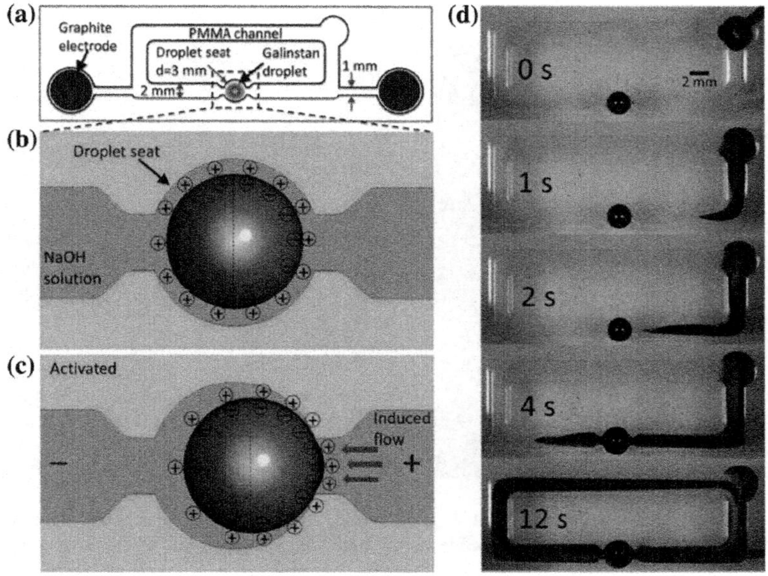

Fig. 2.3 A liquid metal enabled pump. **a** Galinstan droplet in confined channel; **b** schematic of the galinstan droplet surface charge distribution; **c** schematic of the galinstan droplet surface charge distribution when an electric field is applied between the graphite electrodes (the electric field will drive liquid metal in one direction, inducing electrolyte flow in the opposite direction); **d** sequential snapshots for the pumping effect of a galinstan droplet (a droplet of dye is used to demonstrate the pumping effect [33]). All pictures reproduced with permission

describes the continuous pumping effect with the liquid metal droplet ceased by the neck of the chamber under the effect of the external electric field.

Although liquid metal can be actuated via numerous ways, it remains a huge challenge to flexibly control the shape of a liquid metal drop due to its extremely high surface tension. In terms of this issue, Zhang et al. [48] introduced a SCHEME (synthetically chemical electrical mechanism) to regulate the surface tension. It was found that when liquid metal, which had been previously immersed in NaOH solution, touched the anode, gallium oxide with smaller surface tension would be formed. Liquid metal spread out and its surface area increased by 5 times. When the electrode was removed, the liquid metal recovered to spherical shape as the oxide layer gradually dissolved and the surface tension increased (Fig. 2.4).

The non-coalescence phenomenon between a droplet and the same-component liquid surface has been revealed recently [23]. The cathode and the anode were inserted respectively in the liquid metal bulk and the electrolyte. After applying voltage between the electrodes, a bearing electrolyte film filled the gap between the dripped liquid metal droplets and the underneath liquid metal bath, which maintained non-coalescent so long as the electric field existed, as if the droplets were surfing on the interface (Fig. 2.5).

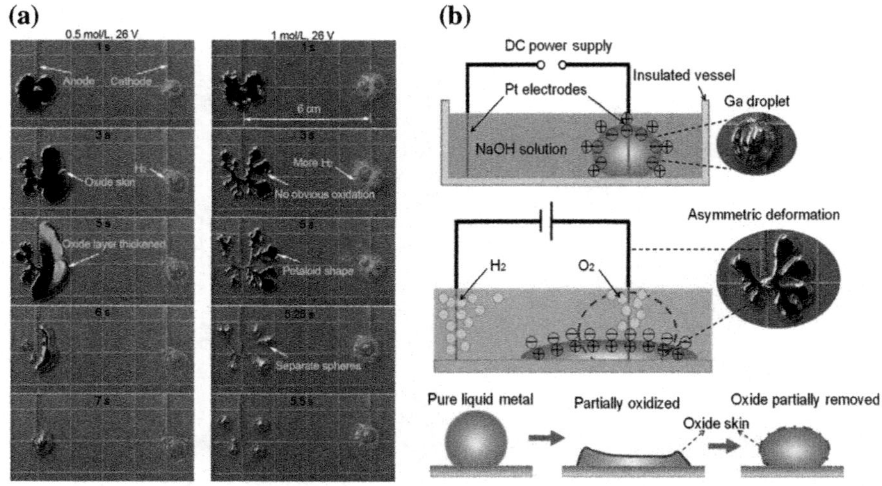

Fig. 2.4 Large scale deformation of liquid metal under electric field [48]. **a** Reversible deformation; **b** mechanism of the reversible liquid metal deformation. All pictures reproduced with permission

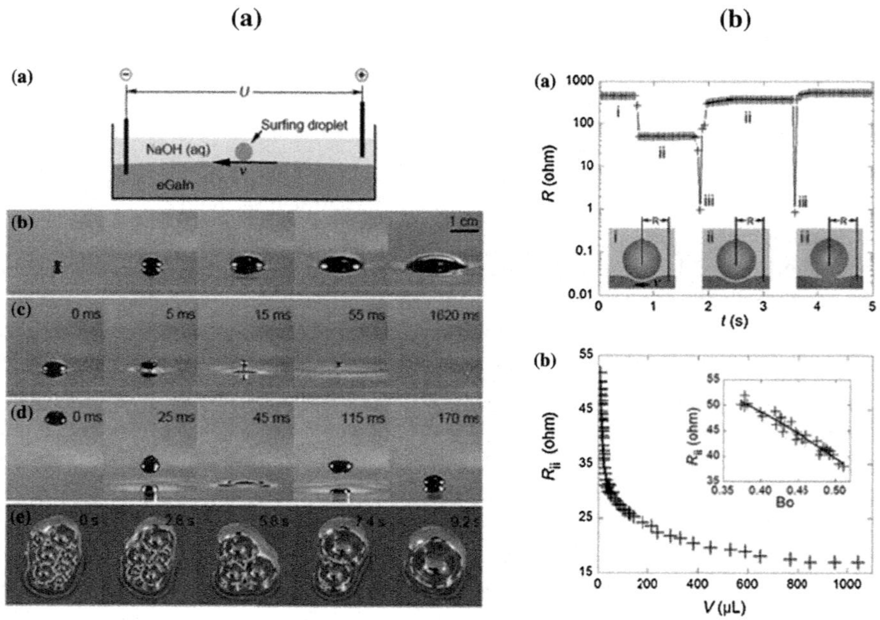

Fig. 2.5 Non-coalescence phenomenon of liquid metal drop. *A* **a**, **b** Surfing droplets with various sizes; **c** a droplet merging with the LM bulk immediately at the switching off of applied voltage; **d** an impacting non-coalescent LMD dropping from a height of 5 cm; **e** a surfing LMD cluster coalescing into a large droplet. *B* Resistance evolution of the solution film before and after cutting off the applied voltage [23]. All pictures reproduced with permission

2.3.2 *Self-driven Motion of Liquid Metal*

A most unconventional discovery on the liquid metal lies in its self-driving effect. For example, eutectic Ga–In alloy droplets can shift spontaneously in NaOH solution through only eating a small piece of aluminum. A milli-/centimeter scaled Ga–In–Al drop is capable of navigating itself to fit in different geometrical spaces where it voyaged at a considerably large velocity of 5 cm/s for more than one hour (Fig. 2.6). The soft machine works just like a biomimetic mollusk which eats Al as food [19], offering inspirations on the future development of bio-robots.

Also interestingly, a self-powered copper wire oscillator was disclosed, as seen in Fig. 2.7 [20]. When contacting a copper wire with the liquid $GaIn_{10}$ alloy pre-fueled with a small piece of aluminum, the copper wire was wetted and then swallowed into the liquid metal body. After a while, it began oscillating across the liquid metal horizontally just like a violin bow.

A fundamental scientific finding was reported that a bouncing bright liquid-metal droplet in an alkaline electrolyte could be transformed to a flat and dull puddle when placed on a graphite surface without the use of electric field. Through the intrinsic interactions between the liquid metal and the graphite, the liquid-metal puddle on the graphite could be manipulated as desired into various stable shapes with sharp angles in a semi-open space via a simple and highly feasible method (Fig. 2.8) [21].

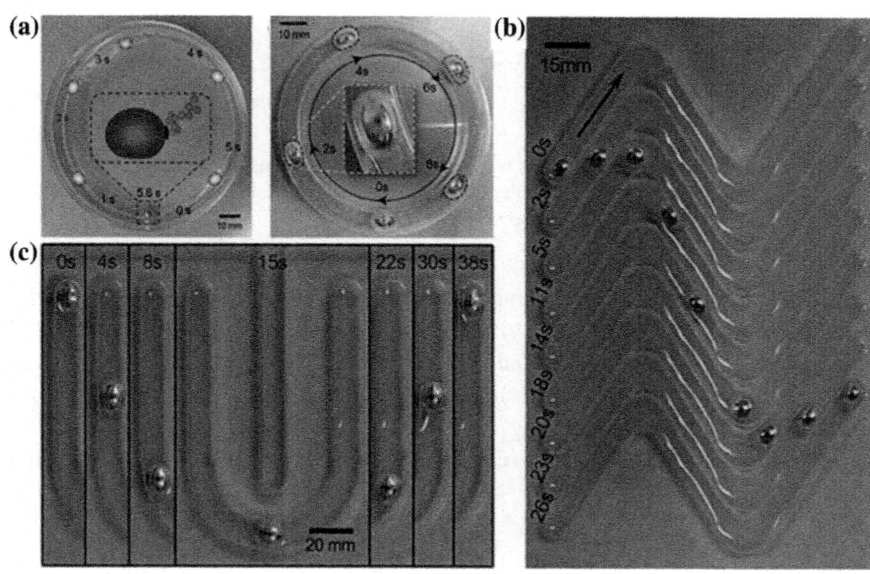

Fig. 2.6 Self-running of liquid Ga–In–Al soft motor along different geometrical space filled with NaOH solution [19]. All pictures reproduced with permission

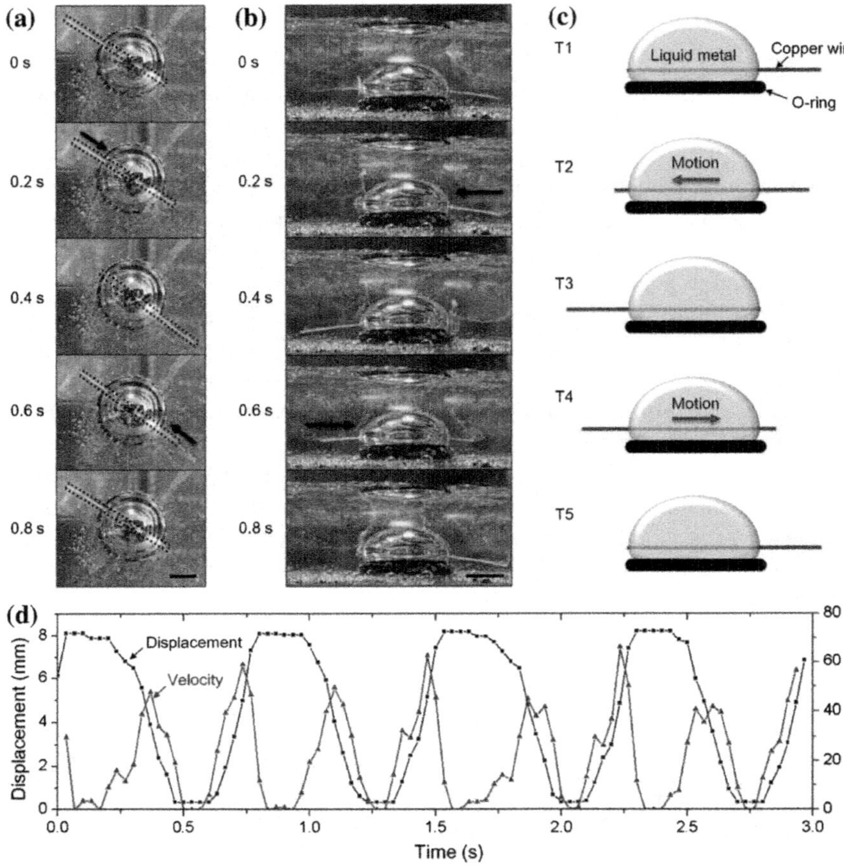

Fig. 2.7 Oscillation behavior of copper wire in liquid metal machine. **a** Top down view; **b** side view; **c** position of the copper wire during one period; **d** time evolution of the copper wire during 3 s [20]. All pictures reproduced with permission

Further, unusual biomimetic amoeba-like behaviors of liquid metal were discovered when amalgamated with Al, with the multi-material system placed on a graphite substrate immersed in the alkaline electrolyte [49]. Systems with varied Al content presented distinctive behaviors, as the less Al involved, the more resembling to the amoeba movement (Fig. 2.9). The underlying mechanism is the surface tension gradient on account of the reductive effect by Al reaction and the oxidative effect by graphite.

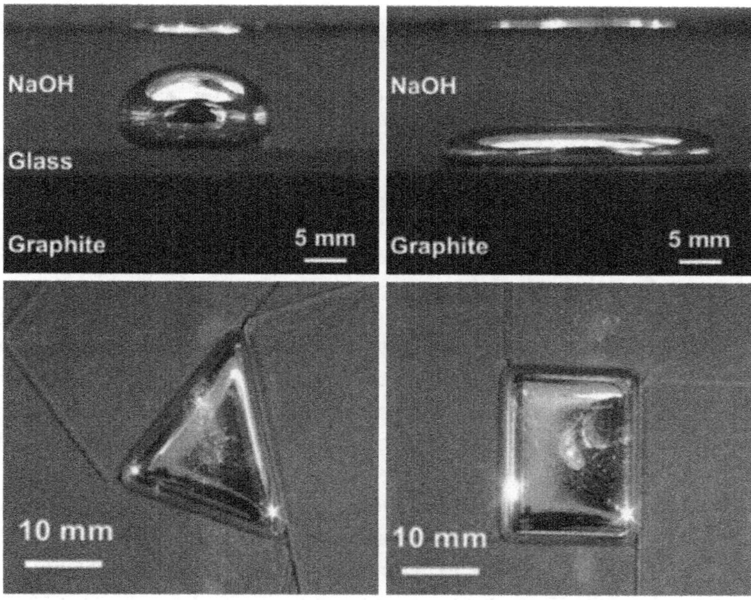

Fig. 2.8 Shape manipulation of the liquid metal droplet on graphite in an electrolyte [21]. Picture reproduced with permission

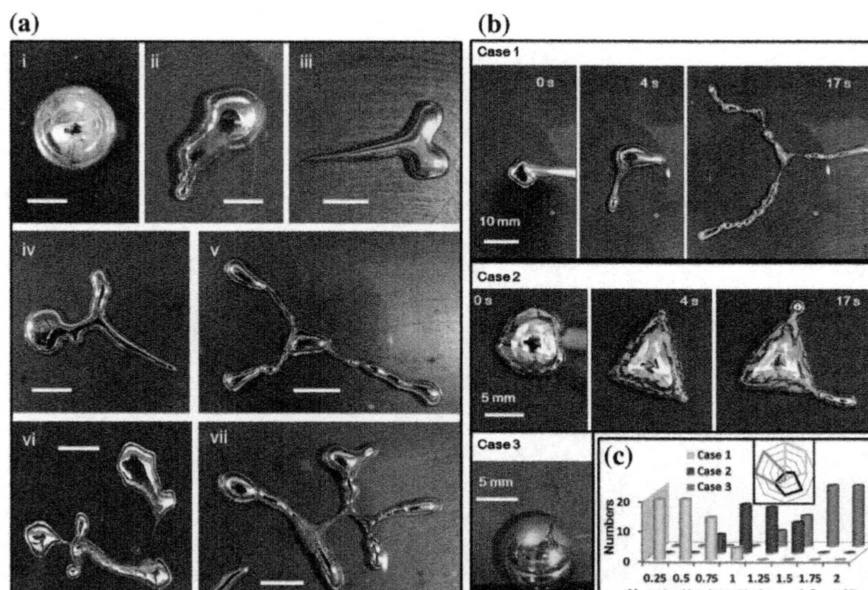

Fig. 2.9 Unusual biomimetic amoeba-like behaviors of liquid metal. **a** Amoeba-like transformations of LM-Al droplet prepared in NaOH in glass petri dish; **b** consecutive snapshots of three typical heteromorphous transformation of LM-Al droplet in Cases 1–3; **c** categorized and numbered LM droplets with various Al contents presenting different behaviors [49]. All pictures reproduced with permission

2.3.3 Coupled Fields on Liquid Metal Machine

Tan et al. [43] reported a phenomenon that the magnetic field could make up a boundary to restrict motion of the aluminum powered liquid metal motor, which was termed as magnetic trap effect. The running of self-propelled Al–Ga–In tiny motors which was achieved via the hydrogen gas generated from the galvanic cell reaction among alloy, aluminum and surrounding electrolyte, is given in Fig. 2.10. Clearly, most of the liquid metal motors were trapped in the interior zone under the effect of magnetic field.

A liquid metal galinstan sphere, along with a NaOH solution, was stimulated to rotate centrifugally around the central electrode, while the rotating speed increases with the voltage. The apparatus and experiment phenomena are illustrated in Fig. 2.11. Here, liquid metal was actuated through the coupled electric field produced by previously arranged electrodes and vertically magnetic field which was produced by magnet underneath [50].

It has been discovered by this lab that adding aluminum to liquid metal droplets will significantly magnify its electric controlling capability, which provides dozens of times of driving force compared to pure $GaIn_{10}$ droplets. After switching on the electrical field, the aluminum powered liquid metal droplet would accelerate to an

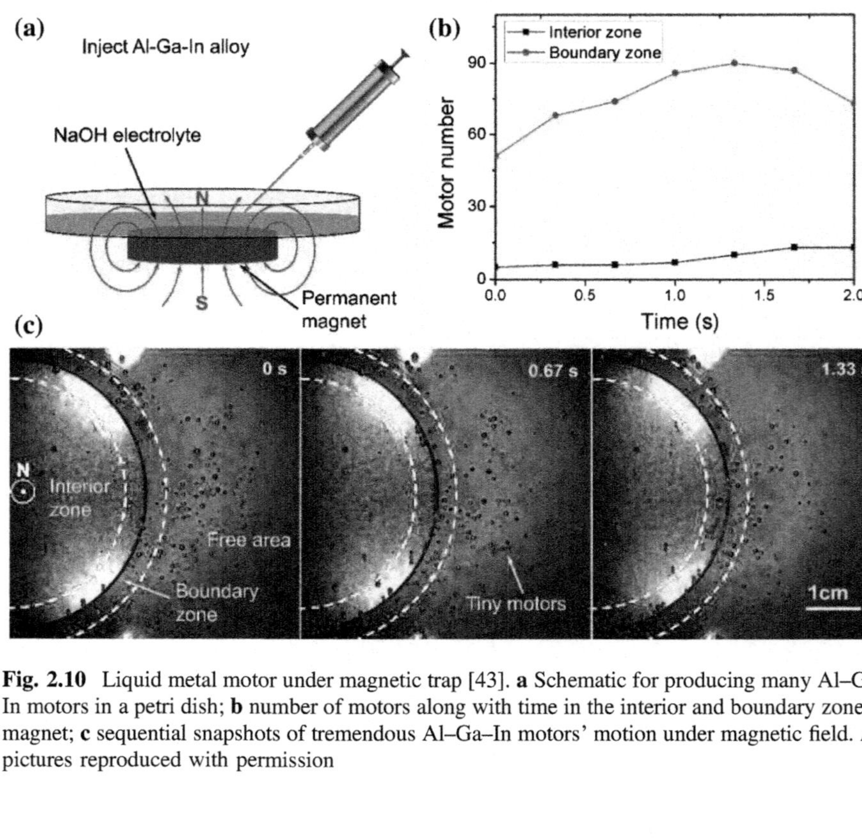

Fig. 2.10 Liquid metal motor under magnetic trap [43]. **a** Schematic for producing many Al–Ga–In motors in a petri dish; **b** number of motors along with time in the interior and boundary zone of magnet; **c** sequential snapshots of tremendous Al–Ga–In motors' motion under magnetic field. All pictures reproduced with permission

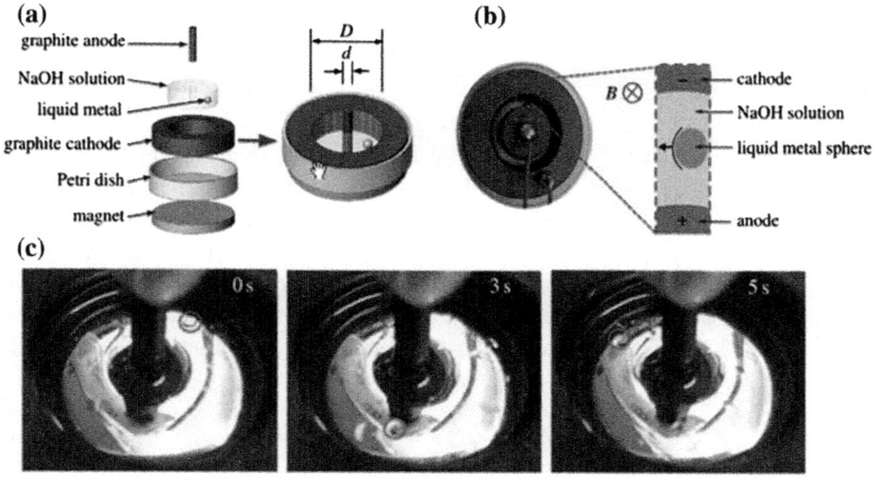

Fig. 2.11 Rotation of liquid metal under the coupled interaction of electric field and magnetic field [50]. **a** Exploded view (left) and side view (right) of a pair of concentric ring electrodes with a permanent magnet underneath; **b** structural diagram of a liquid metal sphere immersed in NaOH solution between a pair of concentric ring electrodes; **c** snapshots of the liquid metal. All pictures reproduced with permission

extremely high velocity [40], as compared in Fig. 2.12a, b. Therefore, the Al–Ga–In motors in a petri dish filled with NaOH solution could be easily controlled to a specific speed and direction, shown in Fig. 2.12c, as desired by an external electric filed.

Overall, these special phenomena indicate that the liquid metal can be actuated by potential fields, which avoids direct contact. These findings have both fundamental and practical significance, e.g., serving as the premise of a generalized way of making a soft machine, collecting discrete metal fluids, as well as flexibly manipulating liquid metal objects.

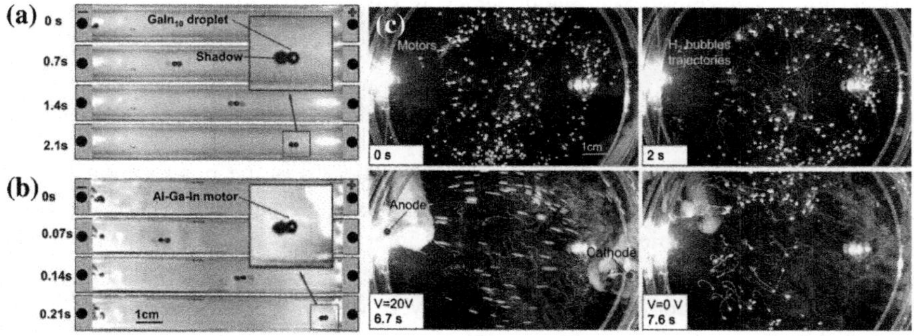

Fig. 2.12 Movement of liquid metal droplets adding aluminum under electric field [40]. **a** Sequential snapshots of motion of a $GaIn_{10}$ droplet; **b** sequential snapshots of motion of an Al–Ga–In motor in a straight channel; **c** sequential snapshots of Al–Ga–In motors shot from bottom up with a black background over the petri dish. All pictures reproduced with permission

2.4 Theoretical Foundation of Liquid Metal

2.4.1 Physical and Chemical Properties of Gallium

Liquid metal is becoming a core material for researchers wishing to combine the advantages of metals, such as high electrical conductivity, thermal conductivity, and reflectivity, with the inherently dynamic nature of fluids [1]. Some physical parameters for several typical liquid metals are listed in Table 2.1. Compared to other liquid metals, gallium and gallium-based alloys are more commonly used in the laboratory, owing to their extremely few toxicity and high stability.

As is well known, liquid gallium is easily oxidized in the air by the chemical formula [55]

$$4Ga + 3O_2 \rightarrow Ga_2O_3 \quad (2.1)$$

which results in a thin layer of gallium oxide on the surface and prevents the continuation of oxidation reaction. Owing to the larger surface tension of gallium than that of gallium oxide which invariably exists on the surface, gallium presents sphere shape in the solution, as shown in Fig. 2.13a.

While the liquid metal is immersed in the NaOH solution, its surface oxide is removed by the electrolyte and the chemical formula can be expressed as [56]

$$Ga_2O_3 + NaOH \rightarrow NaGaO_2 + H_2O \quad (2.2)$$

Therefore, the gallium placed on the glass substrate maintains an ellipsoidal shape in the alkali solution (Fig. 2.13b). Different from gallium in the NaOH solution on the glass substrate, a bouncing bright gallium droplet in NaOH electrolyte can be transformed into a flat and dull puddle when placed on a graphite surface. The special electric double layer (EDL) in the surface of gallium and graphite makes the inhomogeneous distribution of the surface tension around the gallium, which contributes to the transformation (Fig. 2.13c).

Gallium is an amphoteric metal, which is soluble not only in acid generating Ga^{3+}, but also in alkali, generating $[Ga(OH)_4]^-$

$$Ga + OH^- \rightarrow [Ga(OH)_4]^- \quad (2.3)$$

which makes liquid metal negatively charged. Therefore, the positive ions in the solution are electrostatically attracted by these anions and an electric double layer is generated at the liquid metal/electrolyte interface, as shown in Fig. 2.14a. According to the Stern's EDL theory [57, 58], as sketched in Fig. 2.14b, there exist two ion layers, contact layer and diffuse layer, with opposite charges and equal electrical quantity on the interface of two different liquid phases.

Table 2.1 Some physical properties of liquid metals [51–54]

Composition	Melting point (°C)	Boiling point (°C)	Thermal conductivity ($W\ m^{-1}\ K^{-1}$)	Electrical conductivity ($\Omega^{-1}\ m^{-1}$)	Surface tension ($N\ m^{-1}$)	Viscosity ($m^2\ s^{-1}$)	Density ($kg\ m^{-3}$)	Water compatibility
Hg	−38.8	356.65	8.34	1.0	0.455	13.5	1353	Soluble
Ga	29.8	2204.8	29.4	3.7	0.707	2.7	6080	Insoluble
Cs	28.65	2023.8	17.4	4.89	0.248	–	1879	Active
Rb	38.85	756.5	29.3	7.79	0.081	–	1532	Active
$GaIn_{24.5}$	15.5	2000	27.5	4.6	0.624	2.7	6280	Insoluble
$GaIn_{20.5}Sn_{12.5}$	10.5	>1300	–	3.1	0.535	2.98	6360	Insoluble
$NaK_{77.8}$	−12	785	26.2	2.88	0.11	2.4	750	Active

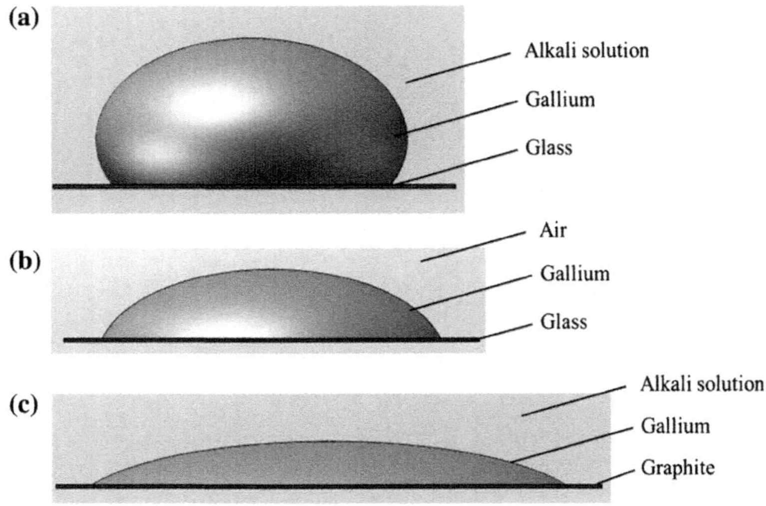

Fig. 2.13 Shape of gallium in different mediums and substrate [1]. **a** Shape of gallium in the air in glass substrate; **b** shape of gallium in aqueous solution in glass substrate; **c** shape of gallium in aqueous solution in graphite substrate. Picture reproduced with permission

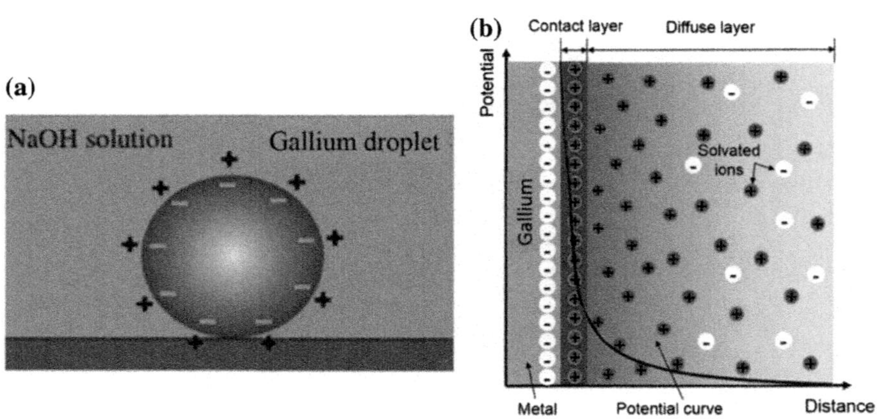

Fig. 2.14 EDL around the liquid metal drop [1]. **a** Schematic of an electrical double layer model of a gallium sphere in alkaline environment; **b** schematic theoretical model of Stern EDL. Picture reproduced with permission

In addition, owing to the larger density of liquid metal, when a droplet of liquid metal is placed in NaOH solution, it presents ellipsoid with an evident boundary. The force of the kinetic friction between liquid metal and the substrate is small because of the few contact areas.

2.4.2 Movement Theory

It is discussed in Sect. 2.2 that when a conducting drop (e.g. gallium) suspended in unbounded electrolyte is exposed to a uniform electric field, it migrates along the field direction and deforms to achieve equilibrium. The electrohydrodynamic effect on the drop is commonly associated with the electrical double layer, which plays a significant role in the interaction between the drop and the electrolyte. Differed by the conductivity, the physical models of drop can be divided into the perfect dielectrics model, the leaky dielectrics model, and the conducting drop model [59].

The development of conducting drop model can be summarized in Table 2.2. Smoluchowski [60] made a tremendous impetus on the theory of electroosmosis and electrophoresis by presenting the formula of the electrophoretic velocity of solid-particle electrophoresis and electrolyte drops. Likewise, Frumkin [61] conducted the first analysis of liquid metal drops in weak applied fields. Booth [62] then studied spherical fluid drops and concluded a same electrophoretic velocity for all dielectrics. In 1962, Levich [63] modified the velocity for highly conducted liquid drops, multiplying the Smoluchowski's scale by δ^{-1}, and confirmed the Frumkin-Levich velocity scaling experimentally.

To acquire the theoretical solution, O'Brien and White [8] put forward the weak-field linearization when studying electrophoretic mobility of colloidal particles, which was applied by Ohshima et al. [64], who made the first systematic analysis of charged liquid metal, independent of Debye thickness and zeta potential. To overcome the limit of weak applied field, Schnitzer [9, 65] simulated the conducting drop using the nonlinear macroscopic model, which was verified in the weak applied field condition.

An uncharged liquid metal drop in unbounded electrolyte in the presence of applied electric field is an equipotential body since electric field is unable to penetrate the drop, resulting in no tangential Maxwell stress exerting on it. Therefore, viscous force arising from the electrolyte is the propulsive force for the drop.

Liquid metal drop suspended in the electrolyte in the presence of an electric field has the following characteristics: (1) The Reynolds numbers of the liquid flows outside and inside the drop are small enough to allow ignorance of inertial terms in

Table 2.2 Developmentof conducting drop model [1]

Year	Name	Breakthroughs
1903	Smoluchowski	The electrophoretic velocity of solid-particle electrophoresis
1946	Frumkin	The first analysis of liquid metal drops in weak applied fields
1951	Booth	A same electrophoretic velocity for all dielectrics
1962	Levich	Multiplying the Smoluchowski's scale by δ^{-1} and confirmed experimentally
1978	O'Brien and White	Weak-field linearization
1984	Ohshima et al.	The first systematic analysis of charged conducting drops
2012	Schnitzer	Nonlinear macroscopic model

the Navier-Stokes equation while the liquids can be regarded as incompressible. (2) Considering the highly polarization of liquid metal drops, it is reasonable to assume that electrostatic charge, field or current do not exist inside the drop and that the drop surface is always equipotential. (3) The drop remains spherical throughout the entire process of motion under the field E. This assumption is satisfied when the surface tension is sufficiently large.

In the study of fluid mechanics, it is crucial to select the proper dimensionless number. Unlike the traditional capillary number used to describe the relationship between the viscosity force and the surface tension, the number of electric capillary number Ca_{E} is put forward to describe the relationship between the electric field stress and the surface tension [66–68], i.e.

$$Ca_{\mathrm{E}} = \frac{a\varepsilon_0 E_{\infty}^2}{\sigma} \tag{2.4}$$

where E_{∞} is applied electric field, σ is the surface tension of gallium, ε_0 is the dielectric constant of gallium in vacuum, a is the diameter of the drop, and Ca_{E} serves as a criterion to predict the possibility of deformation and fracture of dispersed liquid droplets.

The ratio of the density difference between the two phase liquids and the interfacial tension is represented by a non-dimensional parameter Bond number [69–71], which represents the effect of relative gravity of the drop on drop deformation. Bo can be expressed as

$$Bo = \frac{\Delta\rho g R^2}{\sigma} \tag{2.5}$$

where $\Delta\rho$ is the density difference between the two phases, g is acceleration of gravity, and σ represents the interfacial tension coefficient of the two-phase liquid. When the drop radius is smaller than the capillary length ($Bo < 1$), it would be flattened by gravity and form puddles.

Ohnesorge number Oh is used to measure the relationship between viscosity force, inertial force and surface tension [44, 71, 72]. The expression of Oh is

$$Oh = \frac{\mu}{\sqrt{\rho\sigma R}} \tag{2.6}$$

where σ is surface tension, μ is viscosity, ρ is the density of the ball, and R is the diameter of the ball.

The liquid metal drop and the electrolyte inside the electric double layer are considered separately at first and integrated with boundary conditions belatedly. Considering the fact that the liquid metal drop is scaled by millimeters or centimeters and the velocity is less than 1 m/s, the Reynolds numbers of the liquid flows outside and inside the drop are small enough to allow ignorance of inertial terms.

For liquid metal drop, the steady dynamics equations are expressed as

$$\nabla \cdot \boldsymbol{u} = 0 \tag{2.7}$$

$$\nabla \bar{p} = \mu \nabla^2 \boldsymbol{u} + \gamma \tag{2.8}$$

$$\gamma = \gamma_0 - \frac{1}{2} C U^2 \tag{2.9}$$

where $\bar{u}$ is the velocity field of liquid metal, $\bar{p}$ is drop pressure field, γ_0 is maximum surface tension value, γ is the surface tension of the liquid metal under the electric voltage U applied on the liquid metal/solution interface, and C is the capacitance per unit area of the EDL.

For electrolyte, the steady dynamics equations are expressed as

$$\nabla \cdot \boldsymbol{u} = 0 \tag{2.10}$$

$$\nabla p = \nabla^2 \boldsymbol{u} + \nabla^2 \varphi \nabla \varphi \tag{2.11}$$

where φ is electric potential, $\boldsymbol{u}$ is electrolyte velocity field, and p is electrolyte pressure field.

To acquire the electric potential distribution, the electric field equation sets need to be solved:

$$j^{\pm} = -\nabla c^{\pm} \pm c^{\pm} \nabla \varphi \tag{2.12}$$

$$\nabla \cdot j^{\pm} + \alpha u \cdot \nabla c^{\pm} = 0 \tag{2.13}$$

$$-2\delta^2 \nabla^2 \varphi = c^{+} - c^{-} \tag{2.14}$$

in which $j^{\pm}$ are molecular fluxes, $c^{\pm}$ are ionic concentrations, φ is electric potential, α is dimensionless drag coefficient, and δ is dimensionless Debye thickness.

Boundary conditions are also derived to combine the equation sets for liquid metal and electrolyte together. First, the normal ionic fluxes vanish at the interface. Second, the electric potential of liquid metal drop is uniform and the total charge of the drop is conservative. Third, tangential velocities of both liquid medium are equal and radial velocity vanishes to zero. Fourth, tangential-stress is balanced at the interface. Fifth, radial force exerted on the drop vanishes along the surface of liquid metal drop. Finally, at the remote place from the drop, ionic concentration, electric field and electrolyte velocity equal the initial values.

2.4.3 Deformation Theory

The deformation of a drop D can be defined as

$$D = \frac{L - B}{L + B} \tag{2.15}$$

where L represents the length of deformation and B the breadth. The first and second order in Ca_E can describe the small deformation of a spherical drop, put forward by Taylor [73] and later by Ajayi [74]. Taylor's discriminating function F_d can be used to decide whether the drop will deform into a prolate ($F_d > 0$) or an oblate ($F_d < 0$) one, i.e.

$$F_d(R, Q, \lambda) = (1 - R)^2 + R(1 - RQ)\left[2 + \frac{3}{5}\frac{2 + 3\lambda}{1 + \lambda}\right] \tag{2.16}$$

In the electrohydrodynamic analysis of the perfect conducting drop, researchers usually hypothesize that the perfect conducting drop is chemically inertness, which does not react with air or the solution. Another ideal assumption is that the perfect conducting drop is suspended in the solution, ignoring the gravity. The surface tension of the liquid metal is generally considered constant to simplify the analysis. Hence, the capillary number (Eq. 2.4) which is used to identify deformation is small. Therefore, the liquid metal drop remains spherical in the researches as mentioned above, ignoring the fact that surface tension varies with the transformation of the charge distribution on the surface. However, surface tension (Eq. 2.9) remains a significantly important parameter to decide the deformation pattern of the liquid metal. The pressure difference between the electrolyte and the liquid metal droplet p (pressure of Galinstan is higher) can be obtained from the Young-Laplace equation

$$p = 2 \times \frac{\gamma}{r} \tag{2.17}$$

where r is the radius of the liquid metal droplet.

Under applied external electric field, the surface tension changes with the charge redistribution on the surface and subsequently alters the force acting on the liquid metal (Fig. 2.15). The imbalance of the surface tension γ induces a pressure difference Δp between the downstream and upstream hemispheres of the droplet. The unbalanced surface tension will decrease with the increasing voltage, rapidly increasing the dimensionless number Ca to enable evident deformation.

In fact, gallium-based liquid metal is reactive with oxygen, generating a thin layer of gallium oxide with a smaller surface tension and a higher viscosity. Gallium-based liquid metal owns a density six times larger than the aqueous solution, allowing it to sink to the bottom of the container. Therefore, huge discrepancies have been found on the deformation of gallium-based liquid metal and the ideal conducting drop.

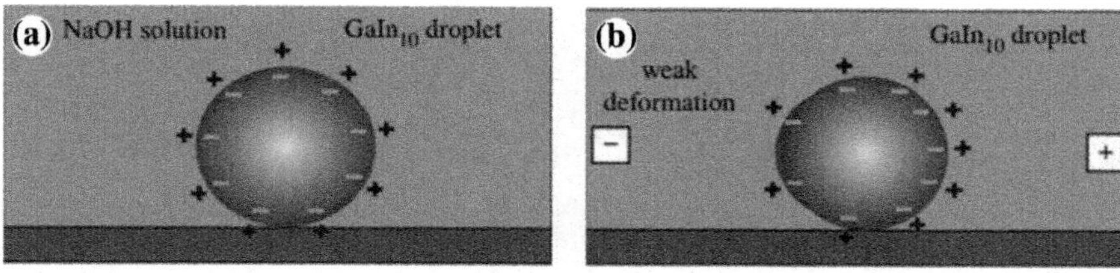

Fig. 2.15 Charge redistribution on surface of liquid metal drop under electric field [40]. **a** Schematic of an EDL model of a liquid metal sphere in alkaline environments; **b** schematic of varied charge distribution of liquid metal droplet and weak shape change under external electric field. Picture reproduced with permission

When the liquid metal contacts with an anode in NaOH solution, electrochemical oxidation occurs and immediately a layer of oxide is formed. The oxide film decreases the surface tension and then alters the contact angle at the interface between liquid metal and electrolyte at once, as Fig. 2.16 depicts [75]. Liquid metal sphere spreads out to an asymmetric layer, as the surface area becomes almost five times that of the original one. The explanation lies in the fact that gallium around the anode loses electrons and reacts with oxygen, generating gallium oxide. Therefore, the surface tension is weaker and the gravity is thus relatively dominant. To retain balance, the liquid metal deforms itself to decrease the effect of gravity. Figure 2.17 suggested that the liquid metal immersed in the alkaline solution placed on the graphite substrate should display a flat pancake without the electric field [21]. The predominant core is the transference of electrons from liquid metal to graphite, leaving liquid metal positively charged and easily oxidized. Sequentially, an oxide film is formed on the surface of the liquid metal, which highly resembles mud.

Although the movement of the gallium-based liquid metal is similar to the conducting drop model, the deformation theory is actually different.

First, the deformation mechanism is different. As shown in Fig. 2.18, the deformation of the gallium-based liquid metal is mainly resulted from the chemical

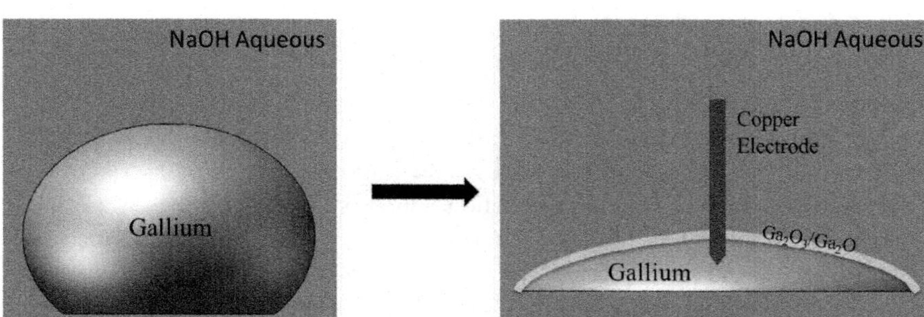

Fig. 2.16 Deformation process of liquid metal based on gallium immersed in the alkaline solution under electric field [1]. Picture reproduced with permission

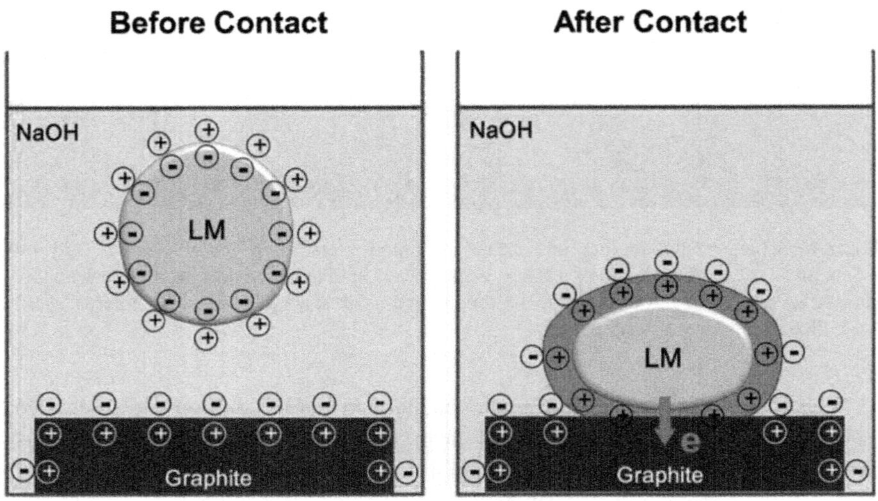

Fig. 2.17 Deformation process of gallium-based liquid metal on the graphite and immersed in the alkaline solution without electric field [21]. Picture reproduced with permission

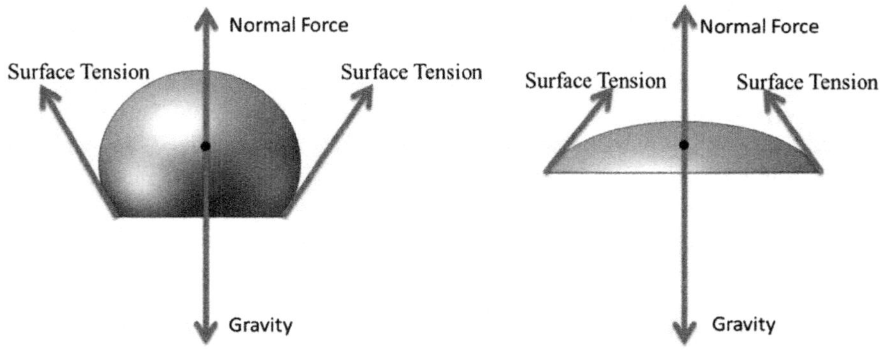

Fig. 2.18 Forces acting on gallium-based liquid metal before and after deformation [1]. Picture reproduced with permission

reaction which evidently decreases the surface tension. Once the surface tension is reduced, liquid metal will expand itself to make more contact with the container. However, the deformation of the ideal conducting drop is mainly ascribed to the inhomogeneous surface charge distribution which is induced by the electric field.

Next, the difficulty to lead to deformation is different. The deformation of gallium-based liquid metal occurs quickly requiring a lower voltage, ascribable to the active chemical oxidation reaction. However, to achieve visible deformation, a high electric field is required to make the Coulomb force at both ends of the ideal conducting drop big enough.

Finally, the deformation scale is different. Liquid metal can transform itself from an ellipsoid to a flat surface under proper electric field, whose surface expands over 1000 times. In contrast, the ideal conducting drop only deforms from sphere to ellipsoid.

2.5 Theoretical Simulation Method

With applied electric field, the fluidic movement contributes to the transport and redistribution of internal charges, which, in turn, affects the electric field distribution in the flow field. For the discrepancy in physical properties of the two-phase fluid, the electric field gradient on the interface is discontinuous under external field. Conductive droplets induce spontaneous electric field, which can be coupled with the original electric field, generating tangential electric force on the interface while inducing fluid motion along the boundary. Under different combinations of the electric field, the net charges and fluid properties, prolate or oblate-shaped deformations as well as circulation flows will be induced. Taylor [73] proposed the well-known leaky-dielectric model, whose accuracy was validated for small deformations. A parameter Ψ was put forward to determine the extent of drop deformation, i.e.

$$\Psi < 0, \quad \text{oblate,} \tag{2.18a}$$

$$\Psi = 0, \quad \text{spherical,} \tag{2.18b}$$

$$\Psi > 0, \quad \text{prolate,} \tag{2.18c}$$

where Ψ is defined as

$$\Psi(R, S, \kappa) = \frac{S}{(R+2)^2} \cdot \left[\frac{R^2+1}{S} - 2 + \frac{3 \cdot \left(\frac{R}{S} - 1\right)(3\kappa + 2)}{5\kappa + 5} \right] \tag{2.18d}$$

where R is conductivity ratio, S is permittivity ratio, and κ is the viscosity ratio of the drop to the surrounding fluid. Taylor also suggested the criteria for the flow direction on the interface, i.e.

$$R < S, \quad \text{from the pole to the equator,} \tag{2.19a}$$

$$R > S, \quad \text{from the equator to the pole,} \tag{2.19b}$$

Torza et al. [76] gave the first quantitative experimental results on a single drop deformation, and extending Taylor's theory to conditions of oscillatory (up to 60 Hz) fields. Alternating fields endowed the deformation an oscillatory part, apart from the steady part. However, disappointing quantitative agreement with Taylor's theory was also reported when large deformation occurred, which boiled down to the electrokinetic effects, demanding more accurate dielectric constants and other properties.

In this chapter, the deformation and movement of conductive droplets are focused on, which are dispersed in immiscible surrounding medium under uniform electric field. Numerous efforts on theoretical studies have been made to simulate the electrohydrodynamic phenomena of two-phase flow and different numerical simulation methods can be developed to mimic the liquid metal/aqueous solution interface, such as the VOF method, the LBM method, the boundary integral method, the finite-element method, and the front-tracking method.

2.5.1 Volume-of-Fluid Method

The volume-of-fluid (VOF) method uses a marker function F to track the fluid volume changes in a computational cell, anywhere between zero and one indicating a free boundary while at either ends representing a single phase. F satisfies [77]

$$\frac{\partial F}{\partial t} + \nabla \cdot (\boldsymbol{U}F) = 0 \tag{2.20}$$

The accuracy and the versatility of the method were verified by Tomar et al. [78], who proposed the coupled level set and volume-of-fluid (CLSVOF) algorithm to simulate the electrohydrodynamic behaviors of two-phase flows, combining the virtues of both schemes. The electric field equations for perfectly dielectric liquids and conducting liquids are

$$\nabla \cdot \boldsymbol{J} = \nabla \cdot (\sigma \boldsymbol{E}) = 0 \tag{2.21}$$

$$\nabla \cdot \boldsymbol{v} = 0 \tag{2.22}$$

respectively, while the hydrodynamic governing equations are

$$\rho(H_\delta)\left(\frac{\partial v}{\partial t} + \boldsymbol{v} \cdot \nabla \boldsymbol{v}\right) = -\nabla p + \nabla \cdot \left[\mu(H_\delta)\left(\nabla \boldsymbol{v} + \nabla \boldsymbol{v}^{\mathrm{T}}\right)\right] + \rho(H_\delta)\boldsymbol{g} + \boldsymbol{f}_v^\gamma + \boldsymbol{f}_v^{\mathrm{E}} \tag{2.23}$$

where $\boldsymbol{J} = \sigma \boldsymbol{E}$ is current density, $\boldsymbol{v} = (u, v)$ is velocity vector, t is time, p is pressure, g is gravitational acceleration, $\boldsymbol{f}_v^\gamma$ is the surface tension force which equals zero except in interfacial transition area, $\boldsymbol{f}_v^{\mathrm{E}}$ is electric field force, $\rho(H_\delta)$ is density, and $\mu(H_\delta)$ is dynamic viscosity,

$$\rho(H_\delta) = \rho_1 H_\delta + (1 - H_\delta)\rho_2 \tag{2.24}$$

$$\mu(H_\delta) = \mu_1 H_\delta + (1 - H_\delta)\mu_2 \tag{2.25}$$

In order to solve the governing equations, $\rho(H_\delta)$ and $\mu(H_\delta)$ are interpolated using a smoothed Heaviside function which indicates different fluids at value 1 or 0 and varies smoothly in the transition region

$$\rho H_\delta(\phi) = \begin{cases} 0 & \text{if } \phi < -\delta, \\ 0.5\left[1 + \frac{\phi}{\delta} + \frac{1}{\pi}\sin\left(\frac{\pi\phi}{\delta}\right)\right] & \text{if } |\phi| < \delta, \\ 1 & \text{if } \phi > \delta, \end{cases} \tag{2.26}$$

where 2δ is transition region thickness and ϕ is a distance function which equals 0 at the interface.

The research shows that under the effect of electric field, the differences of the physical properties between the conducting drop and the surrounding fluid lead to the surface deformation and different forms of free charge redistribution on the interface. As exhibited in Fig. 2.19, for small deformations, the predicted deformation agrees well with the simulation results.

2.5.2 *Lattice Boltzmann Method*

Shan and Chen [79] developed the Lattice Boltzmann Method (LBM) to simulate flows containing multiple phases and components, which was widely employed in further multiphase/multicomponent or interfacial studies. The Lattice Boltzmann method is generally adopted to model complicated boundary conditions and multiphase/multicomponent interfaces, with no need for special treatment on the interface.

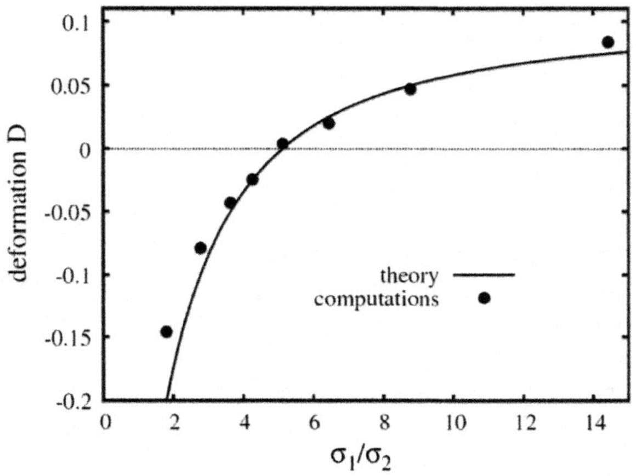

Fig. 2.19 Comparison of deformation factor D between predicted values and computational results for different ratios of the electric conductivities σ_1/σ_2 and $\varepsilon_1/\varepsilon_2 = 10$ [78]. Picture reproduced with permission

Zhang and Kwok [80] applied the 2-dimensional, 9-velocities Lattice Boltzmann method to simulate the drop deformation under electric field with the leaky dielectric theory. They solved the following equation

$$\rho f_i^{(k)}(\boldsymbol{x}+\boldsymbol{e}_i, t+1) - f_i^{(k)}(\boldsymbol{x}, t) = -\frac{f_i^{(k)}(\boldsymbol{x}, t) - \bar{f}_i^{(k)}(\boldsymbol{x}, t)}{\tau^{(k)}}, \tag{2.27}$$

where $f_i^{(k)}(\boldsymbol{x}, t)$ is the number density distribution of the kth component in the ith lattice velocity direction $\boldsymbol{e}_i$ at position $\boldsymbol{x}$ and time t, $\tau^{(k)}$ refers to relaxation time, $\bar{f}_i^{(k)}(\boldsymbol{x}, t)$ is the corresponding equilibrium distribution. The lattice velocities are given by

$$\boldsymbol{e}_0 = 0, \tag{2.28}$$

$$\boldsymbol{e}_i = \left(\cos\frac{i-1}{2}\pi, \sin\frac{i-1}{2}\pi\right) \quad (i = 1\text{–}4), \tag{2.29}$$

$$\boldsymbol{e}_i = \sqrt{2}\left(\cos\frac{2i-9}{4}\pi, \sin\frac{2i-9}{4}\pi\right) \quad (i = 5\text{–}8). \tag{2.30}$$

In order to implement LBM to electrohydrodynamics, it is assumed that the mixed dielectric properties are

$$\varepsilon = \varepsilon^{(1)}\rho^{(1)} + \varepsilon^{(2)}\rho^{(2)} \tag{2.31}$$

$$\sigma = \sigma^{(1)}\rho^{(1)} + \sigma^{(2)}\rho^{(2)} \tag{2.32}$$

where $\varepsilon^{(i)}$, $\sigma^{(i)}$ and $\rho^{(i)}$ are the permittivity, conductivity, and density of different phases. The motion characteristics of the two-phase flow depend on $R = \frac{\sigma_{in}}{\sigma_{out}}$ and $S = \frac{\varepsilon_{in}}{\varepsilon_{out}}$, among which the flow direction is determined only by the relative quantities of R and S, not directly related to drop deformation. The relations of drop deformation, property ratios, and velocity vectors are displayed in Fig. 2.20.

2.5.3 Boundary Integral Method

Miksis [81] developed a boundary integral method to calculate the shape of a suspended dielectric drop immersed in an unbounded medium under the influence of a steady electric field. Similar approach was applied by Sherwood [82] to study deformation and breakup of a single drop under the effect of electric fields, who solved both Laplace's equation for the applied electric field and the Navier-Stokes equations for the fluid motion. Tip-streaming from drops with pointed ends and division of the drop into two blobs connected by a thin thread were observed and

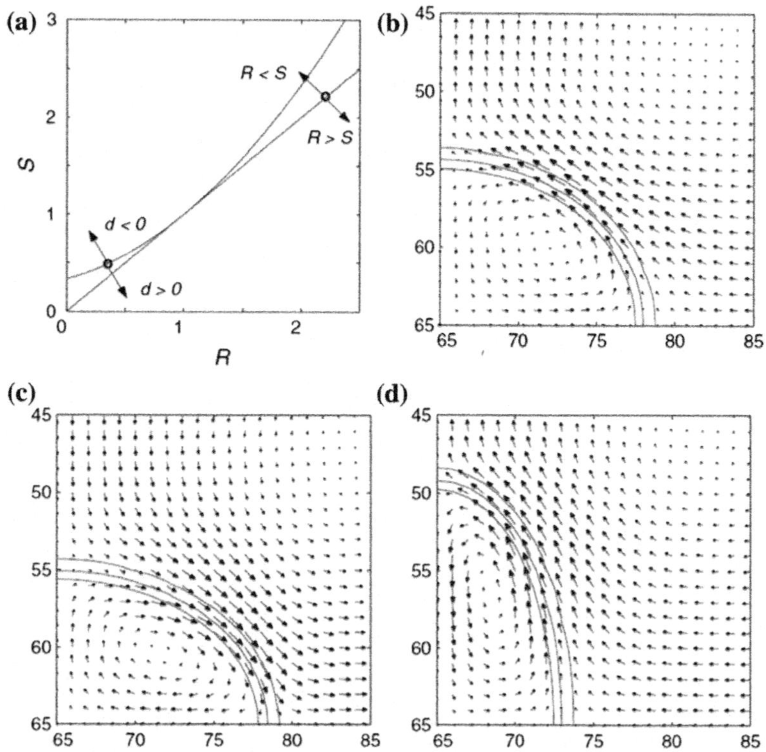

Fig. 2.20 Relations of drop deformation, property ratios, and velocity vectors [80]. **a** Relations of drop deformation factor and induced flow pattern; deformation, velocity vectors, and fluid density contours of the droplet (a quarter of the central region) when **b** $R > S$, $D > 0$; **c** $R < S$, $D > 0$; **d** $R < S$, $D < 0$. All pictures reproduced with permission

predicted by using numerical methods. Baygents et al. [83] employed the same technique to study the motion of two drops with no native charge in a uniform electric field using the leaky dielectric model, giving a boundary integral formulation of the electric field, which is represented as a surface distribution of dipoles.

Applying the boundary integral method to calculate the electric and velocity field, Lac and Homsy [84] studied the deformation and stability of a neutrally buoyant and initially uncharged drop in another solution under the effect of a uniform electric field. To solve hydrodynamic equations for the calculation of the interfacial velocity, stress distribution needs to be determined beforehand, which requires knowledge of the external electric field on the surface of the drop S. Surface distribution of dipoles are extensively used to represent the electric field in the boundary integral method [85] which reads as

$$\boldsymbol{E}^{\infty} + \oint_{S} \frac{\boldsymbol{r}}{4\pi r^3}[E_n(y) - \bar{E}_n(y)]\mathrm{d}S(y) = \begin{cases} \bar{\boldsymbol{E}}(x) & \text{if } x \in V_1, \\ 0.5[\boldsymbol{E}(x) + \bar{\boldsymbol{E}}(x)] & \text{if } x \in S, \\ \boldsymbol{E}(\boldsymbol{x}) & \text{if } x \in V_2. \end{cases} \quad (2.33)$$

Bring in the boundary condition, an integral equation for E_n can be written as

$$\boldsymbol{E}^{\infty} \cdot \boldsymbol{n}(x) + \frac{1-R}{4\pi} \oint_{\varphi} \frac{\boldsymbol{r} \cdot \boldsymbol{n}(x)}{r^3} E_n(y)\mathrm{d}S(y) = \frac{1+R}{2} E_n(x) \quad (2.34)$$

and E_t as

$$\boldsymbol{E}_t = \frac{\boldsymbol{E} + \bar{\boldsymbol{E}}}{2} - \frac{1+R}{2} E_n \boldsymbol{n}. \quad (2.35)$$

2.5.4 Finite-Element Method

Tsukada et al. [86] conducted simulations of the induced circulations inside and outside a stationary suspended deformable dielectric drop with the Galerkin finite-element scheme [87], which subdivided the axisymmetric problem domain into quadrilateral elements (Fig. 2.21). It is found that when $\Psi = 0$, the suspended drop remains spherical even when the dimensionless uniform electric field $E_0^* = 5$. For a silicone oil drop immersed in vegetable-oil mixture, where $\Psi < 0$ and the drop shape is oblate, the inner potential gradient of the drop is larger than the outside potential gradient of the drop. The induced circulation flows from the pole to the equator. For an opposite situation, where $\Psi > 0$ and the drop shape is prolate, the process goes into reverse. The simulation results showed good agreement with the theory of Taylor's [73] for small drop deformations. Conducting the same simulating scheme, Feng and Scott [68] considered a deformable leaky dielectric fluid drop suspended in an immiscible liquid subjected to an electric field and illustrated the deformation phenomena of the drop at finite Reynolds number and different viscosities. The work extended Taylor's linear asymptotic results by introducing nonlinearities which are ascribable to large deformation.

2.5.5 Front-Tracking Method

Front-tracking method is a numerical technique to solve the Stokes equations for the fluid flows, using connected marker points to track the boundary of the fluids, or the front, where generally the deformation and charge redistribution take place. Fernandez et al. [88] studied the effects of an electrostatic field on the distribution of drops in a channel flow using the front tracking method. Tryggvason et al. [89]

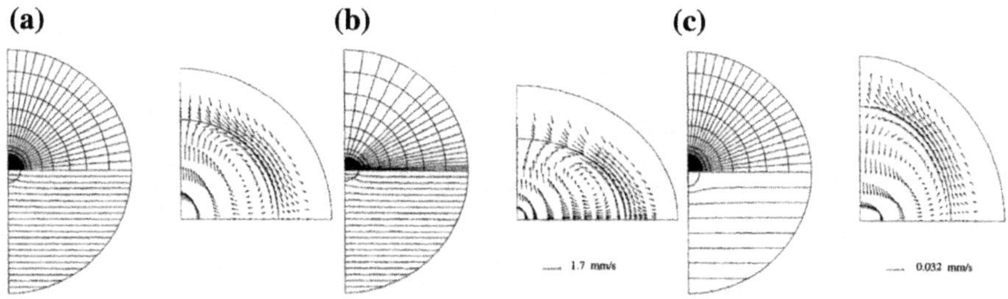

Fig. 2.21 Calculated drop shape, equipotential and velocity vectors [86]. **a** Dimensionless $E_0^* = 5$, ideal fictional system $\Psi = 0$; **b** $E_0^* = 5$, a silicone oil drop immersed in mixed oil; **c** $E_0^* = 2$, a mixed oil drop immersed in silicone oil. All pictures reproduced with permission

combined the front-capturing and front-tracking schemes, applying one set of governing equations while treating different phases as one fluid with different physical properties. It turns out that when conducting surface tension computations, despite its complexity, the front explicitly tracked by marker points is more direct and clearer than reconstructing it from a marker function.

Unverdi and Tryggvason [90] developed the finite-volume/front tracking method for incompressive flows of multi-phases fluids to explicitly track the interface while taking into consideration the surface tension and keeping the density and viscosity field sharp. The identical scheme was conducted by Hua et al. [66] to simulate the deformation and motion of the two-phase drop suspension system. The leaky dielectric model, the perfect dielectric model, and the constant surface charge model were applied, for the comprehensive consideration of the electric field, the net charges, and the properties of the two phases. For leaky dielectric drops, the ratio of electrical conductivity to permittivity decides whether the drops will deform into a prolate or oblate one. The intensity of the electric field-induced circulation flow inside the drop increases with the extent of the drop deformation. However, circulation flows are not obvious in a perfect dielectric drop, which generally deforms into a prolate shape. Drops with constant net charge, which provide resistance to deformation, usually move along the electric field in a prolate shape (Fig. 2.22).

2.6 Challenges and Prospects

Although several theoretical progresses have been made in modeling the movement and deformation mechanism of the liquid metal immersed in solution, there are still many challenges because of the unique characteristics of liquid metal and the complexity of the applied fields. Some of these points can be classified as follows.

(1) Non-uniform potential field. Concerning liquid metal under electric field, a majority of former researches focus on the non-uniform electric field and non-spherical liquid metal, which does not perfectly satisfy existing physical

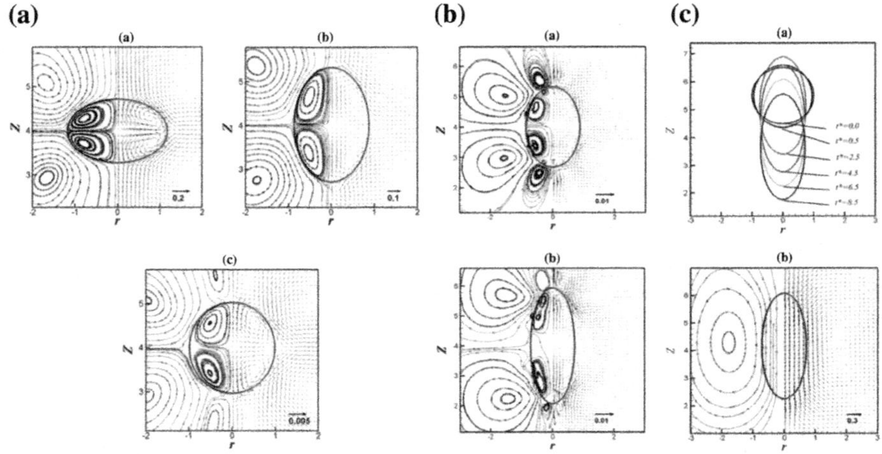

Fig. 2.22 Finite-volume/front tracking simulations of deformation and motion of two-phase drop suspension system, streamline on the left and velocity vector on the right [66]. **a** Simulated flow patterns using a leaky dielectric model for (i) oblate deformation, drop deformation factor $D = -0.09$ under the conditions of conductivity ratio $R = 0.5$, permittivity ratio $S = 2.0$, and electrical capillary number $Ca_{\mathrm{E}} = 0.1$; (ii) prolate deformation, $D = 0.1069$, $R = 50$, $S = 2.0$, and $Ca_{\mathrm{E}} = 0.1$; (iii) prolate deformation, $D = 0.0226$, $R = 0.01$, $S = 0.1$, and $Ca_{\mathrm{E}} = 0.1$, **b** simulated flow pattern using the perfect dielectric model under the conditions of (i) $S = 5$ and $Ca_{\mathrm{E}} = 0.5$; (ii) $S = 5$ and $Ca_{\mathrm{E}} = 1.0$, **c** (i) simulated droplet shape deformation and motion of a charged droplet ($q = 2.5$), $Ca_{\mathrm{E}} = 1.0$, and $S = 5.0$, (ii) snapshot of flow pattern around the charged droplet at $t = 6.5$. All pictures reproduced with permission

models, resulting in the difficulty of predicting the behaviors. The precise equations of the large-scale deformation, rotation, directional movement and merging of liquid metal in the immiscible fluid remain unknown. In order to settle these complex fluidic problems, a promising approach is to use computational fluid mechanics to calculate the hydrodynamics of liquid metal according to its characteristics.

(2) Charged liquid metal. In the experiment mentioned previously, liquid metal has been charged by contacting with the electrode, resulting in partially electrophoresis movement, which is different from the ideal conducting drop model. Meanwhile, the change of the electrical potential distribution on the surface of the charged liquid metal has an indescribable effect on the deformation as well. Therefore, the movement and deformation mechanism of the charged liquid metal needs to be further investigated.

(3) Superpositional potential fields. The theoretical researches on hydrodynamics of liquid metal in aqueous solution have been mainly focusing on situations with electric field exerted. Although the movement and deformation of liquid metal can be calculated by simulating the physical model, it is still tough to quantitate the deformation of the liquid metal, which combines numerous factors, e.g., the electric field, flow field, and chemical field. The specific

mechanisms of acoustic, optic, magnetic, thermal and other potential fields on hydrodynamics of liquid metal still lack sufficient researches. It is highly expected to find a new method to control liquid metal in the aqueous solution to achieve more complex biomedical applications.

(4) Internal flow field image. The observation of the liquid metal internal flow field is significantly important on constructing the movement and deformation mechanism. However, the internal flow field image has not yet been acquired because of the opaque property while only surface changes are visually.

Clearly, the theoretical progresses as made on the hydrodynamics of liquid metal will bring a significant impact on building deformable liquid machines and further on promoting soft robots running inside the biological cavity including blood vessels. Liquid metal is expected to show extraordinary potential in the fields of soft robot, biomedicine, enhanced heat dissipation, and ink-jet printing.

2.7 Conclusion

Liquid metal, endowed with both the outstanding fluidity of fluids and the metallic characteristics [1], has been proven promising in various fields, including both industrial manufacture and scientific studies. This chapter illustrates the unconventional hydrodynamics of the liquid metal immersed in immiscible solution under applied fields. Interesting experimental results are introduced to describe the hydrodynamic phenomena of the liquid metal. Physical models are provided to qualitatively explain the movement and deformation behavior of liquid metal related hybrid fluids under the electric field. Finally, several simulation methods are suggested to solve the physical model. However, it should be emphasized that the issues related to non-uniform potential fields, charged drops, coupled fields, internal streamline, etc., remain unsolved. Tremendous efforts ought to be made to precisely predict the movement and deformation of liquid metal immersed in solution or running inside the biological channel such as blood vessel, natural cavity etc. These would consist of the foundations to develop future biological application devices and technologies.

References

1. Zhang XD, Sun Y, Chen S, Liu J (2018) Unconventional hydrodynamics of hybrid fluid made of liquid metals and aqueous solution under applied fields. Front Energ. https://doi.org/10.1007/s11708-018-0545-3
2. Eow JS, Ghadiri M (2003) Motion, deformation and break-up of aqueous drops in oils under high electric field strengths. Chem Eng Process 42(4):259–272

3. Eow JS, Ghadiri M, Sharif A (2003) Experimental studies of deformation and break-up of aqueous drops in high electric fields. Colloids Surf A Physicochem Eng Aspects 225(1–3): 193–210
4. Tsouris C, Depaoli DW, Feng JQ et al (1994) Electrostatic spraying of nonconductive fluids into conductive fluids. AIChE J 40(11):1920–1923
5. Choi J, Kim YJ, Lee S et al (2008) Drop-on-demand printing of conductive ink by electrostatic field induced inkjet head. Appl Phys Lett 93(19):203
6. Choo RTC, Toguri JM (1992) The electrodynamic behavior of metal and metal sulphide droplets in slags. Can Metall Q 31(2):113–126
7. Mangelsdorf CS, White LR (1992) Electrophoretic mobility of a spherical colloidal particle in an oscillating electric field. J Chem Soc Faraday Trans 88(24):3567–3581
8. O'Brien RW (1978) Electrophoretic mobility of aspherical colloidal particle. J Chem Soc Faraday Trans 74(1):1607–1626
9. Ory S, Itzchak F, Ehud Y (2013) Electrokinetic flows about conducting drops. J Fluid Mech 722:394–423
10. Stone HA (2003) Dynamics of drop deformation and breakup in viscous fluids. Ann Rev Fluid Mech 26(26):65–102
11. Moffatt HK (1980) Rotation of a liquid metal under the action of a rotating magnetic field. MHD-Flows Turbul II(1):45–62
12. Karyappa RB, Deshmukh SD, Thaokar RM (2014) Breakup of a conducting drop in a uniform electric field. J Fluid Mech 754(754):550–589
13. Yang XH, Tan SC, Yuan B et al (2016) Alternating electric field actuated oscillating behavior of liquid metal and its application. Sci China Technol Sci 59(4):597–603
14. Plumlee HR (1964) Effects of electrostatic forces on drop collision and coalescence in air
15. Tryggvason G, Juric D, Nobari MHR et al (1994) Computations of drop collision and coalescence. APS Meeting. APS Meeting Abstracts
16. Gough RC, Morishita M, Dang JH et al (2015) Rapid electrocapillary deformation of liquid metal with reversible shape retention. Micro Nano Syst Lett 3(1):1–9
17. Zhao X, Xu S, Liu J (2017) Surface tension of liquid metal: role, mechanism and application. Front Energ 2:1–33
18. Sheng L, Zhang J, Liu J (2014) Diverse transformations of liquid metals between different morphologies. Adv Mater 26(34):6036–6042
19. Zhang J, Yao Y, Sheng L et al (2015) Self-fueled biomimetic liquid metal mollusk. Adv Mater 27(16):2648–2655
20. Yuan B, Wang L, Yang X, Ding Y, Tan S, Yi L, He Z, Liu J (2016) Liquid metal machine triggered violin-like wire oscillator. Adv Sci 3(10):1600212
21. Hu L, Wang L, Ding Y, Liu J (2016) Manipulation of liquid metals on a graphite surface. Adv Mater 28(41):9210
22. Yi L, Ding Y, Yuan B, Wang L, Tian L, Chen C, Liu F, Lu J, Song S, Liu J (2016) Breathing to harvest energy as a mechanism towards making a liquid metal beating heart. RSC Adv 6:94692–94698
23. Zhao X, Tang J, Liu J (2017) Surfing liquid metal droplet on the same metal bath via electrolyte interface. Appl Phys Lett 111:101603
24. Ma KQ, Liu J (2007) Heat-driven liquid metal cooling device for the thermal management of a computer chip. J Phys D Appl Phys 40(15):4722–4729
25. Ma K, Liu J (2007) Liquid metal cooling in thermal management of computer chips. Front Energy Power Eng Chin 1(4):384–402
26. Ma KQ, Liu J, Xiang SH et al (2009) Study of thawing behavior of liquid metal used as computer chip coolant. Int J Therm Sci 48(5):964–974
27. Deng Y, Liu J (2010) Hybrid liquid metal-water cooling system for heat dissipation of high power density microdevices. Heat Mass Transf 46(11–12):1327–1334
28. Tan SC, Zhou YX, Wang L et al (2016) Electrically driven chip cooling device using hybrid coolants of liquid metal and aqueous solution. Sci China Technol Sci 59(2):301–308

29. Tang J, Wang J, Liu J et al (2016) A volatile fluid assisted thermo-pneumatic liquid metal energy harvester. Appl Phys Lett 108(2):477–650
30. Tang W, Jiang T, Fan FR et al (2015) Liquid-metal electrode for high-performance triboelectric nanogenerator at an instantaneous energy conversion efficiency of 70.6%. Adv Funct Mater 25(24):3718–3725
31. Sánchez S, Soler L, Katuri J (2015) Chemically powered micro-and nanomotors. Angew Chem Int Ed 54(5):1414–1444
32. Gao M, Gui L (2015) Possibility and mechanism study of liquid-metal based micro electroosmotic flow pumps for long-time running purpose. In: ASME 2015, international conference on nanochannels, microchannels, and minichannels collocated with the ASME 2015 international technical conference and exhibition on packaging and integration of electronic and photonic microsystems, p V001T03A002
33. Tang SY, Khoshmanesh K, Vijay S, Phred P, O'Mullane AP, Derek A, Mitchell A, Kalantar-zadeh K (2014) Liquid metal enabled pump. Proc Natl Acad Sci USA 111(9):3304–3309
34. Liu J (2016) Liquid metal machine is evolving to soft robotics. Sci China Technol Sci 59:1793–1794
35. Yu YZ, Lu JR, Liu J (2017) 3D printing for functional electronics by injection and package of liquid metals into channels of mechanical structures. Mater Des 122:80–89
36. Gui H et al (2017) Spraying printing of liquid metal electronics on various clothes to compose wearable functional device. Sci China Technol Sci 60(2):306–316
37. Ge H, Li H, Mei S et al (2013) Low melting point liquid metal as a new class of phase change material: an emerging frontier in energy area. Renew Sustain Energ Rev 21(5):331–346
38. Mei S, Gao Y, Li H, et al (2013) Thermally induced porous structures in printed gallium coating to make transparent conductive film. Appl Phys Lett 102(4):041905-1-4
39. Vazquez G, Alvarez E, Navaza JM (1995) Surface tension of alcohol + water from 20 to 50 C. J Chem Eng Data 40(3):611–614
40. Tan SC, Yuan B, Liu J (2015) Electrical method to control the running direction and speed of self-powered tiny liquid metal motors. Proc Royal Soc A Math Phys Eng Sci 471(2183):32–38
41. Zhang J, Yao Y, Liu J (2015) Autonomous convergence and divergence of the self-powered soft liquid metal vehicles. Sci Bull 60(10):943–951
42. Bojarevičs A, Beinerts T, Sarma M et al (2015) Experiments on liquid metal flow induced by rotating magnetic dipole moment. J Manuf Sci Prod 46(1):4–6
43. Tan SC, Gui H, Yuan B, Liu L (2015) Magnetic trap effect to restrict motion of self-powered tiny liquid metal motors. Appl Phys Lett 18(7):13424
44. Yuan B, He Z, Fang W et al (2015) Liquid metal spring: oscillating coalescence and ejection of contacting liquid metal droplets. Sci Bull 60(6):648–653
45. Yuan B, Tan S, Zhou Y et al (2015) Self-powered macroscopic Brownian motion of spontaneously running liquid metal motors. Sci Bull 60(13):1203–1210
46. Sheng L, He Z, Yao Y et al (2015) Transient state machines: transient state machine enabled from the colliding and coalescence of a swarm of autonomously running liquid metal motors. Small 11(39):5178
47. Fang WQ, He ZZ, Liu J (2014) Electro-hydrodynamic shooting phenomenon of liquid metal stream. Appl Phys Lett 105(13):448
48. Zhang J, Sheng L, Liu J (2014) Synthetically chemical-electrical mechanism for controlling large scale reversible deformation of liquid metal objects. Sci Rep 4:7116
49. Liang H, Yuan B, Jing L (2017) Liquid metal amoeba with spontaneous pseudopodia formation and motion capability. Sci Rep 7(1):7256
50. Wang L, Liu J (2015) Electromagnetic rotation of a liquid metal sphere or pool within a solution. Proc Royal Soc A Math Phys Eng Sci 471(2178):20150177
51. Ma K (2008) Study on liquid metal cooling method for thermal management of computer chip. Dissertation for the doctoral degree. Technical Institute of Physics and Chemistry Chinese Academy of Science, Beijing

52. Xie K (2009) Study on the liquid metal cooling method for thermal management of computer. Dissertation for the master degree. Technical Institute of Physics and Chemistry Chinese Academy of Science, Beijing
53. Morley NB, Burris J, Cadwallader LC et al (2008) GaInSn usage in the research laboratory. Rev Sci Instrum 79(5):112–192
54. Pacio J, Wetzel T (2013) Assessment of liquid metal technology status and research paths for their use as efficient heat transfer fluids in solar central receiver systems. Sol Energy 93(7):11–22
55. Scharmann F, Cherkashinin G, Breternitz V, Knedlik C, Hartung G, Weber T, Schaefer JA (2010) Viscosity effect on GaInSn studied by XPS. Surf Interface Anal 36(8):981–985
56. Gao Y, Liu J (2012) Gallium-based thermal interface material with high compliance and wettability. Appl Phys A 107(3):701–708
57. Gongadze E, Rienen UV, Iglič A (2011) Generalized Stern models of the electric double layer considering the spatial variation of permittivity and finite size of ions in saturation regime. Cell Mol Biol Lett 16(4):576–594
58. Grahame DC (2003) Electrode processes and the electrical double layer. Surfaces, interfaces, and colloids: principles and applications, 2nd ed. Wiley, pp 337–358
59. Saville DA (2003) Electrohydrodynamics: the Taylor-Melcher leaky dielectric model. Ann Rev Fluid Mech 29(29):27–64
60. Smoluchowski MV (1903) Contribution to the theory of electro-osmosis and related phenomena. Bull Int Acad Sci Cracov 3:184–199
61. Frumkin A (1946) New electrocapillary phenomena. J Colloid Sci 1(3):277–291
62. Booth F (1951) The cataphoresis of spherical fluid droplets in electrolytes. J Chem Phys 19 (11):1331–1336
63. Levich VG, Rice SA (1963) Physicochemical hydrodynamics. Phys Today 16(5):75
64. Ohshima H, Healy TW (1984) Electrokinetic phenomena in a dilute suspension of charged mercury drops. J Chem Soc Faraday Trans 80(12):1643–1667
65. Schnitzer O, Yariv E (2013) Nonlinear electrokinetic flow about a polarized conducting drop. Phys Rev E Stat Nonlinear Soft Matter Phys 87(4):76–89
66. Hua J, Liang KL, Wang CH (2008) Numerical simulation of deformation/motion of a drop suspended in viscous liquids under influence of steady electric fields. Phys Fluids 20(11):295
67. Teigen KE, Munkejord ST (2010) Influence of surfactant on drop deformation in an electric field. Phys Fluids 22(11):858
68. Feng JQ, Scott TC (1996) A computational analysis of electrohydrodynamics of a leaky dielectric drop in an electric field. J Fluid Mech 311(311):289–326
69. Lü Y, Tian C, He L et al (2015) Numerical simulations on the double-droplets coalescence under the coupling effects of electric field and shearing field. Acta Petrolei Sinica 36:238–245
70. Melheim JA (2007) Computer simulation of turbulent electrocoalescence. Fakultet for Ingeniørvitenskap Og Teknologi
71. Wang FC, Feng JT, Zhao YP (2008) The head-on colliding process of binary liquid droplets at low velocity: high-speed photography experiments and modeling. J Colloid Interface Sci 326(1):196–200
72. Wang FC, Yang F, Zhao YP (2011) Size effect on the coalescence-induced self-propelled droplet. Appl Phys Lett 98(5):053112-1-3
73. Taylor G (1966) Studies in electrohydrodynamics. I. The circulation produced in a drop by electrical field. Proc Royal Soc A 291(1425):159–166
74. Ajayi OO (1978) A note on Taylor's electrohydrodynamic theory. Proc Royal Soc A 364 (1719):499–507
75. Yuan B, He ZZ, Liu J (2018) Effect of electric field on the wetting behavior of eutectic gallium–indium alloys in aqueous environment. J Electron Mater Interfaces. https://doi.org/10.1007/s11664-018-6134-8
76. Torza S, Cox RG, Mason SG (1971) Electrohydrodynamic deformation and burst of liquid drops. Philos Trans Royal Soc B Biol Sci 269(1198):295–319
77. Nichols BD, Hirt CW, Hotchkiss RS (1980) A fractional volume of fluid method for free boundary dynamics. Lect Notes Phys 141:304–309

78. Tomar G, Gerlach D, Biswas G et al (2007) Two-phase electrohydrodynamic simulations using a volume-of-fluid approach. J Comput Phys 227(2):1267–1285
79. Shan X, Chen H (1993) Lattice Boltzmann model for simulating flows with multiple phases and components. Phys Rev E Stat Phys Plasmas Fluids Relat Interdiscip Topics 47(3):1815–1819
80. Zhang J, Kwok DY (2005) A 2D lattice Boltzmann study on electrohydrodynamic drop deformation with the leaky dielectric theory. J Comput Phys 206(1):150–161
81. Miksis MJ (1981) Shape of a drop in an electric field. Phys Fluids 24(24):1967–1972
82. Sherwood JD (2006) Breakup of fluid droplets in electric and magnetic fields. J Fluid Mech 188(188):133–146
83. Baygents JC, Rivette NJ, Stone HA (1998) Electrohydrodynamic deformation and interaction of drop pairs. J Fluid Mech 368(368):359–375
84. Lac E, Homsy GM (2007) Axisymmetric deformation and stability of a viscous drop in a steady electric field. J Fluid Mech 590(590):239–264
85. Stone HA, Lister JR, Brenner MP (1981) Drops with conical ends in electric and magnetic fields. Proc Royal Soc A 1999(455):329
86. Tsukada T, Katayama T, Ito Y et al (2005) Theoretical and experimental studies of circulations inside and outside a deformed drop under a uniform electric field. J Chem Eng Jpn 26(6):698–703
87. Strang G, Fix GJ (1973) An analysis of the finite element method. Prentice-Hall
88. FernáNdez A, Tryggvason G, Che J et al (2005) The effects of electrostatic forces on the distribution of drops in a channel flow: two-dimensional oblate drops. Phys Fluids 17(9):955
89. Tryggvason G, Bunner B, Esmaeeli A et al (2001) A front-tracking method for the computations of multiphase flow. J Comput Phys 169(2):708–759
90. Unverdi SO, Tryggvason G (1992) A front-tracking method for viscous, incompressible, multi-fluid flows. J Comput Phys 100(1):25–37

Chapter 3
Electrical Properties of Liquid Metal in Making Biomedical Soft Electronics

Abstract This chapter presents an overview on typical electrical properties of liquid metal in making soft or flexible printed biomedical electronics. The core manufacturing material—the room temperature liquid metal was particularly focused for illustration purpose. Meanwhile, a series of recently developed manufacturing technologies spanning from personal electronic circuit printing to 3D room temperature liquid metal printing were comprehensively introduced. Applications of these planar or three-dimensional printing technologies and the related liquid metal alloy inks in making flexible electronics were briefly discussed. The significantly different adhesions of liquid metal inks on various substrates under different oxidation degrees, un-firmness of circuits, difficulty of fabricating high-accuracy device and low rate of good product which challenge current liquid metal flexible printed electronics were interpreted. Prospects of liquid metal electronics to develop ending user biomedical devices and more extensive applications in the coming daily life were given.

Keywords Liquid metal · Electrical property · Soft electronics
Adhesion

3.1 Introduction

Biomedical electronics has played an extremely important role in health care. Traditional electrical devices in the area generally belong to rigid category. That means, most of such hard wares are not so compliant with the human body use purpose. Compared with them, flexible, soft or even stretchable electronics would definitely suit better for various needs in biomedical practices. This chapter presents an overview on typical electrical properties of liquid metal in making soft or flexible printed biomedical electronics [1]. The core manufacturing material—the room temperature liquid metal, currently mainly represented by gallium and its alloys with the properties of excellent resistivity, enormous bendability, low adhesion and large surface tension, was particularly focused for illustration purpose. Meanwhile,

J. Liu and L. Yi, *Liquid Metal Biomaterials*,
Springer Series in Biomaterials Science and Engineering10,
https://doi.org/10.1007/978-981-10-5607-9_3

a series of recently developed manufacturing technologies spanning from personal electronic circuit printing (direct painting or writing, mechanical system printing, mask layer based printing and high-resolution nanoimprinting etc.) to 3D room temperature liquid metal printing were comprehensively introduced. Applications of these planar or three-dimensional printing technologies and the related liquid metal alloy inks in making flexible electronics, such as electronical components, health care sensors and more functional devices were briefly discussed. The significantly different adhesions of liquid metal inks on various substrates under different oxidation degrees, un-firmness of circuits, difficulty of fabricating high-accuracy device and low rate of good product which challenge current liquid metal flexible printed electronics were interpreted. Prospects of liquid metal electronics to develop ending user biomedical devices and more extensive applications in the coming daily life were given.

3.2 Basics About Flexible Printed Electronics

Printed electronics is the technology to fabricate electronic devices based on the principle of printing [2]. Unlike traditional printing technology, the inks used in the printing machine are electronic materials with the properties of being conductive, dielectric, semi-conductive or magnetic. Printed electronics is closely related to rather diverse fields, such as organic electronics, plastic electronics, flexible electronics and paper electronics etc. [3], which indicates that one can not only print circuits on silicon, glass, but also on plastic, paper, and more flexible substrates even human skin. One of the methods to produce flexible electronics is to directly print conductive materials on flexible substrates.

Classical flexible electronics generally refers to the technology that the organic/inorganic electronic devices are deposited on a flexible substrate to form the circuit [4]. Although the rigid circuit board can protect the electronic components from being damaged, it restricts the ductility and flexibility of the electronics. With intriguing properties in softness, ductility and low cost fabrication, the flexible electronics has broad application prospects in information, energy, medicine and defense technology areas through providing smart sensor, actuator, flexible display, organic light emitting diode (OLED) and so on. The most obvious characteristic of soft electronics lies in its flexibility compared with traditional rigid microelectronics, which allows it stretchable, conformal, portable, wearable and easy to print quickly [5–8]. Because of its unique merits in electrical, printable, biomedical and sensing properties, soft or flexible electronics can find rather diverse applications in electronic component [9], implantable device [10] and health monitoring [11], such as antennas [12], eyeball camera [13] and pressure sensor [14] etc. Nowadays, two common strategies have been adopted to improve the softness of the electronics [15]. One is embedding conductive materials, which is stiff and rigid, onto stretchable substrate, such as poly(dimethylsiloxane) (PDMS). Rogers and coworkers introduced a complex wavy structure to keep the circuit stretchable, which can absorb the major tension when stress acts on the soft substrate [16, 17]. The other is using inherently stretchable conductors to form the circuit [18]. Russo and coworkers demonstrated a way to connect circuit using conductive silver ink, which can directly write conductive text to interconnect light emitting diode (LED) arrays and three-dimensional (3D) antennas on paper [12].

Clearly, flexible printed electronics (FPE) combines both features of flexible electronics and printed electronics. In this way, one can quickly manufacture functional flexible electronic devices. Along with the maturation of printing technology, flexible printing has become a hot spot in research area. Several typical printing technologies have been emerging as: tapping mode printing [18], aerosol jet printing, roll-to-roll technology [19], inkjet printing [20], micropen and brush printing [21, 22]. Among them, micropen is perhaps the most straightforward way which is to pump the electrical ink into cartridge to directly write out conductive texts. This makes it possible to draw circuit diagram on an A4 paper. Micropen evidently reduces the complexity of circuit production and improves the efficiency of electronic circuit manufacturing. Extensive coverage makes FPE lots of significant achievements in different fields, such as flexible display devices [23], thin-film solar cells [24, 25], large area sensors and drivers [26, 27], electronic skin [28], wearable electronics and biological prosthetic devices [29], self-charging system [30], self-powered wireless monitoring [31], etc. If a circuit owns the properties of softness, conformability, stretchability and portability, one can call it equipment flectional electronic device. Meanwhile many laboratories have developed electronic devices with flexibility, such as warped display [32], folding battery [9], soft field effect transistor [33], stretchable wire [34] and so on. FPE can also be used in health monitoring, medical examination, vital signs detection, and other daily life needs. Flexible biomedical equipments have been widely utilized in the field of implantable device [10], nerve connection [35, 36], health monitor [11] and wearable medical device. In the meantime, FPE also has been used in biological sensing, the most important one of which is electronic skin (E-skin), such as pressure mapping [37], self-healing sensor [38], prosthesis [39], pressure sensor [14] etc. There are many research organizations working on different materials applied on flexible electronic skin. In Bao's lab, they invented a skin-inspired artificial mechanoreceptor system and the receptor can transform the pressure stimulation into the electrophysiological signal which human neurons can percept [40]. In Rogers' lab, they initiated the wavy structure to realize stretchable epidermal electronics which can maintain its original shape and function after compressing or stretching [16, 41, 42]. In Chiolerio's lab, the researchers invented a printable spin-coated silver nanocomposite ink to manufacture a resistive switching devices for neuromorphic applications and a nanocomposite flexible liquid state device in a synthetic colloidal suspension [43, 44].

Table 3.1 Comparison of the electrical conductivities of several typical conductive inks [54]

Ink type	Ink composition	Conductivity
Carbon conductive ink	Carbon	1.8×10^3 S/m
	CNT	$(5.03 \pm 0.05) \times 10^3$ S/m
Polymer conductive ink	PEDOT: PSS	8.25×10^3 S/m
Nano-silver ink	Ag-DDA	3.45×10^7 S/m
	Ag-PVP	6.25×10^6 S/m
Liquid metal ink	EGaIn	3.4×10^6 S/m
	$Bi_{35}In_{48.6}Sn_{16}Zn_{0.4}$	7.3×10^6 S/m

Generally, traditional nanoparticle-based conductive ink does not have intrinsic conductivity, and needs special post-processing (e.g. sintering, annealing) to remove solvent from the conductive ink to achieve conductive capacity, such as silver nanoparticle, PEDOT: PSS, polyaniline-based ink, nickel and copper conductive ink [45–49]. Unlike this classical way, the newly emerging liquid metal ink intrinsically owns high conductivity which therefore enables it a kind of ideal conductive ink (Table 3.1) (In this chapter, the EGaIn refers to Ga–In which contains the metal elements gallium and indium, which is commonly a mixture of 75.5% gallium and 24.5% indium by weight; while the Galinstan refers to Ga–In–Sn which contains the metal elements gallium, indium and tin, which is commonly a mixture of 62.5% gallium, 21.5% indium and 16% tin by weight.). Liquid metal, just as its name suggests, is a kind of metal which keeps in liquid phase from room temperature until 2000 °C. It is superior to many other liquid materials in thermal conductivity and resistivity at low temperature or around room temperature [50]. Traditional liquid metal—mercury is not accepted on account of its high-toxicity to human body. However, because of the non-toxicity and benign biocompatibility, liquid metal eutectic alloy of gallium indium has made important progresses in biomedical area such as being used as the material of bone cement [51], vascular contrast agent [52] and drug delivery nanomedicine [53]. All of these indicate that liquid metal can be widely used in the fields of electronics, material and biology, which significantly broadens its impacts to flexible printed electronics. Along with the development of material science and technology, liquid metal flexible printed electronics is quickly shaping the area of flexible electronic circuits, biomedical technology and allied machines as a basic way of quickly making functional devices (Fig. 3.1). This chapter is dedicated to integrate the liquid metal alloy inks with flexible printed electronics and focus on interpreting the recently developed typical liquid metal flexible printed electronics.

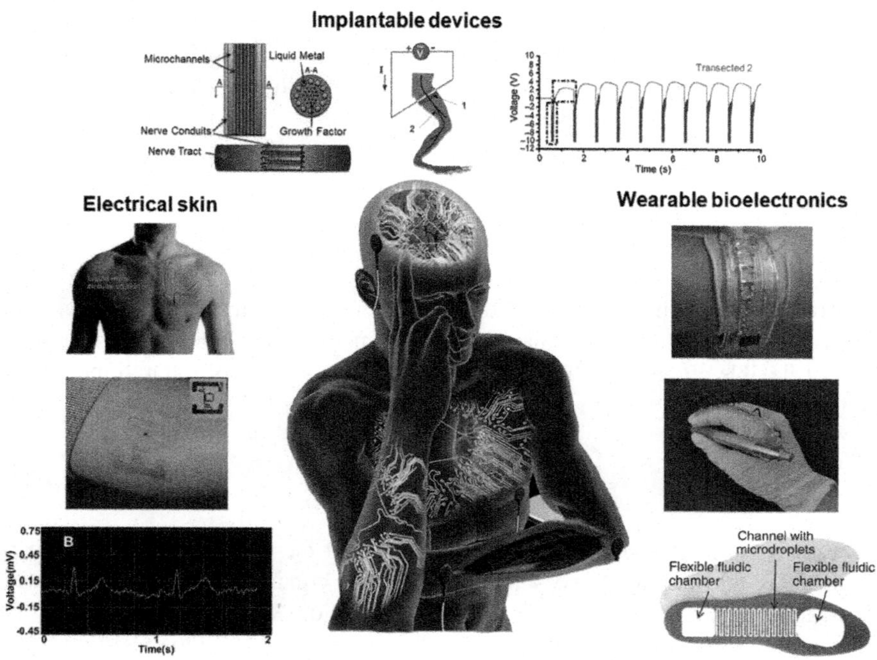

Fig. 3.1 Personalized flexible printed electronics based on liquid metal. 'Implantable devices': liquid metal nerve connection [35]; injectable 3D bioelectrode [55]; electrophysiological measurement of liquid metal reconnected nerve [36]; 'electrical skin': liquid metal circuits on human body [56]; liquid metal tag on human skin [57]; ECG test by liquid metal electrode [58]; 'wearable bioelectronics': liquid metal wristband [59]; a wearable data glove [60]; footwear-embedded microfluidic energy harvest [61]. All pictures reproduced with permission

3.3 Typical Electrical and Allied Behaviors of Liquid Metal

Generally speaking, alloy elements of low melting point include gallium, bismuth, lead, tin, cadmium and indium. Among them $GaIn_{24.5}$ is commonly used, which is a mixture of 75.5% gallium and 24.5% indium by weight. For the same composition, different proportion of the quality may lead to quite varied property of the alloys. Sometimes, even small change of mass ratio would cause strong enough variation of the material behaviors. If loaded with certain microelement, the alloy may also display additional properties accordingly. Therefore, one can change the ratio of chemical materials of alloys or add some microelements to adjust its melting point and more other properties to fulfill various specific needs. Room temperature liquid metal material generally represented by gallium and its alloys offers a unique option to manufacture flexible circuit, due to the combined nature of metallicity and fluidity [62, 63], which makes it especially suitable for printing on the soft substrate. From Ref. [62], one can get the information of the main physical properties of frequently-used liquid metal alloys, such as combination, melting point, density, resistivity and thermal conductivity. In the following, we mainly discussed the electroconductibility and allied behaviors such as flexibility, adhesion and wettability of liquid metal in flexible printed electronics.

3.4 Electrical Resistivity

Resistivity is the ability of an object to conduct an electric current, and generally the conductivity of metal is better than that of non-metal. If the liquid metal is applied to print flexible circuit, we can calculate the resistance value of a liquid metal wire by the formula:

$$R = \frac{\rho \cdot L}{A} \tag{3.1}$$

where R is the resistance. ρ is the resistivity and for the same material ρ is a fixed value. L is the length of measured liquid metal conductive wire and A is the crosssectional area. As it can be seen from the Eq. (3.1), the resistance of the material is directly proportional to the length of the material and the resistivity, and is inversely proportional to its cross-sectional area.

The relationship between the volume and length is:

$$A = \frac{V}{L} \tag{3.2}$$

Therefore, one can get the factors associated with resistance change as:

$$\frac{R}{R_0} = \frac{\frac{\rho \cdot L}{A}}{\frac{\rho_0 \cdot L_0}{A_0}} = \frac{\rho V_0}{\rho_0 V}\left(\frac{L}{L_0}\right)^2 \tag{3.3}$$

The volume of the liquid metal conductor is constant when drawing $V = V_0$; And the resistivity is also considered as constant, $\rho = \rho_0$. Consequently, one can simplify Eq. (3.3) to:

$$\frac{R}{R_0} = \left(\frac{L}{L_0}\right)^2 \tag{3.4}$$

Clearly, the resistance variation of liquid metal conductor takes linear relation with the square of the length change of the conductor before and after stretching, confirming the relationship between resistance and tensile length, which provides theoretical support for the development of liquid metal flexible sensor [56].

However, the resistivity ρ of the liquid metal has significant relationship with the thermal conductivity [64, 65]:

$$\frac{\Lambda}{\rho T} = \frac{\pi^2 \kappa_B^2}{3e^2} = 2.45 \times 10^{-8}\ (\mathrm{W}\ \Omega/\mathrm{K}^2) \tag{3.5}$$

Here, Λ is the thermal conductivity. ρ is the resistivity. T is the thermodynamic temperature, and Fig. 3.2b shows the $\rho - T$ and the $\Lambda - T$ curves for $Bi_{35}In_{48.6}Sn_{16}Zn_{0.4}$. With the increase of temperature from −150 to 50 °C, Λ is similar to a linear increase while ρ to a linear decrease. ρ_B is the Boltzmann constant. e is the electron charge, $e = -1.6 \times 10^{-19} C$. Equation (3.5) is the famous Wiedemann-Franz-Lorenz equation, from which one can deduce that the thermal conductivity of the liquid metal is proportional to the product of the resistivity and the thermodynamic temperature. One can thus get the resistance value of some number of wires connected in parallel by Ohm's Law [66]:

$$R = \left(\sum_{i=1}^{n} \frac{1}{R_i}\right)^{-1} \tag{3.6}$$

Here, n is the number of wires connected in parallel. R_i is the individual resistance values, i.e.

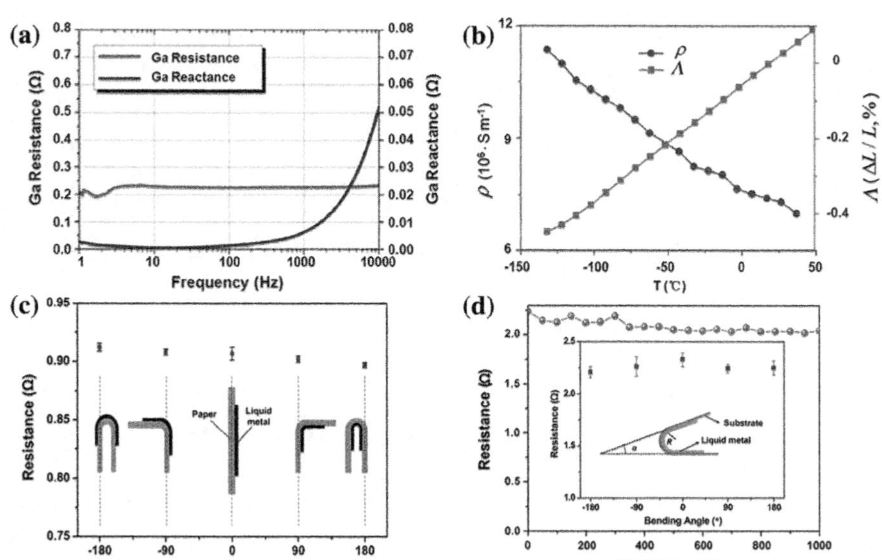

Fig. 3.2 **a** The resistance and reactance curves from 1 to 10 kHz of the liquid metal Ga [58]. **b** ρ (the resistivity)-T (temperature) and Λ (the thermal conductivity)-T (temperature) curves of liquid metal $Bi_{35}In_{48.6}Sn_{16}Zn_{0.4}$ [64]. **c** Resistance values of liquid metal line at five different bending angles [69]. **d** Resistance values of liquid metal line at different bending angles and different bending cycles [70]. All pictures reproduced with permission

$$R_i = \rho \int_0^L \frac{dx}{A_i(x)} \tag{3.7}$$

where, ρ is the resistivity and the resistivity of EGaIn is $29.4 \times 10^{-6}\ \Omega$ cm. Figure 3.3c demonstrates that the measured and predicted resistance values show a high degree of agreement with the number of wires changing [66]. However, there are some non-Ohm's Law phenomena that the current does not linearly vary with the voltage (Fig. 3.3a, b) [67, 68]. In Fig. 3.3a, the liquid metal marble is coated with WO_3 and the substrate is gold. It forms an electrical interface across the n-type semiconducting coating (WO_3) without the native oxide layer on the surface of the liquid metal, and the flow of current is owing to the combination between electron and hole carriers, which forms a n-type semiconductor layer. Therefore the measured current-voltage (I-V) shows the non-Ohm's Law phenomena. There are similar I-V characteristics between Fig. 3.3a, b, however different in theory. In Fig. 3.3b, the electronic device is composed by one gallium droplet and a layer of

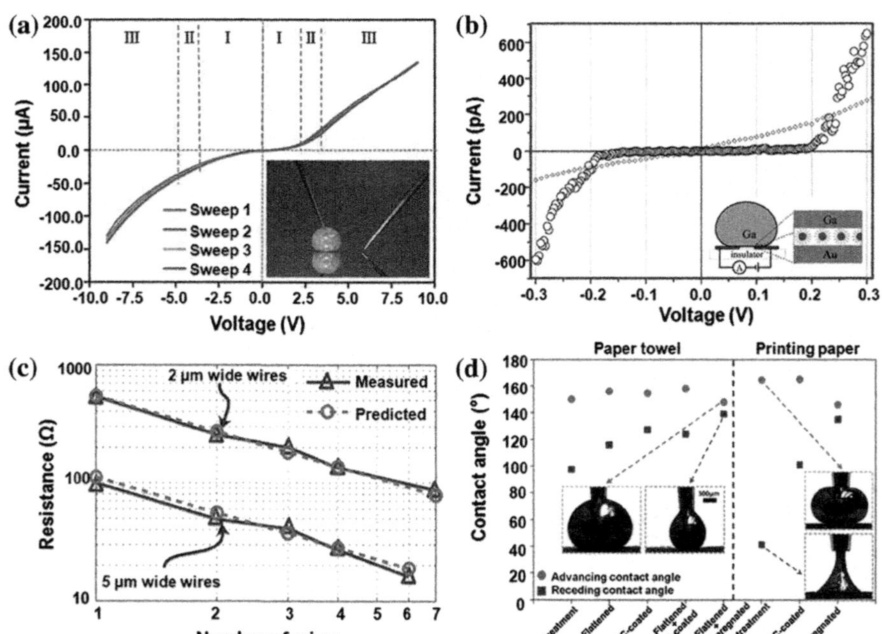

Fig. 3.3 **a** Characteristics between current and voltage of the liquid metal marble coating WO_3 (the substrate is gold) [67]. **b** Plot of the measured current and voltage of the electronic device composed by one gallium droplet and a layer of gold nanoparticles [68]. **c** The measured and predicted resistances of 2 and 5 μm wide wires for different number of wires connected in parallel [66]. **d** The advancing and receding contact angle of the liquid metal droplets on the paper towel and printing paper [71]. All pictures reproduced with permission

gold nanoparticles, and the gallium droplet is the electrode. The nanoparticle and its ligands form a capacitor. This is the process of capacitor charging and discharging. Under the threshold voltage, the circuit is not on and the current is zero. Once up the threshold voltage, the circuit is switched on. Meanwhile, some data demonstrates the relationship among the resistance, the reactance and frequency [58]. Figure 3.2a shows that when frequency changes from 1 to 10 kHz, Ga resistance remains the line at 0.225 Ω. However, Ga reactance closes to 0 Ω from 1 to 100 Hz and keeps analogously exponential growth from 100 to 10 kHz. Liquid metal resistance invariance under different frequency can realize the connection of frequency changing circuit.

3.5 Superior Flexibility

In order to illustrate the feasibility of liquid metal in manufacturing flexible circuit, Zheng et al. carried out a test to study the influence of bending on the stability of the circuit through measuring the resistance value when bending the printed liquid metal wire at −180°, −90°, 0°, 90°, 180°, respectively. Figure 3.2c evidently indicates that resistance variation is very little and the resistance stability of the liquid metal when bending manifests that liquid metal printed wire can be well applied for making flexible electronics [69]. Furthermore, bending the PVC plastic film printed by liquid metal at −180°, −90°, 0°, 90° and 180°, respectively for one cycle, and the resistance value was measured every 50 bending cycles (Fig. 3.2d). The resistance values fluctuated slightly from 1 to 1000 cycles, which demonstrated the stability property of the liquid metal resistor line [70]. Figure 3.4a, b

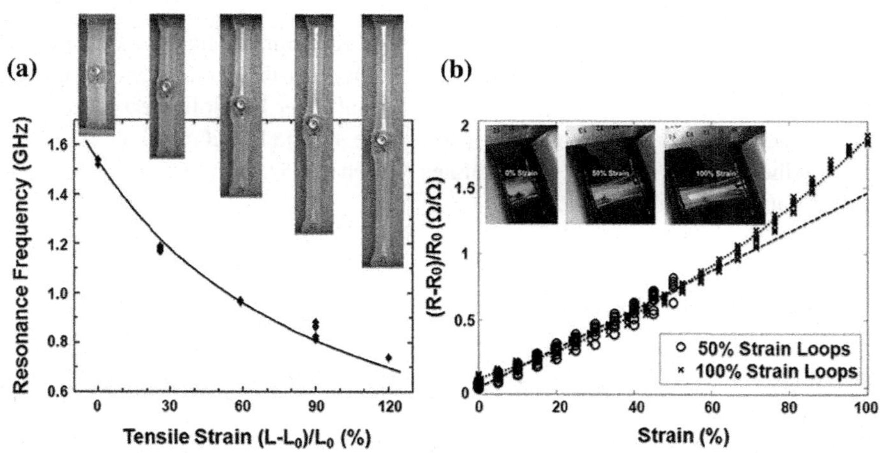

Fig. 3.4 **a** The relationship between the resonance frequency of the antenna and the tensile strain [72]. **b** The relationship between strain and resistance of directly written strain gauge devices [73]. All pictures reproduced with permission

demonstrate that when straining the liquid metal circuits, the resonance frequency and the resistance value can be changed [72, 73]. All the bending and stretching tests suggest that liquid metal printed wire has reliable flexibility when employed in flexible printed electronics.

3.6 Tunable Adhesion

Adhesion is the attraction among different molecules, such as the adhesion between the particle and the substrate [64–66]. When printing circuit, the liquid metal is ejected from the spray gun in the form of droplets [65]. When put in air, the surface of liquid metal droplet may generate a layer of oxide whose composition is Ga_2O_3/Ga_2O [74]. As is disclosed on the proportional relationship between the surface tension of liquid metal droplets and oxide content [75], the smaller the metal droplets, the higher the oxide content, thus the larger the surface tension, and the better the substrate adhesion. Starting from this point, Zhang et al. established a generalized way for ubiquitous printed electronics [65], where through atomized spraying of liquid metal droplets, circuit can be quickly fabricated on almost any desired solid substrate surfaces, whether smooth or rough [65]. Additionally, the greater the oxide content of the metal droplets, the smaller the contact angle between the droplet and substrate [76]. Designing of future printer can take care of such impacts inside.

Based on Young-Dupre equation [77], one has

$$W_{SL} = \gamma_L(1 + \cos\theta) \tag{3.8}$$

where, W_{SL} is the adhesion work of the liquid metal drop, γ_L is its surface tension, θ is the contact angle between the droplet and substrate. The smaller the droplet, the larger the γ_L and the smaller the θ, hence the greater the W_{SL} representing better adhesion. In other words, one can regulate the adhesion of liquid metal ink on substrate by controlling its oxide layer [78]. Another possible strategy would be that of realizing a controlled de-wetting after the metal layer has solidified by a slight temperature increase, as shown in Ref. [79]. However, the liquid metal alloy ink has strong adhesion to a majority of substrates, which makes it a challenge to manufacture micro-precision circuits [80].

3.7 Prominent Wettability

Wettability is the ability that liquid spreads on a solid surface. Contact angle usually expresses the wettability and the smaller the contact angle the better the wettability. The dynamic contact angle is the contact angle of a liquid moving over a surface. The dynamic contact angle (sliding angle and advancing-receding angle) plays an important role to quantify the wetting property of the oxidized Galinstan droplets compared with the static contact angle [81, 82]. And the relation reads as

$$\sin\alpha = \gamma_{LG}\frac{Rk}{mg}[\cos\theta_{rec} - \cos\theta_{adv}] \tag{3.9}$$

Here, α is sliding angle. R is the liquid metal droplet radius. m is the mass of the droplet. θ_{rec} is the receding contact angle. θ_{adv} is the advancing contact angle. The liquid metal droplet on the HCl-impregnated flattened paper has the lowest contact angle while for the non-treated printing paper, it has the highest contact angle (Fig. 3.3d) [71]. Gao et al. has tackled the excellent wettability of liquid metal $GaIn_{10}$ with different substrate materials including smooth polyvinylchloride (Fig. 3.5a), porous rubber (Fig. 3.5b), rough polyvinylchloride (Fig. 3.5c), tree leaf (Fig. 3.5d), epoxy resin board (Fig. 3.5e), typing paper (Fig. 3.5f), glass (Fig. 3.5g), cotton paper (Fig. 3.5h), plastic (Fig. 3.5i), cotton cloth (Fig. 3.5j), silica gel plate (Fig. 3.5k), glass fiber cloth (Fig. 3.5l) and more other substrates with different surface roughness and material properties [63, 75]. Kramer et al. investigated the relationship between the microtextured surface topograghy of the liquid metal marbles and the wetting behaviors [83]. Doudrick et al. tested that the oxide surface of the liquid metal alloy can improve the wettability between the metal material and substrate [80]. When increasing the oxygen content, the resistivity of the liquid metal alloy decreases, the viscosity and the wettability increase. For this reason, we can control the thickness of the oxide layer, and then the wettability of the liquid metal wire on the soft substrate to obtain a more superior performance of the flexible printed circuit.

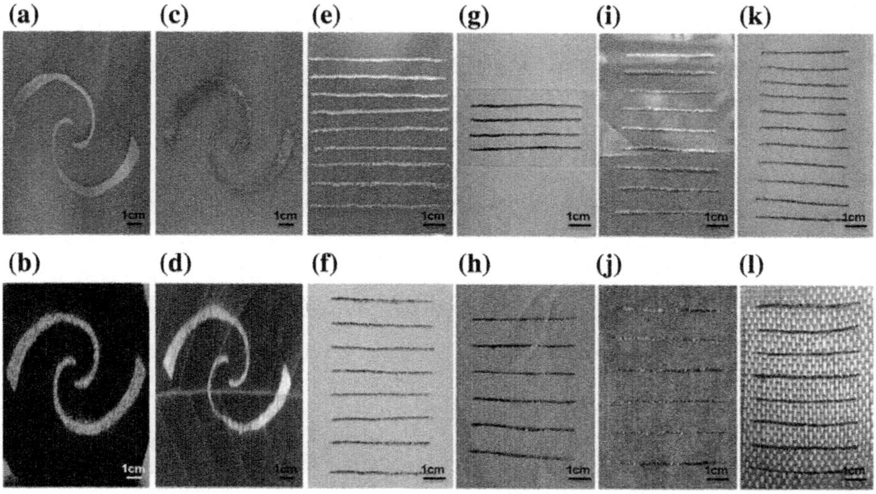

Fig. 3.5 Demonstrated wettability of liquid metal printed on different substrate materials [63, 75]. **a** Smooth polyvinylchloride; **b** porous rubber; **c** rough polyvinylchloride; **d** tree leaf; **e** epoxy resin board; **f** typing paper; **g** glass; **h** cotton paper; **i** plastic; **j** cotton cloth; **k** silica gel plate; **l** glass fiber cloth. All pictures reproduced with permission

3.8 Printing Technologies and Apparatuses

In ancient China, Sheng Bi, a brilliant inventor who lived in the 1041 AD, invented a new-type of printing method: movable type printing, which has brought great convenience for the spread of knowledge and culture. And the basic principle and method of modern letterpress stamping is the same as movable type printing in spite of its incomparable equipment and technical conditions. Clearly, the invention of an excellent printing method and selection of appropriate electronic printing ink has huge impact on human life. Table 3.1 shows conductivity comparison of several typical electroconductive inks [54]. The corrosivity of the liquid metal ink for different substrates (Table 3.2) prevents liquid gallium from being printed on specific flexible substrate.

3.9 Printing of Electronic Circuit

Nowadays, due to high surface tension and good conductive ability of liquid metal, the method to print circuit by liquid metal ink has attracted more and more attentions. The concept of DREAM ink (direct writing or printing of electronics based on alloy and metal ink) [62] as defined by Liu et al. can lead to alternative electronic devices in different fields [63, 85, 86]. So far, there are different methods to print personal electronic circuit: screen printing [70], atomized spraying [75], microcontact printing (μCP) [87], masked deposition [88], and inkjet printing [89].

3.9.1 Direct Painting or Writing

Because of its good wettability with multifarious substrates, room temperature liquid metal (RTLM) can be directly painted or written on paper, glass, cloth as liquid metal ink [63]. Sheng et al. directly painted the liquid metal ink on the

Table 3.2 The corrosion between liquid gallium and other metals [84]

Corrosive behavior	Easy to react with gallium	Better resistance for corrosion	Best resistance for corrosion
Metal	Iron, nickel, cadmium, cerium, copper, aluminum, gold, manganese, platinum, silver, tin and vanadium, zirconium	Titanium, tantalum, niobium, molybdenum, beryllium	Tungsten, rhenium, sintering BeO, Al_2O_3, and fused quartz, graphite
Temperature range	Appearing corrosion at 200 °C or even lower	Appearing corrosion above 400 °C	No corrosion even at 800 °C

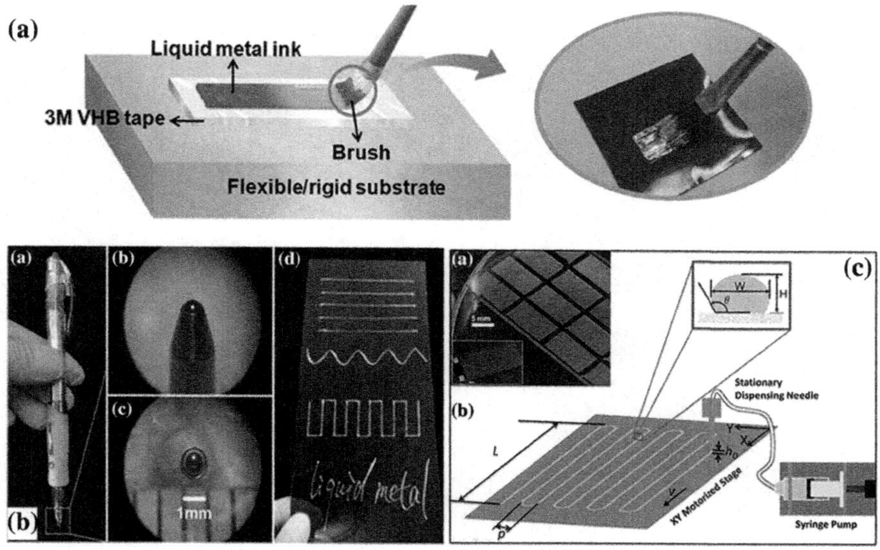

Fig. 3.6 Printing methods of direct painting or writing without machine. **a** Direct painting of the liquid metal ink on the surface of 3 M VHB tape to manufacture capacitor sensor [90]. **b** The liquid metal ink roller-ball pen and conductive tracks thus written [93]. **c** The direct writing system and the high-resolution wires written by it [73]. All pictures reproduced with permission

surface of 3 M VHB tape to manufacture capacitor sensor (Fig. 3.6a) [90]. Because of its gravity and adhesion to substrates, the liquid metal alloy can be directly installed into the refill as a kind of ink to write conductive texts or lines [91, 92]. Zheng et al. developed the liquid metal roller-ball pen (LMRP) which can directly write out conductive lines or electronic devices on soft plates with the tip ball diameters ranging from 200 to 1000 μm (Fig. 3.6b) [93]. Boley et al. illustrated a direct writing system of the liquid metal alloy to fabricate small-scale stretchable electronics (Fig. 3.6c) [73].

3.9.2 Mechanical Printing Methods

Compared to traditional direct painting or writing, mechanical printing methods can realize digital control which makes the liquid metal flexible electronical circuits more accurate and quantitative (Fig. 3.7). Zheng et al. has manufactured and demonstrated a versatile desktop liquid metal printer which can print either plane circuit or 3D metal object. The machine is made up of syringe, nitrogen gas tube, pressure controller, teach pendant, stage, X axis, Y axis, Z axis (Fig. 3.7b) [69]. In order to achieve the matching between different material substrate and printing ink, they have designed a brush like porous needle to print graph files of different types. Such desktop printer can print a variety of electrical patterns via computer software.

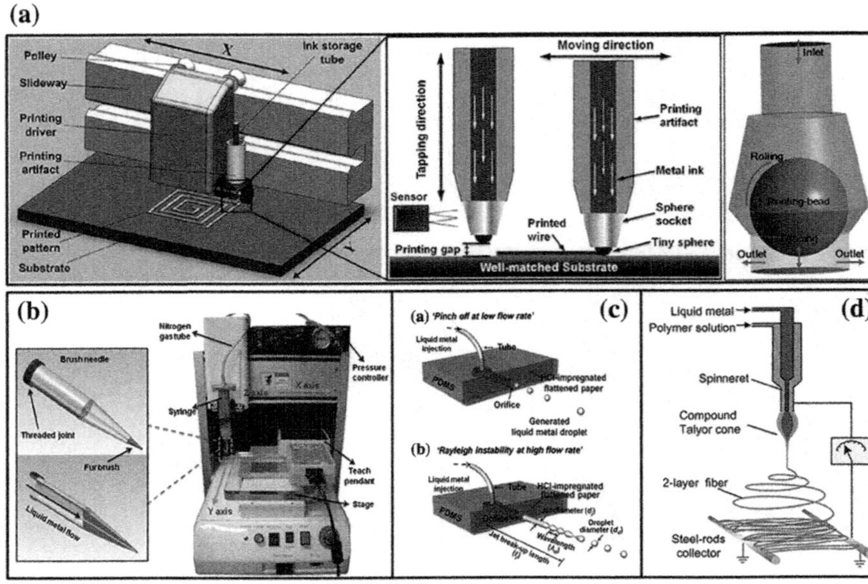

Fig. 3.7 Mechanical printing methods. **a** The tapping mode printer and its printing process [18]. **b** The desktop printer to directly print circuits on paper [69]. **c** Inkjet printing of the liquid metal droplet based on pinch-off and Rayleigh instability [94]. **d** Coelectrospinning to fabricate light-emitting coaxial nanofiber with the liquid metal core and polymer shell [95]. All pictures reproduced with permission

In particular, paper owns characteristics of low-cost and recycling, which makes it the common substrate material and brings in the concept of printed-circuits-on-paper (PCP) [69]. Along with that, the same group invented and created another fully automatic liquid metal printer for pervasive electronic circuit printing [18]. Its theory of tapping mode printing is fixing ink storage tube on printing driver, clamping the driver on the guide rail by sliding wheel, which can make the printer head move along the guide rail in the X direction and drive base plate along the Y direction by motor (Fig. 3.7a). Consequently, one can control the position of the printer head in printing area of the base plate. The tapping mode refers to that the nib can make small distance moving in Z direction. When printing, the printer head falls to contact the base, uplifts a height over printing, so as to avoid the printed line. In the process of printing, the printing header bead rotates due to the interaction with basal friction, which makes the liquid metal ink in the pen container run down. One can use the tapping mode method to manufacture various PCB (printed-circuit-on-board) circuits, antenna and so on. In addition, other mechanical system printing methods to print personal electronic circuit using liquid metal include inkjet printing and coelectrospinning (Fig. 3.7c, d) [89, 94, 95].

3.9.3 Mask Based Printing Method

Printing methods based on mask are the most commonly used method to manufacture the liquid metal flexible electronics in the laboratory. Kramer et al. provided a masked deposition method to fabricate the liquid metal hyperelastic electronic circuits (Fig. 3.8a) [88]. At the same time, Gozen et al. used the masked deposition method to prepare micro-scale high-density soft-matter electronics (Fig. 3.8c) [66]. Wang et al. proposed a rapid fabrication of flexible functional circuits based on liquid metal dual-trans printing, which can be applied to quickly fabricate flexible functional electronic device fitting to any complex surface shape (Fig. 3.8b) [59]. First one can print out liquid metal circuit on PVC membrane, then use polydimethylsiloxane (PDMS) solution to cover the circuit. After a period of time, PDMS solution can be cured and when it is liquid, arbitrary shape objects can be immersed into PDMS solution. Finally cool the whole object to make liquid metal solid and one can completely transfer the initial liquid metal circuit to PDMS flexible substrate. In the process, after PDMS curing, one can peel off the PVC membrane and target object to obtain PDMS device embedded liquid metal flexible circuits. Because the shape of PDMS substrate completely fits with objects, one can

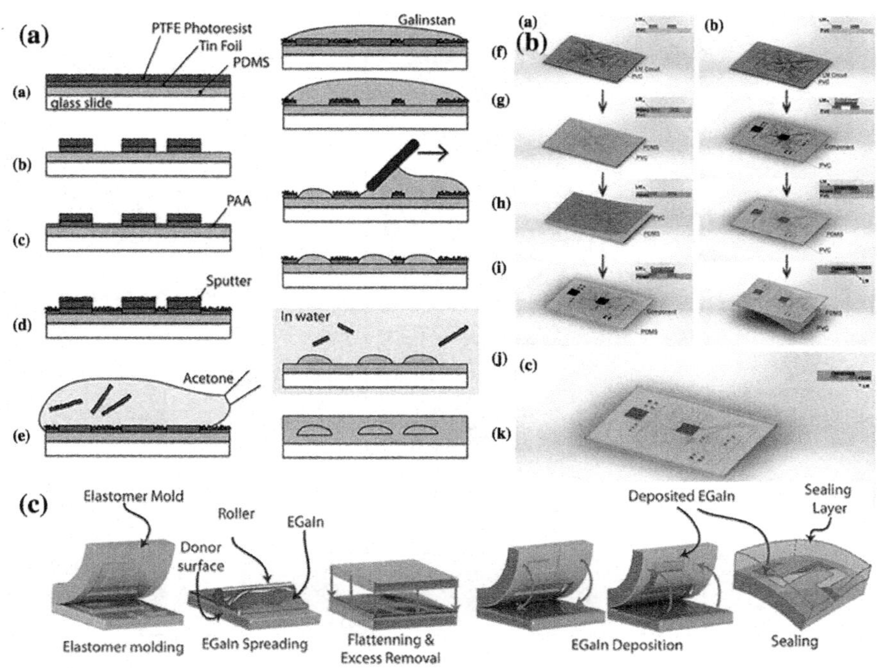

Fig. 3.8 Mask based printing methods. **a** The masked deposition process of gallium-indium alloys for liquid-embedded elastomer conductors [88]. **b** The process of dual-trans printing fabrication [59]. **c** The liquid metal alloy deposition process of micro-scale line [66]. All pictures reproduced with permission

achieve electronic devices highly conformal in manufacturing. This technology has significant implication for sensing, monitoring in health care and household as corresponding device to conduct specific functions. Common methods as mentioned in the literature also included microcontact printing [87], atomized spraying [75], screen printing [70], CO_2 laser ablation [96]. The theory of the atomized spraying and the screen printing methods is that the spraying gun sprays the liquid metal ink onto the substrate through a specific mask to form a circuit processing to the same shape with the mask (Fig. 3.9b, c).

The common method in preparation of liquid metal microfluidic electronics is pouring the liquid metal alloy into a specific shape channel to form the functional circuit. Therefore, from the strict definition, the preparation method of microfluidic electronics can not be classified into the fabrication of the liquid metal flexible printed electronics. However, Fig. 3.10a demonstrates the processing steps of manufacturing liquid alloy microfluidic wireless power transfer in which they employs mask layer and atomization and the power transfer displays large flexibility in rolled state and can attach to human arm [97].

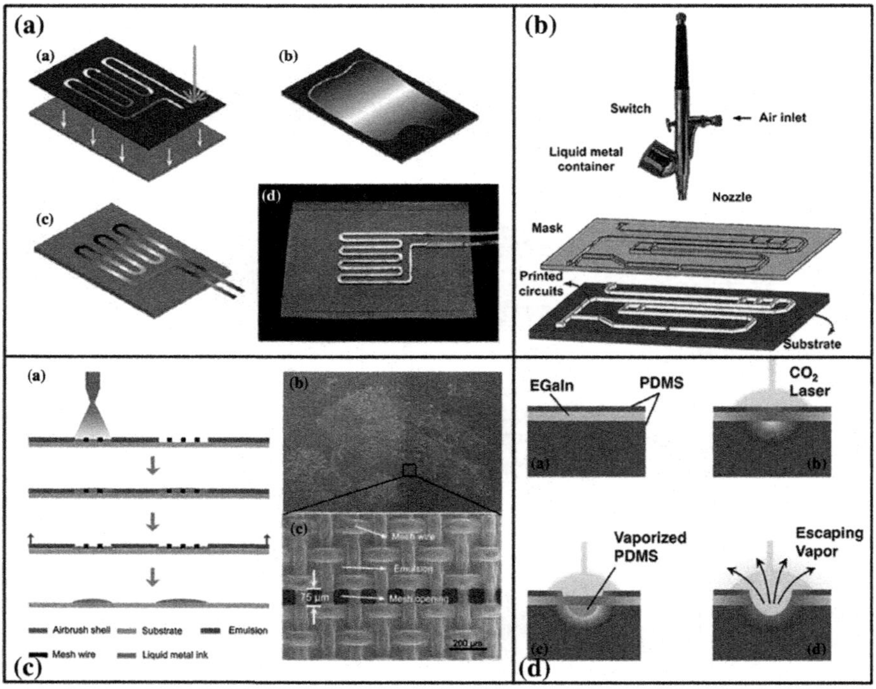

Fig. 3.9 Mask based printing methods. **a** The microcontact printing process to fabricate the liquid metal soft-matter circuit [87]. **b** Atomized spraying of liquid metal droplets to rapid prototype circuits [75]. **c** The screen printing process and scanning electron microscopy image of the screen mesh [70]. **d** Proposed CO_2 laser ablation mechanism of the liquid metal alloy on the PDMS substrate [96]. All pictures reproduced with permission

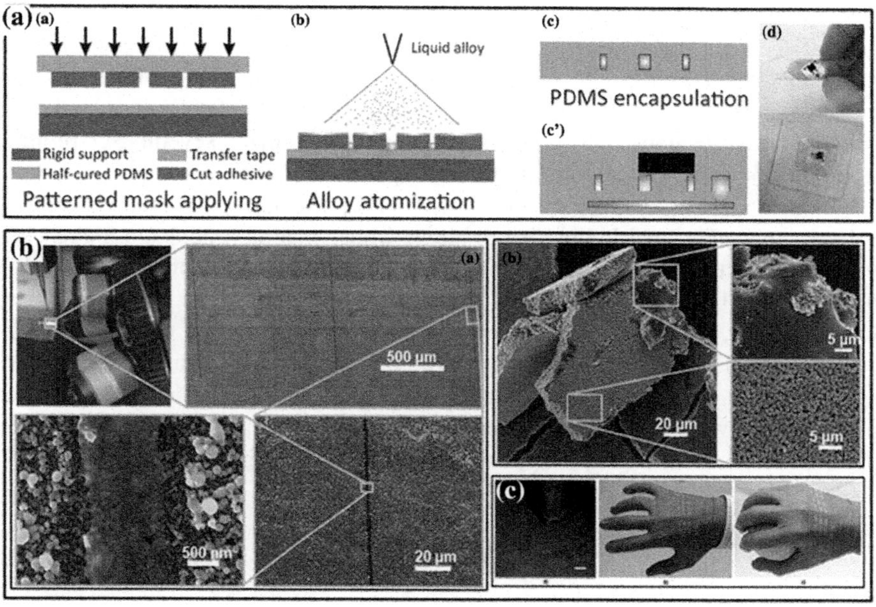

Fig. 3.10 Microfluidic electronics and high-resolution nanoimprint lithography. **a** Processing steps of manufacturing liquid alloy microfluidic wireless power transfer (*a–c*) and in rolled state and attached to human arm (**d**) [97]. **b** (*a*) Small scale line coalescence; (*b*) SEM image of the liquid metal nanoparticles mechanical sintering; (*c*) Process of inkjet printing EGaIn nano-particles and functionalized nitrile glove with stretchable electronics array [98]. All pictures reproduced with permission

3.9.4 High-Resolution Nanoimprint Lithography

Unlike the relatively large size liquid metal droplets, one can also prepare liquid metal nanoparticles to print micro-scale or nano-scale wires. John et al. produces small features through mechanically sintering Gallium-Indium nanoparticles to realize high-resolution nanoimprint lithography [98]. As shown in Fig. 3.10b, 1 μm coalesced EGaIn line arrays were formed by reducing the size of sintering tool. Via inkjet printing EGaIn nanoparticles dispersions on the surface of nitrile glove, the functionalized elastomer glove with liquid metal micro-wire arrays represents excellent stretchability when holding a tennis ball.

3.9.5 3D Printing

3D printing is a technology to construct the object by means of printing layer by layer. In other words, it is a kind of typical additive manufacturing technology. Different from traditional subtractive technology, additive manufacturing is a top-down, layer-by-layer manufacturing process. It can not only avoid corrosion process, achieve green environmental protection, but can also save a lot of raw materials. This significantly reduces the environmental pollution and the cost of materials. Figure 3.11a shows the difference between subtractive and additive manufacturing technologies [99]. Next we will introduce several 3D printing technologies using low melting point metal ink based on the additive mode.

Wang et al. first puts forward the concept of liquid phase 3D printing to employ gallium-, bismuth-, and indium-based alloys whose melting points are higher than room temperature and lower than 300 °C to accomplish printing process [100]. The liquid phase 3D printing is achieved in a liquid environment, and the liquid can be water, ethanol, kerosene, electrolyte solution and so on. However, the melting point of liquid metal ink must be inferior to the liquid environment to ensure printed item against running. In the experiments, Wang et al. introduced $Bi_{35}In_{48.6}Sn_{16}Zn_{0.4}$ as printing ink owing to its littler absorbing/releasing heat than normal metal in the process of phase change [100]. Shortly after, they originated a late-model 3D

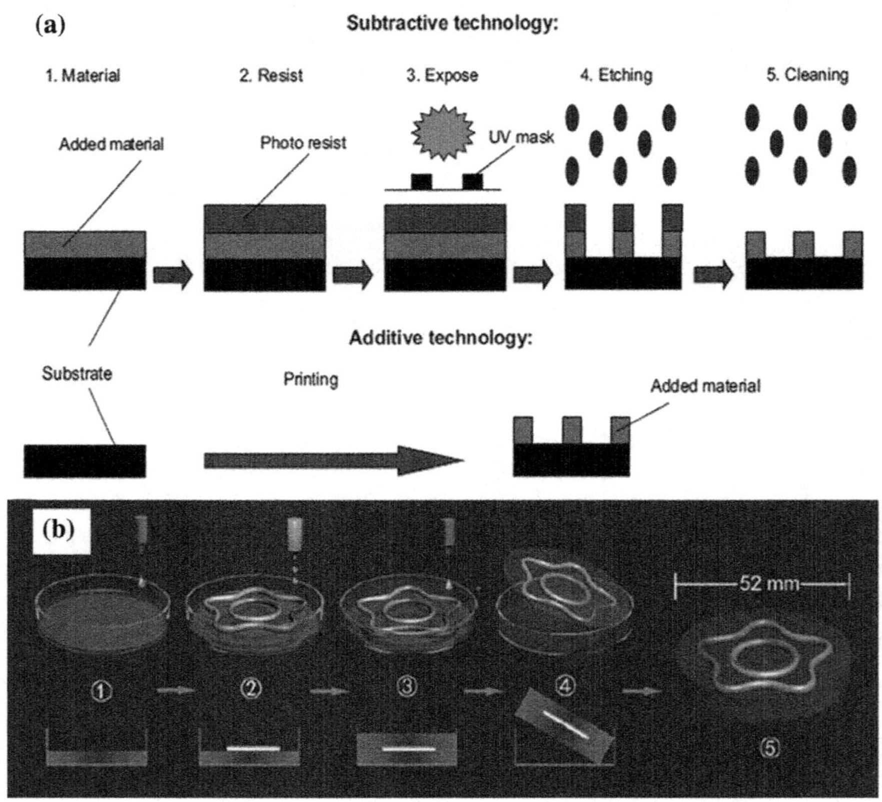

Fig. 3.11 **a** Difference between subtractive and additive manufacturing technologies [99]. **b** Hybrid 3D printing process with $Bi_{35}In_{48.6}Sn_{16}Zn_{0.4}$ and 705 silicone rubber inks [64]. All pictures reproduced with permission

printing technology—hybrid 3D printing, which meant interactive printing of various inks or combination of multiple printing methods. In Fig. 3.11b, the $Bi_{35}In_{48.6}Sn_{16}Zn_{0.4}$ and 705 silicone rubber (nonmetal) inks were adopted to accomplish hybrid 3D printing [64]. 705 silicone rubber serves as a kind of waterproof, anticorrosive, transparent and insulative adhesive, and can be solidified when absorbing water vapor at room temperature. Therefore it is often used as electrical packaging material. First, one can print the bottom layer on the substrate by 705 silicone rubber and print the middle layer on the 705 silicone rubber layer by $Bi_{35}In_{48.6}Sn_{16}Zn_{0.4}$. After that, one can print the top layer using 705 silicone rubber. When solidifying adequately, a sandwich structure can be obtained once taking down the printed item from the basement. Compatible hybrid 3D printing of metal and nonmetal inks fully embodies good mechanical strength and electrical/thermal conductive of metal ink, and excellent insulation of nonmetal ink, which makes the printing circuit applicable in a harsh environment. In fact, except for the above $Bi_{35}In_{48.6}Sn_{16}Zn_{0.4}$ ink, using liquid metal with much lower melting point such as gallium alloy as well as its packaging materials, we can also realize 3D printing of

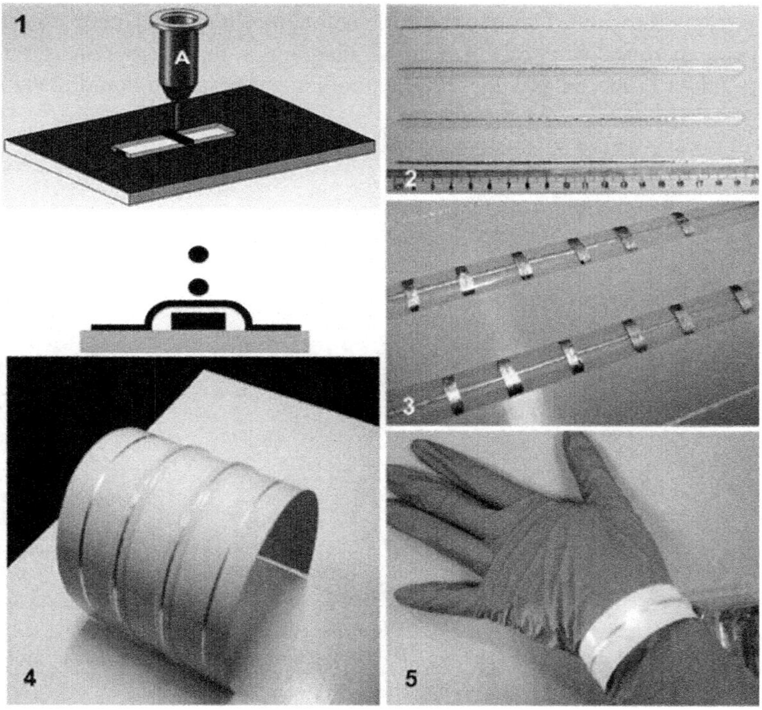

Fig. 3.12 Schematic of hybrid 3D printing of liquid metal electrical circuitry and silicone rubber packaging materials on paper to compose various coated electronics [69]. (1) Printing principle; (2) electrical wires covered with silicone rubber; (3) multi-layer structure or electrical patterns; (4) 3D structure of printed patterns on paper; (5) galvanical annulus wires driven LED. All pictures reproduced with permission

hybrid electro-mechanical device [69]. As depicted in Figs. 3.7b and 3.12, Zheng et al. developed the first ever prototyping machine for the automatic 3D printing of liquid metal which can help quickly compose large scale coated electronics [69]. Fassler and Majidi investigated the freeze casting method to manufacture liquid metal based 3D structures [101]. Ladd et al. tested the case of direct-writing of 3D free-standing liquid metal microstructures at room temperature [102]. The liquid metal can also be employed as injecable 3D bio-electrode to measure the electrocardiograph (ECG) or electroencephalogram (EEG) [55, 58, 103].

3.10 Printing Devices

Aiming at establishing different printing technologies as mentioned above, Liu et al. has delivered printers which now have been put into practical use [18, 100]. Liquid metal circuit printer has completely changed the traditional mode on the principle of technology, breaking the technical bottleneck on personal electronics manufacturing, which makes it a reality to quickly fabricate electronic circuits under extreme low-costing (Table 3.3). Through the computer controlling, even people having no electronic experience can download circuit diagram on the internet and print it out directly. Inkjet Printer is an inkjet printing equipment based on liquid metal screen

Table 3.3 Three kinds of liquid metal printers [18, 69]

Liquid metal Printer	Personal circuit printer	Ubiquitous inkjet printer	3D metal printer
Device type	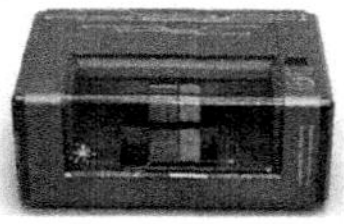	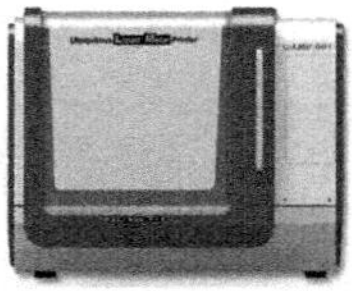	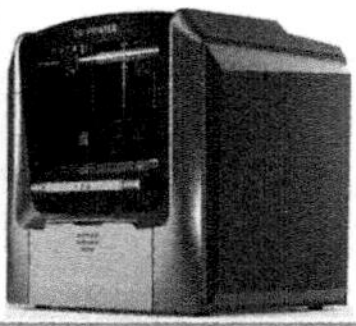
Printed out items	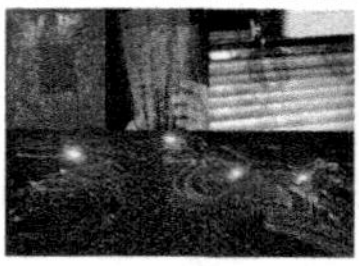	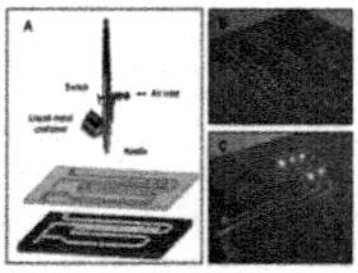	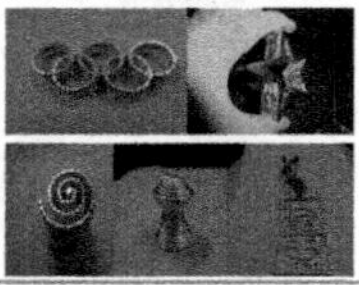
Application fields	Circuit; art; devices; rapid prototyping	Electronic circuit; art; RFID label; antenna	Circuit; radar; antenna; molds

printing process. Through USB cable, the printer can connect with computer to realize online printing, and can also offline print via SD card. Before printing one needs to prepare .gcode files which is to control the nozzle movement. 3D Metal Printer is desktop fused deposition modeling (FDM) device, and it substitutes traditional metal parts processing to prepare metal parts with complex spatial structure.

3.11 Typical Applications

As a novel electronic ink material, the flexibility and shape-preserving of the liquid metal alloy allows it to play an important role in yielding components and soft circuit. Its non-toxicity and benign biocompatibility make it an implant materials in the body, such as the selected low melting point metal skeleton material [51], high-resolution angiography contrast [104], biological micro-droplets [95], nerve connection [35, 36], human exoskeleton [105], and electronical skin [56, 57, 106].

The technology of directly printing liquid metal electronic circuit changes the rigid circuits to flexible desktop manufacturing [107]. With a way to rapidly manufacture various flexible household electronics with different functions, one can envisage that human life will have big changes in the near future. Imaging that quilt with flexible functional circuits containing temperature or pressure sensor can monitor human sleep quality and adjust the quilt temperature according to body temperature to achieve intelligent heating or cooling. In fact, all of these wonderful needs can be implemented by liquid metal flexible circuits. Hereinbefore, we have mentioned that liquid metal flexible printed electronics can be directly printed on many soft substrates, and furthermore produce lots of complex artworks. Zhang et al. demonstrated that even leaves can become circuit board, which provides solid theoretical basis for liquid metal atomized spraying manufacturing flexible electronics with universality [75].

Through the direct-writing method, Li et al. draws liquid metal thermocouple on paper [85]. The liquid metal thermocouple has many special advantages, such as small contact resistance and thermal resistance, no need to weld and the wide working temperature zone. Thermoelectric effect is the theoretical basis of thermocouple temperature measurement. The thermoelectric power produced by the thermocouple has nothing to do with its shape or size, but relates to the composition of the thermoelectric materials and the temperature difference between the two ends. The thermocouple composed of Ga and EGaIn not only has the temperature sensing ability but also the bending capacity.

Fassler et al. prepared two kinds of capacitors—the square wave capacitor (Fig. 3.13a(a)) and the spiral capacitor (Fig. 3.13a(b)) and a square planar spiral inductor (Fig. 3.13a(c)) [108]. They calculated the values of the capacitors or inductor of various shapes via formula derivation. Soft-matter diode, a new-type flexible functional equipment component with liquid metal electrodes is developed

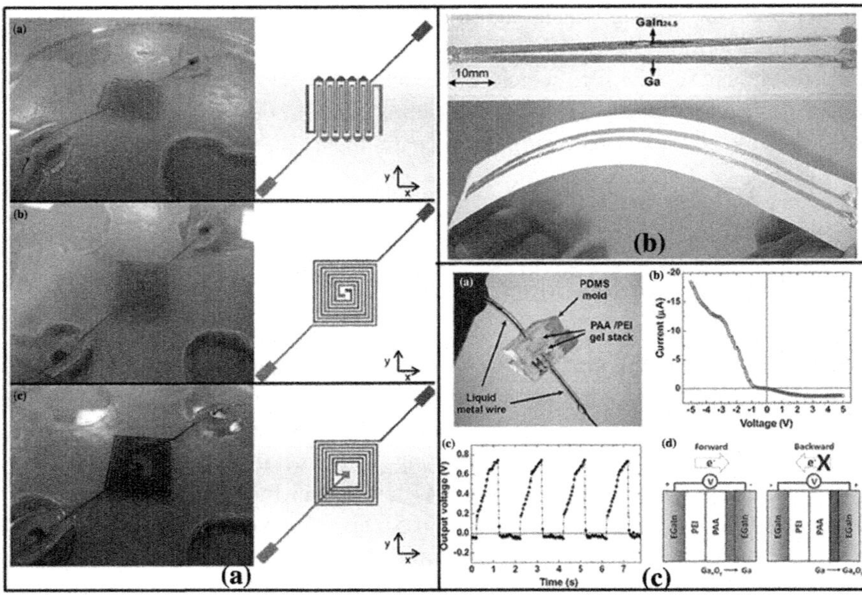

Fig. 3.13 The electronical components based on the liquid metal alloy. **a** The soft-matter capacitors and inductor of the liquid metal alloy embedded in silicone elastomer [108]. **b** The liquid metal thermocouple directly written on paper [85]. **c** (*a*) Soft-matter diodes with liquid metal wire; (*b*) relationship between voltage and current; (*c*) transient voltage response under AC signal of the soft-matter diode; (*d*) schematic diagram of current flow [29]. Pictures reproduced with permission

by So et al. [29] Because the liquid metal EGaIn electrodes sandwich layers are conductive forward from Ga_xO_y to Ga while nonconductive backward from Ga to Ga_xO_y, the soft-matter diode has the function of limiting current and can cause the current one-way through (Fig. 3.13c).

At the same time, because of its flexibility and fluidity, liquid alloy is widely used in sensors and functional devices and Wu's group made important contributions in the field [109]. They revealed a liquid alloy microfluidic stretchable large-area wireless strain antenna, consisting of two layers of liquid metal alloy filled microfluidic channels in a silicone elastomer [110]. A stretchable ultra-high frequency radio frequency identity tag printed on human skin demonstrated that liquid alloy microfluidic electronics can be applied to electronic skin [57]. Liquid alloy microfluidic electronics can also be fabricated as antenna with strong stretchability and rolled space [111, 112] and microfluidic wireless power transfer system [97]. Matsuzaki et al. elaborated a wearable data glove with local strain sensing using GaInSnelestrodes (Fig. 3.14a) [60] and the data glove can judge the degree of the finger bending according to the change of resistance of different monitoring points. Krupenkin et al. showed a footwear-embedded microfluidic

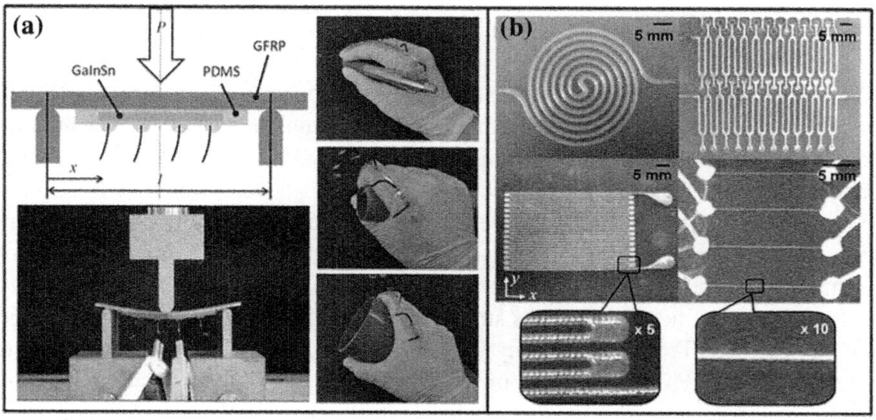

Fig. 3.14 Sensors based on the liquid metal deformation. **a** A wearable data glove with local strain sensing using GaInSn electrodes [60]. **b** Hyperelastic pressure sensors with microchannels of conductive liquid metal alloy [113]. Pictures reproduced with permission

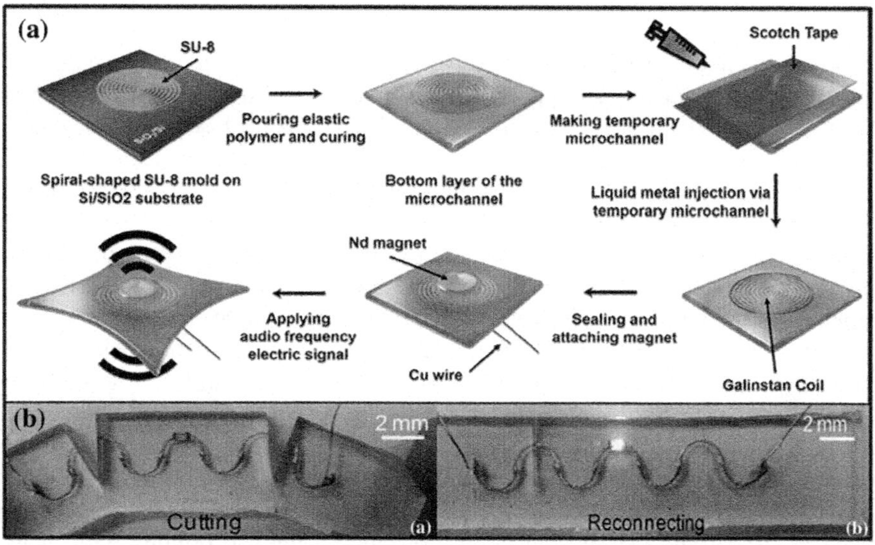

Fig. 3.15 The liquid metal flexible printed electronics functional devices. **a** The fabrication process of the liquid metal stretchable loudspeaker [114]. **b** Physical separation and reconnection of the liquid metal circuit with a LED [115]. All pictures reproduced with permission

energy harvester, which is a novel suitable mechanical-to-electrical energy conversion based on liquid metal microdroplets [61]. Figure 3.15 are several examples for the liquid metal flexible printed electronics functional devices.

3.12 Conclusion

As the new generation inks for realizing flexible printed electronics, the liquid metals possess the outstanding versatile merits in simultaneously owning fluidity, conductivity, metallicity and electromagnetic property [1]. It thus offers tremendous opportunities for making future flectional electronic device which will be very important in health care areas. However, there still exist a group of challenges in preparing, processing and utilizing high performance liquid metal inks. For example, the properties of low adhesion to many substrates, easy oxidation, high surface tension of liquid alloy inks still restrict the realization of high precision and stability circuits. To solve such key issues, one can mix the liquid metal with the materials, which is metal or non-metal. Therefore, new hybrid functional liquid metal materials can be made with desired properties of semiconductor, semi-flexibility, enhanced adhesion and antioxidant ability etc. This would enable the inks to adapt well for more practical situations and more functions. For example, the liquid metal nanocrystallization can improve the printing precision, and one can modify the surface of liquid metal nanoparticles, such as connecting the luminous substance through metal bond to realize the self-luminous colorful printing.

So far, the liquid metal ink has already been able to be printed on a wide range of soft substrates, such as plate, paper, cloth, skin even leaf and so on, which opens many opportunities in making flexible electronical component, sensors or actuators, wearable bioelectronics, electrical skin etc. [1]. The use of such diverse flexible substrates significantly enriches the application field of liquid metal flexible printed electronics, and one can thus expand related practices from human being to other organisms such as animals and plants. For example, one can even print the flexible circuits with features of energy harvesting and light emission on the leaves to capture the energy of swinging leaves to supply light at night.

Various kinds of liquid metal printing technologies are enabling efficient circuit fabrication. At this stage, a series of technological problems still need to be better tackled, such as the precise and reliable connection between the printed liquid metal circuits with the traditional integrated circuits. In addition, multilayer printing including layer-layer interconnection and multilayer softness, high printing precision to achieve the desired liquid metal integrated circuits are also critical for practices. Regarding the specific fabrication, hybrid flexible printing with planar printing and 3D printing are worth of trying. Further, although it is still not so tough, cooling of complex liquid metal circuits should also be taken care of to avoid damage from the "thermal barrier". Meanwhile, encapsulation is often a necessity for making ending user device. For instance, the long lasting liquid metal skin electronics to maintain on the skin mainly depends on the use of the packaging technology. PDMS is often applied to package the liquid metal flexible circuits. However, to various substrates in different environment, one needs to consider diverse encapsulation technology to make the circuit more secure in order to achieve desired functionality. And for the applications in organisms, the non-toxicity and harmless of the packaging materials especially need to be considered. Sometimes, the liquid metal movement and shape-shifting under the electric field can help make more self-configurational operations of the circuits [107, 108]. These unconventional dynamically changing or self-destructive circuits are also worth of pursuing.

In summary, liquid metal flexible printed electronics breaks up the limitation of traditional flexible electronics. The process of circuits manufacturing is rather straightforward, fast, stable and relatively compatible with existing integrated circuit technology. Liquid metal flexible printed electronics would allow making high quality products such as wearable devices, electronic skin, medical implants, flexible display and solar panels which will meet people's many coming demands. The existing liquid metal flexible printed technology is a combination between the liquid metal soft circuit and the rigid components or chips, which is still not the completely flexible electronics in a large sense. At the same time, this kind of semi flexible circuit may partially limit its application. A basic significance of liquid metal flexible printed electronics lies in that with the popularity of liquid metal printing technology, people can discretionarily print their personalized flexible functional devices on any surface, which can significantly expand traditional electronic engineering category. With the overcoming of the problems of high rate of good product, self-repair of damaged circuits, long service life, low environmental pollution and waste recycling, the liquid metal flexible printed electronics would witness a bright future in the coming time.

References

1. Wang XL, Liu J (2016) Recent advancements in liquid metal flexible printed electronics: properties, technologies, and applications. Micromachines 7:206-1–206-124
2. Cui Z (2012) Printed electronics: materials, technologies and applications. Higher Education Press, Beijing
3. Lin Y, Gritsenko D, Liu Q, Lu X, Xu J (2016) Recent advancements in functionalized paper-based electronics. ACS Appl Mater Interfaces 8:20501–20515
4. Yin Z, Huang Y, Bu N, Wang X, Xiong Y (2010) Inkjet printing for flexible electronics: materials, processes and equipments. Chin Sci Bull 55:3383–3407
5. Wong WS, Salleo A (2009) Flexible electronics: materials and applications. Springer, New York
6. Reuss RH, Chalamala BR, Moussessian A, Kane MG, Kumar A, Zhang DC, Rogers JA, Hatalis M, Temple D, Moddel G et al (2005) Macroelectronics: perspectives on technology and applications. Proc IEEE 93:1239–1256
7. Kim DH, Ahn JH, Choi WM, Kim HS, Kim TH, Song J, Huang YY, Liu Z, Lu C, Rogers JA (2008) Stretchable and foldable silicon integrated circuits. Science 320:507–511
8. Stoppa M, Chiolerio A (2014) Wearable electronics and smart textiles: a critical review. Sensors 14:11957
9. Koo M, Park KI, Lee SH, Suh M, Jeon DY, Cho JW, Kang K, Lee KJ (2012) Bendable inorganic thin-film battery for fully flexible electronic systems. NanoLetters 12:4810–4816

10. Reeder J, Kaltenbrunner M, Ware T, Arreaga-Salas D, Avendano-Bolivar A, Yokota T, Inoue Y, Sekino M, Voit W, Sekitani T et al (2014) Mechanically adaptive organic transistors for implantable electronics. Adv Mater 26:4967–4973
11. Kang D, Pikhitsa PV, Choi YW, Lee C, Shin SS, Piao L, Park B, Suh KY, Kim TI, Choi M (2014) Ultrasensitive mechanical crack-based sensor inspired by the spider sensory system. Nature 516:222–226
12. Russo A, Ahn BY, Adams JJ, Duoss EB, Bernhard JT, Lewis JA (2011) Pen-on-paper flexible electronics. Adv Mater 23:3426–3430
13. Jung I, Shin G, Malyarchuk V, Ha JS, Rogers JA (2010) Paraboloid electronic eye cameras using deformable arrays of photodetectors in hexagonal mesh layouts. Appl Phys Lett 96:021110
14. Schwartz G, Tee BCK, Mei J, Appleton AL, Kim DH, Wang H, Bao Z (1859) Flexible polymer transistors with high pressure sensitivity for application in electronic skin and health monitoring. Nat Commun 2013:4
15. Wang X, Dong L, Zhang H, Yu R, Pan C, Wang ZL (2015) Recent progress in electronic skin. Adv Sci 2:1500169
16. Kim DH, Lu N, Ma R, Kim YS, Kim RH, Wang S, Wu J, Won SM, Tao H, Islam A et al (2011) Epidermal Electron. Science 333:838–843
17. Choi WM, Song J, Khang DY, Jiang H, Huang YY, Rogers JA (2007) Biaxially stretchable "wavy" silicon nanomembranes. Nano Lett 7:1655–1663
18. Zheng Y, He ZZ, Yang J, Liu J (2014) Personal electronics printing via tapping mode composite liquid metal ink delivery and adhesion mechanism. Sci Rep 4:4588
19. Ghosh D, Maki SP, Lyons C, Theiss SD, Owings RR (2016) Hybrid dielectric thin films on flexible substrates for embedded capacitor applications. IEEE Trans Compon Packag Manuf Technol 6:941–945
20. Singh M, Haverinen HM, Dhagat P, Jabbour GE (2010) Inkjet printing-process and its applications. Adv Mater 22:673–685
21. http://www.micropen.com/
22. Kim SS, Na SI, Jo J, Tae G, Kim DY (2007) Efficient polymer solar cells fabricated by simple brush painting. Adv Mater 19:4410–4415
23. Jang J (2006) Displays develop a new flexibility. Mater Today 9:46–52
24. Krebs FC (2009) Fabrication and processing of polymer solar cells: a review of printing and coating techniques. Sol Energy Mater Sol Cells 93:394–412
25. Mayer AC, Scully SR, Hardin BE, Rowell MW, McGehee MD (2007) Polymer-based solar cells. Mater Today 10:28–33
26. Someya T, Kato Y, Sekitani T, Iba S, Noguchi Y, Murase Y, Kawaguchi H, Sakurai T (2005) Conformable, flexible, large-area networks of pressure and thermal sensors with organic transistor active matrixes. PNAS 102:12321–12325
27. Madden PGA (2003) Development and modeling of conducting polymer actuators and the fabrication of a conducting polymer based feedback loop. Massachusetts Institute of Technology, Cambridge
28. Hammock ML, Chortos A, Tee BCK, Tok JBH, Bao Z (2013) 25th anniversary article: the evolution of electronic skin (e-skin): a brief history, design considerations, and recent progress. Adv Mater 25:5997–6038
29. So JH, Koo HJ, Dickey MD, Velev OD (2012) Ionic current rectification in soft-matter diodes with liquid-metal electrodes. Adv Func Mater 22:625–631
30. Niu S, Wang X, Yi F, Zhou YS, Wang ZL (2015) A universal self-charging system driven by random biomechanical energy for sustainable operation of mobile electronics. Nat Commun 6:8975
31. Zheng Q, Zhang H, Shi B, Xue X, Liu Z, Jin Y, Ma Y, Zou Y, Wang X, An Z et al (2016) In vivo self-powered wireless cardiac monitoring via implantable triboelectric nanogenerator. ACS Nano 10:6510–6518

32. Rogers JA, Bao Z, Baldwin K, Dodabalapur A, Crone B, Raju VR, Kuck V, Katz H, Amundson K, Ewing J et al (2001) Paper-like electronic displays: large-area rubber-stamped plastic sheets of electronics and microencapsulated electrophoretic inks. PNAS 98:4835–4840
33. Wang X, Tian H, Mohammad MA, Li C, Wu C, Yang Y, Ren TL (2015) A spectrally tunable all-graphene-based flexible field-effect light-emitting device. Nat Commun 6:7767
34. Lessing J, Morin SA, Keplinger C, Tayi AS, Whitesides GM (2015) Stretchable conductive composites based on metal wools for use as electrical vias in soft devices. Adv Func Mater 25:1418–1425
35. Zhang J, Sheng L, Jin C, Liu J (2014) Liquid metal as connecting or functional recovery channel for the transected sciatic nerve. arXiv preprint 2014, arXiv: 1404.5931
36. Liu F, Yu Y, Yi L, Liu J (2016) Liquid metal as reconnection agent for peripheral nerve injury. Sci Bull 61:939–947
37. Wang X, Zhang H, Yu R, Dong L, Peng D, Zhang A, Zhang Y, Liu H, Pan C, Wang ZL (2015) Dynamic pressure mapping of personalized handwriting by a flexible sensor matrix based on the mechanoluminescence process. Adv Mater 27:2324–2331
38. Tee BCK, Wang C, Allen R, Bao Z (2012) An electrically and mechanically self-healing composite with pressure- and flexion-sensitive properties for electronic skin applications. Nat Nanotechnol 7:825–832
39. Kim J, Lee M, Shim HJ, Ghaffari R, Cho HR, Son D, Jung YH, Soh M, Choi C, Jung S et al (2014) Stretchable silicon nanoribbon electronics for skin prosthesis. Nat Commun 5:5747
40. Tee BCK, Chortos A, Berndt A, Nguyen AK, Tom A, McGuire A, Lin ZC, Tien K, Bae WG, Wang H et al (2015) A skin-inspired organic digital mechanoreceptor. Science 350:313–316
41. Wang S, Li M, Wu J, Kim DH, Lu N, Su Y, Kang Z, Huang Y, Rogers JA (2012) Mechanics of epidermal electronics. J Appl Mech 3:031021–031022
42. Webb RC, Ma Y, Krishnan S, Li Y, Yoon S, Guo X, Feng X, Shi Y, Seidel M, Cho NH et al (2015) Epidermal devices for noninvasive, precise, and continuous mapping of macrovascular and microvascular blood flow. Sci Adv 1:e1500701
43. Rajan K, Bocchini S, Chiappone A, Roppolo I, Perrone D, Bejtka K, Ricciardi C, Pirri CF, Chiolerio A (2017) Spin-coated silver nanocomposite resistive switching devices. Microelectron Eng 168:27–31
44. Chiolerio A, Roppolo I, Bejtka K, Asvarov A, Pirri CF (2016) Resistive hysteresis in flexible nanocomposites and colloidal suspensions: interfacial coupling mechanism unveiled. RSC Adv 6:56661–56667
45. Tai YL (2012) Preparation and application of conductive ink for printed electronics. Ph.D. Thesis, Fudan University, Shanghai
46. Rajan K, Roppolo I, Chiappone A, Bocchini S, Perrone D, Chiolerio A (2016) Silver nanoparticle ink technology: state of the art. Nanotechnol Sci Appl 9:1–13
47. Xiong Z, Liu C (2012) Optimization of inkjet printed pedot: Pss thin films through annealing processes. Org Electron 13:1532–1540
48. Alessandro C, Sergio B, Francesco S, Samuele P, Denis P, Davide B, Mario C, Candido Fabrizio P (2015) Synthesis of polyaniline-based inks for inkjet printed devices: electrical characterization highlighting the effect of primary and secondary doping. Semicond Sci Technol 30:104001
49. Petukhov DI, Kirikova MN, Bessonov AA, Bailey MJA (2014) Nickel and copper conductive patterns fabricated by reactive inkjet printing combined with electroless plating. Mater Lett 132:302–306
50. Plevachuk Y, Sklyarchuk V, Yakymovych A, Svec P, Janickovic D, Illekova E (2011) Electrical conductivity and viscosity of liquid sn–sb–cu alloys. J Mater Sci: Mater Electron 22:631–638
51. Yi L, Jin C, Wang L, Liu J (2014) Liquid-solid phase transition alloy as reversible and rapid molding bone cement. Biomaterials 35:9789–9801

52. Wang Q, Yu Y, Pan K, Liu J (2014) Liquid metal angiography for mega contrast x-ray visualization of vascular network in reconstructing in-vitro organ anatomy. IEEE Trans Biomed Eng 61:2161–2166
53. Lu Y, Hu Q, Lin Y, Pacardo DB, Wang C, Sun W, Ligler FS, Dickey MD, Gu Z (2015) Transformable liquid-metal nanomedicine. Nat Commun 6:10066
54. Wang L, Liu J (2014) Research advancement of liquid metal printed electronics ink (in Chinese). Imaging Sci Photochem 4:1674–0475
55. Jin C, Zhang J, Li X, Yang X, Li J, Liu J (2013) Injectable 3-d fabrication of medical electronics at the target biological tissues. Sci Rep 3:3442
56. Guo C, Yu Y, Liu J (2014) Rapidly patterning conductive components on skin substrates as physiological testing devices via liquid metal spraying and pre-designed mask. J Mater Chem B 2:5739–5745
57. Jeong SH, Hagman A, Hjort K, Jobs M, Sundqvist J, Wu Z (2012) Liquid alloy printing of microfluidic stretchable electronics. Lab Chip 12:4657–4664
58. Yu Y, Zhang J, Liu J (2013) Biomedical implementation of liquid metal ink as drawable ecg electrode and skin circuit. PLoS ONE 8:e58771
59. Wang Q, Yu Y, Yang J, Liu J (2015) Fast fabrication of flexible functional circuits based on liquid metal dual-trans printing. Adv Mater 27:7109–7116
60. Matsuzaki R, Tabayashi K (2015) Highly stretchable, global, and distributed local strain sensing line using GaInSn electrodes for wearable electronics. Adv Func Mater 25:3806–3813
61. Krupenkin T, Taylor JA (2011) Reverse electrowetting as a new approach to high-power energy harvesting. Nat Commun 2:448
62. Zhang Q, Zheng Y, Liu J (2012) Direct writing of electronics based on alloy and metal (dream) ink: a newly emerging area and its impact on energy, environment and health sciences. Front Energy 6:311–340
63. Gao Y, Li H, Liu J (2012) Direct writing of flexible electronics through room temperature liquid metal ink. PLoS ONE 7:e45485
64. Wang L, Liu J (2014) Compatible hybrid 3D printing of metal and nonmetal inks for direct manufacture of end functional devices. Sci China Technol Sci 57:2089–2095
65. Tripathi V, Loh YL (2006) Thermal conductivity of a granular metal. Phys Rev Lett 96:046805
66. Gozen BA, Tabatabai A, Ozdoganlar OB, Majidi C (2014) High-density soft-matter electronics with micron-scale line width. Adv Mater 26:5211–5216
67. Sivan V, Tang SY, O'Mullane AP, Petersen P, Eshtiaghi N, Kalantar-zadeh K, Mitchell A (2013) Liquid metal marbles. Adv Func Mater 23:144–152
68. Du K, Glogowski E, Tuominen MT, Emrick T, Russell TP, Dinsmore AD (2013) Self-assembly of gold nanoparticles on gallium droplets: controlling charge transport through microscopic devices. Langmuir 29:13640–13646
69. Zheng Y, He Z, Gao Y, Liu J (2013) Direct desktop printed-circuits-on-paper flexible electronics. Sci Rep 3:1786-1–1786-7
70. Wang L, Liu J (2015) Pressured liquid metal screen printing for rapid manufacture of high resolution electronic patterns. RSC Adv 5:57686–57691
71. Kim D, Lee Y, Lee DW, Choi W, Yoo K, Lee JB (2015) Hydrochloric acid-impregnated paper for gallium-based liquid metal microfluidics. Sens Actuators B: Chem 207:199–205
72. Kubo M, Li X, Kim C, Hashimoto M, Wiley BJ, Ham D, Whitesides GM (2010) Stretchable microfluidic radiofrequency antennas. Adv Mater 22:2749–2752
73. Boley JW, White EL, Chiu GTC, Kramer RK (2014) Direct writing of gallium-indium alloy for stretchable electronics. Adv Func Mater 24:3501–3507
74. Kim D, Thissen P, Viner G, Lee DW, Choi W, Chabal YJ, Lee JB (2013) Recovery of nonwetting characteristics by surface modification of gallium-based liquid metal droplets using hydrochloric acid vapor. ACS Appl Mater Interfaces 5:179–185
75. Zhang Q, Gao Y, Liu J (2014) Atomized spraying of liquid metal droplets on desired substrate surfaces as a generalized way for ubiquitous printed electronics. Appl Phys A 116:1091–1097

76. Xu Q, Oudalov N, Guo Q, Jaeger HM, Brown E (2012) Effect of oxidation on the mechanical properties of liquid gallium and eutectic gallium-indium. Phys Fluids 24:063101
77. Schrader ME (1995) Young-dupre revisited. Langmuir 11:3585–3589
78. Liu Y, Gao M, Mei S, Han Y, Liu J (2013) Ultra-compliant liquid metal electrodes with in-plane self-healing capability for dielectric elastomer actuators. Appl Phys Lett 103:064101
79. Tiberto P, Gupta S, Bianco S, Celegato F, Martino P, Chiolerio A, Tagliaferro A, Allia P (2011) Morphology and magnetic properties of island-like co and ni films obtained by de-wetting. J Nanopart Res 13:245–255
80. Doudrick K, Liu S, Mutunga EM, Klein KL, Damle V, Varanasi KK, Rykaczewski K (2014) Different shades of oxide: From nanoscale wetting mechanisms to contact printing of gallium-based liquid metals. Langmuir 30:6867–6877
81. Li G, Parmar M, Kim D, Lee JB, Lee DW (2014) Pdms based coplanar microfluidic channels for the surface reduction of oxidized Galinstan. Lab Chip 14:200–209
82. Furmidge CGL (1962) Studies at phase interfaces. I. The sliding of liquid drops on solid surfaces and a theory for spray retention. J Colloid Sci 17:309–324
83. Kramer RK, Boley JW, Stone HA, Weaver JC, Wood RJ (2014) Effect of microtextured surface topography on the wetting behavior of eutectic gallium–indium alloys. Langmuir 30:533–539
84. Yi LT (2015) Injectable bone cement based on low-melting-point alloy with liquid-solid phase switchable capability. Ph.D. thesis, Tsinghua University
85. Li H, Yang Y, Liu J (2012) Printable tiny thermocouple by liquid metal gallium and its matching metal. Appl Phys Lett 101:073511
86. Liu J, Li HA (2011) Liquid metal based printed circuit board and its fabrication method. China Patent, 10140156
87. Tabatabai A, Fassler A, Usiak C, Majidi C (2013) Liquid-phase gallium-indium alloy electronics with microcontact printing. Langmuir 29:6194–6200
88. Kramer RK, Majidi C, Wood RJ (2013) Masked deposition of gallium-indium alloys for liquid-embedded elastomer conductors. Adv Func Mater 23:5292–5296
89. Jeong JA, Kim HK (2010) Characteristics of inkjet-printed nano indium tin oxide particles for transparent conducting electrodes. Curr Appl Phys 10:e105–e108
90. Sheng L, Teo S, Liu J (2016) Liquid-metal-painted stretchable capacitor sensors for wearable healthcare electronics. J Med Biol Eng 36:265–272
91. Wang L, Liu J (2014) Printing low-melting-point alloy ink to directly make a solidified circuit or functional device with a heating pen. Proc R Soc A Math Phys Eng Sci 470:0609
92. Yang J, Liu J (2014) Direct printing and assembly of FM radio at the user end via liquid metal printer. Circuit World 40:134–140
93. Zheng Y, Zhang Q, Liu J (2013) Pervasive liquid metal based direct writing electronics with roller-ball pen. AIP Adv 3:112117
94. Kim D, Yoo JH, Lee Y, Choi W, Yoo K, Lee JBJ (2014) In gallium-based liquid metal inkjet printing. In: IEEE 27th international conference on micro electro mechanical systems (MEMS), 26–30 Jan 2014, pp 967–970
95. Yang H, Lightner CR, Dong L (2012) Light-emitting coaxial nanofibers. ACS Nano 6:622–628
96. Lu T, Finkenauer L, Wissman J, Majidi C (2014) Rapid prototyping for soft-matter electronics. Adv Func Mater 24:3351–3356
97. Jeong SH, Hjort K, Wu Z (2015) Tape transfer atomization patterning of liquid alloys for microfluidic stretchable wireless power transfer. Sci Rep 5:8419
98. Boley JW, White EL, Kramer RK (2015) Mechanically sintered gallium-indium nanoparticles. Adv Mater 27:2355–2360
99. Kunnari E, Valkama J, Keskinen M, Mansikkamäki P (2009) Environmental evaluation of new technology: Printed electronics case study. J Clean Prod 17:791–799
100. Wang L, Liu J (2014) Liquid phase 3d printing for quickly manufacturing conductive metal objects with low melting point alloy ink. Sci China Technol Sci 57:1721–1728

101. Fassler A, Majidi C (2013) 3D structures of liquid-phase gain alloy embedded in PDMS with freeze casting. Lab Chip 13:4442–4450
102. Ladd C, So JH, Muth J, Dickey MD (2013) 3D printing of free standing liquid metal microstructures. Adv Mater 25:5081–5085
103. Liu R, Yang X, Jin C, Fu J, Chen W, Liu J (2013) Development of three-dimension microelectrode array for bioelectric measurement using the liquidmetal-micromolding technique. Appl Phys Lett 103:193701
104. Wang Q, Yu Y, Pan K, Liu J (2014) Liquid metal angiography for mega contrast X-ray visualization of vascular network in reconstructing in-vitro organ anatomy. IEEE Trans Biomed Eng 61:2161–2166
105. Deng Y, Liu J (2014) Flexible mechanical joint as human exoskeleton using low-melting-point alloy. J Med Dev 8:044506
106. Li J, Guo C, Wang Z, Gao K, Shi X, Liu J (2016) Electrical stimulation towards melanoma therapy via liquid metal printed electronics on skin. Clin Transl Med 5:21
107. Wang L, Liu J (2015) Ink spraying based liquid metal printed electronics for directly making smart home appliances. ECS J Solid State Sci Technol 4:3057–3062
108. Fassler A, Majidi C (2013) Soft-matter capacitors and inductors for hyperelastic strain sensing and stretchable electronics. Smart Mater Struct 22:055023
109. Cheng S, Wu Z (2012) Microfluidic electronics. Lab Chip 12:2782–2791
110. Cheng S, Wu Z (2011) A microfluidic, reversibly stretchable, large-area wireless strain sensor. Adv Func Mater 21:2282–2290
111. Wu Z, Hjort K, Jeong SH (2015) Microfluidic stretchable radio-frequency devices. Proc IEEE 103:1211–1225
112. Jeong S, Hjort K, Wu Z (2014) Tape transfer printing of a liquid metal alloy for stretchable RF electronics. Sensors 14:16311
113. Park YL, Majidi C, Kramer R, Berard P, Wood RJ (2010) Hyperelastic pressure sensing with a liquid-embedded elastomer. J Micromech Microeng 20:c125029
114. Jin SW, Park J, Hong SY, Park H, Jeong YR, Park J, Lee SS, Ha JS (2015) Stretchable loudspeaker using liquid metal microchannel. Sci Rep 5:11695
115. Li G, Wu X, Lee DW (2016) A galinstan-based inkjet printing system for highly stretchable electronics with self-healing capability. Lab Chip 16:1366–1373

Chapter 4
Mechanical Properties of Liquid Metal After Solidified

Abstract Mechanical properties of liquid metal are significant for various applications in biomedical category. This chapter investigates several classical mechanical issues of bone tissue and typical liquid metal biomaterials. Besides the changes in compositions and ratios of the alloy, representative methods for modifying liquid metal after solidified such as reinforcing with nano particles, casting with different processing technologies etc. are explained. Experimental ways to test mechanical performance and improvement of the low melting point metals were discussed.

Keywords Liquid metal · Low-melting-point alloy · Mechanical property
Solid phase

4.1 Introduction

The liquid metals often present fluid characteristics as other common solutions at room temperature due to their super low melting points. However, for some metals, they own a little higher melting point than those of room temperature liquid metals but much lower than those of common metals. With easily switchable capability between liquid and solid phase, such metal material has unique merit in a group of biomedical applications. In order to distinguish these metals from room temperature liquid metals, the low-melting-point alloys mentioned in this book do not involve room temperature liquid metals if not mentioned. Such alloys are solid under their working conditions. Therefore, apart from the properties introduced in former chapters, their mechanical properties are necessary to be evaluated for the needs of application. The mechanical properties can generally be classified into short-term and long-term characteristics. Short-term properties include performance in tension, hardness, bending, compression and fracture resistance. Long-term properties, such as fatigue, creep and stress-relaxation, their measurement values can be used to predict the behavior of materials in a period of time. Generally, proper mechanical properties are the basic requirements of most biomaterials which are needed to well

J. Liu and L. Yi, *Liquid Metal Biomaterials*,
Springer Series in Biomaterials Science and Engineering10,
https://doi.org/10.1007/978-981-10-5607-9_4

Table 4.1 Mechanical strength of bone tissue and typical metals

Materials	Tensile strength (MPa)	Elastic modulus (GPa)
Cancellous bone	1.5–38	0.01–1.57
Cortical bone	100–200	10–20
Stainless steel	480–834	193–200
Titanium alloys	550–985	100–125
Cobalt alloys	655–1400	195–230
Magnesium	185–232	73–117

Note Data from Refs. [4–8]

match those of natural tissues [1–3]. On the other hand, considering the great potential of low-melting-point alloys in biomedicine, abundant information about this kind of material should be acquired. For example, mechanical properties are significant for special applications in orthopedics. Materials with insufficient mechanical strength cannot achieve the target task. Several known mechanical properties of bone tissue and typical metal biomaterials are listed in Table 4.1 [4–8]. At present, the low-melting-point alloys are widely used in engineering, especially in welding field. In addition to solders, it was reported that the low-melting-point alloys have been investigated as 3D (three dimensional) printing materials and bone cements [9–12]. More studies should be implemented in the near future to understand additional properties of various low-melting-point alloys. Researchers will benefit from the existing mechanical parameters when they are searching for a new biomaterial.

The present group has introduced BiInSnZn alloy as bone cement [12]. The melting point of BiInSnZn alloy is 57.5 °C. It is composed of Bi, In, Sn and Zn with corresponding weight ratio of 35, 48.6, 16 and 0.4%, respectively. Its mechanical properties were tested in comparison with the commonly used hard biomaterial i.e. PMMA (polymethyl methacrylate), including compression strength, bending strength, bending modulus, fatigue performance and fracture toughness etc.

4.2 Compression Test

The compression test has been carried out for BiInSnZn alloy. Before the test, three cylindrical specimens (12 mm in diameter, 15 mm in length) were prepared by casting. Then these samples were cured within molds at room temperature for 24 h. The values of ultimate compressive strength were measured using a universal testing machine MTS-SANS CMT5000 (CMT5000, SANS, MTS Systems Corp., China) under a cross-head speed of 0.5 mm/min at room temperature. The schematic diagram of compression test is shown in Fig. 4.1.

The force was recorded from maximum load during compression. Then the compressive strength was determined through dividing this force by the original

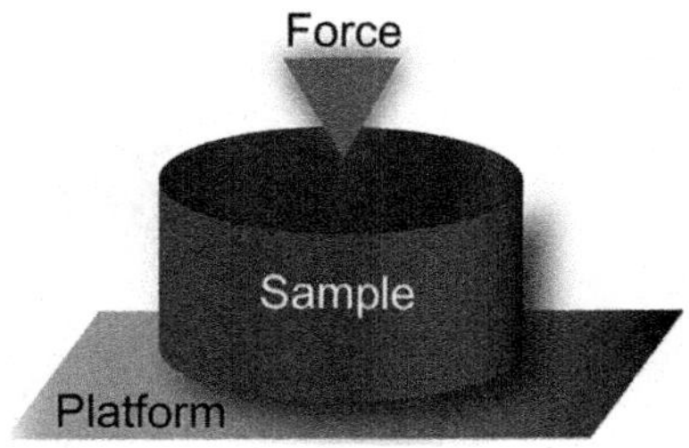

Fig. 4.1 Test method to determine the compressive strength of BiInSnZn alloy

cross-sectional area. The final strength was calculated according to the average value of three cylindrical specimens. The measured magnitude of the compressive strength alloy cement was 37.6 ± 1.56 MPa. In ISO 5833 standard [13], acrylic cement is required with the mean value of compression strength larger than 70 MPa, which is widely utilized in load-bearing applications. In addition, an alternative bone cement, calcium phosphate cement (CPC), has compressive strength of 30 MPa. Such value is larger than that of cancellous bone but lower than that of cortical bone [14–17]. This kind of cement plays a critical role in non-load-bearing applications. In comparison, the compressive strength of BiInSnZn is larger than that of CPC and lower than that of acrylic cement. Consequently, the strength measurement is instructive for application of BiInSnZn alloy in special biomaterial area and could help researchers understand well what property to be improved.

4.3 Bending Test

Bending characteristics are also important mechanical parameters of materials. Based on the different stress loading protocols, the bending modulus and bending strength can be determined by two common means: three-point bend test (Fig. 4.2a) and four-point bend test (Fig. 4.2b). By contrast, the stress loading of three-point test is simpler than that of four-point test. In industry, four-point bend test is seldom used because of its complex structure of fixture. However, the bending stress in four-point bend test can uniformly distribute on samples, which makes the test results more accurate. Therefore, the four-point test is recommended for biomaterials.

According to the International Standard ISO 5833, the bending properties of acrylic resin cements are determined by means of four-point bend test [13]. In the study of BiInSnZn alloy-based bone cement [12], the bending tests were also carried out by this method as follows. The specimens were prepared using rectangular moulds and cured at room temperature for 24 h, with final dimensions of 100 mm length, 20 mm width, and 8 mm thickness, respectively. A universal testing machine MTS-SANS CMT5000 (MTS Systems Corp., China) was employed to measure the bending strength with a cross-head speed of 0.5 mm/min.

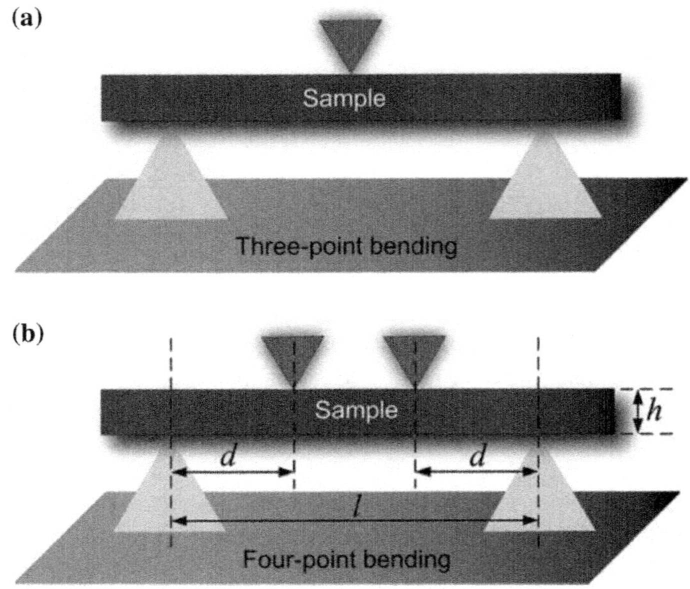

Fig. 4.2 Test method to determine the bending strength of BiInSnZn alloy

The equipped device recorded the deflection of the centre of the specimen in real-time. Notably, when certain force was exerted on their surface, it was found that rectangle specimens were subjected to sever deformation but not broken in the bending tests. Based on the measured data, the bending strength (F_{bend}) was calculated by Eq. (4.1) [13]:

$$F_{bend} = \frac{3Fd}{bh^2} \tag{4.1}$$

where F is the maximum force during the bending process; b and h are the average width and thickness of the specimens, in millimetres respectively; d represents the distance between the inner and the outer loading points (20 mm). Thus, the bending strength of BiInSnZn alloy is 35.31 ± 1.09 MPa. Moreover, the bending modulus of the material is the ratio of stress to corresponding strain within its elastic region. The bending modulus (E_{bend}) can be determined from the expression [13]:

$$E_{bend} = \frac{\Delta Fd}{4fbh^3}\left(3l^2 - 4d^2\right) \tag{4.2}$$

where l is the distance between the outer loading points (60 mm); f denotes the difference between the deflections under two points (90 N and 270 N) which are placed on linear portion of the stress-strain plot and ΔF denotes the load range of corresponding two points (270 N − 90 N = 180 N). Through Eq. (4.2), the bending modulus of BiInSnZn alloy is 6.41 ± 0.81 GPa. In ISO 5833 [13], the minimum requirements of bending strength and bending modulus are 50 and 1 800 MPa for acrylic bone cement. Therefore, the bend test demonstrates that the bending modulus can satisfy the demand but the bending strength of BiInSnZn alloy should be improved when it is applied as acrylic cement.

4.4 Fracture Toughness

Fracture toughness is a characterization of the material's resistance to the combined effects of stress and flaws [18]. For bone cement, it may be broken when the load exceeds its limit, which will lead to severe consequences of surrounding bone tissue and economic lost. Therefore, the fracture toughness of material is of great importance for its application. At present, there are two common kinds of specimens for fracture toughness testing: rectangular compact tension specimen and single edge-notched bend specimen. According to the ISO 12737-2005 standard [19], the fracture toughness of BiInSnZn was carried out using three rectangular compact tension specimens, whose dimensions are shown in Fig. 4.3.

Figure 4.3 gives the specimen's specified geometrical dimensions with a width of 32 mm and a thickness to width (*B*/*W*) ration of 0.5 [20, 21]. The universal testing machine MTS-SANS CMT5000 (CMT5000, SANS, MTS Systems Corp., China) was utilized to perform the crack resistance test with a displacement rate of 2 mm/min at room temperature. The load was applied until the specimen broke apart. Then the fracture surface was measured with the aid of a scanning electron microscope (SEM, FEI Quanta 200, Netherlands).

The conditional value of fracture toughness, i.e. K_Q was calculated by the following equation [19]:

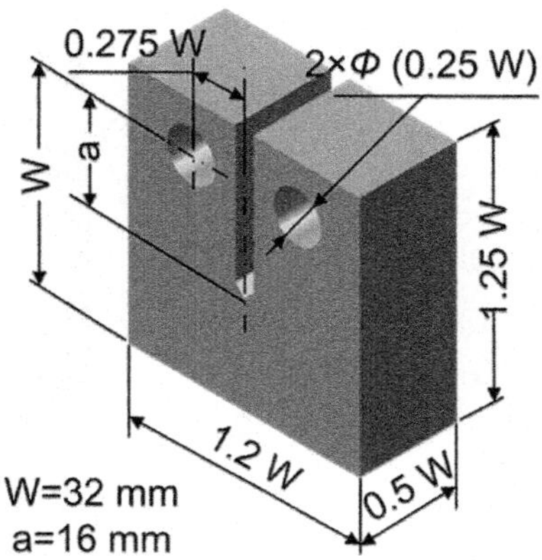

Fig. 4.3 Diagram shows the geometry of rectangular compact tension specimen

$$K_Q = \left(\frac{F_Q}{BW^{1/2}}\right) f\left(\frac{a}{W}\right) \tag{4.3}$$

where, F_Q is the applied load, B and W are the thickness and width of the specimen, respectively, and a is the crack length; $f(a/W)$ is the geometric factor calculated by Eq. (4.3), i.e.

$$f\left(\frac{a}{W}\right) = \left(2 + \frac{a}{W}\right) \frac{0.866 + 4.64\left(\frac{a}{W}\right) - 13.32\left(\frac{a}{W}\right)^2 + 14.72\left(\frac{a}{W}\right)^3 - 5.6\left(\frac{a}{W}\right)^4}{\left(1 - \frac{a}{W}\right)^{3/2}} \tag{4.4}$$

Based on the parameters and measured data, the calculated average value of K_Q is 4.85 ± 0.05 $\mathrm{MPam}^{1/2}$. According to the evaluation of the standard, if the value of F_{max}/F_Q is larger than 1.1, the K_Q is not the effective fracture toughness (K_{IC}). In general, K_{IC} is a standard parameter to evaluate the material's crack resistance, which is related to its composition and structure. On the other hand, K_Q is a condition value that is influenced by the width of specimen. Through the micrographs, see Fig. 4.4, there were massive dimples that can be observed on specimen‘s fracture section. It can be inferred that BiInSnZn is a kind of ductile material. For this kind of material, the specimens with sufficient size are needed to satisfy the plane stain condition for K_{IC} measurement. However, it is hard to prepare the specimens and the corresponding test instrument. Nevertheless, the obtained K_Q can be compared with that of acrylic bone cement with same width. The results demonstrate that alloy cement offers better crack resistance compared to acrylic cement in the width control of 32 mm [21]. The fracture toughness of BiInSnZn should be measured with other effective methods in the near future.

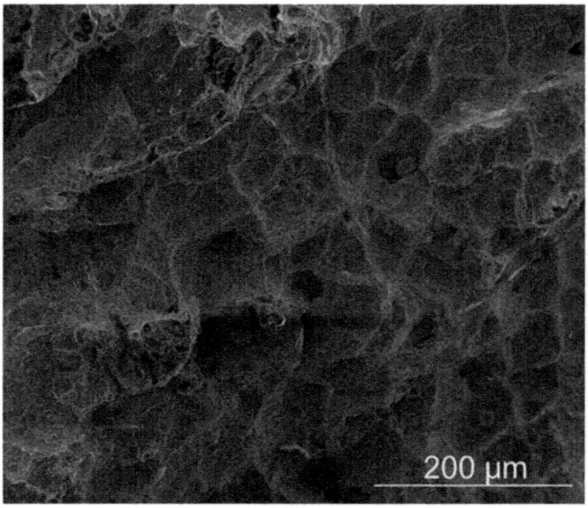

Fig. 4.4 Scanning electron micrograph of the fracture surface [12]. Picture reproduced with permission

4.5 Fatigue Performance

Besides the short-term properties, the long-term performance is also significant for the fatigue life prediction of materials. Fatigue life is a typical parameter which has been frequently tested for evaluating the long-term characteristic. Fatigue tests of BiInSnZn were conducted using a material test machine in air at room temperature (Instron 8874, Instron Corp., Canton, MA) [22]. The specimen was manufactured into a dumbbell type with cylindrical cross-section. Figure 4.5 shows the schematic drawing and the photo of the experimental setup. For comparison, the configuration and its size were prepared the same as those of acrylic specimen in previous studies [23, 24]. It was reported that cement mantle in hip arthroplasty withstands the normal tensile stress ranging from 3 to 11 MPa. [25]. Thus, each BiInSnZn alloy specimen was subjected to a uniaxial constant-amplitude fully reversed (tension-compression) loading with a sinusoidal waveform to a maximum stress of ±15 MPa. The cyclic load was applied at a frequency of 5 Hz. In addition, there are also other test conditions that can be adopted, such as uniaxial tension-tension loading, uniaxial zero-tension loading, three-point flexure, rotating bending and flexure [26]. Fatigue testing continued until the specimen was fractured. Before failure, the maximum number of cycles, N_f (number of cycles to failure) was recorded.

The fatigure specimens with macropores were discarded, since the defects will influence the fatigue performance. Figure 4.6 shows the photos of cross-section of specimen in fracture test. Massive dimples can be observed as well, proving the plasticity of BiInSnZn. Meanwhile, the N_f results of four specimens were recorded as 109 373, 106 549, 78 594 and 76 892. It was found that the number of fatigue stress cycles for alloy specimens are comparable to those of commercial cement such as CMW1, CRX and CXL (Table 4.2) at the same testing conditions with an applied stress of ±15 MPa, at a frequency of 5 Hz [23]. Lewis has reviewed various studies on fatigue life, based on different intrinsic and extrinsic factors [26]. There into, several methods were adopted for processing the fatigue test results: N_f, plot of the Wohler curve, Olgive-type fit to the S-N_f or S-logN_f results, fit of the N_f results to the Weibull relation, etc. All these evaluation methods are effective.

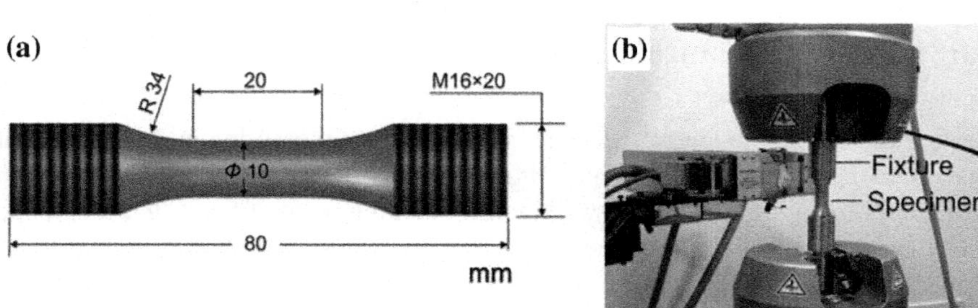

Fig. 4.5 The specimen (**a**) and setup (**b**) of fracture test

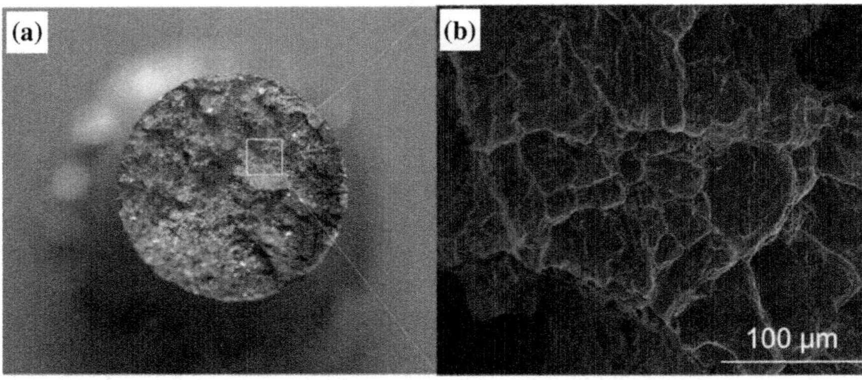

Fig. 4.6 The cross-section of specimen in fracture test. **a** The photo of cross-section; **b** The scanning electron microscope photograph of local part in (**a**)

Table 4.2 The N_f of commercial acrylic bone cements [23]

CMW1	CRX	CXL
3252	25,338	45,549
3476	36,346	51,193
3814	36,604	51,486
6615	38,510	57,554
8075	47,656	59,574
9438	51,628	62,284
10,448	57,655	93,592
26,112	57,978	104,006
28,594	64,363	160,345
31,651		165,590

Notably, a suitable fit to the S-N_f results and the Weibull treatment of the N_f results are recommended for providing more information [26]. However, a large number of specimens and much cost and time are required.

4.6 Other Mechanical Characteristics

Besides the above parameters, there are also studies on measuring other mechanical characteristics of low-melting-point alloys. Yu et al. utilized BiInSnGa alloy (Bi 26%, In 61%, Sn 9%, Ga 4%, by weight) with melting point of 52 °C to achieve the 3D (dimension) printing [11]. They compared the nano-indentation hardness of the printed and cast specimens. The results show that the hardness values of the printed part range from 0.12 to 0.22 GPa, which are higher than those of the cast samples, i.e. 0.04 to 0.07 GPa. It was inferred that such improvement of mechanical properties resulted from the coarse grains' microstructure of printed specimens [27]. The Young's modulus was tested for further evaluation. The Young's modulus values of printed and cast specimens are 17.81 and 15.78 GPa, respectively.

Moreover, the mechanical properties of SnZnBi (Sn-23 wt% Bi-5 wt%) were measured [28], including tests regarding hardness, tensile stress and compressive stress, respectively. Such alloy has the melting point of 175 °C, which has been considered as a kind of lead-free solder material. The researchers investigated the influence of the temperature gradient and growth rate on SnZnBi's mechanical properties. The Vickers hardness (HV) refers to the ratio of a load applied the indenter to the surface area of the indentation, which was determined by using a Future-Tech FM-700 model hardness measuring test device. Using a Shimadzu AG-IS universal testing machine, the tensile and compressive stresses were tested at room temperature. The results show that the values of microhardness, tensile stress and compressive stress all increase with the temperature gradient and growth rate, respectively. With the increase of the temperature gradient from 1.78 to 3.99 K/mm, the values of microhardness, tensile stress and compressive stress would increase from 204.9 to 232.4 MPa, 29.1 to 36.8 and 66.1 to 86.9 MPa, respectively. When the growth rate increases from 8.32 to 478.6 μm/s, the microhardness, tensile stress and compressive stress would increase from 232.4 to 303.0 MPa, 36.8 to 89.1 MPa and 86.9 to 189.9 MPa, respectively.

In addition, the shear strength of InZnGa with melting point of 141.3 °C was investigated [29], which reflects the capacity of solder to withstand shaking. The single lap shear testing was conducted to test the joint strength and the testing specimens were prepared cylindrically. The result shows that the shear strength of such solder alloy is 190.188 MPa.

4.7 Conclusion

Regarding the studies on the mechanical characteristics of low-melting-point alloys, most of them were carried out for providing the basis of their applications in industry. This is mainly because that the biomedical roles of these metals have not been developed widely. In recent years, the researchers have realized their importance of serving as biomaterials. Therefore, it is significant to acquire the knowledge of materials' mechanical properties for particular application. The standards of mechanical properties vary with different applications. Although some mechanical parameters of low-melting-point alloys may not achieve the levels of the replaced biological tissues, there are a great deal of studies on various improving methods due to the rapid development in metallic material field. Some study has reported that the addition of Bi into SnZn alloy can increase the microhardness, tensile strength and elastic modulus, but decrease the elongation [30]. Besides the changes in compositions and ratios of the alloy, common modification methods in engineering, such as reinforcing with nano particles, casting with different processing technologies [31–36] are worthy to be adopted. Both the knowledge acquisition of mechanical performance and improvement of their strength need a lot of efforts in the coming time.

References

1. Hukins DWL, Leahy JC, Mathias KJ (1999) Biomaterials: defining the mechanical properties of natural tissues and selection of replacement materials. J Mater Chem 9(3):629–636
2. Fisher JP, Dean D, Mikos AG (2002) Photocrosslinking characteristics and mechanical properties of diethyl fumarate/poly(propylene fumarate) biomaterials. Biomaterials 23 (22):4333–4343
3. de Guzman RC, Merrill MR, Richter JR et al (2011) Mechanical and biological properties of keratose biomaterials. Biomaterials 32(32):8205–8217
4. Poinern GEJ, Brundavanam S, Fawcett D et al (2012) Biomedical magnesium alloys: a review of material properties, surface modifications and potential as a biodegradable orthopaedic implant. Am J Biomed Eng 2(6):218–240
5. Staiger M, Pietak A, Huadmai J et al (2006) Magnesium and its alloys as orthopedic biomaterials: a review. Biomaterials 27(9):1728–1734
6. Valiathan MS, Krishnan VK (1999) Biomaterials: an overview. Natl Med J India 12(6): 270–274
7. Ridzwan MIZ, Shuib S, Hassan AY et al (2007) Problem of stress shielding and improvement to the hip implant designs: a review. J Med Sci 3:460–467
8. Yi L, Liu J (2017) Liquid metal biomaterials: a newly emerging area to tackle modern biomedical challenges. Int Mater Rev 62(7):415–440
9. Wang L, Liu J (2014) Liquid phase 3D printing for quickly manufacturing conductive metal objects with low melting point alloy ink. Sci Chin Technol Sci 57(9):1721–1728
10. Wang L, Liu J (2014) Compatible hybrid 3D printing of metal and nonmetal inks for direct manufacture of end functional devices. Sci Chin Technol Sci 57(11):2089–2095
11. Yu Y, Liu F, Liu J (2017) Direct 3D printing of low melting point alloy via adhesion mechanism. Rapid Prototyp J 23(3):642–650
12. Yi L, Jin C, Wang L et al (2014) Liquid-solid phase transition alloy as reversible and rapid molding bone cement. Biomaterials 35(37):9789–9801
13. International Organization for Standardization ISO 5833. Implants for surgeryacrylic resin cements (2002)
14. Chow LC, Takagi S (2001) A natural bone cement-A laboratory novelty led to the development of revolutionary new biomaterials. J Res Nat Inst Stand Technol 106 (106):1029–1033
15. Nilsson M, Fernández E, Sarda S et al (2002) Characterization of a novel calcium phosphate/ sulphate bone cement. J Biomed Mater Res 61(4):600–607
16. Fukase Y, Eanes ED, Takagi S et al (1990) Setting reactions and compressive strengths of calcium phosphate cements. J Dent Res 69(12):1852–1856
17. Schmitz JP, Hollinger JO, Milam SB (1999) Reconstruction of bone using calcium phosphate bone cements: a critical review. J Oral Maxillofac Surg (Official Journal of the American Association of Oral & Maxillofacial Surgeons) 57(9):1122–1126
18. Graham J, Pruitt L, Ries M et al (2000) Fracture and fatigue properties of acrylic bone cement: the effects of mixing method, sterilization treatment, and molecular weight. J Arthroplast 15 (8):1028–1035
19. International Organization for Standardization ISO 12737. Metallic materialsdetermination of plane-strain fracture toughness (2005)

20. Lewis G, Nyman JS (2000) Toward standardization of methods of determination of fracture properties of acrylic bone cement and statistical analysis of test results. J Biomed Mater Res 53(6):748–768
21. Lewis G, Mladsi S (2000) Correlation between impact strength and fracture toughness of PMMA-based bone cements. Biomaterials 21(8):775–7781
22. Baleani M, Cristofolini L, Minari C et al (2003) Fatigue strength of PMMA bone cement mixed with gentamicin and barium sulphate vs pure PMMA. Proc Inst Mech Eng [H] 217 (1):9–12
23. Lewis G, Janna S (2003) Effect of test specimen cross-sectional shape on the in vitro fatigue life of acrylic bone cement. Biomaterials 24(23):4315–4321
24. Lewis G, Janna S, Carroll M (2003) Effect of test frequency on the in vitro fatigue life of acrylic bone cement. Biomaterials 24(6):1111–1117
25. Krause W, Mathis RS (1988) Fatigue properties of acrylic bone cements: review of the literature. J Biomed Mater Res 22(A1 Suppl):37–53
26. Lewis G (2003) Fatigue testing and performance of acrylic bone-cement materials: state-of-the-art review. J Biomed Mater Res B Appl Biomater 66(1):457–486
27. Felton LE, Raeder CH, Knorr DB (1993) The properties of tin-bismuth alloy solders. J Miner Met Mater Soc 45(7):28–32
28. Çadırlı E, Böyük U, Kaya H et al (2011) Determination of mechanical, electrical and thermal properties of the Sn-Bi-Zn ternary alloy. J Non-Cryst Solids 357(15):2876–2881
29. Efzan MNE, Faziera MNN, Abdullah MMAB (2016) Mechanical and physical properties of In-Zn-Ga lead-free solder alloy for low energy consumption. IOP Conf Ser Mater Sci Eng 133 (1):012048
30. Wadud MA, Gafur MA, Qadir MR et al (2015) Effect of bismuth sddition on structure and mechanical properties of tin-9zinc soldering alloy. Mater Sci Appl 6(6):792–798
31. Kuzumaki T, Miyazawa K, Ichinose H, Kuzumaki T et al (1998) Processing of carbon nanotube reinforced aluminum composite. J Mater Res 13(9):2445–2449
32. Kwon H, Estili M, Takagi K et al (2009) Combination of hot extrusion and spark plasma sintering for producing carbon nanotube reinforced aluminum matrix composites. Carbon 47 (3):570–577
33. Dong SR, Tu JP, Zhang XB (2001) An investigation of the sliding wear behavior of Cu-matrix composite reinforced by carbon nanotubes. Mater Sci Eng A 313(1):83–87
34. Kim KT, Cha SI, Hong SH et al (2006) Microstructures and tensile behavior of carbon nanotube reinforced Cu matrix nanocomposites. Mater Sci Eng A 430(1–2):27–33
35. Chu K, Wu Q, Jia C et al (2010) Fabrication and effective thermal conductivity of multi-walled carbon nanotubes reinforced Cu matrix composites for heat sink applications. Compos Sci Technol 70(2):298–304
36. Esawi AMK, Borady MAE (2008) Carbon nanotube-reinforced aluminium strips. Compos Sci Technol 68(2):486–492

Chapter 5
Preparations and Characterizations of Functional Liquid Metal Materials

Abstract This chapter summarizes the fabrication methods and characterizations of the functional liquid metal biomaterials. The future outlooks, including challenges, routes and related efforts, were illustrated and interpreted.

Keywords Functional liquid metal · Fabrication method · Preparations
Characterization

5.1 Introduction

As new generation functional materials, the preparations of low-melting liquid metals become more and more increasingly important. So far, various methods, such as alloying, oxidizing, adding metals or non-metallic materials and so on, have been developed to prepare desirable functional materials based on the gallium or more other metals [1]. These methods could not only change the form of the materials, but also endow the original liquid metals with rather diversified performances, which have further expanded the application range of the low-melting liquid metals to meet various needs. This chapter summarizes on the fabrication methods and characterizations of the functional liquid metal materials. The future outlook, including challenges, routes and related efforts, will be illustrated and interpreted.

Clearly, the low-melting liquid metals have kept attracting great attentions over a wide variety of important areas owing to their excellent rheological properties at around room temperature. It is well known that the pure metals which present liquid state at low temperatures are mercury (Hg, −39 °C), cesium (Cs, 28.40 °C), gallium (Ga, 29.8 °C) and rubidium (Rb, 38.89 °C). Among them, mercury, cesium and rubidium cannot be widely used because of their unavoidable toxicity or high chemical activity. Therefore, more and more studies have centered on gallium, which is non-toxic and stable in air and water, and many distinctive findings have revealed a series of novel properties of this material in various areas [1, 2].

J. Liu and L. Yi, *Liquid Metal Biomaterials*,
Springer Series in Biomaterials Science and Engineering10,
https://doi.org/10.1007/978-981-10-5607-9_5

Gallium element is widely distributed in the earth's crust. It does not exist in pure metal, but is usually found in the ores including bauxite and sphalerite. Therefore, it is often extracted as a by-product during processing the ores of other metals. Starting from its low-melting point character, other properties of the gallium are also distinctive from the traditional rigid metals. It is used commonly in the analog integrated circuits, high temperature thermometers, nuclear reactors, focused ion beam, biomedical sensors and so on. What's more, based on this fundamental element, it becomes possible to fabricate the liquid metal into different forms and characteristics.

So far, there are already quite a few methods available to deal with the liquid metals through which the material characteristics including melting point, thermal and electrical conductivity, viscosity, fluidity and plasticity could be adjusted to meet different needs. These low-melting alloys and materials derived from the room temperature liquid metals could collectively be called functional liquid metal materials which will clearly be next big wave research.

5.2 Preparation Methods

5.2.1 Alloying

Gallium could readily alloy with most metals. So as an ingredient, it could be used to form many low-melting alloys with other metals, such as indium (In), bismuth (Bi), tin (Sn), lead (Pb), zinc (Zn), aluminum (Al) and so on [3]. The melting points of the alloys are different depending on the constituent and the proportion. EGaIn (78.6% Ga and 21.4% In by weight) and Galinstan (68.5% Ga, 21.5% In, and 10.0% Sn by weight) are commonly available. Since Galinstan is liquid below room temperature, it is often used as a better substitute for mercury. These low-melting alloys could be fabricated by stirring in liquid state, and some raw metals still require heating slightly. Taking EGaIn as an example, it is fabricated by placing 78.6 wt% gallium and 21.4 wt% indium in a container, then heating and mixing them with a magnetic stirring apparatus or a glass pipette until thoroughly combined. Similar to gallium, bismuth could also comprise a series of low-melting alloys with Pb, Sn, Cd, Zn and In, etc. [4, 5]

In addition, NaK alloy [6] which is formed from the alloying of potassium and sodium, is also one of the most common low-melting alloy (eutectic composition: 22% Na and 78% K by weight, −12.8 °C). Taking a certain amount of Na and K metals and placing them in the reaction container under the protection of nitrogen, the NaK alloy could be achieved quickly by shaking. The NaK alloy containing 40–90% K by weight usually retains liquid state at room temperature. Since the NaK alloy is rather active, it is often stored under organic solvents such as hexane and oil without oxygen, or inert gases such as dry argon and dry nitrogen, in order to prevent the chemical reactions with water and air. Besides, in the alkali metal family, NaCs and NaRb are also low-melting alloys [7].

5.2.2 Oxidizing

Oxidizing is an effective method to change the properties of the liquid metal. Once exposed to the air, the liquid metal could spontaneously form trace amounts of oxide layer on the surface. As is well known, the easily-formed oxide layer prevents the liquid metal to be oxidized further. However, the oxide layer could be broken via the vigorous stirring so that more and more metals are further oxidized, by which a uniformly-dispersed mixture of liquid metal and its oxide is achieved, as shown in Fig. 5.1a. The control in the extent of oxidation through stirring could change the thermal conductivity, interface resistance and viscosity of the material, consequently obtain various targeted functional liquid metal materials [8]. For example, as the viscosity of the mixture increased gradually with the amount of liquid metal oxides, it offers a possible approach to obtain the functional liquid metal with a suitable viscosity by vigorously stirring for a certain period of time.

Besides, the surface gallium oxide itself is a promising functional material with great possibilities for broad application fields. It could be disturbed by the sonication and then form “liquid metal” / “metal oxides” structures (Fig. 5.1b) [9, 10], or harvested as nanoflakes by further sonication in DI water and subsequent annealing (Fig. 5.1c) [11].

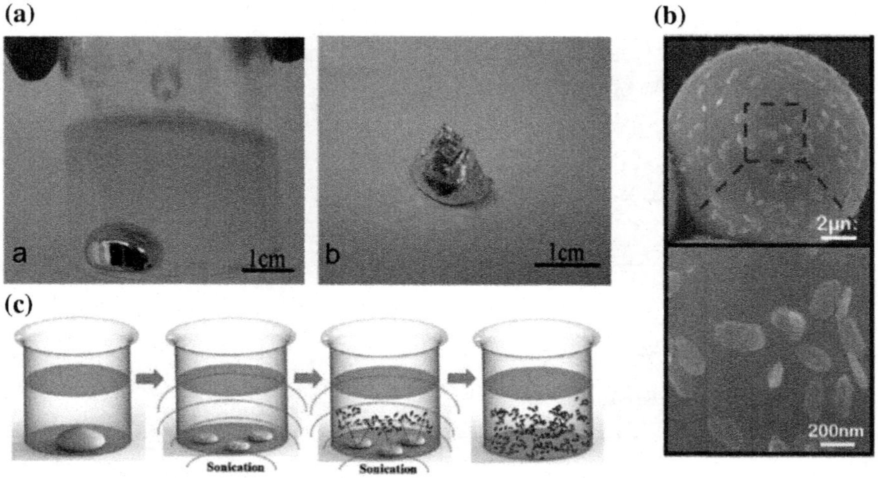

Fig. 5.1 **a** The morphology contrasts between *a* pure liquid gallium and *b* oxidized gallium achieved after the vigorous stirring [8]. **b** The SEM image of LM/MO spherical structures assembly after sonication for 20 min [9]. **c** Schematic of the synthesis process converting gallium metal into gallium oxide nanoflakes during sonication [11]. All pictures reproduced with permission

5.2.3 *Fabrication of Liquid Metal Droplets*

The morphological change is also an aspect of the liquid metal-based functional materials. When the liquid metal is fabricated into small droplets, they could achieve specific functions and have been utilized in wide applications.

In recent years, many fabrication means of the liquid metal micro-droplets have been developed, and among them, the microfluidic approach is the most common one. Figure 5.2a shows the production process and the monodisperse spherical microdroplets droplets take shapes by flow focusing using a PDMS-based microfluidic device filled with an aqueous polyethylene glycol (PEG) solution or deoxygenated silicone oil. Here, both the PEG solution and the silicone oil are used to create a high viscosity fluid in the fabrication process. The size mainly depends on the channel dimension and flow rate applied [12]. Hutter et al. even created non-spherical droplets by filling the channel with oxygenated silicone oil to instantaneously form oxide layers on the droplets [13]. It is worth mentioning that during this method, these solutions are all mixed with sufactant sodium dodecyl sulfate (SDS), which plays the role of surfactant to stabilize these produced droplets.

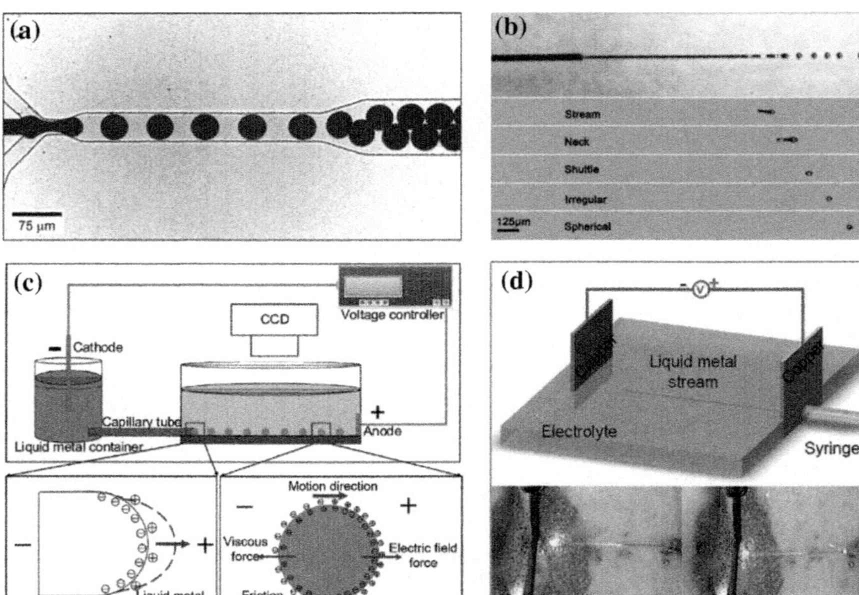

Fig. 5.2 **a** The microscopy image of liquid-metal droplets formation in the flow-focusing microfluidic device [13]. **b** The detailed processes of droplets channelless fabrication [16]. **c** The experimental set up for the electro-hydrodynamic shooting phenomenon of liquid metal stream [17]. **d** The Platform structure and phenomenon for triggering discharge plasma in liquid with the liquid metal stream electrode [18]. All pictures reproduced with permission

Considering that it is still costly and technically complex in the fabrication of the micro-fluidic channels, another alternative and much simpler way to produce micro-droplets is to directly jet the liquid metal flow into another fluid from a small hole [14, 15]. Yu et al. proposed a channelless fabrication method based on self-breaking up mechanisms of the liquid metal. As shown in Fig. 5.2b, the liquid metal with a certain velocity was jetted from the syringe needle into the SDS solution, then it automatically split into multiple droplets with hundreds of micrometers in diameter rapidly, along with five shape stages including stream, neck appearing, shuttle shape, irregular shape and spherical droplet. For further process, these liquid metal droplets could be cooled down so as to freeze them into solid particles. Various typical factors, such as the pinhole size of the injection needle, density, viscosity of the fluid and surfactants added, would influence the liquid metal droplets generation behavior [16]. Further, as presented in Fig. 5.2c, Fang et al. applied a small direct current (DC) voltage, then the liquid metal inside the capillary tube was spontaneously injected into the SDS solution to form discrete droplets. The shooting velocity was proportional to the applied voltage while the droplet size depended on the aperture diameter of the capillary nozzle [17]. Afterwards, in order to obtain liquid metal droplets with smaller size, Wang et al. improved the liquid metal channelless fabrication device by shooting the liquid metal stream into an electrode plate under the electrical field, as shown in Fig. 5.2d. As a result, accompanied by the blue-violet light, quantities of non-uniform droplets sized in a range from several micrometers to hundreds of nanometers were available [18].

5.2.4 Preparation of Liquid Metal Nanoparticles

The liquid metal could even be made into nanoparticles to obtain multiple functions, which could be achieved via a simple ultrasonication approach in the presence of organic solvents [19]. During a typical synthesis process, as shown in Fig. 5.3a, a certain amount of liquid metal bulk is first added in a container filled with the ethanolic solution of thiol first of all. And then, an ultrasonic probe is applied to introduce cavitation in the solution, leading to local extremes of pressure and temperature within an ultrashort time. In this case, the liquid metal bulk stabilized by the oxidation layer is rapidly fractured into some liquid metal nanoparticles under the oscillating shear force. Meanwhile, thiolated ligands can be readily and strongly assembled onto the surface of the new-born liquid metal nanoparticls, competing with the reoxidation process. Finally, spherical liquid metal nanoparticles form under continuous sonication and are stable owing to the protection from the thiolate ligands and rapid oxidation on the surface. After sonication, these liquid metal nanoparticles need to be removed from the container and resuspended in water, then the grey slurry is obtained as shown in the right image of Fig. 5.3b, which could remain suspended up for several weeks [20–22].

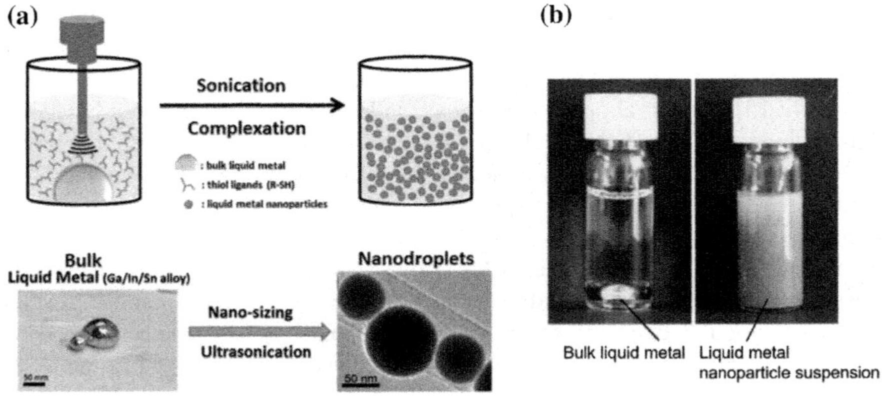

Fig. 5.3 **a** Schematic illustration of the preparation route for liquid metal nanodroplets [20]. **b** The comparison of liquid metal bulk before ultrasonication and nanodroplets after ultrasonication [21]. All pictures reproduced with permission

5.2.5 Coating Surface

When liquid metal droplets or nanoparticles are coated by micro- or nanoparticles, they are called liquid metal marbles, which not only maintain both the flexible reconfigurability offered by the fluid and other attractive properties of the liquid metals, but also prevent the liquid metal from adhering to their environment or corroding their metal contacts [23]. There are two methods to embed the liquid metal droplets with non-metal particles due to the strong cohesive forces between them. One of the methods is to roll the liquid metal on a powder bed (as shown in Fig. 5.4a), and another approach is to submerge the liquid metal in a colloidal suspension of micro or nano size powders (as shown in Fig. 5.4b). With the two different methods, Sivan et al. created some liquid metal marbles by coating small Galinstan droplets within a coating of insulators (including Teflon and silica) and semiconductors (including WO_3, TiO_2, MoO_3, In_2O_3 and carbon nanotubes) respectively, and it was found that the coating formed through the submerging approach was more uniform [24]. To maintain a high surface tension, Chen et al. pretreated the liquid metal droplets with the NaOH aqueous solution for about 3 s before rolling the liquid metal droplets on the powder bed, then fabricated the NaOH-treated GaInSn alloy droplets coated with polytetrafluoroethylene (PTFE) particles [25]. Zhang et al. presented the liquid metal marbles incorporated Ga_2O_3 or WO_3 nanoparticles via sonication, and it was found that sonication duration is important to determine the dimension of the liquid metal marbles [9, 10]. Fig. 5.4c presents the morphology of some liquid metal marbles.

The nanoparticle coatings offer the marbles with additional dimensions of control. Tang et al. has fabricated liquid metal marbles consisting of a galinstan core

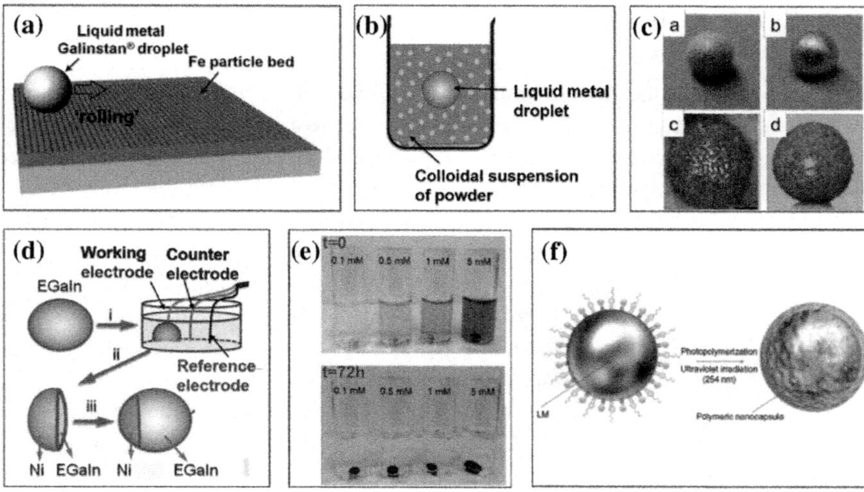

Fig. 5.4 **a** Schematic for rolling a liquid metal droplet on the powder bed [29]. **b** Schematic for submerging a liquid metal droplet in the powder colloidal suspension. **c** Optical images of several liquid metal marbles coated with *a* PTFE particles [25], *b* silica particles [25], *c* Fe particles [29], *d* WO_3 powders [24]. **d** Sketch for the fabrication of the magnetic soft liquid metal by electroplating method [31]. **e** Formation of Au–GaInSn via sonication in $KauBr_4$ solutions of varied concentrations after 0 and 72 h [32]. **f** Schematic illustration of a liquid metal nanocapsule fabricated by crosslinking of butadiyne moieties [33]. All pictures reproduced with permission

coated with tungsten oxide nanoparticles, and demonstrated that these liquid metal marbles could move in aqueous media when an electrical current is applied as a result of asymmetry in the surface tension created by these nanoparticles [26]. In addition to electrochemical manipulation, the liquid metal marbles could also be manipulated through photochemical reactions [27] or magnetic field [28–30].

Besides, the metal surfaces or metallic nanoparticles could be coated on the liquid metal droplets via electroplating or sonication. Figure 5.4d shows the electroplating process mentioned in Zhang et al's work [31]. A copper wire connected with a liquid metal in the nickel plating solution was the working electrode, and a Pt wire and a Ag/AgCl electrode served as the counter electrode and reference electrode, respectively. When applying a voltage to this device, the Ni layer was coated on the upper surface of the liquid metal droplet. Hoshyargar et al. proposed another elegant approach to create a liquid metal marble with a solid metal shell [32]. As shown in Fig. 5.4), the liquid metal droplets were placed in the $KAuCl_4$ for some time and sonicated in the solution, then the metallic silver layers were formed. This method is also possible with other metals, such as Ag.

In addition, the liquid metal nanopaticles are facile to be modified by some functional radical groups and to be encapsulated as a nanocapsule. As shown in Fig. 5.4f, the polymeric core-shell structure encapsulating liquid metal is fabricated by crosslinking of butadiyne moieties with 254 nm ultraviolet irradiation [33].

5.2.6 Adding Nanomaterials

The performance of the liquid metals could be changed by loading a small amount of other metal or non-metal nanoparticles for new features. Liu and Ma proposed for the first time the concept of the nano liquid-metal fluids [34], which are prepared through adding nonmaterials (nanoparticles, nanofibers, nanotubes, and nanowires) into the liquid metal fluids. These nanomaterials generally comprise metals including gold, silver, copper, aluminum, iron and nickel, and non-metal such as copper oxide, titanium oxide, silicon oxide as well as carbon nanotubes [35].

For water, it is effortless to mix nanomaterials into the fluid [36]. While for various liquid metal fluids, this issue is challenging due to the unique features of the liquid metal such as high surface tension. The widely used method for preparing nano liquid metal fluids is similar to the traditional nanofluids. The nano-sized dry powders can be dispersed into the liquid gallium, Ga–In, or other liquid metal fluids with the aid of mechanical mixing, magnetic force agitation or ultrasonic agitation for a certain time [37]. During the stirring course, the wettability and compatibility of liquid metal with various materials could be improved due to oxidization (Fig. 5.5a). If the metal is solid in the room temperature, it is necessary to heat the metal sufficiently and melt it into liquid before adding nanoparticles.

However, due to the high surface tension, the easy surface oxidation and the poor wettability of the liquid metal, the nanomaterials would be precipitated out of

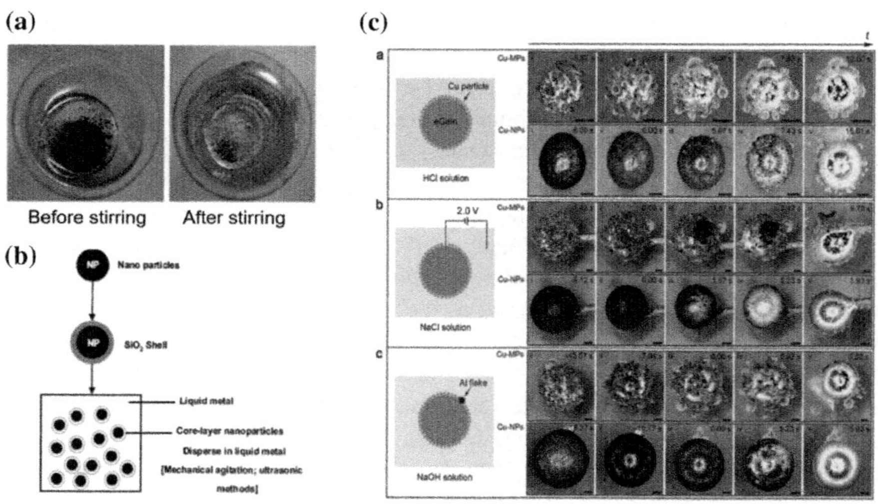

Fig. 5.5 **a** Appearances of gallium and Ni particles before and after stirring [37]. **b** The modification procedure for preparation the liquid metal nanoparticle fluid by coating the metal nanoparticles in advance with silica [35]. **c** Methods to realize liquid metal composite fluid with copper particles in *a* acidic solution with no additional assistance, *b* neutral solution assisted by an electrical polarization and *c* alkaline solution assisted by an aluminum flake. Scale bars: 200 μm [40]. All pictures reproduced with permission

the surface gradually. Therefore, how to enhance the stability of the nanomaterials in the liquid metal fluids is very important in preparing metal nanofluids. As shown in Fig. 5.5b, in order to improve the dispersion stability, one method is to coat the metal nanoparticles in advance with silica, which can also protect the core of the particles from oxidation and corrosion [35]. Iron alloys [38], micron, submicron and nanometer Ni particles [37, 39] have been successfully suspended in the liquid gallium or gallium–indium alloy in some reports.

Tang et al. discovered another highly efficient way to prepare liquid metal composite fluid with copper microparticles and nanoparticles in acidic solution (HCl), neutral solution (NaCl) or alkaline solution (NaOH), respectively [40]. Figure 5.5c shows the preparation process. In this method, the droplets of the EGaIn were coated with micro- and nanoparticles by rolling the droplets on the copper particle beds. Then, these droplets were submerged under HCl solution. After a while, the copper particles on the surface would be quickly swallowed into the EGaIn droplets, accompanied with bubble generation. For NaCl solution, similar particle-eating behavior could also be observed with the help of a cathode polarization voltage of 2 V or more. While for NaOH solution, this method could be realized by placing metals such as aluminum and magnesium in the alkaline solution.

5.2.7 Compositing with Other Materials

When the liquid metal is homogeneously dispersed inside some base materials, such as methyl silicone oil, polydimethylsiloxane (PDMS), its original properties would have some changes, including weaker electrical conductivity, higher thermal conductivity, higher viscosity and lower surface energy. The common methods to fabricate the composite liquid metal material is to mix the two materials and stir them using a magnetic stirrer for some time. For example, as shown in Fig. 5.6a, Mei et al. obtained the liquid metal grease by adding methyl silicone oil and the galinstan into the beaker and stirred at room temperature using a magnetic stirrer for 20 min at the speed of 200 rounds per min [41]. With the volume fraction of liquid metal increased, the concentration of liquid metal droplets also increased, resulting in more liquid metal droplets connected with each other. From the plain-view SEM images shown in Fig. 5.6b, it could be observed that the liquid metal droplets in the liquid metal grease were irregularly shaped.

Afterwards, Lin et al. proposed another method to fabricate a kind of liquid metal matrix composite material, by stretching viscoelastic polymer substrates supporting a drop of gallium-based liquid metal [42]. Figure 5.6c illustrates the fabrication process. During the stretching process, the liquid metal would also be elongated because of the adhesion between it and the polymer substrate.

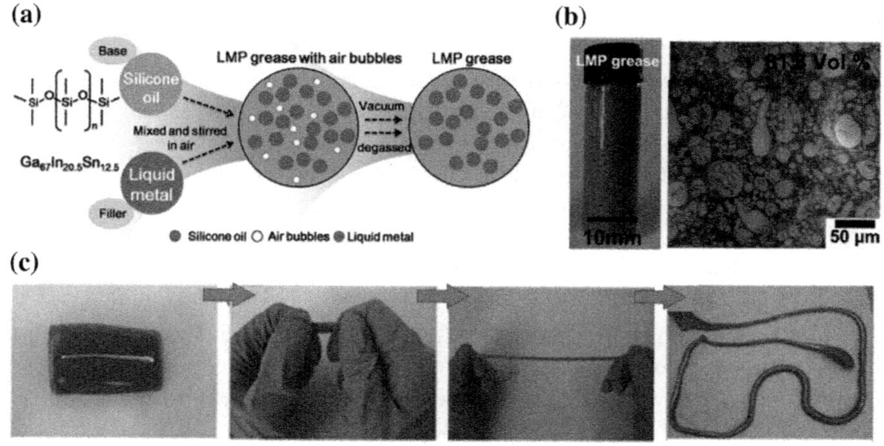

Fig. 5.6 **a** The schematic diagram for the fabrication process of the LMP grease. **b** The optical image and plain-view ESEM image of liquid metal grease [41]. **c** The process of drawing of EGaIn wires by hand at room temperature [42]. All pictures reproduced with permission

5.3 Characterizations of Functional Liquid Metal Materials

Generally, the metal materials with melting points below 200 °C are called low melting point liquid metal, including gallium, gallium-based alloys, bismuth-based alloys, and so on. With different composition and proportion, the liquid metal alloys have different properties, to meet different application needs. Table 5.1 compares the properties of several typical liquid metals and water, including melting point, thermal conductivity, electrical conductivity, surface tension, etc [43–50].

Besides alloying, other fabrication approaches could also make the characteristics of the functional liquid metal materials vary from those of original liquid metals. For example, adding nanoparicles into the liquid metals will change the thermal and electrical conductivities. Modification on the surface of the liquid metals could offer new optical or magnetic properties.

5.3.1 Regulation of Thermal Properties

The melting point is a basic property of the functional liquid metal materials. If some trace elements are added to the liquid metals, the characteristics of the alloys would correspondingly change. Therefore, the melting point and other properties can be adjusted by changing the chemical ratio of the alloy or adding other trace elements in it according to the specific needs. For example, the melting point of Sn–Zn–Ga alloy could be approximately considered as a positive linear function of the

Table 5.1 Basic properties of water and several typical liquid metal materials

	Water	Pure Ga	$Ga_{75.5}In_{24.5}$	$Ga_{68.5}In_{21.5}Sn_{10}$	$Ga_{67}In_{20.5}Sn_{12.5}$
Melting point (°C)	0	29.8	15.5	−19	10.35
Density (g cm^{-3})	1	6.05	6.28	6.4	6.54
Thermal conductivity (W m^{-1} K^{-1})	0.599	29.28			39
Heat capacity (J Kg^{-1} K^{-1})	4183	409.9			366.5
Electrical conductivity (10^7 S m^{-1})	5.5×10^{-13}	0.22	0.34	0.38	0.31
Surface tension (N m^{-1})	0.072	0.72	0.435	0.535	0.533
Viscosity (cSt)	1.002	0.23	0.32	0.37	0.0023

gallium content. Furthermore, the boiling points of the liquid metals are higher, and the liquid metals could keep liquid state from the room temperature to above two thousand degrees, so that their working temperature ranges are rather wide.

In addition to the melting point, the thermal conductivity is also an important index for the low-melting liquid metals. The thermal conductivity of the gallium is about 29.4 W/(m °C), much higher than that of the water [0.6 W/(m °C)]. After oxidation treatment, the adding of gallium oxide could obviously decrease its thermal conductivity and the value is reduced to about 13.07 W/(m °C) at room temperature. Even so, it is still significantly higher than that of currently commercialized thermal grease which has the best thermal conductivity of 7 W/(m °C) when filled with some metal nanoparticles [8]. Not only that, but the thermal conductivity of liquid metal could also be improved by adding other nanomaterials, such as carbon nanotube, gold, silver and copper.

Further, it is found that adding SiO_2 nanoparticles to the pure gallium can enhance the supercooling of gallium. In Cao et al's study, the liquid gallium with the weight of 5 g still remained liquid at 276–277 K after adding 1.0 wt% 10 nm-diameter SiO_2 particles, and was able to hold about 400 days without solidification [51].

Besides, thermal interface resistance is also an important property for liquid metal. The thermal interface resistance is lower, the heat transfer process proceeds more smoothly. Usually, the metal nanoparticles can be added into the liquid metal to decrease the thermal interface resistance. The better wetting performance of liquid metal after oxidizing treatment can also reduce effectively the thermal contact resistance at the interface.

5.3.2 Regulation of Electrical Properties

Generally, the electrical conductivity of the metal is superior than that of nonmetal, and could decrease with the increase of the temperature. Different contents of metal in alloys can lead to different conductances. In addition to the alloy methods, adding nanoparticles into the liquid metals could also change the electrical properties, which greatly depends on the dispersed phases, additive species, morphology, size and concentration, as well as the presence of surfactants or dispersants. Not only that, oxidation treatment is also an efficient approach to increase the electrical resistivity of liquid metal [52].

Besides, Ga is facile to form a native oxide on the surface which has special semiconductor properties. Ga_2O_3 has a wide energy bandgap (4.8 eV), and its valence band edge is located at −7.75 eV vs vacuum [53]. In addition, other compounds such as GaAs, GaN and GaS, also have special electrical characteristics [54, 55]. For instance, GaAs possesses higher saturation electron rate and higher electron mobility.

5.3.3 Regulation of Magnetic Properties

Gallium itself is non-magnetic, but is an excellent magnetic nanoparticle carrier. The liquid metal magnetic fluid could be synthesized by dispersing ferromagnetic nano powders in a liquid gallium. And in the case of a magnetic field, the fluid will show magnetism. Under action of the magnetic field gradient, the magnetic particles dispersed in the base fluid will drag the entire fluid flow under magnetic force [56]. Micro- or nano-sized iron, nickle, chromic metal powders and their alloys are common magnetic substances used in the liquid metal [57–59]. The magnetization intensity of the magnetic fluid is directly proportional to that of the magnetic material. In addition, the liquid metal marbles coated with ferromagnetic micro/nano materials could also become magnetic, and could be manipulated by the outside magnetic field.

5.3.4 Regulation of Fluidic Properties

As a kind of fluid, the wettability of the liquid metal plays a key role in its applications, which mainly depends on the viscosity and surface tension. The liquid gallium has low viscosity and high surface tension, and both parameters decrease with the increase of temperature.

Oxidation treatment will significantly improve the viscosity, and the existence of the gallium oxide could change the surface tension of the liquid metal. For example, the surface tension of pure EGaIn liquid drop is about 435 mN/m, while that of the EGaIn liquid drop coated oxide films could be adjusted to 624 mN/m. Therefore

Table 5.2 The corrosive properties of gallium with various metals

Corrosive properties	Poor corrosion resistance	Better corrosion resistance	Anti-corrosion
Metal	Iron, nickel, cadmium, cerium, copper, aluminum, gold, manganese, platinum, silver, tin, vanadium, zirconium	Titanium, tantalum, niobium, molybdenum, beryllium	Tungsten, rhenium, sintered BeO, Al_2O_3 and fused silica, graphite
Temperature range	200 °C and lower	Higher than 400 °C	Uncorroded at 800 °C

this method influences the wettability of the liquid metal. It has been demonstrated that with the increase of oxide content in the liquid metal, the wettability of the liquid metal gradually improves on different substrates including paper, silica gel plate and rubber sheet [52]. Besides, given extra pressure, the wettability could also be improved [60].

The morphological change is also a factor to affect the wettability of the liquid metal. For instance, the EGaInSn nanoparticle dispersions could exhibit more excellent wettability than liquid metal bulk on the substrates.

5.3.5 *Chemical Properties*

The pure gallium is stable in water or air, and can be eaten by concentrated HCl. What's more, gallium has a strong corrosive effect on some metals such as aluminum [61, 62]. Table 5.2 lists the corrosive properties of gallium with various metals. Lu et al. even fabricated quickly complex patterns on aluminum based on liquid metal corrosion property [63]. Liquid metal encapsulated with semiconducting and insulating coatings could effectively prevent the corrosion behavior.

5.4 Liquid Metal as Energy Harvesting or Conversion Medium

In the field of energy, liquid metal has also shown potential for harvesting mechanical energy based on various principles and technologies, such as electromagnetic induction, magnetohydrodynamic power generation, piezoelectric effect and so on. For instance, the liquid metal has been studied as a liquid triboelectric nanogenerator to generate high power through conversion of mechanical energy in recent studies [64]. Figure 5.7a shows the device configuration and working principle of this technology. Compared with the solid materials, the liquid metal has larger contact surface up to 100%, which greatly improves the total energy conversion efficiency.

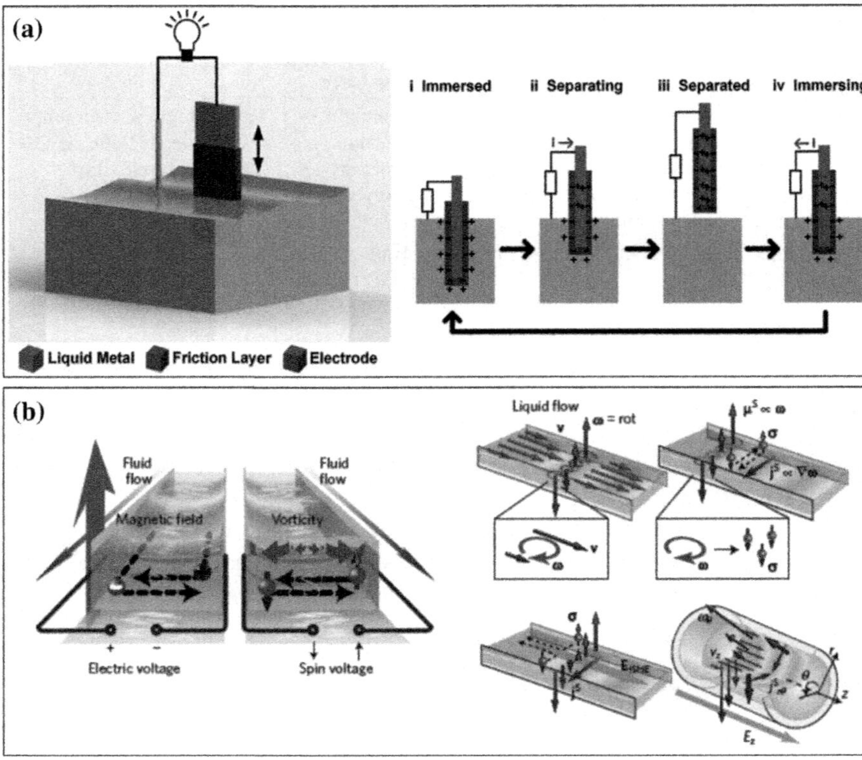

Fig. 5.7 **a** The device configuration and working principle of the liquid-metal-based triboelectric nanogenerator [64]. **b** Schematic of conventional magnetohydrodynamic generation (left) and spin hydrodynamic generation (right) [65]. All pictures reproduced with permission

There is another application case for the generation of energy. As shown in Fig. 5.7b, when the liquid metal flows in a narrow channel, the velocity gradually decreases from the inner wall to the center due to friction. As a result, the spin motion generates and the spin electrons of liquid metal flow to the center. Then a faint longitudinal current is formed in the liquid, which is proportional to the velocity of the liquid metal [65]. This phenomenon supplies a new method to generate mechanical spin-current and electric generators without using magnets, and is beneficial to realize super miniaturization of power generation devices.

5.5 Liquid Metal as Catalysts

The liquid metal could be used as catalysts in some chemical reactions. One typical application is to generate hydrogen based on GaAl alloy. Aluminum is the preferred material for hydrogen production with water in terms of its low cost, abundant reserve and environment-friendliness [66]. However, since the aluminum is easy to be oxidized, it is difficult for pure aluminum to react with water continually. One effective way reported is to ameliorate the aluminum through alloying treatment. Some works have tried to activate the aluminum with the addition of gallium and gallium-based alloys, which would constantly etch the aluminum and destroy the oxide layer [67–76]. Another application reported recently is to form an active catalyst with Pb for alkane dehydrogenation. It is proven that the liquid state of gallium-rich Pd–Ga mixture behaves a higher activity than Pd-rich compounds, because the former proceeds as homogeneously distributed metal atoms at surface of the liquid metallic phase [77].

Gallium-based catalysts decomposed into a mixture of Ga, GaN, Ga_2O_3 under the growth conditions could also be applied for the growth of GaN nanowires [78]. Unlike other foreign metal catalysts, gallium-based catalysts are beneficial to eliminate the risk of contamination from foreign metals. Beyond that, liquid metal is facile to prepare catalytically active materials. For instance, In/Sn rich microspheres (the ratio of In:Sn is 2:1) with a trace of Ga could be achieved by sonicating galinstan alloy in alkaline solution or treated the alloy with reducing agents such as $NaBH_4$. This material has high catalytic activity in the reduction of ferricyanide and nitrophenol [79].

Besides, the existence of the native oxide on the surface endows the liquid metal with a better photocatalytic ability which could be improved by the incorporation of additional Ga_2O_3 [9–11]. The photocatalytic performance is applicable for the decomposition of various organic pollutants under UV and visible-light irradiation.

5.6 Two-Dimensional Materials

Two-dimensional (2D) materials are very different from their bulk and play important roles on a wide range of application due to their unique properties [80]. The atomically thin oxide layer on the surface of gallium is considered as a naturally occurring 2D material, which is suitable for sensing gases including NO_2, CH_4 and NH_3 [81].

In a recent report, the gallium-based liquid metal has been utilized as a reaction solvent to achieve more variety of 2D materials at the room temperature. Some metals could be alloyed into the liquid metal, and the composition of self-limiting interfacial oxide, such as HfO_2, Al_2O_3, and Gd_2O_3. Then these surface oxides can be exfoliated as a 2D layer using the van der Waals exfoliation technique or gas injection method, as shown in Fig. 5.8a [82].

In addition, the gallium oxide layer is valuable as a substrate to grow other 2D semiconductors, such as 2D GaS [55, 83]. As shown in Fig. 5.8b, by placing the liquid metal with its oxide layer on silica substrate and squeegeeing the metal, the pure gallium could be removed readily and the oxide layer sticks to the silica substrate. Then the 2D GaS is produced by exposing it to hydrochloric acid vapour and sulfur gas exposition in succession.

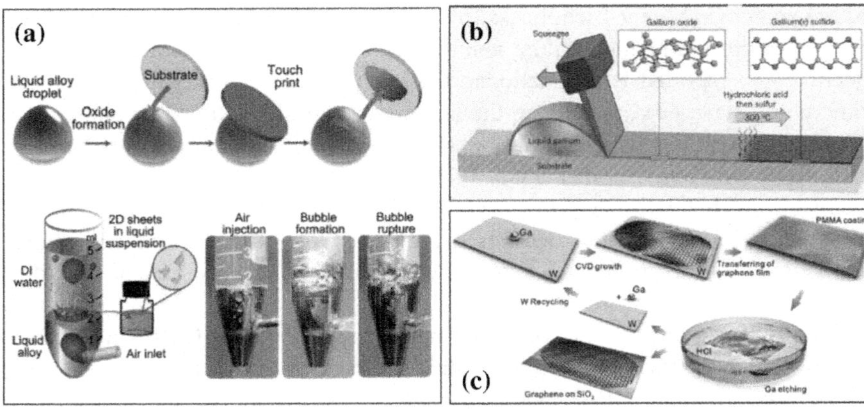

Fig. 5.8 **a** Schematic of *a* the van der Waals exfoliation technique and *b* the gas injection method [82]. **b** Schematic for making atomically thin layers of GaS using liquid metal substrate [83]. **c** Schematic illustrates graphene growth and transfer over liquid Ga supported on a W substrate [84]. All pictures reproduced with permission

Besides, the gallium has also been demonstrated to be a good substrate during the growth assembly, and transfer behavior of uniform graphene and other graphene-like two dimensional materials, which could be illustrated by Fig. 5.8c [84]. Compared to the traditional solid substrates, the liquid gallium oxide substrate has a smooth and isotropic surface, and has advantages of strict self-limitation, ultra-fast growth and smooth stitching of grains.

5.7 Future Outlook

In the above, several mature methods to prepare various functional liquid metal materials with different properties have been summarized [1]. In addition to these, ion implantation technology is possible to be drawn on to obtain another new-type functional material. Ion implantation is an effective physical method for material surface modification, by which the ions of one element are accelerated into the target, thereby changing the physical, chemical, or electrical properties of the target [85]. The targets used at present are common in solid state, and the crystal structure of the target can be damaged in the process. If the ion implantation method is used for the low-melting liquid metals, it is worth studying that how such interactions occur between the ions and the surface of the liquid metals in liquid state. Besides, the low-melting liquid metal with porous structure is also a trend to prepare new functional liquid metal materials, which could be realized through introducing chemical reaction mechanism [86], possibly by adding foaming agent or directly injecting gas into a whole liquid metal bulk, or accumulating and solidifying the liquid metal droplets under high pressure. This porous liquid metal has higher specific surface area, which is potential to play new roles in some applications.

Looking at all the functional liquid metal materials presented above, one will notice that most of them have only a single silver-white color. For the solid metals such as copper and silver, they can wear colorful clothes through various mature technologies including anodizing [87, 88], chemical immersion [89], electroplating [90], direct brushing, etc. While the coloring methods of the liquid metal are still scarce. Liang et al. have first put the basic idea of "colorful liquid metal printed electronics" forward, and tried to make colorful liquid metal utilizing the adhesion mechanism of the mineral pigments [91] as well as fluorescent particles [92] on the liquid metal oxide layer. Besides, it is possible to reflect colorful light if the liquid metal is modified by some periodic nanostructures on the surface [93, 94]. Gorgeous colors are easily appreciated by most people, and it is believed that colorful liquid metal will add new elements to the liquid metal family and open more novel applications. Therefore, it is a matter of considerable interest to develop mature technology to fabricate colorful liquid metals.

Naturally, there are still some issues waiting to be better addressed in current technologies. For instance, with the increase of the metal nanoparticles dispersed in the liquid metal, the electricity or magnetic properties could be enhanced, but the fluidity of the functional liquid metal material would evidently reduce. Another confusing problem is that there are no suitable devices to evaluate the distribution of the nanoparticles in the liquid metal bulk since the liquid metal is not transparent like water.

5.8 Conclusion

In summary, for the recently emerging functional liquid metal materials, their preparation methods, and characterizations in various fields have been systematically interpreted. Low-melting liquid metal materials own a group of unique merits in many aspects, such as favorable fluidity, super compliance, high electrical conductivity, and so on. Until now, there have been many methods to fabricate various functional liquid metal materials, including alloying, oxidizing, fabricating liquid metal micro-droplets and nanoparticles, coating surface, adding nanomaterials and mixing the liquid metal with other soft materials [1]. These new functional materials could influence the properties of original liquid metals on the thermal, electrical, magnetic, fluidic, chemical performances. The diverse functional liquid metal materials have enriched the application range of the low-melting liquid metal, and they have played significant roles in the fields such as biomedical electronics, thermal management, printed electronics, 3D printing, bioelectrode, drug delivery, tumor treatment, soft robot, microfluidics, energy, catalyst, etc. Admittedly, there are still many remaining challenges around the functional liquid metal materials. Nevertheless, the new-generation materials have also opened broader academic and technologic views, and we believe that this will be the next big wave research.

References

1. Wang Q, Yu Y, Liu J (2017) Preparations, characteristics and applications of the functional liquid metal materials. Adv Eng Mat 20:1700781
2. Moskalyk RR (2003) Gallium: the backbone of the electronics industry. Miner Eng 16 (10):921–929
3. Cheng J, Steckl AJ (2001) Mg–Ga liquid metal ion source for implantation doping of GaN. J Vac Sci Technol, B 19(6):2551–2554
4. FeltonL E, RaederC H, Knorr DB (1993) The properties of tin-bismuth alloy solders. JOM 45 (7):28–32
5. Ge H, Li H, Mei S et al (2013) Low melting point liquid metal as a new class of phase change material: An emerging frontier in energy area. Renew Sustain Energy Rev 21(5):331–346
6. Koirala RP, Singh BP, Jha IS, Adhikari D (2015) Viscosity of liquid Na–K alloy. Bibechana 12:135–144
7. Berghout A, Knider F, Hugel J et al (2007) Partial resistivity analysis of the NaK, NaRb and NaCs liquid alloys. J Non-Cryst Solids 353(32):3226–3230
8. Gao Y, Liu J (2012) Gallium-based thermal interface material with high compliance and wettability. Appl Phys A 107(3):701–708
9. Zhang W, Ou JZ, Tang S, Sivan V, Yao DD, Latham K, Khoshmanesh K, Mitchell A, Omullane AP, Kalantarzadeh K (2014) Liquid metal/metal oxide frameworks. Adv Func Mat 24(24):3799–3807
10. Zhang W, Naidu BS, Ou JZ, Omullane AP, Chrimes AF, Carey BJ, Wang Y, Tang S, Sivan V, Mitchell A, Bhargava SK, Kalantarzadeh K (2015) Liquid metal/metal oxide frameworks with incorporated Ga_2O_3 for photocatalysis. ACS Appl Mater Interf 7(3):1943–1950
11. Syed N, Zavabeti A, Mohiuddin M, Zhang B, Wang Y, Datta RS et al (2017) Sonication-assisted synthesis of gallium oxide suspensions featuring trap state absorption: test of photochemistry. Adv Funct Mater 27:1702295
12. Thlelen J, Dickey MD, Ward TA (2012) study of the production and reversible stability of EGaln liquid metal microspheres using flow focusing. Lab Chip 12(20):3961–3967
13. Hutter T, Bauer WAC, Elliott SR, Huck WTS (2012) Formation of spherical and non-spherical eutectic gallium-indium liquid-metal microdroplets in microfluidic channels at room temperature. Adv Funct Mater 22(12):2624–2631
14. Utada AS, Fernandez-Nieves A, Stone AHA, Weitz DA (2007) Dripping to jetting transitions in coflowing liquid streams. Phys Rev Lett 99(9):094502
15. Utada AS, Fernandez-Nieves A, Gordillo JM, Weitz DA (2008) Absolute instability of a liquid jet in a coflowing stream. Phys Rev Lett 100(1):014502
16. Yu Y, Wang Q, Yi L, Liu Y (2014) Channelless fabrication for large-scale preparation of room temperature liquid metal droplets. Adv Eng Mater 16(2):255–262
17. Fang W, He Z, Liu J et al (2014) Electro-hydrodynamic shooting phenomenon of liquid metal stream. Appl Phys Lett 105(13):134104
18. Yu Y, Wang Q, Wang XL, Wu YH, Liu J (2016) Liquid metal soft electrode triggered discharge plasma in aqueous solution. RSC Adv 6(115):11477
19. Zhang W, Srichan N, Chrimes AF, Taylor M, Berean KJ, Ou JZ et al (2016) Sonication synthesis of micro-sized silver nanoparticle/oleic acid liquid marbles: a novel SERS sensing platform. Sens Actuators B Chemical 223:52–58
20. Ren L, Zhuang J, Casillas G, Feng H, Liu Y, Xu X et al (2016) Nanodroplets for stretchable superconducting circuits. Adv Func Mater 26:8111
21. Lu Y, Hu Q, Lin Y et al (2015) Transformable liquid-metal nanomedicine. Nat Commun 32 (6):10066
22. Yamaguchi A, Mashima Y, Iyoda T (2015) Reversible size control of liquid metal nanoparticles under ultrasonication. Angew Chem 54(43):12809–12813

23. Bormashenko E (2011) Liquid marbles: properties and applications. Curr Opin Colloid Interf Sci 16(4):266–271
24. Sivan V, Tang S, Omullane AP et al (2013) Liquid metal marbles. Adv Func Mater 23 (2):144–152
25. Chen Y, Liu Z, Zhu D, Wang SH, Liang S, Yang J et al (2017) Liquid metal droplets with high elasticity, mobility and mechanical robustness. Mater Horiz 4:591
26. Tang S, Sivan V, Khoshmanesh K et al (2013) Electrochemically induced actuation of liquid metal marbles. Nanoscale 5(13):5949–5957
27. Tang X, Tang S, Sivan V et al (2013) Photochemically induced motion of liquid metal marbles. Appl Phys Lett 103(17):174104-1–174104-4
28. Zhao Y, Fang J, Wang H et al (2010) Magnetic liquid marbles: manipulation of liquid droplets using highly hydrophobic Fe3O4 nanoparticles. Adv Mater 22(6):707–710
29. Kim D, Lee J (2015) Magnetic-field-induced liquid metal droplet manipulation. J Korean Phys Soc 66(2):282–286
30. Jeon J, Lee J, Chung SK et al (2016) Magnetic liquid metal marble: characterization of lyophobicity and magnetic manipulation for switching applications. IEEE/ASME J Microelectromechanical Syst 25(6):1050–1057
31. Zhang J, Guo R, Liu J et al (2016) Self-propelled liquid metal motors steered by a magnetic or electrical field for drug delivery. J Mater Chem B 4(32):5349–5357
32. Hoshyargar F, Crawford J, Mullane AP (2017) Galvanic replacement of the liquid metal galinstan. J Am Chem Soc 139:1464–1471
33. Chechetka SA, Yu Y, Zhen X, Pramanik M, Pu K, Miyako E (2017) Light-driven liquid metal nanotransformers for biomedical theranostics. Nat Commun 8:15432
34. Ma K, Liu J (2007) Nano liquid-metal fluid as ultimate coolant. Phys Lett A 361(3):252–256
35. Zhang Q, Liu J (2013) Nano liquid metal as an emerging functional material in energy management, conversion and storage. Nano Energy 2:863–872
36. Yu W, Xie H (2012) A review on nanofluids: preparation, stability mechanisms, and applications. J Nanomater 1–17
37. Xiong M, Gao Y, Liu J et al (2014) Fabrication of magnetic nano liquid metal fluid through loading of Ni nanoparticles into gallium or its alloy. J Magn Magn Mater 354:279–283
38. Dodbiba G, Ono K, Park HS, Matsuo S, Fujita T (2011) FeNbVB alloy particles suspended in liquid gallium: investigating the magnetic properties of the MR suspension. Int J Mod Phys B 25(7):329–337
39. Ito R, Dodbiba G, Fujita T (2012) MR fluid of liquid gallium dispersing magnetic particles. Int J Mod Phys B 19:1430–1436
40. Tang JB, Zhao X, Li J, Zhou Y, Liu J (2017) Liquid metal phagocytosis: Intermetallic wetting induced particle internalization. Adv Sci 4(5):1700024
41. Mei SF, Gao YX, Deng ZS, Liu J (2014) Thermally conductive and highly electrically resistive grease through homogeneously dispersing liquid metal droplets inside methyl silicone oil. J Electron Packag 136:011009
42. Lin Y, Ladd C, Wang S, Martin A, Genzer J, Khan SA, Dickey MD (2016) Drawing liquid metal wires at room temperature. Extreme Mech Lett 7:55–63
43. Li P, Liu J (2011) Self-driven electronic cooling based on thermosyphon effect of room temperature liquid metal. ASME J Electron Packag 133(4):041009
44. Alchagirov BB, Mozgovoi AG (2005) The surface tension of molten gallium at high temperatures. High Temp 43(5):791–792
45. Assael MJ, Armyra IJ, Brillo J, Stankus SV, Wu JT, Wakeham WA (2012) Reference data for the density and viscosity of liquid cadmium, cobalt, gallium, indium, mercury, silicon. J Phys Chem Ref Data 41(3):285
46. Larsen RJ, Dickey MD, Whitesides GM, Weitz DA (2009) Viscoelastic properties of oxide-coated liquid metals. J Rheol 53(6):1305–1326
47. Dickey MD, Chiechi RC, Larsen RJ, Weiss EA, Weitz DA, Whitesides GM (2008) Eutectic gallium-indium (EGaIn): A liquid metal alloy for the formation of stable structures in microchannels at room temperature. Adv Func Mater 18(7):1097–1104

48. Liu T, Sen P, Kim C (2012) Characterization of nontoxic liquid-metal alloy galinstan for applications in microdevices. IEEE/ASME J Microelectromech Syst 21(2):443–450
49. Surmann P, Zeyat H (2005) Voltammetric analysis using a self-renewable non-mercury electrode. Anal Bioanal Chem 383(6):1009–1013
50. Morley NB, Burris J, Cadwallader LC, Nornberg MD (2008) GaInSn usage in the research laboratory. Rev Sci Instrum 79(5):112–192
51. Cao L, Park H, Dodbiba G et al (2011) Keeping gallium metal to liquid state under the freezing point by using silica nanoparticles. Appl Phys Lett 99(14):143120-1–143120-3
52. GaoY X, Li H, Liu J (2012) Direct writing of flexible electronics through room temperature liquid metal ink. PLoS One 7:e45485
53. Qiao L, Su F, Bi H, Girault HH, Liu B (2011) Ga_2O_3 photocatalyzed on-line tagging of cysteine to facilitate peptide mass fingerprinting. Proteomics 11(17):3501–3509
54. Suo G, Jiang S, Zhang J et al (2014) Synthetic strategies and applications of GaN nanowires. Adv Condens Matter Phys 2014:1–11
55. Carey BJ, Ou JZ, Clark RM, Berean KJ, Zavabeti A, Chesman ASR et al (2017) Wafer-scale two-dimensional semiconductors from printed oxide skin of liquid metals. Nat Commun 8:14482
56. Hartshorne H, Backhouse CJ, Lee WE (2004) Ferrofluid-based microchip pump and valve. Sens Actuators B: Chem 99(2):592–600
57. Raj K, Moskowitz B, Casciari R (1995) Advances in ferrofluid technology. J Magn Magn Mater 149(1):174–180
58. Pankhurst QA, Connolly J, Jones SK, Dobson J (2003) Applications of magnetic nanoparticles in biomedicine. J Phys D Appl Phys 36(13):R167
59. Tsai TH, Kuo LS, Chen PH, Lee D, Yang C (2010) Applications of ferro-nanofluid on a micro-transformer. Sensors 10(9):8161–8172
60. Zheng Y, He ZZ, Yang J, Liu J (2014) Personal electronics printing via tapping mode composite liquid metal ink delivery and adhesion mechanism. Sci Rep 4:4588
61. Deng Y, Liu J (2009) Corrosion development between liquid gallium and four typical metal substrates used in chip cooling device. Appl Phys A 95:907–915
62. Surmann P, Zeyat H (2005) Voltammetric analysis using a self-renewable non-mercury electrode. Anal Bioanal Chem 383:1009–1013
63. Lu J, Yi L, Wang L, Tan S, Gui H, Liu J (2016) Liquid metal corrosion sculpture to fabricate quickly complex patterns on aluminum. Sci China Technol Sci 60:65–70
64. Tang W, Jiang T, Fan FR et al (2015) Liquidmetal electrode for high performance triboelectric nanogenerator at an instantaneous energy conversion efficiency of 70.6%. Adv Func Mater 25(24):3718–3725
65. Takahashi R, Matsuo M, Ono M, Harii K, Chudo H, Okayasu S, Ieda JI, Takahashi S, Maekawa S, Saitoh E (2016) Spin hydrodynamic generation. Nat Phys 12(1):52
66. Wang H, Leung DY, Leung MK, Ni M (2009) A review on hydrogen production using aluminum and aluminum alloys. Renew Sustain Energy Rev 13(4):845–853
67. Yang W, Zhang TY, Liu JZ, Wang XH, Zhou JH, Cen KF (2015) Experimental researches on hydrogen generation by aluminum with adding lithium at high temperature. Energy 93 (1):451–457
68. Ho C, Huang C (2016) Enhancement of hydrogen generation using waste aluminum cans hydrolysis in low alkaline de-ionized water. Int J Hydrogen Energy 41(6):3741–3747
69. Wu D, Ouyang L, Wu C, Wang H, Liu J, Sun L, Zhu M (2015) Phase transition and hydrogen storage properties of Mg–Ga alloy. J Alloy Compd 642:180–184
70. Ilyukhina AV, Kravchenko OV, Bulychev BM, Shkolnikov EI (2010) Mechanochemical activation of aluminum with gallams for hydrogen evolution from water. Int J Hydrogen Energy 35(5):1905–1910
71. Baniamerian MJ, Moradi SE (2011) Al–Ga doped nanostructured carbon as a novel material for hydrogen production in water. J Alloy Compd 509(21):6307–6310
72. Kravchenko OV, Semenenko KN, Bulychev BM, Kalmykov KB (2005) Activation of aluminum metal and its reaction with water. J Alloy Compd 397(1):58–62

73. Wang W, Zhao X, Chen DM, Yang K (2012) Insight into the reactivity of AL–Ga–In–Sn alloy with water. Int J Hydrogen Energy 37(3):2187–2194
74. Parmuzina AV, Kravchenko OV (2008) Activation of aluminium metal to evolve hydrogen from water. Int J Hydrogen Energy 33(12):3073–3076
75. Fan MQ, Xu F, Sun LX (2007) Studies on hydrogen generation characteristics of hydrolysis of the ball milling Al-based materials in pure water. Int J Hydrogen Energy 32(14):2809–2815
76. Yuan B, Tan S, Liu J (2016) Dynamic hydrogen generation phenomenon of aluminum fed liquid phase Ga–In alloy inside NaOH electrolyte. Int J Hydrogen Energy 41(3):1453–1459
77. Taccardi N, Grabau M, Debuschewitz J, Distaso M, Brandl M, Hock R, Maier F, Papp C, Erhard J, Neiss C, Peukert W, Görling A, Steinrück HP, Wasserscheid P (2017) Gallium-rich Pd–Ga phases as supported liquid metal catalysts. Nat Chem 9(9):862
78. Simpkins BS, Ericson LM, Stroud RM et al (2006) Gallium-based catalysts for growth of GaN nanowires. J Cryst Growth 290(1):115–120
79. Hoshyargar F, Khan H, Kalantar-zadeh K, Omullane AP (2015) Generation of catalytically active materials from a liquid metal precursor. Chem Commun 51:14026–14029
80. Kalantar-zadeh K, Ou JZ, Daeneke T, Mitchell A, Sasaki T, Fuhrer MS (2016) Two dimensional and layered transition metal oxides. Appl Mater Today 5:73–89
81. Shafiei M, Hoshyargar F, Motta N, O'Mullane AP (2017) Utilizing p-type native oxide on liquid metal microdroplets for low temperature gas sensing. Mater Des 122:288–295
82. Zavabeti A, OuJ Z, Carey BJ, Syed N, Orrell-Trigg R, Mayes ELH et al (2017) A liquid metal reaction environment for the room-temperature synthesis of atomically thin metal oxides. Science 358:332–335
83. Kim YD, Hone J (2017) Screen printing of 2D semiconductors. Nature 544:167
84. Wang J, Zeng M, Tan L, Dai B, Deng Y, Rümmeli M et al (2013) High-mobility graphene on liquid p-block elements by ultra-low-loss CVD growth. Sci Rep 3(3):2670
85. Liu X, Chu PK, Ding C et al (2004) Surface modification of titanium, titanium alloys, and related materials for biomedical applications. Mater Sci Eng R-reports 47(3):49–121
86. Wang H, Yuan B, Liang S, Guo R, Wang X, Chang H, Ding Y, Liu J, Wang L (2018) PLUS-material: porous liquid-metal enabled ubiquitous soft material. Mater Horiz. https://doi.org/10.1039/C7MH00989E
87. Donahue CJ, Exline JA (2014) Anodizing and coloring aluminum alloys. J Chem Educ 91 (5):711–715
88. Diamanti MV, Curto BD, Masconale V et al (2012) Anodic coloring of titanium and its alloy for jewels production. Color Research and Application 37(5):384–390
89. John S, Perumal AS, Shenoi BA et al (1984) Chemical colouring of aluminium. Surf Technol 22(1):15–20
90. Wahab HA, Noordin MY, Izman S et al (2013) Quantitative analysis of electroplated nickel coating on hard metal. Sci World J 2013:631936
91. Liang S, Liu J (2017) Colorful liquid metal printed electronics. DOI/, Sci China Technol Sci. https://doi.org/10.1007/s11431-017-9116-9
92. Liang S, Rao W, Song K, Liu J (2017) Fluorescent liquid metal as transformable biomimetic chameleon. ACS Appl Mater Interfaces. https://doi.org/10.1021/acsami.7b17233
93. Yablonovitch E (1987) Inhibited spontaneous emission in solid-state physics and electronics. Phys Rev Lett 58(20):2059–2062
94. Sajeev J (1987) Strong localization of photons in certain disordered dielectric superlattices. Phys Rev Lett 58(23):2486–2489

Chapter 6
Liquid Metal Image Contrast Agent in Angiography

Abstract This chapter is to illustrate the use of liquid metal as a high quality image contrast agent for the coming angiography. Characteristics of liquid metal as vascular contrast agent were evaluated. Typical examples of liquid metal angiography and its applications in reconstruction of vascular network were presented. Quantitative comparison regarding the practices between traditional and liquid metal contrast agents was performed.

Keywords Image contrast agent · Angiography · Liquid metal

6.1 Introduction

This chapter is to illustrate the use of liquid metal as a high quality image contrast agent for the coming angiography. As is well known, blood vessels are distributed throughout the biological body, which are vital channels to and from tissues. These vessels constitute networks that branch frequently to continuously transit blood. The blood that flows in the circulatory system involving heart, lung, arteries, veins and capillaries, brings oxygen, nutrients to organs and tissues and takes away carbon-dioxide and metabolic wastes. By virtue of such unique vascular system, vertebrates can efficiently implement various complex tasks. The health of vessels is crucial for the body to realize physical function. Serious diseases even death can be induced once some problems occur in vessels, especially a series cardiovascular disease. Typically, cardiovascular disease can cause mass disability. According to statistical data, it was estimated that the disability-adjusted life years (DALYs) will increase from a loss of 85 million DALYs in 1990 to a loss of $\sim$150 million DALYs globally in 2020 [1]. Moreover, it was reported that coronary artery disease has been the leading cause of death in the United States [2].

Considering the significance of vessels, physicians and scientists have devoted great efforts to understand their structures and physiological mechanism sand reveal the relationship between vascular system and diseases for centuries, thereby providing the basis for prevention, diagnosis and therapy of such diseases. As is well

J. Liu and L. Yi, *Liquid Metal Biomaterials*,
Springer Series in Biomaterials Science and Engineering10,
https://doi.org/10.1007/978-981-10-5607-9_6

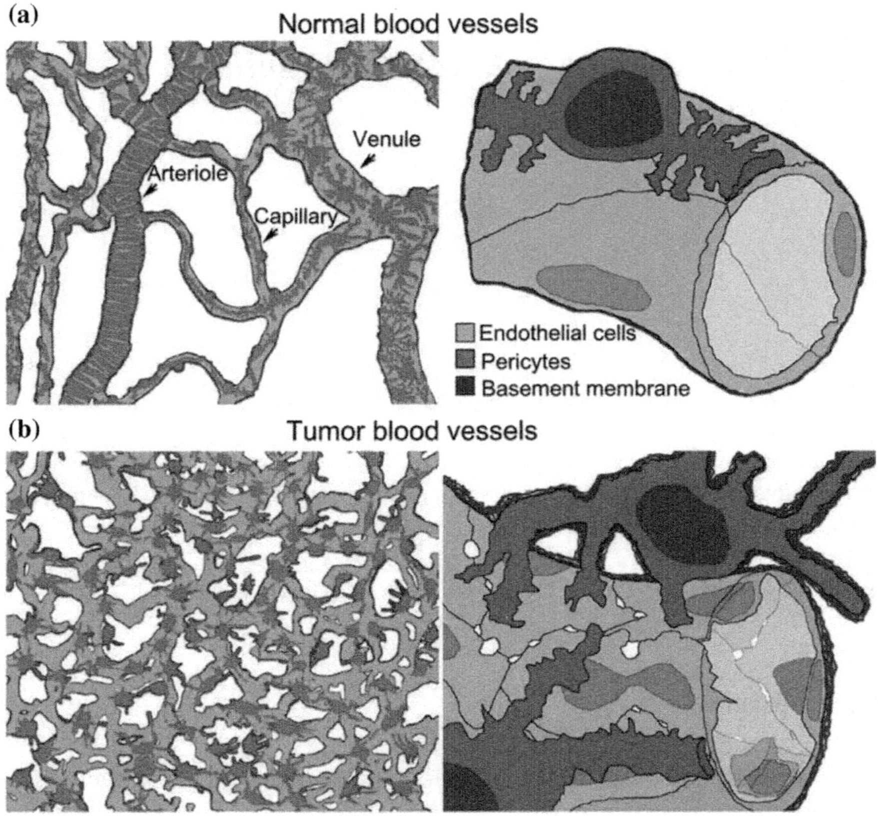

Fig. 6.1 Typical vasculatures for a normal organ or a tumor at two magnifications [4]. All blood vessels consist of endothelial cells (green), mural cells (red) and vascular basement membrane (blue). **a** Normal blood vessels generally own hierarchy vasculature of arterioles, capillaries and venules with characteristic size, shape and wall structure, respectively. **b** Tumor blood vessels present distinctive characteristics of disorganized, lacking of conventional hierarchy. It is difficult to distinguish arterioles, capillaries and venules. All pictures reproduced with permission

known, cancer is an unsolved global issue puzzling human beings. Based on estimates from GLOBOCAN, about 14.1 million new cancer cases and 8.2 million deaths occurred in 2012 worldwide [3]. It has been clarified that tumor blood vessels often display multiple structural and functional abnormalities [4], which are irregularly shaped, tortuous, and lack the normal hierarchical arrangement of arterioles, capillaries and venules (Fig. 6.1). For these vessels, they tend to be abundant in the regions of active growth, often at periphery, but absent in necrosis area of tumor. These abnormal characteristics can also be employed to help distinguish the progress of tumor conversely [5, 6]. There is convincing evidence that angiogenesis provides nutrition to the growth of tumor. In this sense, interpreting the blood supply may lead to tumor regression. However, limited knowledge about abnormalities of tumor blood vessels restricts the development of this research. Overall, it is well worth taking great efforts to visualize the distributions and fine structures of blood vessels in the physiological and pathological research. It can be said that the vascular medical image has become an essential foundation for interpreting life sciences.

6.2 Angiography

Clinically, angiography is a common method based on vascular reconstruction that helps physicians diagnose vascular disease, which greatly benefits the determination of appropriate clinical management. Compared to direct conventional angiography, other indirect evaluation methods, such as stress testing, have limited ability in diagnostics which restrict their applications. By virtue of angiography, the vascular situation including presence, extent, location, and severity of lesions can be clearly presented. As an invasive technology, angiography remains the standard for the diagnosis of vascular disease [7].

Angiography plays important roles not only in living tissues for direct diagnosis but also in postmortem investigations. As an indispensable part of forensic medicine, postmortem angiography turns out to be an important tool for characterizing the vascular system which is becoming more and more sophisticated. The reason of the increasing impact of postmortem angiography lies in that it offers an rapid evaluation on vascular pattern of organ, its alteration under pathologic or physiologic conditions, and tissue variation caused by artificial or unnatural factors [8]. The obtained information from postmortem angiography contributes to a better understanding of complex disease, thus establishing analytic model for medical research and clinical treatment. Therefore, further improvements such as visualizing the vascular system of the entire body in detail will serve as a valuable supplement for evaluation of the vascular system, enriching the postmortem anatomic, pathologic, and forensic diagnostic knowledge.

6.3 Clinical Solutions of Angiography

Actually, angiography required to be performed in combination with various imaging methods, such as ultrasonography, magnetic resonance imaging (MRI), computed tomography (CT) and X-rays etc. [9–11]. These modern imaging technologies have already found their way into anatomy and pathology. Taking account of the scale of vessels and resolution of imaging equipment, large vessels can be observed using ultrasonography and MRI with clarity, but smaller ones cannot. To improve the imaging quality, contrast agents with higher density have been introduced to modify the density in the vessels, which are to enhance the difference between vessels and surrounding tissues for CT and X-ray imaging. Although numerous contrast agents have been proposed and studied in the past, only few of them were proven feasible and effective, such as barium sulfate and iodinated agents [12], which have survived in the present time. Nowadays, vascular-enhanced radiological angiography in fact establishes the foundation for advanced CT and 3D vasculature reconstruction [13–15]. Moreover, it can be operated as a standard reference for evaluating other contrast-enhanced imaging methods [16–18].

Generally, X-ray is essential for obtaining good contrast image of vessels. However, it has always been a difficulty to visualize the vascular system, especially for those complex networks made up of tiny capillaries. If the energy of X-ray is raised to solve this problem, the contrast efficacy of iodine would decrease. Additionally, most of the existing contrast agents are solutions adding solute with high density. The resembling property of solution limits the contrast between tiny capillaries and tissues in medical images. Although various metal materials like lead, bismuth, rose metal or Wood's metal were previously investigated as contrast materials, their high melting point, shrinkage during hardening and output problems are inevitable disadvantages [8]. Consequently, it remains a big challenge to clearly display the vessels for current materials and technologies up to now.

6.4 Liquid Metal Contrast Agent

Given the imaging problem with solution contrast agent, there is a need for high contrast material for angiography. Thus, innovative contrast agents, i.e. liquid metals with distinctive characteristics have been introduced by Wang et al. for improvement of imaging quality [19].

6.4.1 Characteristics of Liquid Metal as Vascular Contrast Agent

Considering the low density restricting by the essence of solution, metal material with higher density can be an alternative contrast agent. Common metals are solid at room or body temperature. Their extraordinarily high melting points make their injection into vessels impossible. It is noteworthy that a kind of liquid metals have managed to address this problem. Gallium is one of such liquid metals with melting point of 29.78 °C, which is close to the room temperature. Remarkably, such metals endowed with property of supercooling, ensuring its liquid state even when the temperature decreases to its melting point in a period of time. The low viscosity and high fluidity makes liquid gallium reach everywhere of vessels connecting in the network system. Moreover, gallium is much safer than the typical liquid metal mercury, and is a sort of environment friendly material which offers convenience for operation. The concerned density of gallium is 5.9 g cm^{-3} which is several times of that of solution. Generally, liquid metals have superior visibility under X-ray irradiation and are able to make a fluent and conformal filling throughout the target vessels. Therefore, there are sufficient reasons to progress an attempt using liquid metals as contrast medium.

6.4.2 Imaging Organ Vessel Using Liquid Metal

To verify the imaging quality of liquid metal, gallium has been introduced and investigated as a vascular contrast agent [19]. With respect to the abundance of vessels, heart is an appropriate organ with complex capillary network which can be studied as experimental model. Besides, kidney as another important organ has large amount of vessels as well, which plays an important role of blood filter. Therefore, the isolated heart and kidney can serve as the typical and suitable experimental targets for angiography. The porcine heart and kidney were prepared for injection with the blood drained clean. Meanwhile, traditional contrast agent, iohexol, was selected as a comparison to evaluate the performance and to investigate the basic imaging principle of liquid metal based radiological angiography. In experiments, iohexol (35 g (I)/100 mL) and liquid metal gallium (purity, 99.999%) were infused to the main branches of the vessels within these two organs respectively. The angiograms of isolated organs were taken by X-ray and the results are shown in Fig. 6.2. It is obvious that liquid metal has much higher contrast than iohexol. As depicted in Fig. 6.2a, b, vessels of heart infused with liquid metal (Fig. 6.2a) are highly clear to visualize compared to that of heart infused with iohexol. It can be observed that gallium makes whole coronary network outstanding while only several relatively large vessels filling with iohexol can be distinguished from angiograms.

Similar situation occurs in the X-ray imaging of kidney. The renal artery of the kidney infused with gallium and relevant X-ray images are displayed in Fig. 6.2c. With the addition of irradiation intensity, the contrast between the vessels containing gallium and surrounding soft tissues increases evidently. From angiogram, it is found that liquid metal can spread all over the renal artery network, resulting in the dramatic demonstration, even making some capillaries visible. Under high

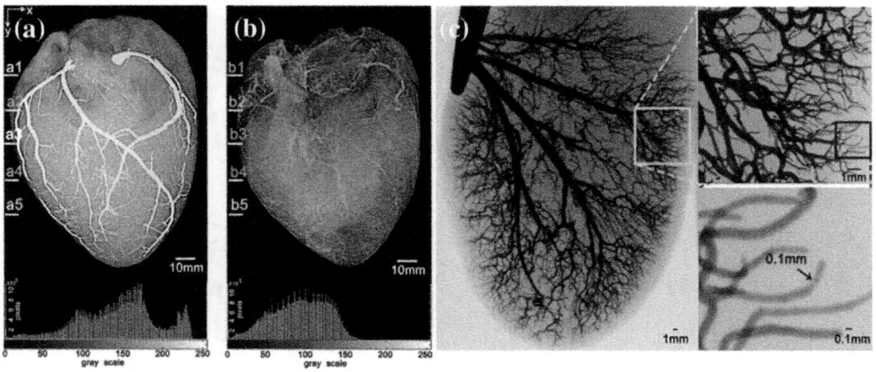

Fig. 6.2 Liquid metal angiography. X-ray angiogram of heart filled with liquid metal gallium (**a**) and iohexol (**b**), respectively. The working parameters for the X-ray in both (**a**) and (**b**) are 55 kV and 25 mAs. The resolution is 0.1 mm/pixel. **c** Angiogram of a whole pig kidney with one branch of its arterial network filled with gallium at three magnifications. The X-ray parameters for this angiogram are 70 kV and 3.2 mAs [19]. All pictures reproduced with permission

magnification, the thinnest tube of vessel ending shown in the images can reach 0.1 mm. In the previous studies, liposomes were utilized to visualize details in width of 100–200 μm, and the nano-emulsions enabled the detection of tumors smaller than 300 μm with a targeting ability [12]. On this basis, liquid metal with high contrast can be applied to substitute traditional contrast agent for improvement of imaging quality.

Figure 6.3 reveals the effects of X-ray irradiation intensity on the image quality of heart filled with liquid metal gallium. With the same exposure parameter (10 mAs), the contrast between the vessels (gallium) and the other soft tissues increases along

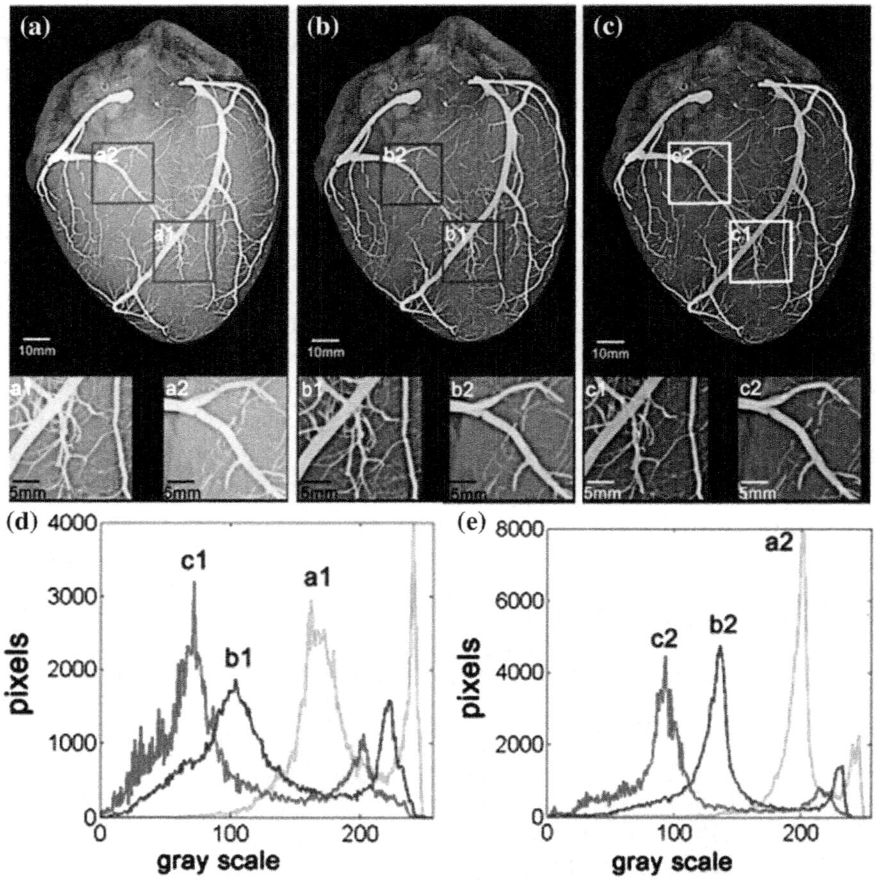

Fig. 6.3 Effect of X-ray irradiation intensity on image contrast of heart filled with liquid metal gallium. **a** Image of the heart at 80 kV. **b** Image of the heart at 100 kV. **c** Image of the heart at 120 kV. The exposure parameter in all 3 images is set as 10 mAs identically. The square labeled with a1, a2, b1, b2, c1, c2 is zoomed in and presented below the image **a**, **b**, **c**, respectively. **d** Comparison of the histogram for three sub-images labeled with a1, b1, c1 in **a**, **b** and **c**. **e** Comparison of the histogram for three sub-images labeled with a2, b2, c2 in **a**, **b** and **c**. All pictures reproduced with permission

with the addition of the X-ray intensity (Fig. 6.3a, 80 kV; Fig. 6.3b, 100 kV; and Fig. 6.3c, 120 kV). However, the increasing penetrability also makes some capillaries invisible, which can be seen in the sub-images in a1–a3 and b1–b3. The plots of the sub-images' grayscale histograms in Fig. 6.3d, e have given proofs in quantity. In both plots, there exist two peaks for the sub-images, which can be generally seen as one representing the enhanced vessels and the other representing the background tissues. The distance between the two peaks becomes longer when the X-ray gets stronger, indicating a higher contrast; while the height of the vessel peak decreases at the same time, which means the vessels become darker.

6.5 Quantitative Comparison Between Traditional and Liquid Metal Contrast Agents

The angiograms have embodied the superiority of liquid metal in radiological imaging. Furthermore, the quantitative analysis can provide more information about the difference between liquid metal and traditional contrast agent.

6.5.1 Grayscale Comparison

Grayscale is a significant parameter which directly reflects the contrast effect in angiogram. Therefore, in the study of liquid metal angiography [19], grayscale was employed to describe the comparison between gallium and iohexol. The grayscale curves were calculated along the horizontal lines at five different heights labeled in Fig. 6.2a, b. The obtained grayscale curves are shown in Fig. 6.4. The a1–a5 curves representing the gallium-based angiography cases all show more significantly steep peeks than b1–b5 curves of the iohexol enhanced image cases.

6.5.2 Numerical Index

The evaluation given by gray level is still a rough method, which is a simple expression of image contrast. Additionally, numerical index can be used for further description of the contrast discrepancy between the angiograms of liquid metal and iohexol. Such contrast indicating gray-level distribution considers the dynamic range of the gray-levels and the ratio of black and white areas as the factor for contrast [20], and the equation was expressed as:

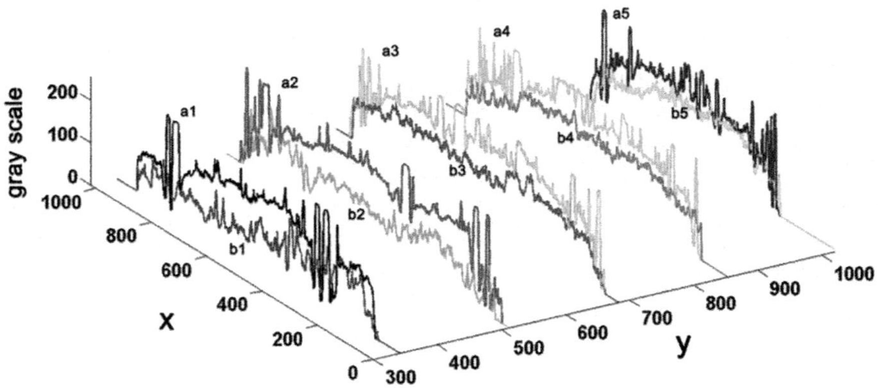

Fig. 6.4 Grayscale analysis between X-ray angiogram of heart filled with liquid metal gallium and iohexol. Plots (a1–a5, b1–b5) indicate the grayscale along the horizontal lines at five different heights labelled in Fig. 6.2**a**, **b** [19]. Picture reproduced with permission

$$F_{contrast} = \frac{\sigma}{(\alpha_4)^{0.25}} \tag{6.1}$$

where, σ denotes standard deviation of the grayscale probabilistic distribution and α_4 denotes the kurtosis. The Kurtosis based on the mean μ_4 and the variance σ^2 can be defined as:

$$\alpha_4 = \frac{\mu_4}{(\sigma^2)^2} \tag{6.2}$$

The numerical indexes can be calculated for different regions of interest, such as lines or squares. In the cases of liquid metal- and iohexol-based angiograms in Fig. 6.2a, b, numerical indexes of a1–a5, b1–b5 and whole pictures were calculated through Eqs. (6.1) and (6.2) respectively, and the results were listed in Table 6.1. Obviously, the contrast value of liquid metal group is much higher than that of iohexol group, which also revealed that gallium has much higher contrast ability than iohexol under the same radiological conditions.

Table 6.1 Numerical indexes calculated for Fig. 6.2a, b [19]

Region of interest	Figure 6.2a	Figure 6.2b
Whole heart	38.75	28.05
a1 and b1	34.43	22.84
a2 and b2	34.54	20.29
a3 and b3	30.47	17.12
a4 and b4	33.30	20.19
a5 and b5	34.54	22.92

6.6 Optimization of Irradiation Intensity

Irradiation intensity plays a key role in the X-ray imaging quality. As has been disclosed above, to obtain optimal angiogram, appropriate irradiation intensity should be determined for liquid metal serving as an innovative contrast agent. It has been known that with the same exposure parameter (10 mAs), the contrast between the vessels full of gallium and the other soft tissues increases along with the addition of the X-ray intensity (80, 100 and 120 kV) [19]. However, the increasing penetrability may also make some capillaries invisible. Consequently, the quantitative method can be demonstrated using grayscale histograms to analyze the interested area. Generally, there exist two peaks as one representing the enhanced vessels and the other representing the background tissues. The distance between the two peaks becomes longer when the X-ray gets stronger, indicating a higher contrast; while the height of the vascular peak decreases at the same time, which means that the vessels become darker. In practice, for physicians and clinicians, they can select optimum and suitable irradiation intensity for getting more information according conditions of actual object.

Due to the high density, gallium has extremely large X-ray attenuation coefficient. The contrast of vessel in the whole image C can be expressed as:

$$C = 1 - \exp[-(\mu_2 - \mu_1)] \tag{6.3}$$

where, μ_2 and μ_1 denote the X-ray attenuation coefficient of the contrast agent filled in the vessels and that of the surrounding tissues respectively, and l denotes the diameter of a vessel. It means that the larger the difference between μ_2 and μ_1, the clearer the vascular imaging can be observed under the same contrast condition. Therefore, the high X-ray attenuation coefficient of the gallium makes it a mega contrast X-ray agent, which indicates that vessels can be more distinctive in the radiological image. Nevertheless, the high attenuation property always requires strong X-ray irradiation intensity, otherwise the X-ray cannot penetrate the whole objective. Generally, the attenuation is mainly caused by Compton scattering when the X-ray energy is high, then the attenuation factors of the contrast agent and the surrounding tissues will have small differences. Naturally, the corresponding image will produce poor contrast. However, for gallium angiography, this problem does not exist as reflected in the above discussion.

6.7 Reconstruction of Vascular Network Based on Liquid Metal

Although X-ray photo is the main imaging method in angiography, it simply reflects the 2-D (dimension) information which sometimes is insufficient to master the whole structure of vessels. So, the CT method can be carried out to reconstruct the vascular model for further investigation. Generally, the artifacts of metal in CT severely decrease the image quality. But the results are different for liquid metal gallium which shows clear edges. Given the imaging apparatus with high enough resolution, the fine structures of 3D heart and kidney vasculature with gallium are capable of being presented through the reconstructed models from CT slices (Fig. 6.5) [19]. Therefore, segmentation of the renal artery becomes rather easy now by the new method. In such sense, the application of liquid metal on angiography is promising in helping people understand more about vascular disease, which is rather meaningful for pathology evaluation, especially for forensic medicine. In addition to the in vitro research, the in vivo study of liquid metals on angiography will be of great significance in the near future.

In order to offer more evidence of the ability of the liquid metal alloy enhancement, Fig. 6.6 provides the closer X-ray photographs of two areas with plenty of even tinier vessels. Figure 6.6a is the vascular network in the digestive organs, while Fig. 6.6b demonstrates the main branches spreading in the head. For both figures, the sensor focused in a square field with each side 6.6 mm long, and the resolution is thus set as 13 μm/pixel. Accordingly, it can be referred that the thinnest vessel can be seen is less than 30 μm wide, which means a tremendous improvement of the blood vessel visualization was obtained.

This result indicates that the liquid metal alloy performs quite well in the vascular image enhancement. Thanks to its liquid phase, the material is able to flow throughout the whole body to obtain fine angiograms at multiple scales, including the capillaries whose diameter is at a scale of micrometers. Such a feature makes the

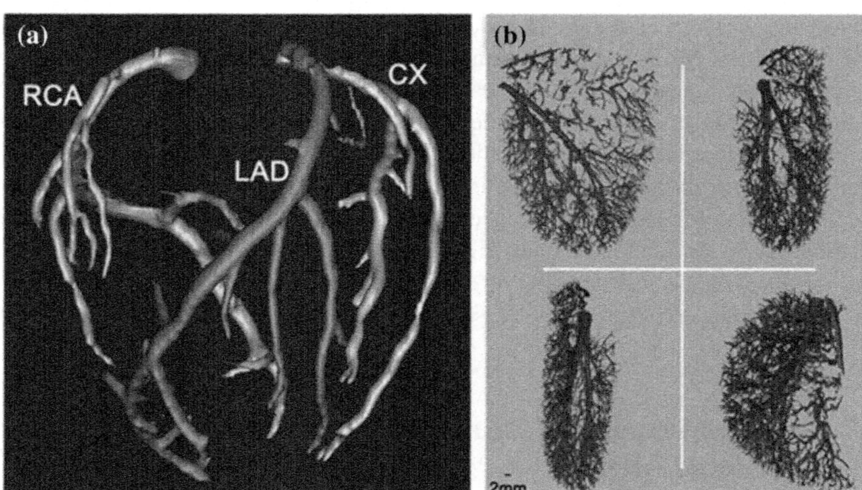

Fig. 6.5 Gallium enhanced 3D vasculature of the heart and kidney. **a** The right coronary artery (RCA), the left anterior descending (LAD) and the circumflex (CX) are demonstrated in blue, magenta and yellow, respectively. **b** Gallium enhanced kidney 3D vasculature viewed in various directions [19]. All pictures reproduced with permission

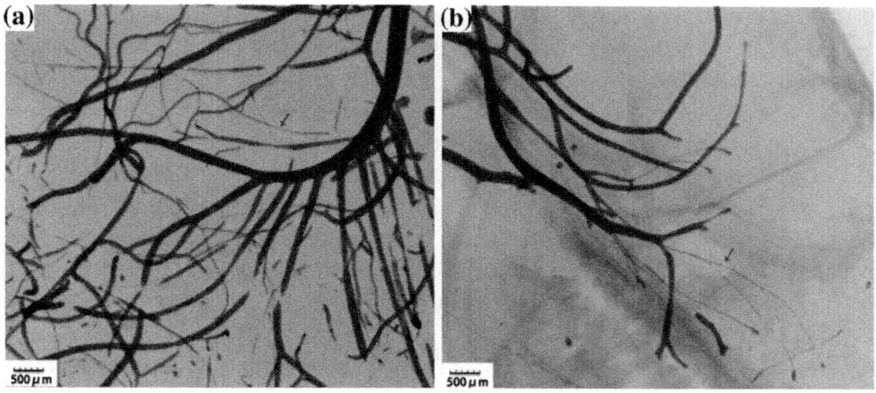

Fig. 6.6 X-ray image of localized areas in the mouse with higher resolution. **a** The image of vessels in the abdomen. **b** The image of vessels in the head. In both images, the resolution is 13 μm/pixel, and capillaries with a diameter less than 30 μm can be found easily, which are pointed out with blue arrows in the images. All pictures reproduced with permission

liquid metal an ideal tool for the vasculature observation, especially for many research on small animals. The liquid metal is endowed with plenty of merits like softness, quickness and easy-to-use. The high contrast of the angiogram and 3D reconstruction provides the possibility to see and evaluate vascular changes and damages, while it is more valuable in observing tiny capillaries since blur does not happen in the image of a localized field though the agent's amount decreases a lot, which suggests a promising application in the study of vessel growth in tumor or other tissues.

Compared to other existing contrast agents, the liquid metal alloy is inexpensive and easy to prepare. Actually, the material used in the experiments represents a series of galinstan room temperature liquid metal alloy, even including the simple substance of gallium itself. These alloys differ in constituent and proportion, which control their physical and chemical characters such as melting point and viscosity [6, 7]. Taking advantages of the diversity, the liquid metal infused for angiography may achieve additional complementary effects in diagnostics and treatments.

6.8 Conclusion

Overall, it has been found that gallium demonstrates significant values in serving as contrast agent in angiography. Such material is much simpler than traditional agents who need further preparation or processing. By virtue of the low melting point, this liquid metal material displays similar characteristics to solution, such as low viscosity and good fluidity, enabling the conformal filling of vessels with various scales and structures. The filling and freezing of the liquid metal would keep the shapes of the targets. Meanwhile, high density of metal significantly improves the contrast between vessels and their surrounding tissues under X-ray imaging, which is obvious in the grayscale histograms. Based on this, liquid metal contrast agent can greatly reflect the actual information of vessels and clearly display the image in angiograms. Moreover, liquid metal can be provided as a highly convenient and useful tool for reconstructing the distribution of the fine vessel networks in tissues and organs, especially in computational tomography and 3D modeling, which is quite important for studying visual animal vasculature including human subjects in the near future. With all the above merits, the metal flow performs much better than those conventional contrast agents for visualizing vessel networks, which suggests that gallium could serve as an ideal contrast agent for in vitro vascular-enhanced radiological imaging.

Currently, only a few liquid metals have been investigated as contrast agents in several experimental examples. However, liquid metals include a series of metals with low melting points, such as GaIn alloy or GaInSn alloy. In addition, the imaging quality is affected by the precision of imaging apparatus to some extent. It is entirely feasible to map further smaller vessels using the present method on condition that the resolution of the imaging device is precise enough like the X-ray micro-CT [21, 22]. Meanwhile, the basic idea of the present investigation is pretty generalized. Besides vessels, the characterized research objects can be extended to more other cavities spanning from animals' digestive tracts to plants' tube structures, even including insects' holes. Verification of such liquid metal based channel mapping may reveal more secrets in unexpected discoveries. With respect to liquid metal contrast agent, more studies need to be implemented for fulfilling their potential in abundant applications.

Liquid metal agents overcome the problem that capillaries are hard to clearly distinguish using traditional agents. It opens a new way for revolutionizing the current radiological imaging, providing the nonsurgical method for characterizing the fine distribution and variation of the biological vasculature system. Liquid metal material establishes a highly efficient way to quickly reconstruct high resolution spatial channel network for scientific research or engineering applications where complicated and time-consuming resections are no longer needed. Besides, since the liquid metal will overflow through the orifices, the infusion may help find out some unnoticeable wounds on or beneath the surface, which can be useful when applied in forensic detection.

References

1. Torbicki A (2012) European guidelines on cardiovascular disease prevention in clinical practice (version 2012), Pharmacokinetics in clinical practice. W.B. Saunders Company, Philadelphia, pp 1635–1701
2. Rosamond W, Flegal K, Furie K et al (2008) Heart disease and stroke statistics–2008 update: a report from the American heart association statistics committee and stroke statistics subcommittee. Circulation 125(1):188–197

3. Torre LA, Bray F, Siegel RL et al (2015) Global cancer statistics, 2012. CA Cancer J Clin 65 (2):87–108
4. Baluk P, Hashizume H, Mcdonald DM (2005) Cellular abnormalities of blood vessels as targets in cancer. Curr Opin Genet Dev 15(1):102–111
5. Fait E (2001) 3D microvascular architecture of pre-cancerous lesions and invasive carcinomas of the colon. Br J Cancer 84(10):1354–1362
6. Carmeliet P, Jain RK (2011) Principles and mechanisms of vessel normalization for cancer and other angiogenic diseases. Nat Rev Drug Discovery 10(6):417–427
7. Miller JM, Rochitte CE, Dewey M et al (2008) Diagnostic performance of coronary angiography by 64-row CT. N Engl J Med 359(359):2324–2336
8. Grabherr S, Djonov V, Yen K et al (2007) Postmortem angiography: review of former and current methods. Am J Roentgenol 188(3):832–838
9. Zhang Z, Wang H, Zhou Y et al (2013) Computed tomographic angiography of anterior spinal artery in acute cervical spinal cord injury. Spinal cord 51(6):442–447
10. Anderson CM, Saloner D, Lee RE et al (1992) Assessment of carotid artery stenosis by MR angiography: comparison with x-ray angiography and color-coded Doppler ultrasound. AJNR Am J Neuroradiol 13(3):989–1003
11. Knowles J (2003) Seeing is believing. Science 299(5615):2002–2003
12. Hallouard F, Anton N, Choquet P et al (2010) Iodinated blood pool contrast media for preclinical X-ray imaging applications -a review. Biomaterials 31(24):6249–6268
13. Ananda S, Marsden V, Vekemans K et al (2006) The visualization of hepatic vasculature by X-ray micro-computed tomography. J Electron Microsc 55(3):151–155
14. Van JP, Schwarz JC, Van HP et al (2013) 3D Imaging of vascular networks for biophysical modeling of perfusion distribution within the heart. J Biomech 46(2):229–239
15. Jorgensen SM, Demirkaya O, Ritman EL (1998) Three-dimensional imaging of vasculature and parenchyma in intact rodent organs with X-ray micro-CT. Am J Phys-Heart Circ Physiol 275:H1103–H1114
16. Yang Q, Li K, Liu X et al (2009) Contrast-enhanced whole-heart coronary magnetic resonance angiography at 3.0-T: a comparative study with X-ray angiography in a single center. J Am Coll Cardiol 54(1):69–76
17. Froeling V, Diekmann F, Renz DM et al (2013) Correlation of contrast agent kinetics between iodinated contrast-enhanced spectral tomosynthesis and gadolinium-enhanced MRI of breast lesions. Eur Radiol 23(6):1528–1536
18. Khilnani NM, Winchester PA, Prince MR et al (2002) Peripheral vascular disease: combined 3D bolus chase and dynamic 2D MR angiography compared with X-ray angiography for treatment planning. Radiology 224(1):63–74
19. Wang Q, Yu Y, Pan K et al (2014) Liquid metal angiography for mega contrast X-ray visualization of vascular network in reconstructing in-vitro organ anatomy. IEEE Trans Bio-Med Eng 61(7):2161–2166
20. Tamura H, Mori S, Yamawaki T (1978) Textural features corresponding to visual perception. IEEE Trans Syst Man Cybern 8(6):460–473
21. Ananda S, Marsden V, Vekemans K et al (2006) The visualization of hepatic vasculature by X-ray micro-computed tomography. J Electron Microsc 55(3):151–155
22. Plouraboue F, Cloetens P, Fonta C et al (2004) X-ray high-resolution vascular network imaging. J Microsc 215(2):139–148

Chapter 7
Liquid Metal as Vascular Embolic Agent in Tumor Therapy

Abstract This chapter illustrates a new conceptual vascular embolization therapy enabled by the liquid metal materials. Several typical experiments on in vivo animal vasculatures were presented to illustrate the evidences of the method in destroying the targeted tissues. Through appropriate administration, the liquid metal embolization is able to destruct the target regions which might starve the tumors to death through a relatively easy way. Meanwhile, theoretical valuation regarding the tumor growth with zero, partial or complete filling of the metal agent inside the vessels were also given to evaluate the liquid metal starvation therapy effects.

Keywords Vascular embolic agent · Tumor therapy · Liquid metal

7.1 Introduction

It is well known that tumor growth relies heavily on the continuous supply of blood and nutrients. Theoretically, vascular embolization would serve well for the killing of tumor. This in fact offers an important therapeutic way for tumor clinics. Unfortunately, most of the currently available vascular embolic agents are still rather insufficient to fulfill the real clinical need. Typical reasons can generally be attributed as: incomplete filling of target vasculature, being easily washed away by blood or body solution, or just producing toxicity to tissues. From an alternative way, Wang et al. [1] had ever proposed the body temperature liquid metal, a kind of soft and highly compliant fluidic material, as blood vessel embolization agent for tumor physical therapy. With its unique capability of easy phase transition between liquid and solid state and sub-cooling behavior, such material can be fluently injected into the tiny vessels including ending capillaries and fully block them. The in vitro cytotoxicity experiments showed that treating localized diseased tissues through liquid metal embolic agent is acceptable. As an additional advantage, the liquid metal in vessels showed high image contrast under the X-ray scan. Endowed with a high density, the liquid metal-filled vessels are highly visible under the CT scan, which offers the potential of diagnosis-treatment integration. These evidences

J. Liu and L. Yi, *Liquid Metal Biomaterials*,
Springer Series in Biomaterials Science and Engineering10,
https://doi.org/10.1007/978-981-10-5607-9_7

suggest a potential tumor therapy for the coming clinics. In the present chapter, this new conceptual vascular embolization therapy enabled by the liquid metal materials will be interpreted. Several typical experiments on in vivo animal vasculatures will be presented to illustrate the evidences of the method in destroying the targeted tissues. Through appropriate administration, the liquid metal embolization is able to destruct the target regions which might starve the tumors to death through a relatively easy way. Meanwhile, theoretical valuation regarding the tumor growth with zero, partial or complete filling of the metal agent inside the vessels will also be given to evaluate the liquid metal starvation therapy effects.

7.2 Growing Behavior of Tumors and Conventional Embolization Ways

Originated from somatic mutations, the tumor cells generally proliferate and differentiate continuously under the regulation of various growth factors as well as the oxygen and nutrients provided throughout the blood vessels [2–4]. At the early stage when the death and the regeneration of tumor cells are nearly balanced, the existing vascular network near the tumor tissues supplies nutrients and carries away metabolites (Fig. 7.1). Afterwards, a new tumor vascular network generates around the tumor tissues due to the vascular endothelial growth factor secreted by the tumor cells [5]. Then, the rapidly increasing tumor cells would diffuse to other parts via the tumor-induced angiogenesis. Clearly, the blood vessels play a significant role on the growth and metastasis of the tumor [6].

Considering the dependency of the tumor growth on the blood vessels, the treatment of vascular targeting therapy for starving the tumors to death has increasingly attracted the attentions of researchers across the world [7, 8]. One of such strategies is to prevent the tumor-induced angiogenesis by the angiogenesis inhibitors, which was originally proposed by Folkman in the early 1970s [9]. Ever since then, various inhibitive drugs have been developed [10–13], and such embolization therapy has also been combined with chemotherapy or radiotherapy

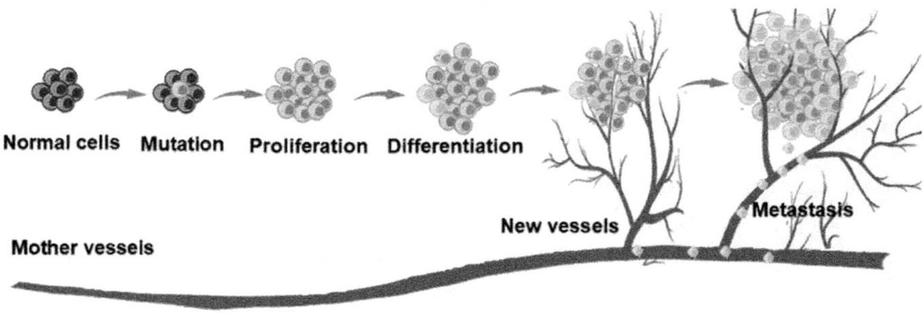

Fig. 7.1 Process for tumor occurrence and progress

for better treatment [14]. However, the angiogenesis inhibitors have to be used for a long time. And some studies found that within this period, the tumor itself would gradually generate resistance to these drugs, which makes it not as effective as expected [15]. As another approach focusing on blocking the existing vessels, colchicine was reported to destroy the vessels, yet with rather high toxicity [16]. Afterwards, some other vascular disrupting agents were studied including small molecular agents [17, 18].

Except for these drugs, there are some other physical embolization ways to offer the possibility of starving the tissues or tumor to death by means of embolic agents, such as autologous clots, coils, gelfoam, balloons, glue, nanoparticles, microspheres embolic agents and so on [19–23]. However, the failure to embolize the vessels may often occur. One key reason lies in that some solid embolic agents cannot conform well to the vessels, leaving certain space at the interface for nutrients to leak in. Another existing issue is that some embolic agents are easily rushed away by the blood flow, such as the balloons. What's more, the catheters or other more complex equipments are needed in order to place some of the embolic agents into the target positions. Different from these approaches, gas embolotherapy uses gas bubbles to occlude the blood flow [24]. The bubbles originate as small diameter liquid droplets of dodecafluoropentane (DDFP) mixed in saline and albumin. After injected into the vascular system, these droplets are small enough to pass through the capillary beds. At the strategic location, the droplets are vaporized into larger bubbles through acoustic wave to occlude flow. However, the entry of gas into the vessel system is a risk in virtually all areas of clinical care [25].

In view of the above tumor treatment situations, Wang et al. [1] proposed and preliminarily demonstrated an alternative vascular embolization therapy, through introducing the body temperature liquid metal as a kind of unconventional vessel embolic agent for starving the target tissues or tumors to death.

7.3 Basic Feature of Liquid Metal Vascular Embolic Therapy

As a soft, compliant and fluidic material, the liquid metal can be easily injected and filled into the vessels and capillaries sufficiently, which stops the blood flow and all the related physiological events thus enabled because of its high density and fluidity. Figure 7.2 illustrates the basic principle of the liquid metal embolization therapy and surgical operation of its injection and removal [1]. As is widely known, tissues acquire oxygen and nutrition from the nearby feeding vessels (Fig. 7.2a). Though the vascular blockage can shut down the blood supply, yet the stream is still able to pass through the vessels interior when the embolic agent fails to completely occlude the vessels. As a result, the reduction of blood flow does not guarantee a strong enough effect on starving the necrotic cells (Fig. 7.2b) and the

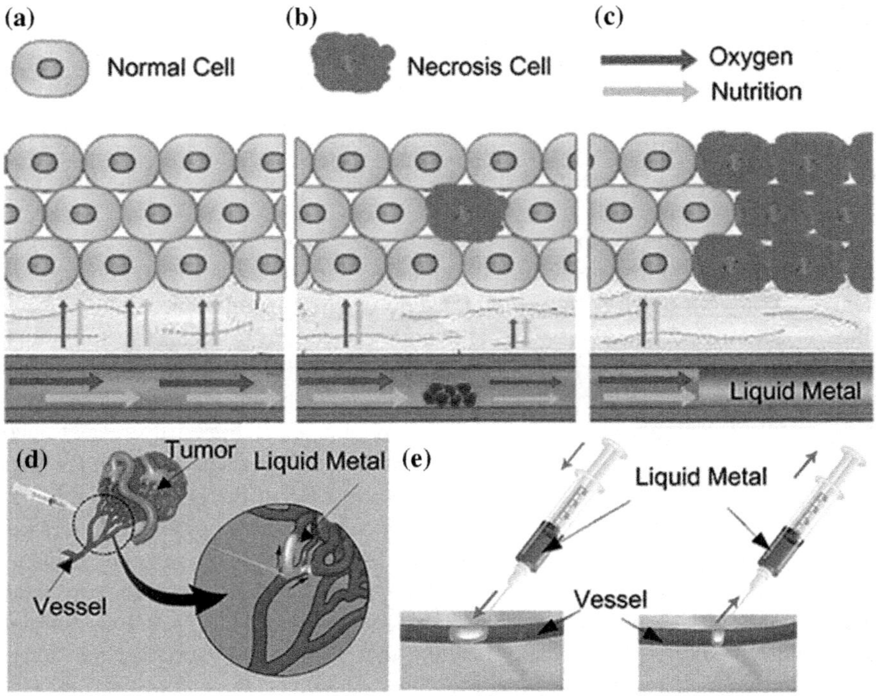

Fig. 7.2 The principle illustration of liquid metal based tumor vascular embolization therapy [1]. **a** The oxygen and nutrition supplies from the vessels to tissues without any embolic agents. **b** The incomplete occlusion. **c** The complete occlusion by the liquid metal. **d** The physical occlusion of the blood supply to tumor. **e** The liquid metal could be injected into or sucked out of the vessel in case of need. All pictures reproduced with permission

embolic agent can even possibly be rushed away within a short period after it was injected. Being able to maintain in liquid state at body temperature, the liquid metal agent can easily shape itself along the vessels and fully occlude the channels due to its perfect compliance (Fig. 7.2c). Compared with the normal tissues, the tumor is more dependent on the nutrients supplies from the surrounding vessels. After injected into the vessels, the liquid metal results in a physical occlusion and thus leads to tumor regressions (Fig. 7.2d). Another merit of the current therapy still lies in that, theoretically, the liquid metal could also be well sucked out in case of need after completing its treatment role (Fig. 7.2e).

7.4 Deliverable Properties of the Liquid Metal Agents

Clearly, plenty of liquid metal candidates can serve as the treatment agents. But for brief, Wang et al. just focused their point on the pure gallium and $Ga_{75.5}In_{24.5}$ alloy as the illustration examples [1]. To characterize the physical behaviors of such metal agent, they measured the thermal property of pure gallium with the differential scanning calorimetry device (DSC 200 F3 Maia, Netzsch Scientific Instrument Trading Co. Ltd, Germany). The 14.63 mg of gallium was put into the alumina crucible with another empty one as the reference, which were both placed in a heating furnace. The test temperature range included three cycles, which were set as 40 °C → 60 °C for 1 min → −60 °C for 1 min → 60 °C for 1 min −60 °C for 1 min → 60 °C for 1 min → −60 °C for 1 min → 60 °C for 1 min → 45 °C → 70 °C, and the heating and cooling rates were both prescribed at 10 °C/min. The results were analyzed by the software of NETZSCH Proteus Thermal Analysis. The works revealed the thermal properties of the gallium and verified its feasibility for the delivery of therapy.

Figure 7.3 depicts the DSC curves of the gallium in reciprocally reverse processes. In either the cooling or the heating process, the measurement goes for three trials and the results are almost identical. There is a very sharp exothermic peak over the cooling process, and the freezing temperature is 4.5 °C, while the endothermic peak is also steep in the heating process and the melting point is 28.3 °C. The curves indicate an easy transition between the solid and liquid phase of the gallium, which is an excellent property for the phase control. What's more, owing to its sub-cooling effect, the material is able to maintain in the liquid state for a long time at the body temperature. Thanks to its liquid phase, compliance and fluidity, the material is able to fluently flow into and fill the tiny vessels including the capillaries whose diameter is at a scale of micrometers.

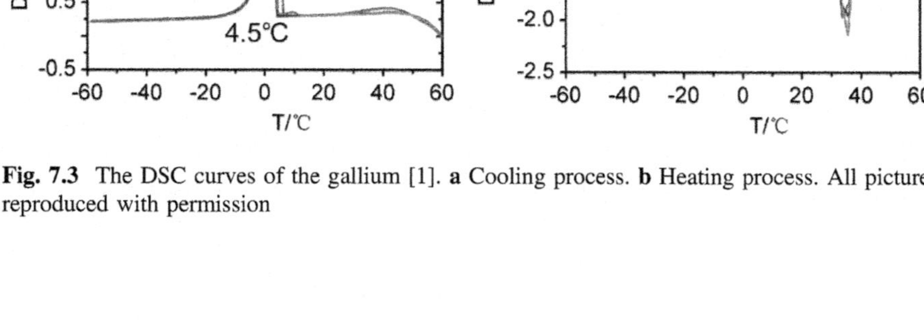

Fig. 7.3 The DSC curves of the gallium [1]. **a** Cooling process. **b** Heating process. All pictures reproduced with permission

7.5 Cytotoxicity of Liquid Metal Agents In Vitro

Two tests including the cell counting kit-8 (CCK-8) and the flow cytometry were applied on the mouse embryonic fibroblast cells (NIH3T3) to evaluate the cytotoxicity of the liquid metal.

A drop of the gallium was put on the six-well plates filled with culture solution, soaking for 24 and 48 h in the incubator. Meanwhile, a piece of polished and sterilized indium and copper were soaked under the same condition.

CCK-8 method: Cells at logarithmic growth phase were treated by trypsin and tuned into single cell suspension with a concentration of 50,000/ml, then seeded in a 96-well plate with 100 μL in each well. After being cultured for 24 h, the cells were observed under the microscope and the samples in bad state were eliminated. The original culture solution was removed and the wells were washed with PBS solution. Then, the soaked solution of gallium, indium, copper and the original culture solution (control group) were added into the wells with 5 parallel samples in each group. After being cultured for 24 h, each well was washed and added with a mixture of 100 μL fresh culture solution and 10 μL CCK-8. The 96-well plates were put into the incubator for 2 h, then optical density (OD) at 450 nm wavelength were measured with multifunctional microplate reader (EnVision, USA PerkinElmer). The cell viability was calculated according to the following equation:

$$\text{Cell viability} = (\text{OD} - \text{OD}_0)/(\text{OD}_c - \text{OD}_0) \tag{7.1}$$

where, OD_c was the OD value of the control group and OD_0 was the OD value of black wells without any cells.

Flow cytometry method: The cells were seeded into the sterile dish of 60 mm diameter with 300,000 cells each. After cultured for 24 h in the incubator, the original culture medium was removed and the wells were then washed with PBS solution. The three soaked solutions and the original culture solution were added separately. After cultured for another 24 h, the cells in each dish were collected into the centrifuge tubes. Through centrifuge at 1500 r/min for 5 min, the supernatant was removed and 1 mL cell staining buffer and 5 μL PI staining solution were added, then a 30-min ice bath followed. Finally, the cell solutions were placed in the flow cytometer, detecting the red fluorescence by flow cytometry (BD Calibur, the USA BD).

Figure 7.4a shows the viability of the cells after cultured in different metal soaked solutions with CCK-8 method. The cell viability in the copper soaked solution in 24 h was measured as 7%, and almost all died in 48 h. The cell viability of the gallium soaked solution in 24 and 48 h were 100.6 and 75.7%, and that of indium were 107 and 79.7%, respectively. According to the cytotoxicity evaluation criteria of the national standard, cell viability above 75% is qualified and safe. The viability of the cells can also be visually demonstrated through the microscope, which is shown in Fig. 7.4b. The cells of the gallium, indium soaked solution and original culture solution were exactly of the right size and shape large, while those

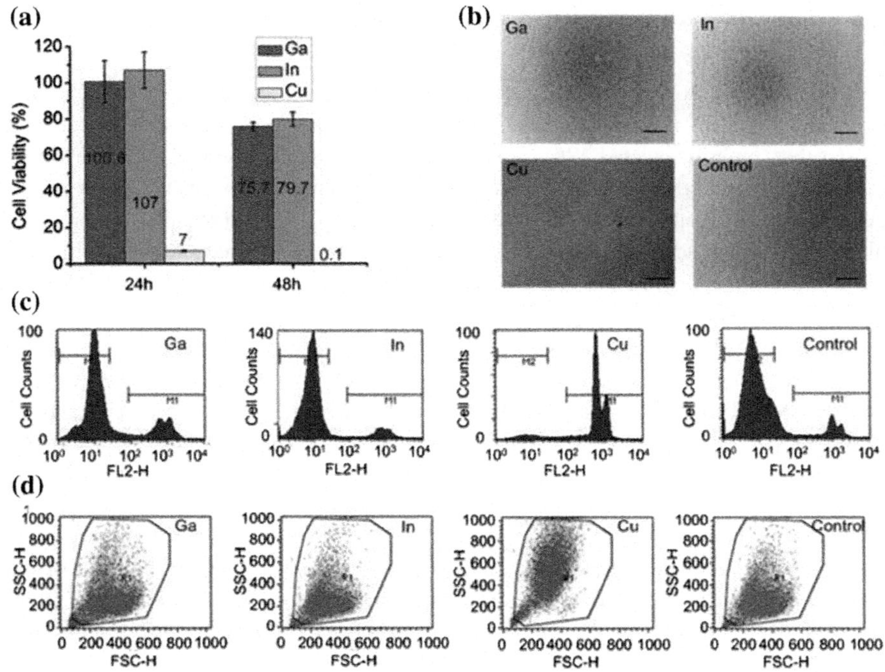

Fig. 7.4 Cytotoxicity in vitro [1]. **a** The cell viability after cultured in different metal soaking solution with CCK-8 method. **b** The cellular morphology in each experimental group observed under the microscope. **c** The cell apoptosis with flow cytometry method. **d** The scatter images with flow cytometry method. All pictures reproduced with permission

in the copper soaked solution distributed sparsely and the shapes were relatively round, which means most of them were dead.

Figure 7.4c indicates cell apoptosis of each experimental group. In the PI fluorescence intensity histograms, M1 stands for apoptosis cells while M2 represents living cells. Compared with the control group, the relative apoptosis rates of gallium and indium group was 10.18 and 7.9% respectively while 78.44% for the copper group. In the scatter images in Fig. 7.4d, it can be further found that the strength of forward scattered light reduced and the one side scattered light increased in the copper soaked solution, which also indicated that there were more apoptosis and necrosis cells. However, the gallium and indium group showed tiny difference with the control group.

These experiments have revealed that the cytotoxicity of the gallium and indium ion are relatively low and their applications on localized severe disease treatment are clinically acceptable, given its unique values as will be revealed in later sections.

7.6 Image Guidance for Delivering the Liquid Metal

As explained in former chapter, unlike other embolic agents, liquid metal has excellent visibility under the X-ray, which is a unique advantage compared with most other embolic agents [26]. Thus the tumor vessels injected with the liquid metal could be highly visualized under CT scan. This serves an idealistic image guidance to distribute the liquid metal into the site of the target vasculatures. To illustrate this characteristic, cases on several representative objects such as in vitro swine kidney, a healthy 8-week-old female CD1 mice and an 8-week-old female Barb/c nude mice with a tumor are presented as follows.

About 0.8 mL liquid metal gallium was infused into the artery branches of the swine kidney. Then the filled kidney was X-ray photographed by a micro-CT scanner (XM-Tracer-130, from Institute of High Energy Physics, Chinese Academy of Sciences).

The mouse has both arteries broad enough for liquid metal $Ga_{75.5}In_{24.5}$ alloy infusion and thin capillaries to display the alloy's high contrast. First, the mouse was excessively anesthetized to death, then the heart was exposed by cutting open its chest. A thin syringe needle was used to penetrate into the left ventricle of the mouse heart and it was clamped to prevent leakage and reverse flow. With a slight cut near the right atrium, the liquid metal alloy could finally be infused into the circulatory tunnels and flow throughout the body. When the silvery alloy flows to the right heart, it was supposed to finish the infusion and that the sample had been stuffed with the contrast agent. Then the sample was taken to the imaging instrument (Super Nova CT, from Technical Institute of Physics and Chemistry, Chinese Academy of Sciences). Images with higher resolution were obtained from the micro-CT (XM-Tracer-130, from Institute of High Energy Physics, Chinese Academy of Sciences).

The structures of the vessels in the tumor tissues and normal tissues may be different. In order to provide more evidences on various tissue vasculatures, the present lab also managed to infuse the liquid metal $Ga_{75.5}In_{24.5}$ alloy into the tumor vessels [1]. The mouse breast cancer cells (EMT6, 1×10^6 cells) were injected directly into the subcutaneous at the back of the nude mice. The tumor reached approximately a diameter of 5 mm in two weeks and the vessels were visible on the skin. After the mice was anesthetized with intraperitoneal injection of 0.2 mL 1% (g/L) sodium pentobarbital (Nembutal), the liquid metal was injected directly into a tumor vessel via a special syringe needle with an inner diameter of 0.3 mm. Afterwards, the tumor region went under a CT scan (Super Nova CT, from Technical Institute of Physics and Chemistry, Chinese Academy of Sciences) for visualizing the vessels injected with liquid metal.

The X-ray images of renal artery of the in vitro swine kidney are presented in Fig. 7.5a. Clearly, a whole branch of the renal artery network is intact and the texture of the small vessels is rather clear. As shown in Fig. 7.5b, the vessels are separated with the other tissues obviously in highlight in the CT scan reconstruction of a whole-body infused mouse. In the image, it is easy to identify the liquid metal's

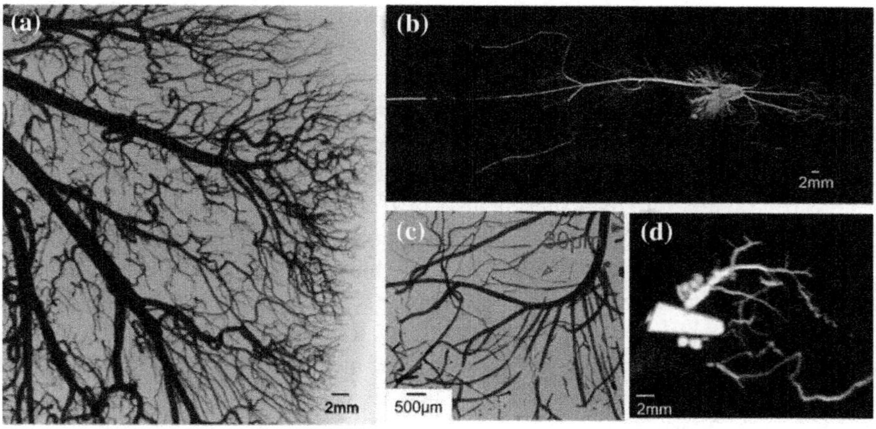

Fig. 7.5 The images of vessels filled with the liquid metal under the X-ray. **a** The X-ray image of renal artery of the in vitro swine kidney. **b** The top view of a liquid metal infused mouse in a whole-body CT scan and 3D reconstruction. **c** The X-ray image of vessels in the mouse abdomen with higher resolution. **d** 3D reconstruction image of tumor vessels. All pictures reproduced with permission

flow path throughout the carotid, limb and tail vessels even to the end tips. Besides, the branches in the lung, head and abdominal organs can also be distinguished with ultra-high contrast and clarity. In order to offer more evidences of the image guidance ability of the liquid metal alloy enhancement, Fig. 7.5c provides the closer X-ray photographs of vascular network in the abdomen of the mouse which has plenty of even tinier vessels. In the figure, the sensor focused in a square field with each side 6.6 mm long, and the resolution is thus set as 13 μm/pixel. Accordingly, it can be referred to that the thinnest visible vessel is less than 30 μm wide, which means a tremendous improvement of the blood vessel visualization. Besides, the tumor vessels filled with liquid metal are highly visible under the CT scan as expected. As can be seen, the tumarized vasculature appeares somewhat irregular (Fig. 7.5d) as compared with normal tissue vessels (Fig. 7.5a). This clearly reflected the growth behavior of such diseased vessels.

7.7 Liquid Metal as Embolic Agents of Blood Vessels In Vivo

In Wang et al.'s work [1], a two-month-old male New Zealand rabbit (purchased from the Center of Biomedical Analysis of Tsinghua University), weighted about 2.2 kg, were used as the experimental subject, because the vessels in the ears are broad and visible. Anesthetized with intraperitoneal injection of 4% (g/L) sodium pentobarbital (Nembutal) by the standard of 1 ml/kg, the rabbit was injected with liquid metal gallium into the vein of one ear. It was observed that the material filled the vessels at the rim and the tip of the ear quickly. The other ear was used for contrast. The infrared camera (Thermovision A40, FLIR, Wilsonville, OR) was adopted to record the temperature changes of the rabbit ear during the operational process. Afterwards, the rabbit was observed for half an hour and then put back to the caring center. The rabbit continued to be observed every day. Blood analysis were carried out before the experiments and 1 day, 3 days, 7 days afterwards with the automatic hematology analyzer (BM800), each time with 3 repeated trials. After the occurrence of necrosis at the ear tip, the rabbit was sacrificed through standard procedure. Then the tissues of both the necrotic region and the same position of the other ear were surgically cut and immediately restored in formalin for 24 h. The samples were then sectioned, stained with HE methods (Hematoxylin-eosin) and observed under the microscope.

Afterwards, Wang et al. injected the liquid metal gallium into the vessels of the mouse tail and the rabbit leg in the same way [1]. Such experiments all have been approved by the Ethics Committee of Tsinghua University, Beijing, China under contract [SYXK (Jing) 2009-0022].

As shown in Fig. 7.6a, the liquid metal has filled the rabbit ear vein at the rim and the tip. Without abnormal reactions, the rabbit showed obvious symptoms of necrosis only in the ear tip in three weeks, which finally come out like a dry leaf. The necrotic changes appeared not so serious at the rim of the ear, which might be due to the supply of certain surrounding tiny vessels. However, the very side of the ear had been crimped, which was a reflection of the liquid metal obstruction.

As an attendant phenomenon, the temperature of the liquid metal obstructed region would decrease due to stop of the blood flow. As a special evaluation of the material's influence, the temperature distributions in 0, 24, 48 and 72 h from the thermal infrared images are depicted in Fig. 7.6b. Clearly, at the moment of the injection, the blood was immediately blocked, causing the temperature rise in the upstream and decrease in the downstream regions. With the time went on, the area of the low temperature region shrunk gradually, which indicated the concentration of the material to the tip.

In order to provide a biological inspection, Fig. 7.6c displays the sections of both the necrotic and normal tissues. It can be seen that near the liquid metal blocked vessels, the surrounding area tends to be emptier and the cells are much smaller than the situation in the similar region in a normal tissue. This shows the damage effect of the liquid metal embolization treatment.

Other than the morphologic analysis, blood tests were also carried out in a week and seven parameters including WBC, LYM%, MON%, GPA%, HGB, RBC and PLT are shown in Fig. 7.6d. Figure 7.6e shows the WBC, RBC and PLT dynamic histograms distribution, respectively. As can be seen from the figure, the second peak of WBC distribution was lowered after one day but returned to normal after 3 days, which indicated the reduction of the neutrophil granulocytes. These blood analysis results demonstrated that the blood parameters would soon return to normal level after the liquid metal gallium was injected into the blood.

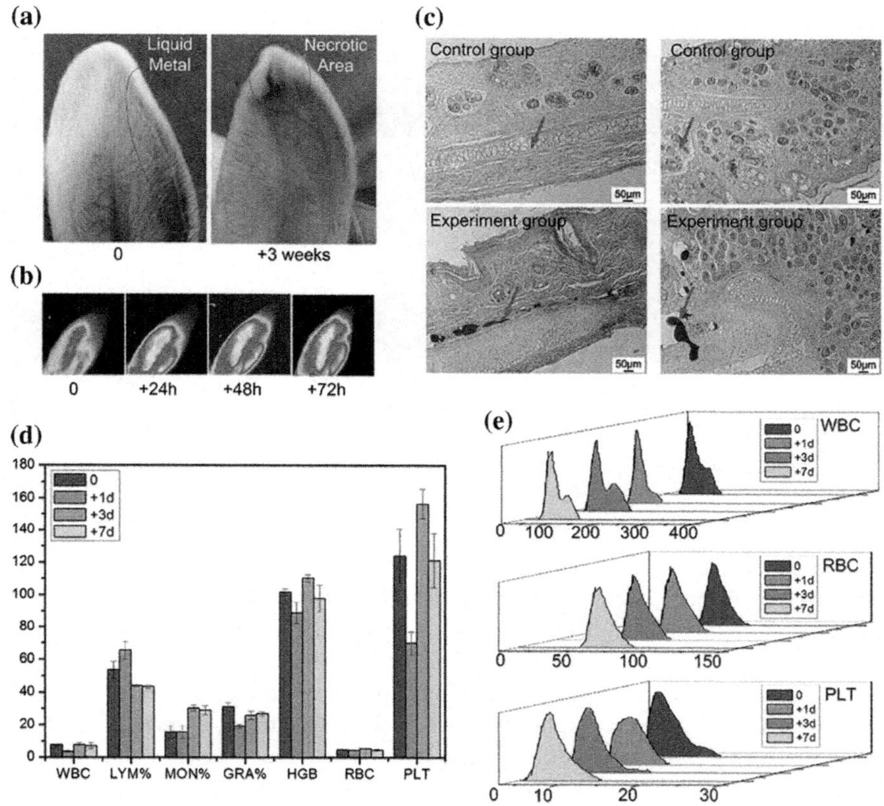

Fig. 7.6 The effects of liquid metal embolization at the rabbit ears [1]. **a** The symptoms of necrosis in the ear. **b** The temperature distribution changes after 0, 24, 48 and 72 h. **c** Comparison between the necrosis tissue sections and control normal tissue section. **d** The results of WBC, LYM%, MON%, GRA%, HGB, RBC and PLT* changed over time. **e** WBC, RBC and PLT dynamic histograms distribution. *WBC: white blood cell; LYM: lymphocyte; MON: monocyte; GRA: granulocyte; HGB: hemoglobin; RBC: red blood cell; PLT: platelet. All pictures reproduced with permission

It should be pointed out that, not all the injections will be able to completely fill the vessels and thus lead to damage of the target tissues. The output in fact depends on the specific surgical injection and delivery way of liquid metal. To explain this point, the present group selected the tail vessels of the mice as an additional test object to evaluate the blockage effect of liquid metal embolization on the tissues in vivo. As shown in Fig. 7.7a, three tail vessels of the mice were filled with liquid metal gallium. However, there was no visible necrosis after three weeks later. Moreover, certain new small blood vessels were even observed to regenerate (Fig. 7.7b). The reason can be interpreted as follows. With a single flow direction and different from former cases, it was more difficult in current situation to fully block the femoral vessels at the tail of the mice. This led some of the liquid metal to

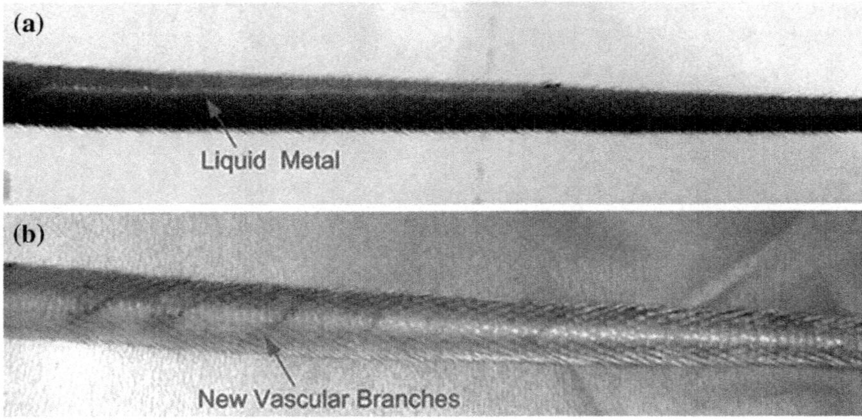

Fig. 7.7 The effects of liquid metal embolization at the mice tail [1]. **a** The liquid metal injected into the tail vein. **b** The regenerated vascular branches. All pictures reproduced with permission

flow away and no visible necrosis occurs at the target tissues over the whole experiments. Besides, these regenerated blood vessels near the tail vessels have further contributed to the nutrition and oxygen supply. This reminds us that, without appropriate administration of injecting the liquid metal agent, the embolization effect as anticipated before may not always necessarily be guaranteed. Therefore, for therapeutic purpose, careful treatment planning should be made in advance to surgically deliver liquid metal into the target vessels along specific directions. Lastly, it was also worth mentioning that these mice filled with liquid metal were kept alive for a rather long time like several weeks. Such findings indicate the safety and non-toxicity of the liquid metal materials staying inside the vessels on condition that they will not cause physically physiological danger.

7.8 Theoretical Evaluation on Tumor Growth with Liquid Metal Embolization

Although the liquid metal embolization of blood vessels in vivo was implemented on the vessels of rabbit ears and legs, a case of tumor might be more illustrative. In this section, a theoretical modeling and simulation of tumor growth affected by the metal blockage of blood vessels nearby (see Fig. 7.8) was carried out to interpret the starvation effect of the current therapy.

Without losing any generality, there are generally four dependent variables to dominate the tumor growth model, including cancer cell density, oxygen density, extracellular matrix density and matrix degrading enzymes. The functions of each variable (further details about the functions could be seen in Alexander's work [27]) in non-dimensional are expressed as

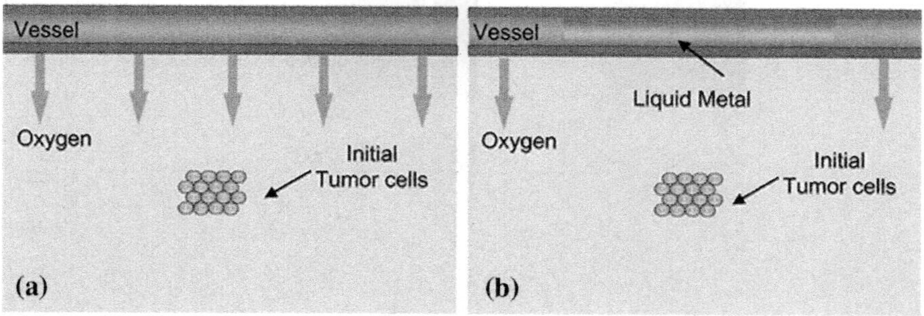

Fig. 7.8 Illustration of the theoretical tumor growth model [1]. **a** Without the liquid metal in the vessel. **b** With the liquid metal embolic agent in the vessel. All pictures reproduced with permission

$$\frac{\partial n}{\partial t} = d_n \nabla^2 n - \rho \nabla \cdot (n \nabla f) \tag{7.2}$$

$$\frac{\partial o}{\partial t} = d_o \nabla^2 o + \nu f - \omega n - \varphi o \tag{7.3}$$

$$\frac{\partial f}{\partial t} = -\eta m f \tag{7.4}$$

$$\frac{\partial m}{\partial t} = d_m \nabla^2 m + \kappa n - \sigma m \tag{7.5}$$

where n, o, f denote the density of cells, oxygen and extracellular matrix respectively, and m denotes the matrix degrading enzymes.

The oxygen is supplied by the vessel and one can make the assumption that the oxygen concentration is zero at the metal blockage position. The probabilities of movement of an individual cell are generated by discretizing Eq. (7.2).

Besides, it is assumed that the cancer cells migrate through a combination of diffusion and haptotaxis as well as undergoing proliferation. And each cell is allowed to migrate when the number of neighbor cells is more than one. Cell death can occur due to lack of oxygen. In the model, we also make the assumption that each cell produces two daughter cells when the cell has reached maturity. If no empty space around the parent cell exists, the cell becomes quiescent until space appears. We assume that quiescent cells only consume half amount of oxygen of the active tumor cells. The tumor cells would not only maintain one phenotype, but also becomes more unstable and more aggressive phenotypes due to mutations. In the model, we mainly consider three phenotypes. The irreversible mutations occur at the mitosis stage.

The computation domain is divided by 200 × 200 grids with a space step of $h = 0.005$ and a time step of $k = 0.0001$. Initially, 36 tumor cells are in the center. The initial value of oxygen density, extracellular matrix density and matrix

Table 7.1 The non-dimensional parameter values used in the simulations

Parameters	Value	Parameters	Value
d_n	0.0005	κ	1
d_0 (out of/in the tumors)	0.05/ 0.025	σ	0
d_m	0.0005	ν	0.5
ρ	0.01	ω	0.57
η	50	φ	0.025

degrading enzymes are 1, 1 and 0, respectively. The non-dimensional parameter values used in the simulations are listed in Table 7.1 [27].

Theoretical simulations on the two cases with and without liquid metal embolic agents in the vessels near the tumor have been implemented to interpret and evaluate the performance of tumor growth suppression by the liquid metal embolization therapy. Figure 7.9 depicts the changes of oxygen concentration near the tumor at six times (5 days, 9 days, 11 days, 13 days, 15 days and 17 days later). The tumor growth consumes oxygen and the oxygen concentration in tumor center is the lowest. In order to maintain growth, the tumor needs adequate oxygen supply by the vessel. However, as a result of liquid metal blockage in the vessel, the oxygen concentrations of the nearby tissues are decreasing. Figure 7.10 shows the predicted results for tumor growth. Different color represents different phenotype cells, and red is the most aggressive cells. The tumor grows towards the vessel since there exists only one single vessel on one side. The tumor cell distribution shows a dead central region, which is due to lack of the oxygen as shown in Fig. 7.9. For the case without liquid metal embolic agent, the dead central region occures after the 17 days, while for the case with liquid metal embolic agent, the dead central region occurs after the 11 days. As the time goes on, the dead central regions continue to enlarge.

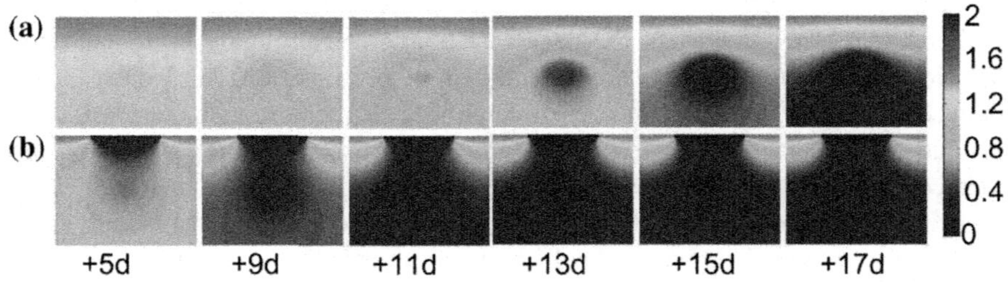

Fig. 7.9 The oxygen distribution with the change of time [1]. **a** Without the liquid metal in the vessel. **b** With the liquid metal embolic agent in the vessel. Picture reproduced with permission

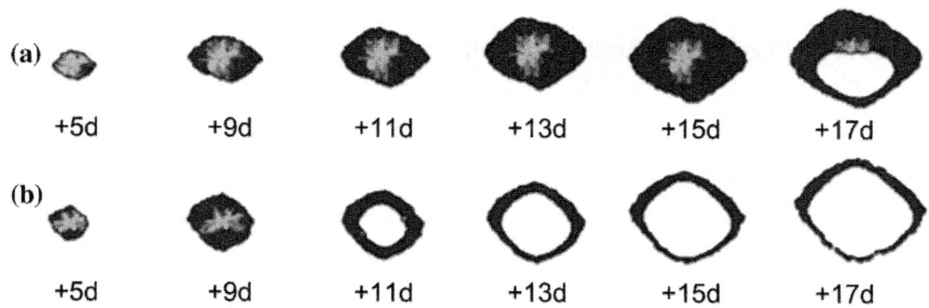

Fig. 7.10 Spatial distribution of tumor cells with the time [1]. **a** Without the liquid metal in the vessel. **b** With the liquid metal embolic agent in the vessel. Picture reproduced with permission

7.9 Challenges and Opportunities

As is well known, the abundant vessels in the tumor tissues make it difficult for tumor treatment. Curatie surgery can easily lead to a massive hemorrhage, and large blood vessels would produce localized cooling in heated tissues during tumor hyperthermia, for instance. As explained above, the body temperature liquid metal yields a promising injectable tumor therapy. With its easy phase conversion, such material owns the capability to flow into tiny vessels at liquid state and stay at the target tissues at the solid state. Once the liquid metal was injected into the vessels, the nearby tissues would be possibly starved to death due to cutting off the feeding route of the nutrition and oxygen supplies.

Though the unprecedented application of the liquid metal on the tumor treatment seems to be beyond imagination, there remains a wide range for the further utilization of the material. In the above experiments, only gallium and $Ga_{75.5}In_{24.5}$ alloy were tested for brief. In fact, the melting points of the liquid metal could be modified through adding some other metals into alloys and adjusting the compounds ratio.

As a metal, the gallium is endowed with good electrical and thermal conductivity. Hence on the base of the blocking therapy, newer treatment might still be developed through combining the electrical and thermal stimulation together. One could even add certain substances into the liquid metal to obtain or enhance specific properties. The present lab had ever proposed a method to fabricate liquid metal with desired properties by loading with nanoparticles [28]. These nanoparticles include magnetic oxides such as Fe_3O_4, metallic particles and some other semi-conductive particles, which further expands the application of liquid metal as the embolic agents. What's more, it is possible to combine this approach with chemotherapy or radiotherapy by injecting mixed liquid metal with chemotherapy and radiotherapy substances.

It is worth emphasizing the role of the liquid metal angiography, which reveals an extra advantage of the vessel blocking therapy. The visibility of the material under the X-ray has provided the possibility for monitoring the flow process along the gallium injection and evaluating vascular changes and damages. The combination of the liquid metal blocking and the X-ray imaging even opens a promising approach to the investigation of the tumor vessel growth and distribution, which also indicates a great potential of the diagnosis-treatment integration.

However, there still exist many issues to be solved in order to further improve the efficiency of the liquid metal embolization. Considering the difficulties to inject the liquid metal into the artery due to fast blood flow there and deep position in the tissues, the currently available experiments so far were mainly administrated on the veins. However, as we all know, the blood in artery flows into the capillary vessel, while that in vein blood flows out of the capillary vessel. Therefore, it is better to inject the liquid metal into the artery to occlude the vessel. Besides, the regeneration of the tumor vessel network under the obstructive condition is also a common challenge in the blocking therapy.

The safety is another non-negligible issue in this new conceptual blood vessel embolization strategy. As mentioned above, some of the liquid metal could be washed away from the target tissues since injection from the veins. As is shown in Fig. 7.11, the liquid metal has entered the heart and lungs of the rabbit in the experiments of leg infusion yet the rabbit is still alive. Therefore, it is very important to adopt measures to prevent this problem from happening in further studies. One possible solution is to apply proper pressure on the proximal end to slow the blood flow velocity. Another method to decrease the blood flow is to reduce the temperature of the blood in the target tissues, which could also speed up the solidification of the liquid metal. It also indicates that the in vivo application is highly sophisticated due to safety control and thus skilled surgical operation is required as well. In former trials [1], Wang et al. only used gallium and $Ga_{75.5}In_{24.5}$ alloy as the embolic agents, whose melting point are both under the 37 °C. Next, one needs to try to synthetize more other liquid metal alloys with a little higher melting point than 37 °C and test their embolization effects. In addition, a comprehensive evaluation of long-term toxicity still requests further research.

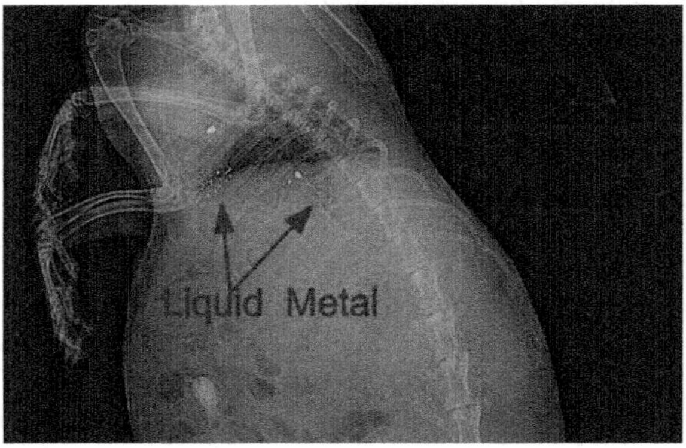

Fig. 7.11 Traces of the liquid metal in the heart and lungs of the rabbit [1]. Picture reproduced with permission

7.10 Conclusion

In summary, the liquid metal, as an unconventional fluidic material at body temperature, opens a new blood vessel embolic agent to starve the necrotic tissues or target tumors to death. With its merits of easy phase transition and sub-cooling, such kind of material can be conveniently injected into the vessels with relatively easy operations. A series of in vitro experiments on the material cytotoxicity have been implemented to evaluate its safety and the results have indicated that both gallium and indium irons show low toxicity on normal cell growth. On considering its application against tumor or other severe diseases, such a performance is quite acceptable. As an extra advantage, the liquid metal is endowed with excellent contrast under the X-ray over the tissues, which provided a powerful soft tool for tumor vascular research and offered promising potential to realize the diagnosis-treatment integration. Furthermore, both in vivo experiments and theoretical model simulations have preliminarily demonstrated the performance of the liquid metal to starve the target tissues or tumors to death. Though still facing many challenges, the unprecedented utilization of the liquid metal agent offers new opportunity for future tumor vessel blocking therapy.

References

1. Wang Q, Yu Y, Liu J (2014) Delivery of liquid metal to the target vessels as vascular embolic agent to starve diseased tissues or tumors to death. arXiv: 1408.0989
2. Esther W, Michael S, Yosef Y (2010) Roles for growth factors in cancer progression. Physiology 25(2):85–101
3. Zhimin L, Guo J, Peter B, Tony H (2001) Epidermal growth factor-induced tumor cell invasion and metastasis initiated by dephosphorylation and downregulation of focal adhesion kinase. Mol Cell Biol 21(12):4016–4031
4. Wells A (2000) Tumor invasion: role of growth factor-induced cell motility. Adv Cancer Res 78:31–101
5. Folkman J (1974) Tumor angiogenesis factor. Can Res 34(8):2109–2113
6. Jain RK (1990) Vascular and interstitial barriers to delivery of therapeutic agents in tumors. Cancer Metastasis Rev 9(3):253–266
7. Eichhorn ME, Strieth S, Dellian M (2004) Anti-vascular tumor therapy: recent advances, pitfalls and clinical perspectives. Drug Resist Updates Rev Commentaries Antimicrob Anticancer Chemother 7(2):125–138
8. Thorpe PE (2004) Vascular targeting agents as cancer therapeutics. Clin Cancer Res (An Official Journal of the American Association for Cancer Research) 10(2):415–427
9. Folkman J (1990) What is the evidence that tumors are angiogenesis dependent? J Natl Cancer Inst 82(1):4–7
10. Kerbel RS (2000) Tumor angiogenesis: past, present and the near future. Carcinogenesis 21 (3):505–515
11. John A, Tuszynski G (2001) The role of matrix metalloproteinases in tumor angiogenesis and tumor metastasis. Pathol Oncol Res 7(1):14–23

12. Kim KJ, Li B, Winer J, Armanini M, Gillett N, Philips HS, Ferrara N (1993) Inhibition of vascular endothelial growth factor-induced angiogenesis suppresses tumour growth in vivo. Nature 362(6423):841–844
13. O'Reilly MS, Boehm T, Shing Y, Fukai N, Vasios G, Lane WS, Flynn E, Birkhead JR, Olsen BR, Folkman J (1997) Endostatin: an endogenous inhibitor of angiogenesis and tumor growth. Cell 88(2):277–285
14. Feldman AL, Libutti SK (2000) Progress in antiangiogenic gene therapy of cancer. Cancer 89 (6):1181–1194
15. Quesada AR, Medina MA, Alba E (2007) Playing only one instrument may be not enough: limitations and future of the antiangiogenic treatment of cancer. BioEssays 29(11):1159–1168
16. Philip ET, David JC, David CB (2003) The first international conference on vascular targeting: meeting overview. Can Res 63(5):1144–1147
17. Denekamp J (1999) The tumour microcirculation as a target in cancer therapy: a clearer perspective. Eur J Clin Invest 29(9):733–736
18. Hori K, Saito S, Kubota K (2002) A novel combretastatin A-4 derivative, AC7700, strongly stanches tumour blood flow and inhibits growth of tumours developing in various tissues and organs. Br J Cancer 86(10):1604–1614
19. Lovet JM, Bruix J (2003) Systematic review of randomized trials for unrespectable hepatocellular carcinoma: chemoembolization improves survival. Hepatology 37(2):429–442
20. Liu LX, Zhang WH, Jiang HC (2003) Current treatment for liver metastases from colorectal cancer. World J Gastroenterol 9(2):193–200
21. Yu H, Zhu G, Xu R et al (2011) Arterial embolization hyperthermia using As_2O_3 nanoparticles in VX2 carcinoma-induced liver tumors. PLoS ONE 6(3):e17926
22. Chen X, Lv H, Ye M, Wang S, Ni E, Zeng F, Cap C, Luo F, Yan J (2012) Novel superparamagnetic iron oxide nanoparticles for tumor embolization application: preparation, characterization and double targeting. Int J Pharm 426(1–2):248–255
23. Teng MM, Chang CY, Chiang JH, Lirng JF, Luo CB, Chen SS, Chang FC, Guo WY (2000) Double-balloon technique for embolization of carotid cavernous fistulas. Am J Neuroradiol 21 (9):1753–1756
24. Joseph LB (2005) Cardiovascular bubble dynamics. Crit Rev Biomed Eng 33(4):299–346
25. Claus MM, Erik SS (2000) Gas embolism. N Engl J Med 342(7):476–482
26. Wang Q, Yu Y, Pan K, Liu J (2014) Liquid metal angiography for mega contrast X-ray visualization of vascular network in reconstructing in-vitro organ anatomy. IEEE Trans Biomed Eng 61(7):2161–2166
27. Anderson ARA (2005) A hybrid mathematical model of solid tumour invasion: the importance of cell adhesion. Math Med Biol 22(2):163–186
28. Ma KQ, Liu J (2007) Nano liquid-metal fluid as ultimate coolant. Phys Lett A 361(3):252–256

Chapter 8
Liquid Metal Enabled Injectable Biomedical Electronics

Abstract In clinics, a medical device is defined as implantable if it is either partly or totally introduced, surgically or medically into the human body and is intended to remain there after the procedure. By virtue of characteristics of well controlled wettability, high electrical conductivity, low cost and easy operation, liquid metal materials have been developed into above area in recent years. In this chapter, representative strategies to develop liquid metals as implantable or injectable medical electronics were introduced and discussed.

Keywords Injectable electronics · Implantable medical electronics
Liquid metal

8.1 Implantable Medical Devices

With the ageing of population and elevation of the incidence rate of neurological and cardiovascular diseases, the rapid increase of patients cannot be ceased simply via conventional medication. Facing such situation, implantable medical devices are often required in healthcare applications, which would aid to monitor and treat serious diseases inside the biological body. Over the past few decades, they have contributed significantly in restoring body functions, enhancing the quality of life and the survival rate of patients globally [1]. It was reported that 8–10% of the population in America and 5–6% of people in industrialized countries have experienced and benefited from implantable medical devices [2]. In addition, implantable electronic systems have helped us understand the complex mechanisms of biological processes taking place within the human body, such as neural communication or control, and significantly enhanced the knowledge of how these are affected by various diseases and treatments [3].

In clinics, a medical device is defined as implantable if it is either partly or totally introduced, surgically or medically into the human body and is intended to remain there after the procedure [4]. Such device can be attached directly to an internal organ, which is considered as an alternative system for clinically

J. Liu and L. Yi, *Liquid Metal Biomaterials*,
Springer Series in Biomaterials Science and Engineering10,
https://doi.org/10.1007/978-981-10-5607-9_8

monitoring electric signals from the inner body [1, 5, 6]. Over the past few decades, scientists have taken honorable efforts to improve the performance of various medical devices. During this period, implantable electronic systems and devices have undergone great development in science and engineering, especially in microelectronics, biotechnology, and materials. The developed typical devices range from sensors, gastric and cardiac pacemakers, cardioverter defibrillators, cochlear implants, artificial vision prostheses, neuromuscular stimulators, to deep brain and bone stimulators, drug monitoring and delivery systems, which efficiently participate in the management of a wide spectrum of diseases, such as Parkinson's disease, hearing disorders, diabetes, cardiac arrhythmia and so on [7–13]. For instance, monitoring electric activity is of great importance in terms of diagnosing and treating in the case of heart disease, such as cardiac arrhythmias [5, 14]. Moreover, another well-known medical device pacemaker has revolutionized the implantable electronics systems since it emerged. In combination with the micro and nano technology, the miniaturization of implant components will enable on-organ monitoring and highly-specific treatment delivery, without compromising normal function of surrounding organs and tissues [3]. These implantable medical devices have been widely employed as valuable biomedical tools to sense a physiological response in vivo or to actuate the function of organs. Nevertheless, more studies on implantable medical devices are still necessary and being continuously conducted for further optimization.

8.2 Typical Requirements of Implantable Devices

In human body, implants have to get along with the surrounding environment with special pressure, temperature, humidity, pH and various ions in different concentrations. An eligible design of implantable medical device should meet multiple requirements to deal with complicated internal conditions. These typical items generally include good biocompatibility, reliable sealing, reasonable structure design and simple delivery system.

8.2.1 Biocompatibility

Undoubtedly, biocompatibility of implantable medical device should be firstly taken into account. It is because that the implanted device directly contacts with the body tissue and interact with them. When the device is initially located in the body, nonspecific blood and tissue fluid proteins cling to or penetrate its materials. Afterwards, nearby immune and inflammatory cells, such as monocytes, leukocytes, and platelets, gather and react to defend the body from the foreign specimen [15–17]. In case of the bad compatibility with biological system, the implant material should be eliminated even though it performs well in other aspects. In addition, sterilization of the material surface is necessary in order to prevent the harm from microorganisms before the implantation of device. Generally, the purpose of applying medical device is to improve the patients' health instead of bringing about new damage to body. Therefore, the biocompatibility of the chosen implant material should be verified by a series of experiments according to corresponding international standard (ISO 10993-1 [18]), including initial and supplementary evaluation tests. Concretely, the standard gives the detailed items of initial evaluation tests, i.e. cytotoxicity, sensitization, irritation, intracutaneous reactivity, systemic toxicity, subacute and subchronic toxicity, genotoxicity, implantation and haemocompatibility. Meanwhile, the supplementary biological evaluation tests shall be considered in chronic toxicity, carcinogenicity, reproductive and developmental toxicity and biodegradation. In conclusion, these tests comprehensively guarantee the biological safety of implant materials and should be carried out before their application in practice.

8.2.2 Packaging

Generally, implantable medical devices contain electrodes or sensors as functional parts. To ensure the quality and reliability of the devices and protect the healthy tissue, a protective barrier is needed for device to separate inner body elements such as cells, proteins, platelets, and chemical gases. Packaging is a common method for providing the protective layer. It can not only effectively prevent the injury from inner electrical and rigid components, but also trap the outgas of the inner materials [19]. Thus, material selection is significant for the functional realization of packages. As mentioned above, the packages for implantable components are required to be biocompatible and hermetic. If gas, liquid or moisture penetrates the encapsulant, it may result in device failure [20]. As the increasing knowledge of current materials and technologies, the packaging materials are developed diversely, such as polymers, metals, quartz and ceramics [21–24]. Among them, polymer encapsulation materials, taking advantages of their good biocompatibility, chemical resistivity, optical transparency, have been widely studied, which meet the basic criteria of implantable packaging materials [25]. Besides, such materials are soft, light-weight, low-cost and easy-to-process compared with metals and ceramics. Conventional implantable polymers include epoxies, silicones, polyurethanes, polyimides, silicon-polyimides, parylenes, polycyclic-olefins, and liquid crystal polymers. Their distinctive properties enable them to be utilized in different applications. For example, silicon rubber is used to encapsulate artery line pressure sensors, epoxies is used to cover the feedthrough connections in implantable cardioverter defibrillators, and recently developed high-performance liquid crystal polymers (LCPs) have been used to encapsulate flexible radio frequency integrated circuits [26–28]. The existing materials have provided numerous choices for implantable medical device. When a new implant sensor or electrode is proposed, the suitable packaging material should be synthetically screened by multiple tests according to practical situation.

8.2.3 Structure Design and Delivery

The structure design of implantable medical devices is another critical issue which should be paid with great attention. The human body is a complex environment that different parts of body may present different chemical, biological and mechanical features. Medical devices implanted into particular position need serious consideration of corresponding local situation. Hence, the structure of medical devices should be well designed in shapes, sizes, placement, functionality, and reactions accordingly. Specifically, an appropriate implantable device owns advantages of soft, minimal size and light weight, which result in rapid healing, less invasion, pain and discomfort, thus affording high quality life of the patients. In addition, the electrode structure is capable of inducing the desired stimulation which is low as not to damage the surrounding tissues and the electrode itself. To achieve these goals, the design requires abundant multidisciplinary knowledge and has to experience various research stages, including mathematical simulations, animal studies and clinical trials.

The delivery methods of implantable medical device also raise serious concerns of scientists and engineers. Common devices are rigid and in the scale of centimeter, whose delivery needs implantation surgery including process of incision, device implantation and suture. Notably, some action sites such as neural system require sophisticated surgical skills.

8.2.4 Current Challenges

As the development of implantable medical devices, there still remain challenges restraining their widespread applications. Traditional electrode materials are inherently characterized by their stiffness, unchangeable shape and insufficient spatial density, which may damage adjacent soft tissue and bring about physical pain and emotional stress to patients [29–31]. Moreover, the complicated implantation surgery including surgical placement, orientation, extraction and follow-up maintenance of the electrodes is intricate, and thus lead great physiological and economic burden. Clearly, the features of less rigidness, minimally invasion, low cost and easy-operation feature are urgently required for implantable medical devices. Great efforts should be made to resolve these issues.

8.3 Liquid Metal Enabled Injectable Electronics

Liquid metals are a kind of metal materials with low melting points which have attracted considerable interests in industrial and medical fields. By virtue of characteristics of well controlled wettability, high electrical conductivity, low cost and easy operation, such materials have been developed as printed electronics in recent years [32–35]. For the earliest trials, our group manages to propose liquid metals as implantable or injectable medical electronics which will be introduced and discussed in the following sections [36].

8.3.1 Injectable Fabrication of 3-D Electronics

The typical liquid metal, GaInSn alloy (weight percent, Ga 67.0%, In 20.5%, Sn 12.5%) can be adopted as electronic material. Its melting point is as low as 10.5 °C. Such alloy presents liquid state at room and body temperature. Its low viscosity and good fluidity enable the direct injection during operation. With respect to the packaging material, gelatin can be selected owning to its biocompatible, bio-degradable and injectable characteristics. Here, to improve the visual effect, gelatin was dyed with green color during the experiment.

The fabrication of liquid metal electrode is simple which can be operated by a common syringe. Firstly, gelatin solution (mass fraction of 25.0%) with 5 mL is injected into the target position within the body at a rate of 1 mL/s. Then insert the syringe needle along the injection direction to produce a channel for making liquid metal electrode. After 3 $\sim$ 5 min, the channel becomes stable and remove the needle, then a three-dimensional (3-D) packaging domain is formed. Next, 2 mL GaInSn alloy is injected into the empty channel at a rate of 0.5 mL/s. Finally, the liquid metal electrode is fabricated simply with ordinary syringe. It is noted that the packaging material should completely wrap the non-working part of electrode. This fabrication method provides an embodiment of implantable electrode. The selection of specific volume of gelatin and liquid metal, the syringe type, and the configuration of the electrode relies on the final object in the body. All these can be easily realized through adjustment. Consequently, various shapes of functional electronic devices or components can be manufactured, such as electric wire network, node-shaped electronic component and 3D triangle frame electronic component.

8.3.2 Electrical Performance of Injected Liquid Metal

To obtain the basic electrical properties, the liquid metal 3-D electrode was fabricated in a 1 mL pipette tip according to the method described in 8.3.1 (Fig. 8.1a). The tests show that the formed electrode has an overall electrical resistance of

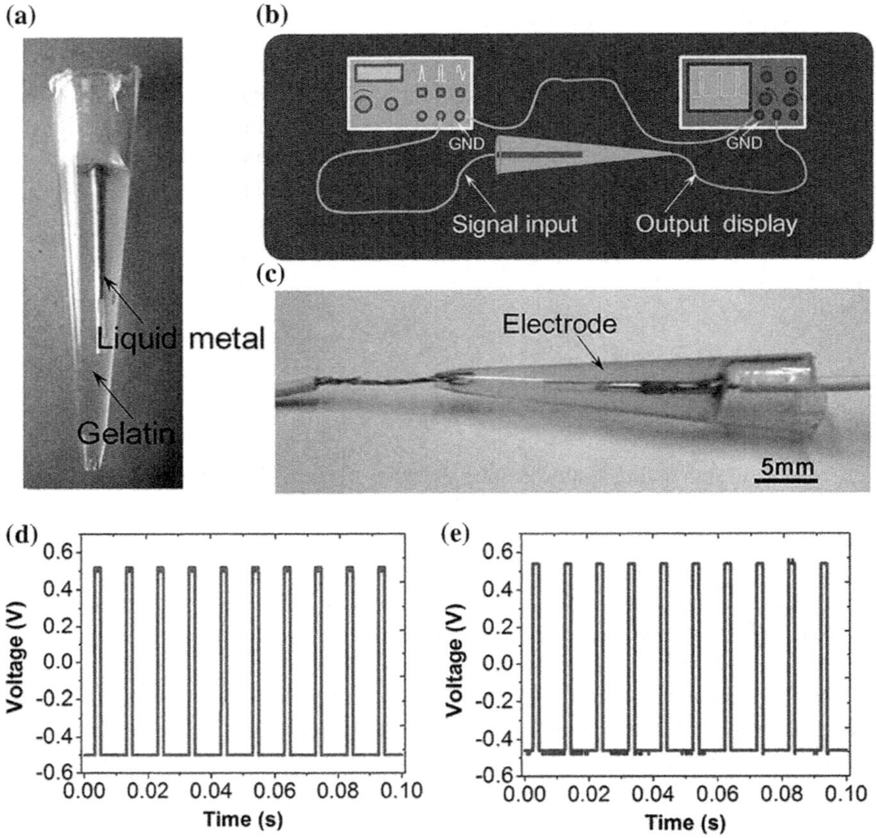

Fig. 8.1 Characteristics of injectable packaged electrode in a transparent pipette tip [36]. **a** Photograph of liquid metal electrode packaged by gelatin in a 1 mL pipette tip. Schematics **b** and photograph **c** are for electronic tests of the electrode. **d**, **e** The input signal and the output result, respectively. All pictures reproduced with permission

16×10^3 Ω, whereas the resistivity of the liquid metal is only about 200 Ω. It is concluded that the packaging material with large resistivity can effectively protect the surrounding tissue from electronic stimulation. Moreover, it has been reported that the impedance of deep brain stimulation (DBS) electrodes in clinic ranges from 500 to 1500 Ω [37]. From this point of view, liquid metal electrode satisfies the requirement of DBS in conducting the electrical signals.

Additionally, more experiments were implemented to further evaluate the electrical performance of the injectable electrode. The experimental setup is shown in Fig. 8.1a, c. The connecting wire is made of copper with a diameter of 0.5 mm. The digital signal generator was employed to provide input stimulation signal, i.e. typical wave square voltage with amplitude of 1 V, frequency of 100 Hz and duty ratio of 20% respectively, as shown in Fig. 8.1d. The positive and negative pole of digital signal generator connected to the liquid metal electrode and GND (counter electrode), respectively. The other side of the electrode connected to the digital oscilloscope to display the output signal. The recorded output signal in Fig. 8.1e indicates a good electrical conduction performance of electrode. Such curve appears to have certain faint noises and a slight baseline drift which may result from the electrode structure and the used packaging material. Overall, the current experimental results demonstrate the feasibility and effectiveness of injectable medical electronics based on liquid metal and in situ packaging.

8.4 Injectable Electrode Within In Vitro Porcine Tissues

After validating the feasibility of injectable liquid metal electronics, experiments in vitro and in vivo were carried out for further evaluation.

According to the manufacture method as explained above, the liquid metal electrode was injected into the porcine tissue in vitro. The difference is that the syringe needle with a diameter of 1 mm was utilized to make the electrode mold in gelatin. Thus, the liquid metal electrode with diameter of 1 mm was obtained. The status of the electrode can be observed through the cross-sectional photograph (see Fig. 8.2a). The liquid metal electrode is a proximate cylinder with length of 12 mm and radius of 0.5 mm, meeting the standards of DBS electrode, e.g. cylindrical Medtronic 3387/3389 DBS electrode with a radius of 0.64 mm [37]. By macroscopic observation, the packaging material and liquid metal continuously distributed along the inner tissue which ensures the integrity of electrode. It has been proven by SEM (scanning electron microscope) photos as well. Figure 8.2b, c display the interface between gelatin and liquid metal, gelatin and pock tissues, respectively. The boundary between the packaging material and the pock tissues

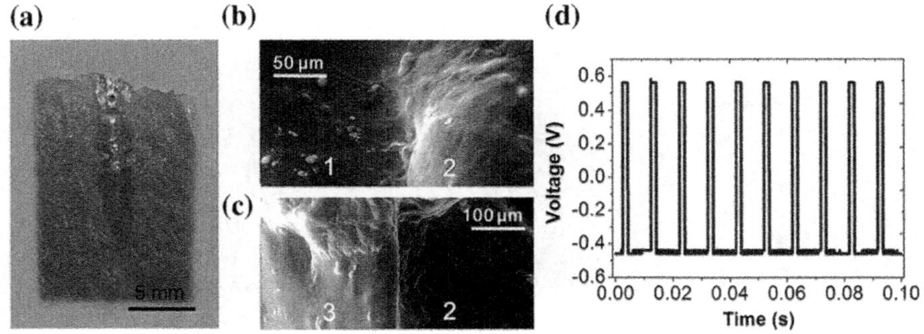

Fig. 8.2 The injectable liquid metal electrode fabricated in porcine tissues in vitro [36]. **a** The cross-sectional photograph of the shaped injected electrode. The micro-boundary SEM images (**b** and **c**) Here, symbols 1, 2, 3 denote the pock tissues, packaging material and liquid metal ink, respectively. **d** The electronic test results for the formed electrode. All pictures reproduced with permission

was irregular due to their mechanical interaction. However, liquid metal showed uniform distribution in the packaging material which guaranteed the function of electrode. Importantly, the electrical signal can be effectively transmitted within tissues in vitro (Fig. 8.2d). All these provide a basis for the following investigation and application.

8.5 Injectable Electrode in Mouse

The animal experiments were carried out and some electrophysiological applications of injectable electronics were performed. It is well known that electrocardiogram (ECG) is a common method for reflecting the electrical activity of heart. It is an essential physiological parameter for both clinical diagnostics and health monitoring. Therefore, the liquid metal electrode with length of 5 mm was tested as an ECG electrode implanted in mouse (weighting 20.0 g). The incision caused by injecting electronics is minor, so that it was hard to observe. Figure 8.3a presents the schematic illustration for the testing procedure. After anesthetizing experimental mouse, the electronic system involving liquid metal and gelatin were injected inside the left side of the thorax near the left upper limb (Fig. 8.3b). A low-pass filter with the cutoff frequency of 150 Hz was adopted to improve the SNR (signal to noise ratio) of the recorded signal. Figure 8.3d demonstrates the recorded ECG signals through liquid metal electrode at 5 and 10 min after the mouse was anesthesia. Such

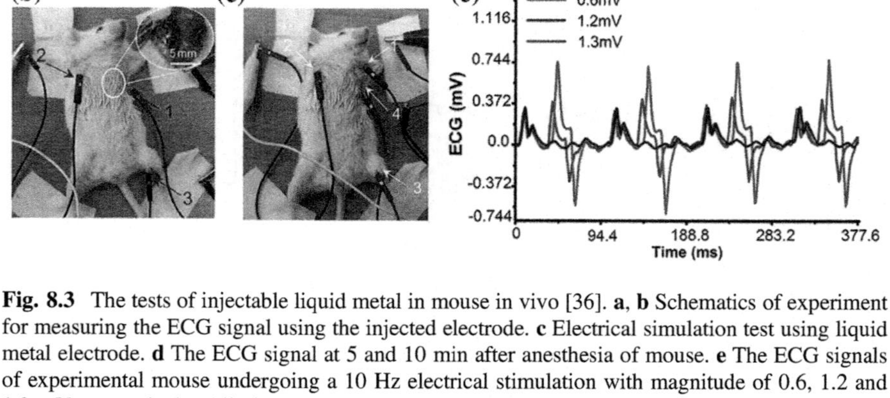

Fig. 8.3 The tests of injectable liquid metal in mouse in vivo [36]. **a**, **b** Schematics of experiment for measuring the ECG signal using the injected electrode. **c** Electrical simulation test using liquid metal electrode. **d** The ECG signal at 5 and 10 min after anesthesia of mouse. **e** The ECG signals of experimental mouse undergoing a 10 Hz electrical stimulation with magnitude of 0.6, 1.2 and 1.3 mV, respectively. All pictures reproduced with permission

signals show very similar features with a typical mouse ECG, including a P wave, a QRS complex and a ST segment [38, 39]. The magnitude of 0.3 mV appears somewhat slightly weak which may be caused by two primary factors, i.e. the electronic properties and lead mode of the injected electrode. In addition, some typical indexes were measured that the heart rate and QT interval were 630 bpm and 66.0 ms, respectively. The existing results have proven that the injectable electronics based on liquid metal were in good accordance with the results of mouse ECG in previous research [38, 39].

The injected liquid metal electrode was also applied to introduce an electrical stimulation in the same mouse model. The experimental setup was shown in Fig. 8.3c. A series of square wave signals with varying magnitudes (the default constants of signal frequency and duty ratio are 10 Hz and 20%, respectively) were provided as electrical stimulation. Meanwhile, the transient ECG signals were recorded to monitor the responses. As shown in Fig. 8.3c, the injected liquid metal (i.e. label 4) was employed as the stimulator electrode to introduce the electrical stimulation into the mouse body. A lead-II mode was utilized to measure the mouse ECG. And two implanted electrodes (i.e. label 1 and 2) served as positive and negative port, respectively; while the third electrode (i.e. label 3) was in the left lower limb, which was an active ground electrode. Through the recorded data, it can be found that the mouse ECG evidently changed when the magnitude of the stimulation signal was 0.6 mV, as displayed in Fig. 8.3e. Besides, the electrical stimulation mainly appeared at the PQ interval of the mouse ECG, resulting in an increase of heart rate. When the stimulating voltage increased to 1.2 mV, similar response can be observed. However, when the magnitude increased to 1.3 mV, the physiologic response induced by the electrical stimulation seems disappeared according to the record. It can be concluded that the higher electrical stimulation may cause the spasm of the mouse muscle which prevents the stimulation signal conduction to the body.

8.6 Electrical Stimulation to the Sciatic Nerves

A key application of implantable electrodes is the treatment of neurologic diseases. The sciatic nerve of frog is commonly used as experimental model for neurologic diseases research. Therefore, frog was selected for investigating the diverse performances of injectable liquid metal electrodes in conducting the electrical-stimuli signals to nerves.

In experiment, an interceptive lower part of a bullfrog body was prepared. Two liquid metal electrodes were fabricated as described in the above test, and injected to the left and right side of the sciatic nerve near the femur, respectively (Fig. 8.4a, b). In terms of the unique advantage of liquid metal in radiography, it is easy to monitor the molding effect of fabricated injectable electrodes (Fig. 8.4c). For the sake of contrastive analysis, the electric-stimuli signal was connected to the target tissue (group 1), packaging material gelatin (group 2) and liquid metal electrodes

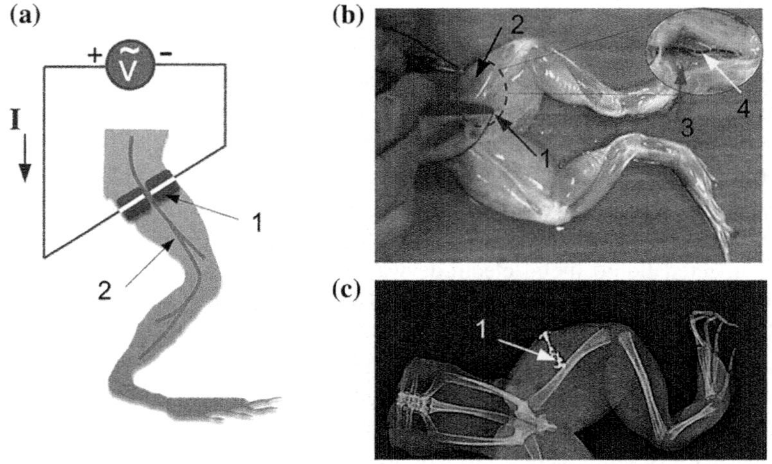

Fig. 8.4 Nervous electrical stimulations using injectable liquid metal electrode [36]. **a** Schematic of experimental setup for loading the electrical stimulations to the sciatic nerve of a frog in vivo; here symbols 1, 2 denote the fabricated electrode and sciatic nerve, respectively. **b** Photo of electrical stimulation operation; the inset is the topography of the frog's tissue with sciatic nerve and injectable electrode; here symbols 1 and 2 are respectively the positive and negative leads of the electrical input signal, symbols 3 and 4 respectively denote the injectable electrode and sciatic nerve. **c** X-ray image of frog's leg implanted with liquid metal electrode; symbol 1 represents the liquid metal electrode. All pictures reproduced with permission

(group 3) respectively. Similar response was found in group 1 and group 2. In these two groups, the contraction of local muscles occurred when the input signal was 2 V. Such contraction would be stronger when the amplitude increases to 4 V. It suggests the good insulativity of the used gelatin. In group 3, the contraction of the gastrocnemius muscle was induced and can be obviously observed, indicating the availability of injectable electrode in conducting electrical stimulations to the sciatic nerve.

8.7 Liquid Metal Enabled Injectable Conformable Electrochemical Therapy

8.7.1 Background

Electrochemical treatment of tumors (EChT) has recently been identified as a very effective way for local tumor therapy. However, hindered by the limited effective area of a single rigid electrode, multiple electrodes are often recruited when tackling large tumors, where too many electrodes not only complicate the clinical procedures but also aggravate patients' pain. To improve this situation, Sun et al. [40] proposed a new conceptual electric stimulation tumor therapy through introducing the injectable liquid metal electrodes, which can adapt to complex tumor shapes so as to achieve desired therapeutic performance. Such approach can offer evident merits for dealing with the complex physiological situations, especially for those irregular body cavities like stomach, colon, rectum or even blood vessel etc., which are hard to tackle otherwise. As it was disclosed from the conceptual experiments that, unlike traditional rigid and uncomfortable electrodes, liquid metal possesses high flexibility to attach to any crooked biological position to deliver and adjust targeted electric field to fulfill anticipated tumor destruction. And such amorphous electrodes exhibit rather enhanced treatment effect of tumors. Further, it can be found that EChT with liquid metal electrodes would produce more electrochemical products during electrolysis. If needed, transformations with the shapes of liquid metal additionally provided an easily regulatable strategy to improve EChT efficiency, which can conveniently aid to achieve better output compared to multiple electrodes. In vivo EChT of tumors clarified the effect of liquid metal electrodes in retarding tumor growth and increasing life spans.

8.7.2 Basics of Electrochemical Treatment of Tumors

The past few decades has witnessed tremendous endeavours in tumor therapy. Electrochemical treatment (EChT) of tumors, a minimal invasive strategy, together with other methods, such as radio-frequency ablation, microwave ablation, laser ablation and irreversible electroporation etc., is rapidly developing as an effective tumor therapy [41–45]. It has been introduced to China and demonstrated its powerful role in treating both malignant and benign tumors through millions of clinical trials [46–48]. Studies in more other countries also observed remarkable tumor regression rate and achieved rather promising cases [49]. Overall, EChT ablation has relatively local destruction range and less systemic side effects compared to those chemical drug therapies. In principle, EChT is defined to impose direct electric current or voltage on tumors after electrodes were inserted to the tumor area, where the solid neoplasms or liquid electrolytes begin to electrolysis and produce various electrochemical toxic products subjected to the electric action. The main mechanism underlying this process depends on the drastic change of pH around and adjuvant to the electrode, which has been proven both in experiments and theoretical models [50, 51].

Normally, when the tumor has an abnormal shape or large size, more than two electrodes will be adopted in the therapy. Challenge in the electrochemical treatment of tumors lies in the electrode number and configuration. Such administration is extremely important for clinical surgery which so far still remains much debate [52–55]. However, empirical principle is prevailing in this field. Multiple insertions of electrodes are prevailing which however not only complicate the operations but also add extra discomfort and pain to patients. Till now, disputes on the standardization of electrode displacement and therapeutic dose stay controversial and need urgent improvement.

Recently, the room temperature liquid metal alloy, such as EGaIn (75% gallium and 25% indium), owning unique characteristics, such as favourable electrical conductivity, high flexibility and low toxicity, enables itself a superior candidate as the biological electric-transmitting materials for the new generation utilizations. Benefited from its soft nature, liquid metal could conformably attach to various surface areas or any kind of cavity regarding electric transmission, which is otherwise difficult for the conventional rigid electrodes to accomplish and in turn could promote individualized medical treatment via a much easier way. Specially, liquid metal electrodes through syringe injection [56] offers additional application modality with shape transformable and dose controllable flexible electronics [57–59], besides skin electronics in bioelectronics field. However, so far, few trails were ever reported to apply the liquid metal electrode for EChT of tumors, which should own particular virtue for future practices.

It was from the above consideration, Sun et al. [40] proposed a new conceptual injectable electrode EChT modality based on liquid metal and its transformable capability with various shapes through injection to achieve individualized therapy and alleviate patient's suffering. Aided with different modules, various shapes of liquid metal electrodes were shown to have similar or even better therapeutic results compared to multiply electrodes. In vitro EChT was performed with injected liquid metal electrodes and better antitumor result demonstrates its feasibility to tackle tumor cells compared with platinum electrodes. In addition, what's beyond one's expectation is that liquid metal also serves as a highly efficient electron-transferring material in the electrochemical reaction. The electrical current is expected to be twice as big as that with inert electrodes. The electrochemical toxic products of electrolysis with liquid metal electrodes exhibited better tumor destruction effect in both anode and cathode sites. What's more, conformable liquid metal electrodes are also expected to achieve better performance for the malignant melanoma in vivo. It can be anticipated that, the liquid metal soft electrodes will help mold new generation whole electronic medical therapy.

8.8 Liquid Metal Electrode Enhanced EChT of In Vitro Tumor Cells

In vitro cytotoxicity of EChT experiment is first adopted as vital evaluation index of tumor therapy. In Sun et al.'s experiments [40], $EGaIn_{24.5}$ alloy with a melt point of 15.5 °C is employed (Fig. 8.5). As heavy in mass and fluidic character for liquid metals in cell culture medium, an EChT platform with small bowel-like container (Fig. 8.6a) can be fist designed to isolate liquid metal from cultured cells. Polydimethylsiloxane (PDMS), owing to their fine biocompatibility, low toxicity to cell and easy fabrication property, was adopted to make the container. Then one can put the container in specific location of the cell culture dish before seeding and fixing them with no voluntary movement. The cell seeding procedure is of great

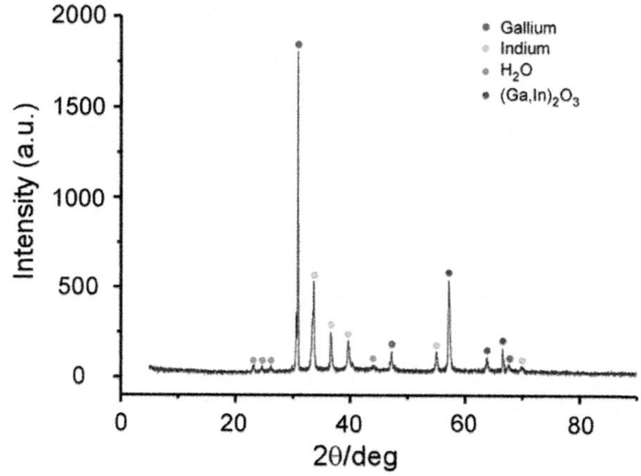

Fig. 8.5 The XRD patterns of the EGaIn24.5 alloy [40]. Picture reproduced with permission

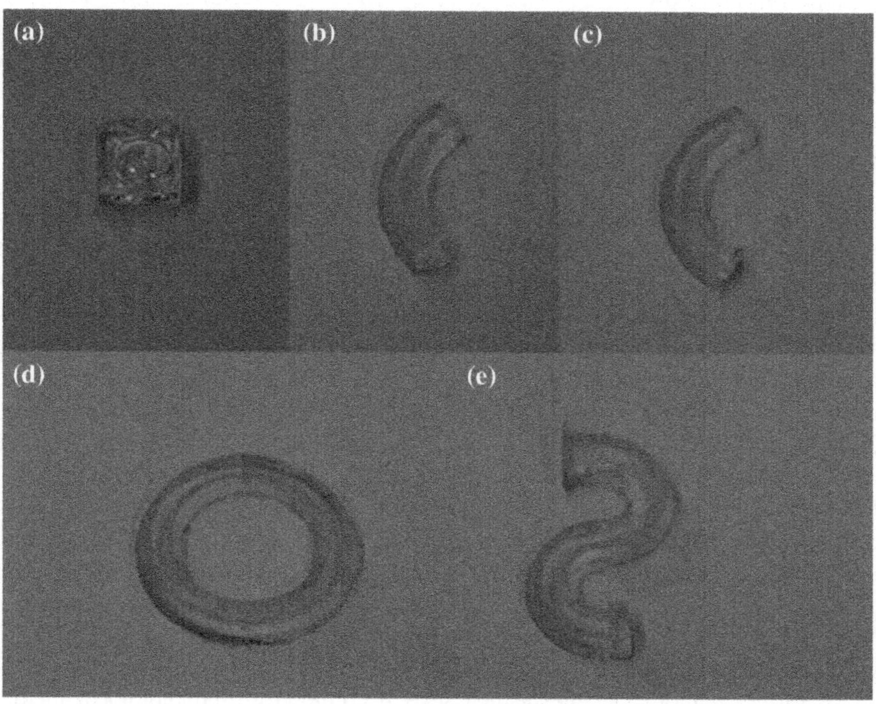

Fig. 8.6 Modules of PDMS container [40]. Molds composed of PDMS are made into different shapes, such as bowl-like (**a**), 90° annulus (**b**), 120° annulus (**c**), full circle annulus (**d**) and S shape (**e**). All pictures reproduced with permission

care to avoid decrease in cell number and to make sure that the prepared cells all attached to the bottom of the culture flask. For the preparation, two symmetrical holes were punched in the center of the lid with a distance of 1 cm to appropriate the platinum electrodes insertion vertically. EChT experiments were performed one day after cell seeding. On the experimental day, all cell culture medium was changed with 3 mL Hank's solution before EChT. Although there is no direct contact between liquid metal and tumor cells, the cell culture medium works as a connector and current flow path bonding them together (Fig. 8.7a).

Experiments were divided into four different groups [40]: control, EChT_Pt, LM and EChT_LM groups. No operation was performed on the control group. EChT_Pt group is to electrolysis with 5 V direct voltage stimulation for 5 min through two platinum electrodes with a diameter of 0.5 mm vertically inserted to the PDMS bowl. LM group is just to add two droplets of liquid metal (about 200 uL) to the PDMS container and without any other operation. EChT_LM group is to stimulate with 5 V direct voltage for 5 min with liquid metal electrodes which were connected to the power via the platinum electrodes.

When current flows through the Hank's solution, ion began to move under the electric force and electrolysis happened [51] (Fig. 8.7a), where serious change of pH around the electrodes occurred as evidenced by the instantaneous solution color alterations for the existence of phenolphthalein indicator. After treatment, cells were cultured for another 4 h to accomplish the EChT procedure. The cell destruction effect was assessed via a standard (3-[4,5-dimethylthiazol-2-yl]-2,5-diphenyltetrazolium bromide) MTT assay. As expected, EChT exhibited distinctive tumor cell killing effect in both EChT_Pt and EChT_LM groups (Fig. 8.7b). Without electric stimulation, the liquid metal alone in the medium or the operation of adding liquid metal exhibited no harm and toxicity to the tumor cells ($105.13 \pm 9.19\%$). However, what's beyond ones' expectation lies in that, EChT of tumors with liquid metal electrodes showed significantly stronger tumor destruction effects ($10.25 \pm 1.78\%$) than the platinum electrodes group ($19.65 \pm 1.90\%$). To further clarify the above findings and identify cell viability around the electrode, Sun et al. [40] stained the tumor cells with propidium iodide (PI) to detect and visualize the dead cells (red) and the effective area of the EChT. After removal of the PDMS container, clear boundary could be observed from the fluorescence images, which demonstrated in number the successful seeding of the tumor cells without damage. As is shown in Figs. 8.7c, d, from the confocal imaging, large areas of dead cells (red) near the anode and cathode electrodes were detected in the EChT_LM group as compared with the relatively limited destruction effect in EChT_Pt group of both ends, which strongly indicated the lethality of EChT with liquid metal electrodes.

To further demonstrate the results, several commonly used biological media, such as PBS (phosphate buffered saline) buffer solution, 0.9% NaCl solution, cell culture medium (short for CCM, including DMEM-F12 with 10% FBS and 2% PS) and tyrode solution were adopted [40]. Quantitative data was shown in Fig. 8.7e. Similarly, PBS solution and saline solution showed significant cell destruction effect as with Hank's solution, in which liquid metal electrodes demonstrated better performance than the inert platinum electrodes. Moreover, severe cell death around

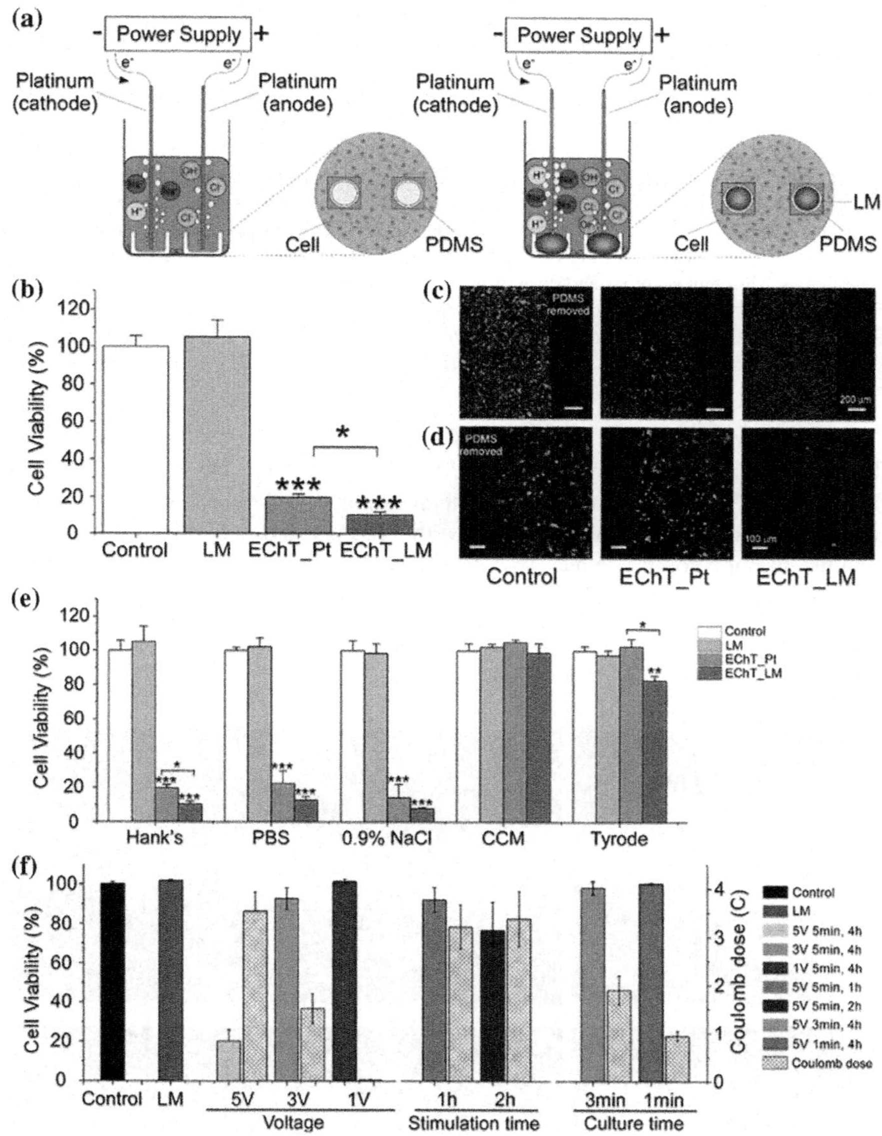
(a)
- Power Supply +
Platinum (cathode)
Platinum (anode)
Cell
PDMS
LM
(b)
Cell Viability (%)
Control LM EChT_Pt EChT_LM
(c)
PDMS removed
200 μm
(d)
100 μm
Control EChT_Pt EChT_LM
(e)
Hank's PBS 0.9% NaCl CCM Tyrode
Control
LM
EChT_Pt
EChT_LM
(f)
Coulomb dose (C)
Control LM 5V 3V 1V
Voltage
1h 2h
Stimulation time
3min 1min
Culture time
Control
LM
5V 5min, 4h
3V 5min, 4h
1V 5min, 4h
5V 5min, 1h
5V 5min, 2h
5V 3min, 4h
5V 1min, 4h
Coulomb dose

◂**Fig. 8.7** Liquid metal electrode enhanced EChT of tumors in vitro [40]. **a** Schematic design of EChT with platinum (left) or liquid metal electrodes (right) in vitro. **b** Cell viability of EChT in Hank's solution by MTT assay. Error bars indicate s.e.m. (n = 4), $*P < 0.05$, $***P < 0.001$ compared with the control group (two-tailed Student's t-test). Representative confocal fluorescence images around the anode (**c**) and cathode (**d**) after EChT. The C8161 tumor cells were cultured for 4 h after EChT with Hank's solution, then incubated with PI (red). *Note* The C8161 cell line was a C8161-GFP cell line. Left, control group without treatment, middle, EChT with platinum electrodes, right, EChT with liquid metal electrodes. **e** C8161 tumor cells were exposed to different solutions: Hank's solution, PBS buffer solution, 0.9% NaCl solution, cell culture medium (CCM) and Tyrode solution during EChT. Platinum or liquid metal electrodes were used over the experiments. Different schemes and dose of EChT through liquid metal electrode. **f** Specially, 5 V 5 min, 4 h indicate electric stimuli is 5 V direct voltage last for 5 min and then cultured for another 4 h before test. Error bars indicate s.e.m. (n = 4), $*P < 0.05$, $**P < 0.01$ and $***P < 0.001$ compared with the control group (two-tailed Student's t-test). All pictures reproduced with permission

the electrodes indicated by the visible massive red dots was shown from the fluorescence images, where cells lost their original cell morphology, turned to round dead bodies and finally stained with PI (Figs. 8.8 and 8.9). However, no obvious tumor shooting effect was found with cell culture medium or tyrode solution undergoing the same treatment process. The electrolyte was considered to play an important role for tumor shooting. Besides, EChT effectiveness was

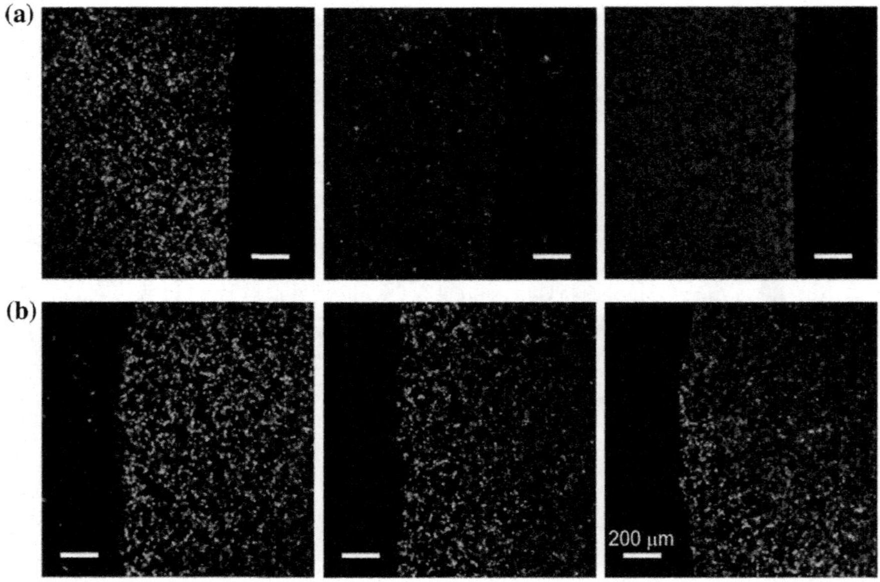

Fig. 8.8 Representative confocal fluorescence images around the anode (**a**) and cathode (**b**) [40]. The C8161 tumor cells were cultured for 4 h after EChT treatment with PBS solution, then incubated with PI (red). Left, control group without treatment, middle, EChT with platinum electrode, right, EChT with liquid metal electrode. All pictures reproduced with permission

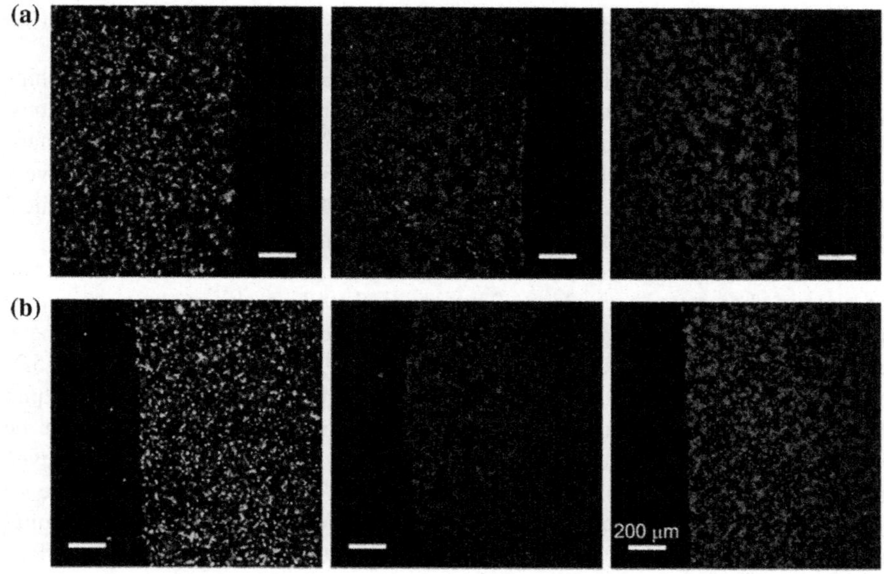

Fig. 8.9 Representative confocal fluorescence images around the anode (**a**) and cathode (**b**) [40]. The C8161 tumor cells were cultured for 4 h after EChT treatment with 0.9% NaCl solution, then incubated with PI (red). Left, control group without treatment, middle, EChT with platinum electrode, right, EChT with liquid metal electrode. All pictures reproduced with permission

explored through changing stimulation scheme. Over the work, Sun et al. [40] found three key factors for the administration of EChT which are: voltage amplitude, stimulation time and culture time, respectively (Fig. 8.7f). The destructive effect of EChT with liquid metal electrodes increased with voltage value and stimulation time, which serve as main factors of the total charge. Although coulomb dose has already been demonstrated as the determinants of EChT, sufficient dose was a necessary condition, but not the guarantee of strong lethality in EChT and a certain time of cell culture in the altered chemical environment is crucial for the electrolysis to exert cytotoxicity on tumor cells (Fig. 8.7f).

8.9 Anodic and Cathodic Morphology Alterations of Liquid Metal During EChT

Liquid metals would display diverse morphology transformation when an electric field is applied to its surface [60, 61], which makes it different from those inert electrodes. Usually, high surface tension of liquid metal makes a huge difference to be distingue from water. Thus, they kept at the original spherical or oval shape while emerging under the water. The electrical double layer (EDL) is formed around the surface of liquid metal, which works as a charged capacitor [61] according to the integrated Lippmann's equation.

The Young-Laplace equation [62] could be adopted to explain the relationships between the pressure difference and the shape change. From the two equations, when inserting an anode and exerting a small voltage to the liquid metal, the surface tension would change with the external potential [61]. However, when relatively high voltage was imposed to the liquid metal which induced electrochemical reaction, large scaled transformation would be observed.

When an external power was applied to the droplets, the number and distribution of electric charge on the surface of liquid metal will be altered, as is shown in Fig. 8.10a. In Sun et al.'s experiments [40], the anode and cathode of liquid metal electrodes exhibited distinctly different phenomenon under the exposure to the 5 V direct voltage external electricity. In the cathode, the negatively charged liquid metal surface will recruit many cations, such as sodium and potassium ions in the Hank's solution. The increase of surface tension induced by cathode would even make the surface area reduce to one tenth [60, 61]. The layer of gallium oxide on the original surface will be depleted. The elimination of the oxide on the liquid metal surface removed the pressure to the liquid metal, thus increasing the surface tension of the droplet. Then the increased surface tension altered the shape of liquid metal to a more spherical form (Fig. 8.10b). Whereas, this changed the contact point of liquid metal with the external power, which regulated the surface tension afterwards. The non-uniform external electric field is probably another explanation for this continuous oscillating liquid metal droplet [60]. The imbalanced surface tension of liquid metal not only made the liquid metal itself swaying but also stirred the solution around (Fig. 8.10b). The external electricity seemed to show a combined attractive and repulsive force to the liquid metal but can not reach a stable state. Besides, numerous cations accumulated around the cathode and produced reduction reaction with products like hydroxyl and hydrogen. What's more, hydrogen occurred on the edge of liquid metal and attached on the surface of PDMS, then growing bigger with time as shown in video. However, the influence of bubbled hydrogen on the imbalanced metal is negligible. When the power switches on, the surface area change under sudden input of the electric field in the cathode is as much as 13.372% (Fig. 8.10e). Then the surface tension induced surface area change went ups and downs through time. What's more, a layer of water solution attracted and tightly surrounded by the liquid metal also waggled with the movement of the liquid metal probably due to the Marangoni effect [63, 64], enhancing the flowability of the content in the water. The interesting phenomenon is when the power switches off, the trend for the increased surface tension to induce surface area decrease did not cease immediately. Like the inertial effect, the rise and fall last for several seconds, as shown in Fig. 8.10e.

Despite the ups and downs, the whole trend under revocation of the power supply induced surface area increase is obvious in the enlarged figure of Fig. 8.10e. Resulted from the imbalanced electrical field, the drastic waggle of liquid metal not only stirred the whole electrolyte solution but also induced water swirl by recruiting more ions to accelerate electrolyte electrochemistry reaction.

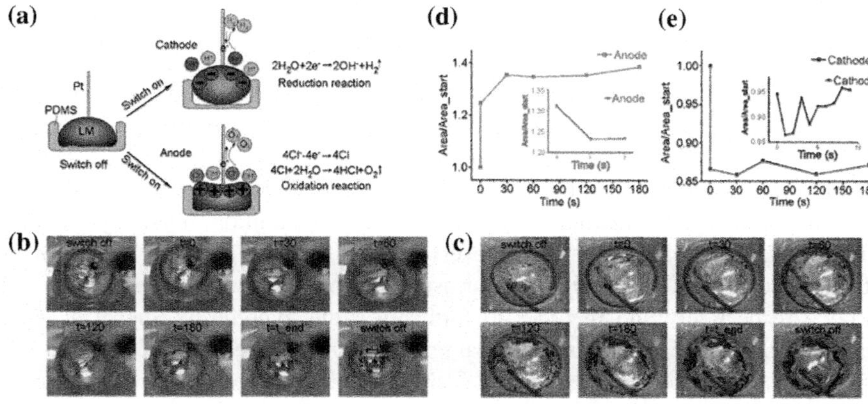

Fig. 8.10 Anodic and cathodic morphology alterations of liquid metal electrodes during EChT [40]. **a** Schematic description of liquid metal morphology change under the external electricity during EChT. The sequential snapshots of the cathode (**b**) and anode (**c**) under the external voltage of 5 V lasting for about 200 s. The relative surface area changes of liquid metal in the anode (**d**) and cathode (**e**) under external electricity along with time. The symbol Area and Area_start respectively refer to the real time surface area of liquid metal and the start surface area without electricity stimulation. The insets in (**d** and **e**) display the surface area change when the external power is off. All pictures reproduced with permission

For the anode, the situation seems totally opposite [40]. A large amount of negative ions represented by chloridion aggregate on the surface of the liquid metal, lose electrons and produce chlorine and oxygen (Fig. 8.10a). Then the liquid metal oxide appeared as small dark particles on the edge of the metal surface in Fig. 8.10c. The production of the oxide stems from the electrolytic oxidation, while the movement of the dark particles is probably due to the Marangoni flow effect [64]. The produced oxygen adhered as small bubble to the PDMS surface (Fig. 8.10c). Different from the cathodic phenomenon, a slim of oxide could be observed on the surface of the liquid metal, the formation of the solid oxide would decrease the surface tension dramatically [61]. The superficial area reaches to 24.62% higher as compared to no electricity case. Further increase of surface area to 35.5% higher was obtained due to surface tension decline. When the power switched off, the obvious change of surface area from about 1.31–1.23 is dramatic. However, no matter it was anode or cathode, due to interaction with electric field the surface tension alteration can not go back to its original state. Generally, the surface area of cathode decreased to 0.95 due to increased surface tension while increase of the anode surface area to about 1.23 is resulted from the decreased surface tension. What's more, the whole solution color changes to light pink or even colorless due to that various redox products were also obtained during the experiments.

8.10 Anodic and Cathodic Cytotoxicity During EChT

Motivated by the above findings that EChT efficiency was improved by liquid metal electrodes as well as the phenomenon of the drastic sway of liquid metal and the furious agitation of the surrounding solution, Sun et al. [40] hypothesized that the liquid metal electrodes could be used as highly efficient electron-transferring materials in the electrochemical reaction procedure. In addition, relatively different effects of anode and cathode were observed from the EChT_Pt and EhT_LM in PBS solutions (Fig. 8.8). With the curiosity of what happened in the anode and cathode respectively and in order to further test the hypothesis, Sun et al. [40] managed to separate the electrochemical reaction of the two ends. A KCl-based salt bridge was employed to complete the circuit and keep ion balance. The main mechanism of tumor cell destruction is the acidic and alkaline production around electrodes during the process of electrolysis. Especially, the acid environment could lead to cell destruction through activating lysosome reaction and preventing protein formation [65–67]. Cell superoxide caused by these oxidizing agents around cathode also increases the susceptibility of tumors. The instant pH change and the ultimate uniform pH for both the anodic and the cathodic ends are vital evaluation index of electrochemical reaction speed and efficiency of EChT. The configuration, as is shown in Fig. 8.11a, makes it possible to not only qualitatively but also quantitatively monitor electrochemical reaction speed under different circumstances, with platinum electrodes or liquid metal electrodes. 2 mL treatment solution was added to two culture dishes separately. Salt bridge made of saturated KCl solution along with a DC power composed the full circle (Fig. 8.11a). Then the solution was charged with 4 V direct voltage. Serious pH change indicated by obvious color change of Hank's solution was detected during electrochemical reaction. One can also feel an acidic smell during the stimulation. After 5 min, pH paper can be immediately taken to detect the immediate pH change around anode or cathode electrode respectively, recording as EC_NE for platinum electrodes and EC_LM_NE for liquid metal electrodes. The final uniform solution pH was then measured with pH meter, recording as EC_WS and EC_LM_WS respectively.

Overall, the instant pH value could reach 10–13 in the cathode and 1–3 in the anode regardless of the type of electrodes. However, among those solutions, the ultimate pH value of the EChT_LM group is much higher in the cathode and much lower in the anode than the EChT_Pt group, which indicated that liquid metal electrode could produce more hydroxyl or hydrion to increase or decrease the pH value. The results demonstrated that the liquid metal could accelerate the electrochemical reaction efficiency. To further prove the results, electric current was then measured. Surprisingly, under the 5 V direct voltage, the average current of the EChT_LM group was determined to be about 4 mA, which is 2-fold higher than that of EChT_Pt group (2 mA). The recorded coulomb dose of the EChT_LM group was also twice as much as that of EChT_Pt group. So in order to transmit the same amount of electric charge of 0.6 and 0.3 C respectively, liquid metal electrodes take only half of the time that Pt electrode may need (Fig. 8.12). Result from

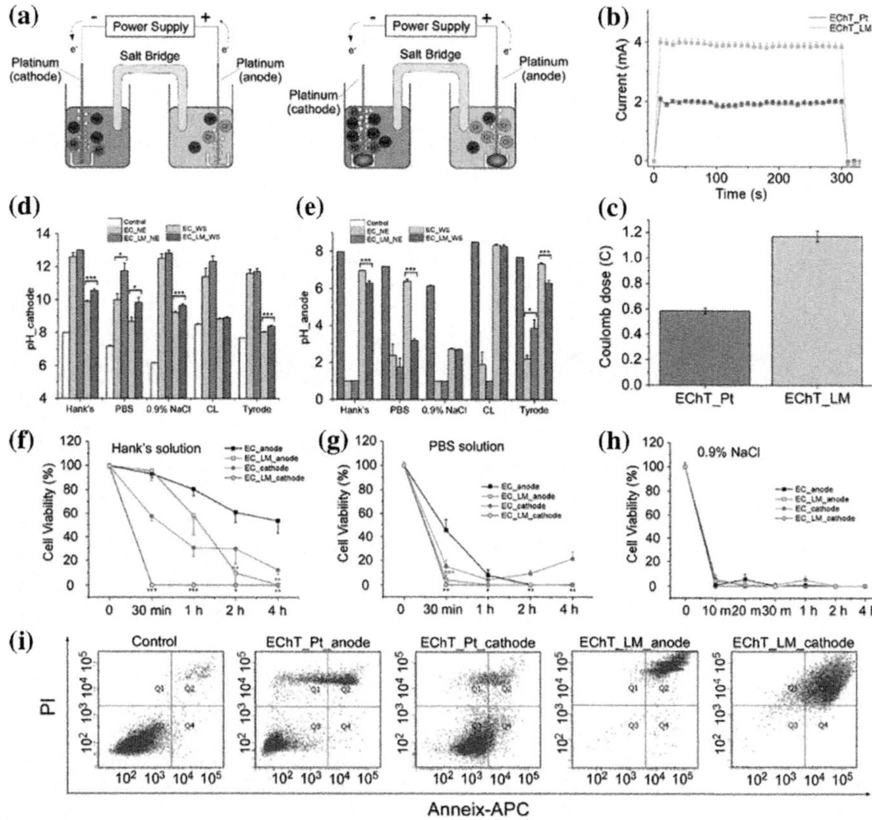

Fig. 8.11 Characterization of anodic and cathodic cytotoxicity during EChT [40]. **a** The experimental framework for separation of electrochemical reaction in anode and cathode with platinum (left) or liquid metal electrodes (right). The salt bridge adopted here was to keep ion balance. The average current (**b**) and coulomb dose (**c**) under external 5 V voltage. Error bars indicate s.e.m. (n = 6). pH change of cathode (**d**) and anode (**e**) with different solutions. The immediate pH change near electrode after EChT was recorded as EC_NE, EC_LM_NE for EChT_Pt and EChT_LM group respectively. The pH of the final uniform whole solution was then measured with pH meter, recording as EC_WS and EC_LM_WS for EChT_Pt and EChT_LM group respectively. Error bars indicate s.e.m. (n = 4), $*P < 0.05$, $***P < 0.001$. Cell cytotoxicity was measured by exposure to the electrolysis of Hank's (**f**), PBS solution (**g**) and 0.9% NaCl solution (**h**). EC_anode, EC_LM_anode, EC_cathode, EC_LM_cathode stands for electrolysis from either anode or cathode with EChT_Pt or EChT_LM respectively. Error bars indicate s.e.m. (n = 4), $**P < 0.01$ and $***P < 0.001$ compared with when the initial cell viability before treatment (two-tailed Student's t-test). **i** Representative apoptosis analysis of c8161 tumor cells induced by the electrolysis of PBS solution using the Annexin V-APC/PI staining for 10 and 45 min of the cathode and anode electrolysis group respectively. All pictures reproduced with permission

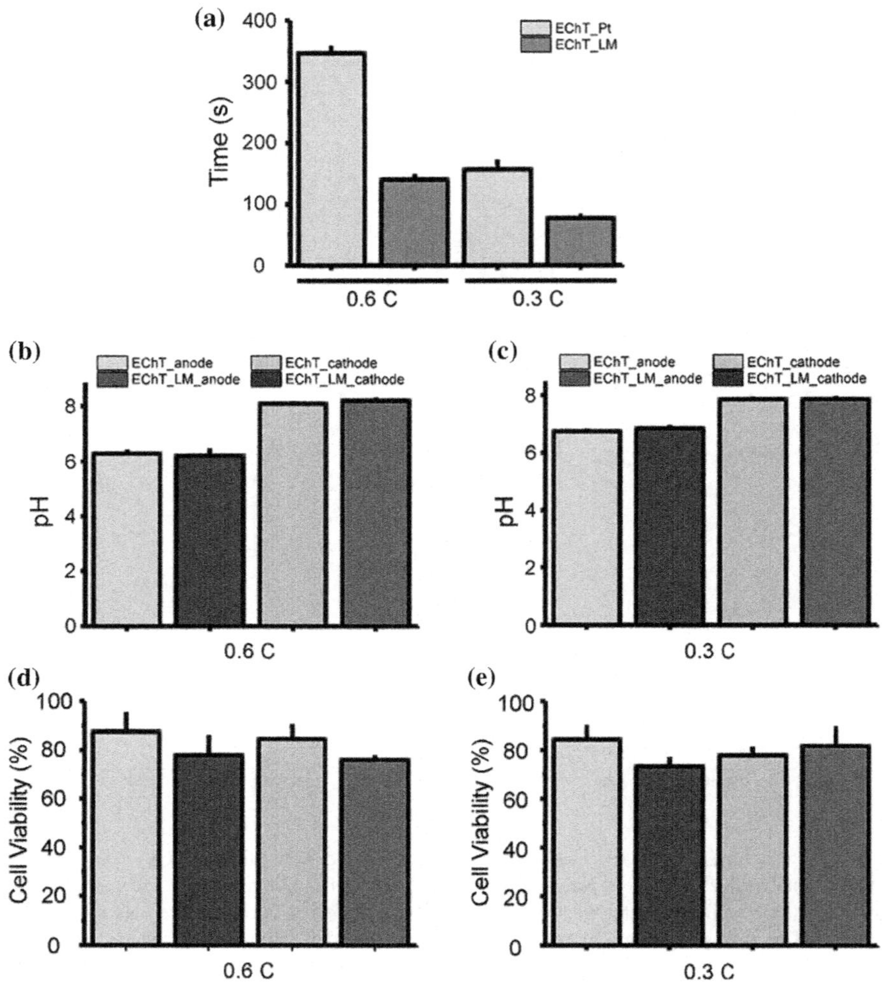

Fig. 8.12 The influence of different electric dose on EChT [40]. **A** The time consumed to deliver 0.6 and 0.3 C with Pt or LM electrodes. **b** pH change with different electrolysis under the electricity of 0.6 C. **c** pH change with different electrolysis under the electricity of 0.3 C. **d** Cell cytotoxicity with the electrolysis from **b**. **e** Cell cytotoxicity with the electrolysis from **c**. EChT_anode, EChT_cathode, EChT_LM_anode, EChT_LM_cathode stands for electrolysis from either anode or cathode with Pt electrodes or liquid metal electrodes respectively. All pictures reproduced with permission

the identical charge shows no difference in tumor cells destructive ability between the two groups. Therefore, the distinct cell destructive phenomenon from liquid metal group should be attributed to its fast electron-transferring speed resulted from the unique interaction between liquid metal and the external electric field.

Such electrolytes can be used to culture tumor cells with different exposure durations and adopted MTT assay to test the cytotoxicity. These reagents were considered to exhibit distinct cell destruction function and the cell toxicity is stronger with longer exposure time (Fig. 8.11f, g, h). In all, the liquid metal group had significantly high cytotoxicity in both ends. In both Hank's solution and PBS solution, the cathode had relatively strong cell damage effect than the anode and the cell damage ratio increased with the culture time in both electrodes. However, the cathodic electrolyte of liquid metal group had phenomenal cytotoxicity that 30 min culture of tumor cells in the Hank's electrolysis is enough to kill all the cells to death, while the cell lethality was only 42.271% in platinum group. However, in PBS solution, short time culture of tumor cells in electrolyte of liquid metal group significantly reduced the cell viability to 0 and 0.04 ± 0.04 in cathode and anode respectively compared to 0.15 ± 0.05 and 0.46 ± 0.09 in platinum group attributed to the accelerated electrochemical reaction efficiency by liquid metal. To further understand the mechanism of tumor destruction of EChT, the Annexin V-APC and PI apoptosis detection was performed to evaluate the apoptosis level induced by these electrolytes. The flow cytometry was utilized to determine the proportion of viable cells (both Annexin V and PI negative, bottom left, Q3), early apoptosis (only Annexin V positive, bottom right, Q4), late apoptosis (both Annexin V and PI positive, up right, Q2) and necrosis (only PI positive, Q1). The representative flow cytometry data were shown in Fig. 8.11i. 10 min culture of the cathodic electrolyte and 45 min culture of the anodic electrolyte of PBS solutions significantly destroyed the tumor cells in both groups.

The proportion of early and late apoptosis in EChT_LM group is more than two and a half times than that in EChT_Pt group (Fig. 8.13), which was in good agreement with the MTT test.

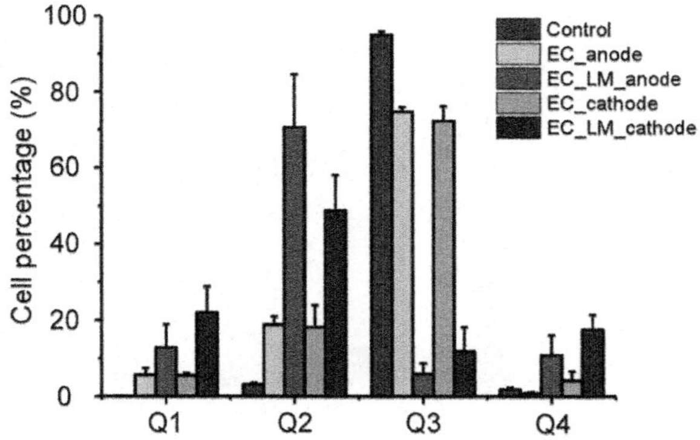

Fig. 8.13 Cell percentage analysis of flow cytometry data [40]. Tumor cells were cultured in the cathodic and anodic electrolysis of PBS solution for 10 and 45 min respectively then stained with Annexin V-APC and PI. Q1 represented the part of necrosis cells. Q2 represented the cell of late apoptosis cells. Q3 represented the percentage of live cells. Q4 represented the percentage of early apoptosis cells. All pictures reproduced with permission

The electrolyte of the common physiological solution was determined to exhibit higher cell destruction effect, where all the cells were killed within 10 min cell culture. The cytotoxicity of the electrolysis from Tyrode solution and cell culture medium were also tested (Figs. 8.14 and 8.15). Positive relationship was found between the final pH value and the cytotoxicity under short time exposure. This is the first ever time to obtain the quantitative relationship of cell viability with separate electrolysis products via liquid metal soft electrodes or inert platinum electrodes.

In order to exclude the influence factor of the surface areas, the Pt electrodes can be artificially fabricated with almost identical surface area by adding a platinum plate with a radius of 4 mm (Fig. 8.16a). The current from liquid metal groups was more than 2-fold bigger than its identical counterpart Pt electrode group. The pH change also shows a 4-fold bigger in the anode (Fig. 8.16c). The electrolysis from liquid metal group exhibits a stronger toxicity (Fig. 8.16d). So other than the surface area, the liquid metal material itself accounts for this unique phenomenon.

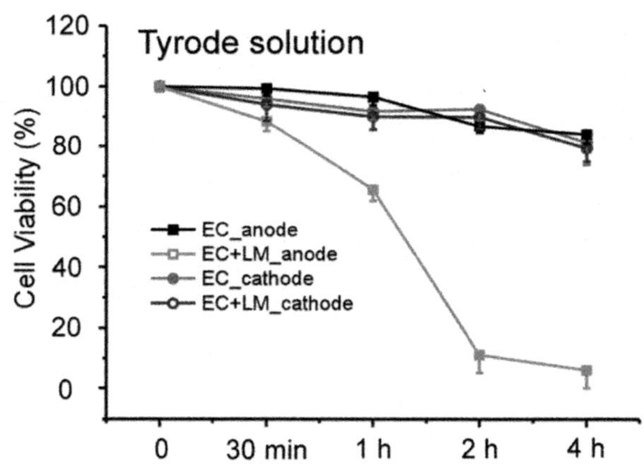

Fig. 8.14 Cell viability of exposure to electrolysis of Tyrode solution [40]. Picture reproduced with permission

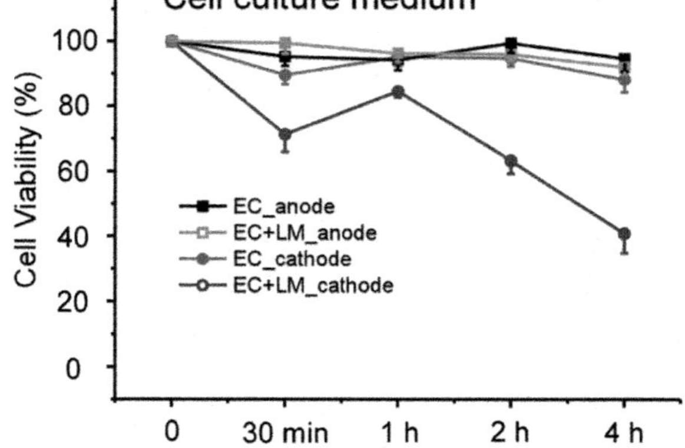

Fig. 8.15 Cell viability of exposure to electrolysis of cell culture medium [40]. Picture reproduced with permission

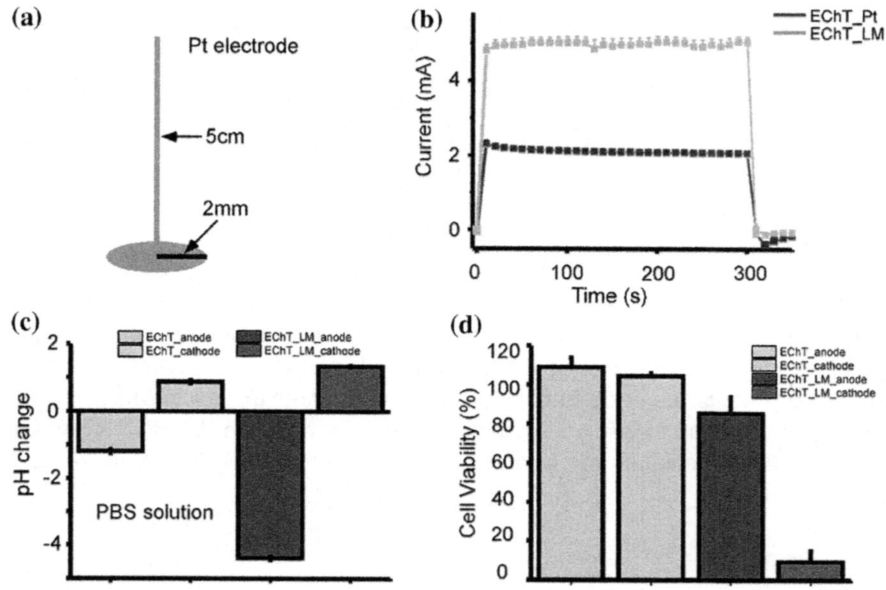

Fig. 8.16 EChT effect comparison between Pt electrode and liquid metal electrode under the same surface area [40]. **a** Pt electrode with identical surface area to liquid metal electrode. **b** The average current under external 5 V. **c** pH change with different electrolysis. **d** Cell cytotoxicity from these different electrolysis. EChT_anode, EChT_cathode, EChT_LM_anode, EChT_LM_cathode stands for electrolysis from either anode or cathode with Pt electrodes or liquid metal electrodes respectively. All pictures reproduced with permission

What's more, compared to the inert electrode, the formation and depletion of oxide on liquid metal surface would cause ions to dissolve into the electrolyte. The results from the ICP-MS demonstrate that the anodic electrolysis would dissolve almost 76 times of gallium and more than 8.8 times of In than that of cathode. A small amount of gallium and indium was also detected in the intracellular area (Table 8.1). The Indium compounds were considered to cause lung lesions on animals. Exposure to InAs (7.7 mg/kg) and InP (3 mg/kg) was discovered to cause

Table 8.1 Concentration of gallium and indium in the anodic and cathodic electrolysis

	Concentration of the electrolysis after 5 V 5 min stimulation		Intracellular ion concentration after a certain time of cultivation			
	Cathode (μg/mL)	Anode (μg/mL)	Cathode (1 h) (ng/mL)	Anode (1 h) (μg/mL)	Cathode (30 min) (ng/mL)	Anode (30 min) (μg/mL)
Ga	2.925	222.1	48.62	8.924	46.97	1.996
In	5.382	47.74	62.73	0.3659	13.69	0.06403

inflammatory response as well as body weight loss, while this electrochemically induced dissolution may cause further destructive effect to tumor cells.

Previous studies have shown dispute conclusions towards whether anode or cathode would have pronounced power of tumor collapse [68, 69]. The above results with quantitative analysis could partly explain such phenomenon. The microenvironment and surrounding ingredient varies a lot to different tumor types or even the same kind formed close to different organs or regions. It is possible that cytotoxicity of the electrolysis products varies when facing different kinds of malignance. At the same time, electrolysis products with different degrees of toxicity were generated from different tumor types or around different electrodes of the same tumor. On the other hand, malignant tumors of various toxic tolerances make them exhibit varying degrees of lesions. Thus it is plausible that anode or cathode displayed stronger tumor destruction power in different malignance. Moreover, the compositions of the electrolyte reveal a strong influence with the effectiveness of EChT, in which amounts of chloride containing and buffered ions lead to better treatment effect.

8.11 Shape Influence of Liquid Metal Electrode on EChT Efficiency

The inherent flexibility and plasticity of liquid metal electrodes serve as unique superiority compared to the complicated fabrication process by other inert electrodes. The conformability to any complex surface and its fast fabrication merits to any forms just by injection make it possible to simply accomplish any shapes of electrodes in two or even three dimensions [56]. To further explore the influence of the electrode shape on the effect of EChT, Sun et al. [40] designed several molds as container of liquid metal, including 90° annulus, 120° annulus, full circle annulus and a special S shape mold (Fig. 8.6b–e). Different shapes of liquid metal electrodes could be obtained via simple injection by syringe. Through arrangement and combination, they achieved five kinds of treatments as shown in Fig. 8.17a, b. Upon the same treatment of EChT to a certain number of cells through different electrode arrays, the cell EChT effect was compared within groups. The cell destruction effect varies with the electrode shapes. One could easily achieve better performance of EChT by changing the shape of liquid metal through injection. Specifically, the similar cell viability is resulted from the three electrode configurations of the S shape group and the two electrodes configuration of the O shape group, indicating similar therapeutic effect. From the above result, one could completely achieve similar or even better results via the way of transforming liquid metal electrode morphology, which would offer huge benefit to patient of EChT.

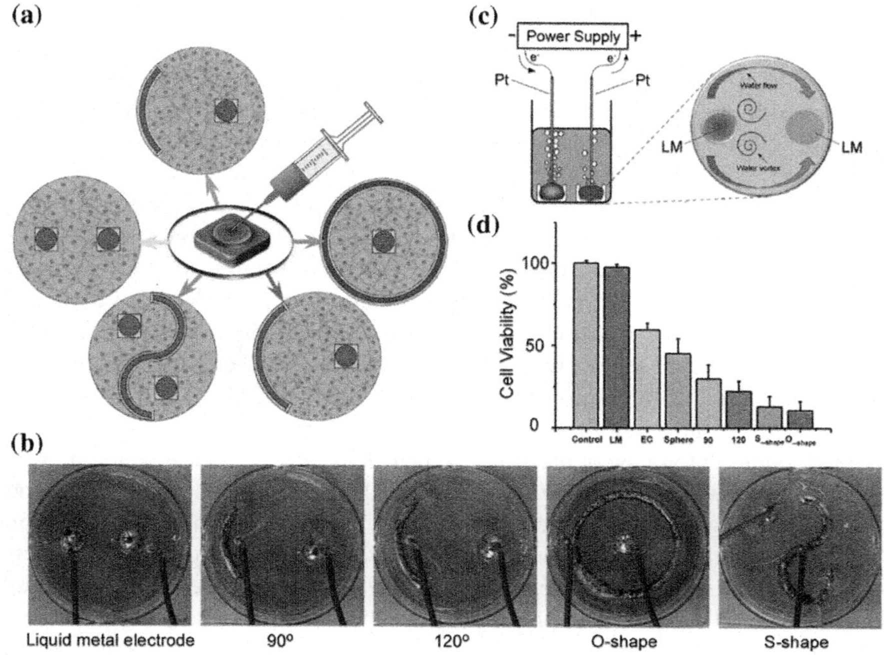

Fig. 8.17 Transformed liquid metal electrodes enhanced the efficiency of EChT [40]. **a** Five therapeutic method configurations of liquid metal electrode in different shapes. **b** The snapshots at 200 s during EChT under the external voltage of 5 V with different electrode shapes, from left to right are small bowl, 90° annulus, 120° annulus, full circle annulus and S shape electrodes, which were simplified as sphere, 90, 120, O_shape and S_shape respectively. **c** The schematic water flow and water vortex induced by liquid metal under electric field. **d** The cell viability of EChT under different configurations of liquid metal electrodes. The cells were cultured for another 2 h after EChT. All pictures reproduced with permission

8.12 Animal Tests on Antitumor Efficacy of EChT with Liquid Metal Electrode

The antitumor efficacy of EChT through liquid metal electrode was further assessed in the tumor-bearing mice [40]. When direct current flows through the tumor tissue, EChT will produce electrolysis, electroosmosis and electrophoresis effects. Under the electrolysis, EChT produces chlorine and hydrion in the anode along with excitant gas in the air, and hydrogen and hydroxyl in the cathode. Serve pH change would cause tumor cells to death.

In addition, the water molecular flows from anode to cathode causing dehydration in anode and edema in cathode and further changing the microenvironment in tumors. What's more, under the electric field force, big molecules movement from cathode to anode leads to denaturation and coagulation of proteins. Moreover, due to the electrolysis and electroosmosis, ionic concentration change outside the cell membrane became another favorable factor to destruct tumor cells. All nude mice completed the experiments and none died due to the anaesthesia or the procedure of EChT. No significant change of mice body weights was observed after the treatment (Fig. 8.18). The EChT therapy with either platinum or liquid metal electrode displayed remarkably higher melanoma tumor growth retardation as compared to the control group (Figs. 8.19a, and 8.20). Particularly, in EChT_LM group, all the tumors were effectively ablated at the first five days after the EChT therapy, which shows a noticeable difference from the EChT_Pt group, where the incomplete tumor regression is obvious, further demonstrating the advantage of liquid metal electrode. No complete regression of tumors was observed in the EChT_Pt group after the therapy mainly because of the big volume of tumor. In addition, obvious life spans prolongation associated with the tumor growth inhibition were obtained in both of the EChT groups (Fig. 8.19d). Liquid metal electrode attached to the tumor surface connected with the anode, while the cathode was inserted to the central area of the tumor. When charged with 15 V direct voltage to the local tumor, the impedance was smaller and the current was bigger in the liquid metal group (Fig. 8.21). The recorded current showed an exponential decrease in both experimental groups. A typical acidity excitant smell was produced in less than 1 min and gas formation was also observed in both of the anode and the cathode. The cathodic showed phenomenal edema while the anodic lesion became hard and firm during the procedure. The first day after EChT, the solid tumor tissue was almost eliminated, while the lesion remained edematous. After two to three days, black scars were left at the tumor sites (Fig. 8.20). The complete inhibition of tumor in the EChT_LM group was obvious as compared to the EChT_Pt group at the sixth day after therapy, where obvious recurrences of tumor were seen in the platinum group (Fig. 8.19b). The survival time of the control group was

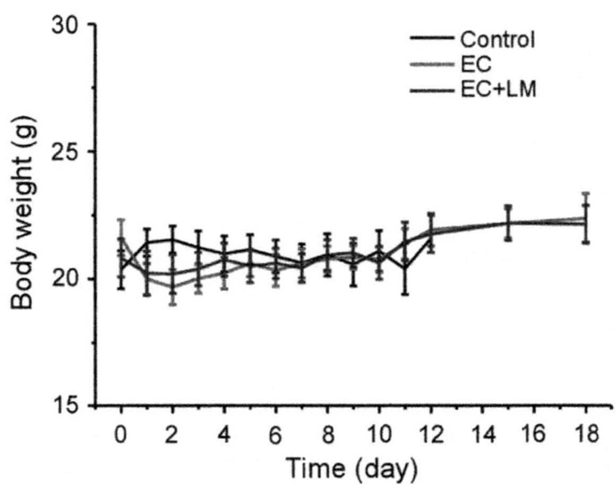

Fig. 8.18 The change of body weight of tumor-bearing mice in different groups after treatment [40]. Picture reproduced with permission

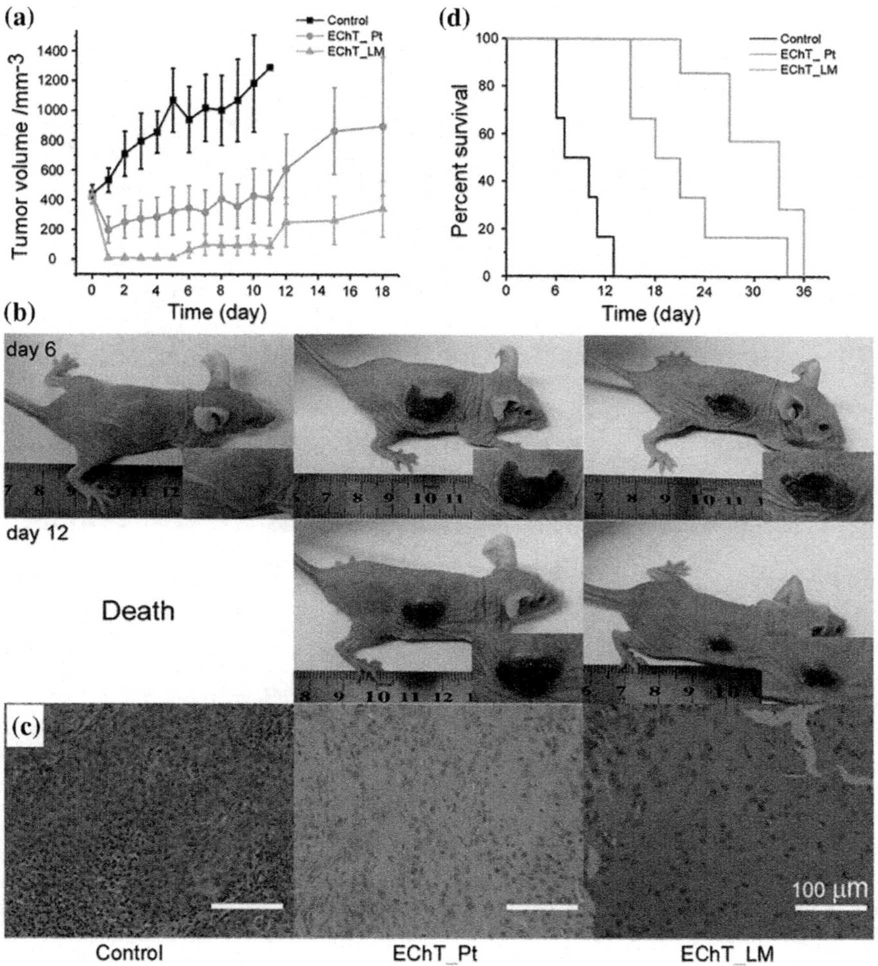

Fig. 8.19 The antitumor efficacy of EChT with liquid metal electrode [40]. **a** Tumor growth curves of different groups of melanin tumor-bearing mice. **b** The 6th (upper) and 12th (lower) days photograph of melanin tumor-bearing mice after treatments. **c** HE stained tumor slices from different groups after EChT. From left to right, control, EChT_Pt, EChT_LM group respectively. **d** Survival curves of melanin tumor-bearing mice after EChT. Error bars indicate s.e.m for control group (n = 6), EChT_Pt group (n = 6), EChT_LM group (n = 7). All pictures reproduced with permission

8.8 ± 1.2 days. In contrast, the EChT_LM group prolonged the survival time to 29.1 ± 1.9 days, which is much higher than that (21.2 ± 2.9) of EChT_Pt group. EChT_LM group showed significant life spans prolongation of mice. The histological images using haematoxylin and eosin staining (Fig. 8.19c) indicated

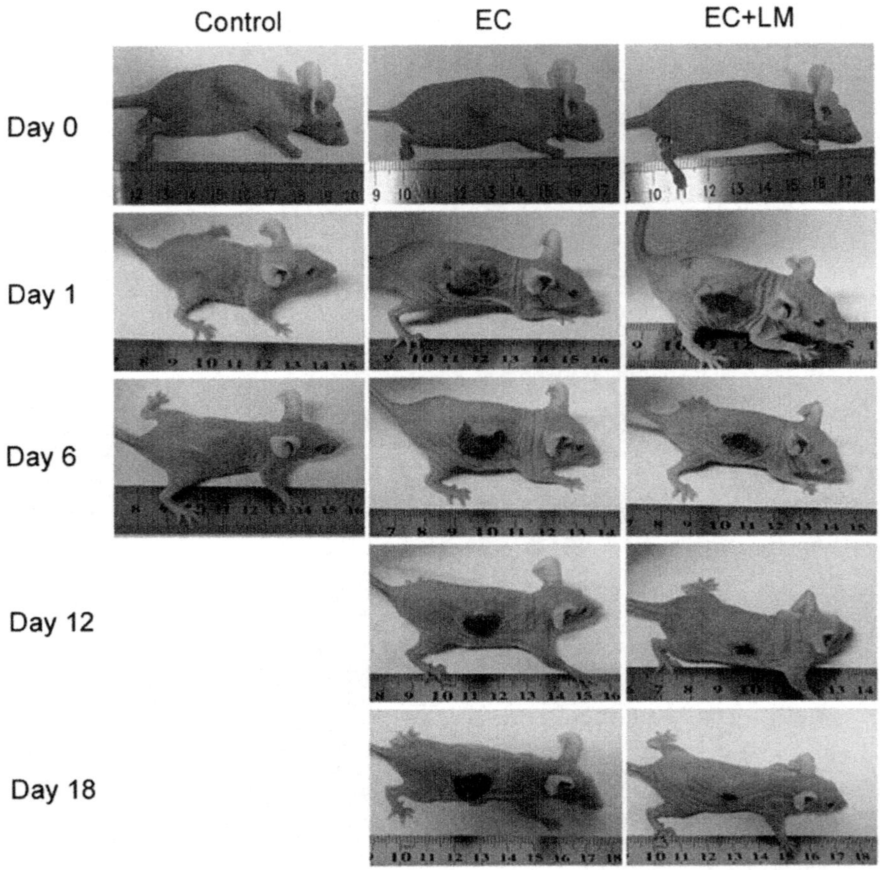

Fig. 8.20 EChT in vivo. Representative photos of tumor-bearing mice for different groups [40]. EChT_LM group showed significant tumor growth suppression. Picture reproduced with permission

obvious cancer cell remission in both groups. However, the delivered coulomb dose from the EChT_LM is lower than the EChT_Pt group (Fig. 8.22), which is probably associated with the way of electric delivery and demonstrating the unique advantage of liquid metal in tumor destruction with low dose therapy. Collectively, these results demonstrated that EChT with liquid metal electrode not only inhibited the tumor growth but also prolonged the life span, which is very effective for EChT of tumors in vivo.

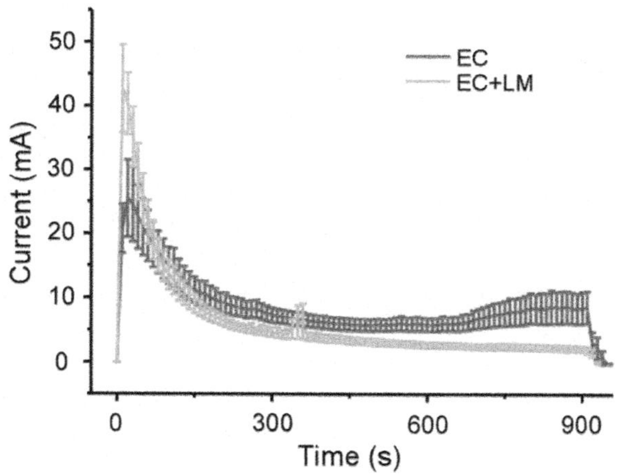

Fig. 8.21 The average current stimulation for EChT_Pt and EChT_LM groups [40]. The current was recorded continuously when stimulated with 15 V voltage for 15 min.
Picture reproduced with permission

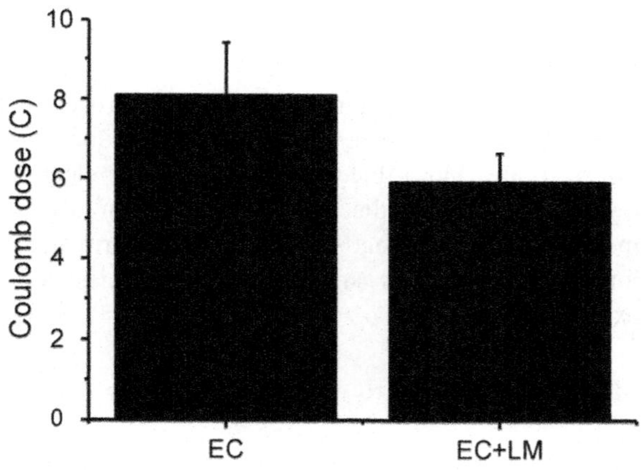

Fig. 8.22 The coulomb dose for EChT and EChT_LM groups [40].
Picture reproduced with permission

8.13 Prospects of Injectable Liquid Metal Soft Electronics in EChT

Electrodes and electronics as smart biomedical electronic materials are extremely important in electric and electrochemical stimulator fields to treat various disorders. Clearly, metals with high conductivity as well as other newly emerging organic polymers with novel characteristics are critical to deliver constant current or couples of electric pulses. However, limitations of those highly conductive metal materials are also evident, such as poor elasticity, low reconfigurability and difficult fabrications etc. These restrict their flexible applications in conformable clinical use. Graphene, carbon nanotube, carbon fiber and various carbon-based materials have excellent physical properties and possess basic flexible and easy-processing merits.

When combined with other nanomaterials, its conductivity is highly increased. However, the conductivity of those carbon-based materials is still 100–1000 times less than their metal counterparty. As an alternative, liquid metal integrates advantages of metal and non-metal materials together with both high conductivity and natural soft traits which is molding it as wonderful biomedical injectable soft electronics medium. For illustration purpose, a schematic description of the conceptual applications of such injectable liquid metal can be depicted in Fig. 8.23. To substitute surgical operation, this flexible liquid metal electrode could be easily injected and filled to the intestinal neoplasms parts, then linked to the outside power through two flexible liquid metal wires. The wires are also composed of soft robber hose filled with liquid metal to make up a whole flexible system. Under the stimulation of the power, hydrion and hydroxyl would be produced around anode and cathode respectively. Damage of the plasma membrane would further cause about tumor cells apoptosis and necrosis. What's more, through multi-injections, liquid metal soft electronics could be distributed in the solid tumors, such as lung cancer, for further electric or electrochemical treatments. For tumors of digestive organs like stomach or intestine, the flexible liquid metal could also flexibly stick to the inner surface of the tissue to perform individualized electrochemical treatment that a conventional electrode is hard to approach. Through injection, liquid metal flows with the blood stream to the lesion location to impose electric fields on diseased site. Multi-injections with the soft electronics provide new modality to regulate and adjust the electric distribution of those malignant carcinoma and metastatic tumors. What's more, better performance in the combined application of injectable electronics and dermal electronics for tumor therapy can also be expected.

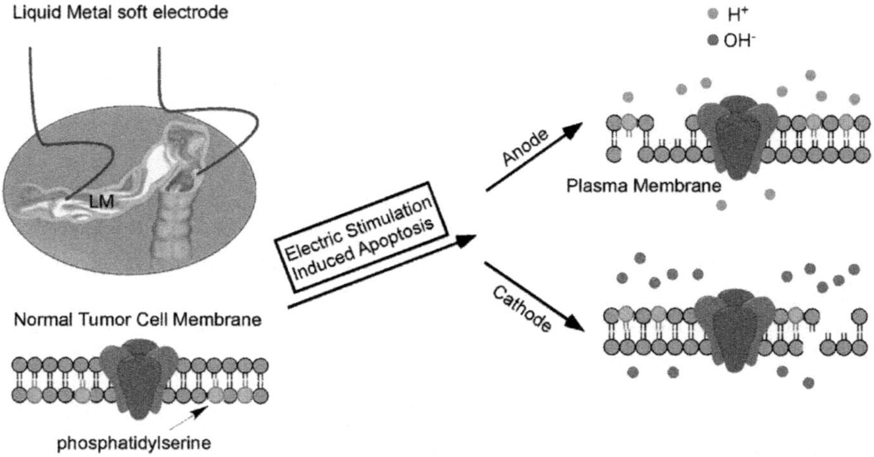

Fig. 8.23 A schematic illustration of the conceptual application and the mechanism induced by injectable liquid metal soft electronics in EChT [40]. Picture reproduced with permission

8.14 Liquid Metal Enabled Electrobiology Towards Generalized Health Care

Except for the above illustrated cases, liquid metal electronics can in fact play more roles in a wide range of disease therapy category and health care issues. It is based on this consideration, we had ever proposed a generalized biomedical strategy which can be termed as liquid metal enabled electrobiology [74]. This easy going way is based on the physiological fact that specially administrated electricity would induce a series of subsequent desired biological effects, either shortly, transitional or permanently. Just as explained before, owing high compliance within any part of the biological tissues, the liquid metal would aid to mold a pervasive way to treat various physiological or psychological diseases. As highly conductive, printable or injectable and non-toxic multifunctional flexible materials, such liquid metals (LMs) consist of the core to generate any requested electric treating fields (ETFields) which can adapt to various sites of the human body. From this way, a group of typical disease challenges can be tackled by liquid metal electrobiology, which include but are not limited to: tissue electronics enhancement, brain disorder repairing, immunotherapy, neural functional recovery, muscle stimulation, skin rejuvenation, improved cosmetology and dieting, serving as artificial organs, cardiac pacing and cancer therapy including psychological interpretation etc. Readers are referred to [74] for more detailed discussion.

8.15 Conclusion

So far, the liquid metal based injectable or implantable medical electronics has been established on principle stage. Nevertheless, more fundamental and practical investigations are still urgently needed along this direction. The liquid metal as electrode displays outstanding characteristics of electrical conductivity, easy operation and low cost. Meanwhile, gelatin meets the requirements of packaging materials for liquid metal. Both liquid metal and gelatin materials are liquid at body temperature, which enables the injectability of such implantable system. The advantages of injectability are evident, such as reducing the difficult in surgery, optimizing the size of incision and improving the recovery effect. Remarkably, the extraction of electrodes may be easily operated by syringe or self-priming pump under the guidance of medical image system. Moreover, liquid metal electrode and gelatin packaging materials are soft, enhancing the comfortability of medical device inside the body, thus lightening the physical pain and emotional stress to patients. Such features overcome the challenges of traditional materials as mentioned above.

The currently performed experiments have proven the feasibility of injectable liquid metal electrodes no matter in vitro or in vivo. It provides the basis for further research advancing the development. Meanwhile, it should also be noted that the accuracy and effect can be significantly promoted by practicing or using mechanizing the injection and fabrication methods.

Notably, safety is an important concern of implantable medical devices. In previous chapter, the biocompatibility of liquid metal has been discussed. However, more experiments should be implemented for further confirmation according to ISO standards. Besides, packaging material plays a role in isolating electrode from tissues. Therefore, the biocompatibility of injectable electrode system mainly depends on the performance of packaging materials. As is well known, gelatin is a commonly used biocompatible material with biodegradability. It can be concluded that the biocompatibility will not become a safety problem of the biological body within injected liquid metal electrode.

Moreover, liquid metal demonstrates high contrast in biological tissue by X ray imaging. In contrast to some typical metals, liquid metal material based on Ga, In and Sn also behaves non-magnetic which is capable of imaging under MRI (Magnetic Resonance Imaging). This provides flexible choices for the practices of medical examination.

Overall, a fundamentally innovative method has been established for directly making 3-D compliant medical electronics inside the biological tissues through direct injection of liquid metal and the allied packaging material to the target area. Different from the conventional surgical principles, such injected fabrication technique opens the way for minimally invasive medical implantation. Both in vitro tissue and in vivo animal experiments provide strong evidences for the excellent performances of the injectable electrodes. In addition, the formed liquid metal electrode can serve as highly efficient ECG electrode and stimulator electrode. These findings clarified the unique features and practicability of the implantable liquid metal electronics. This strategy provides the way for directly manufacturing electrophysiological sensors or therapeutic devices in situ via a truly minimally invasive approach and offers new understandings on biomedical transplantation science, which is expected to be well adopted for future research and practices.

With respect to injectable electrodes, there are various kinds of liquid metals composed of different elements for selection. Thus, more investigations should be carried out to explore distinctive characteristics of these liquid metals for diverse purposes, such as monitoring or diagnosis in different targets in vivo. Considering packaging materials, their solidification has evident influence on performance of the injected electrode. The packaging material used for liquid metal, i.e. gelatin is one kind material which satisfies the basic requirements. Notably, gelatin is degradable which can be utilized for short term use [70]. Abundant materials have been validated available as packaging materials. Besides gelatin, some other materials can be attempts as packaging materials for liquid metal to achieve different effects. For example, chemically crosslinking gelatin (e.g. mixed with genipin) takes a longer time than gelatin to degrade [71–73]. Such material will remain in body in a period of time for a longer term use. Additionally, the fabrication method can be effectively improved through adopting special tools and normalized manufacture. An injector with two-layer concentric circles structure can be designed to simultaneously inject liquid metal and packaging material into target area. The operation of injector can be controlled by program and mechanical device, which will guarantee the machining accuracy of electrodes. Overall, the injectable liquid metal electronic system is promising in refreshing the implantable medical devices, meanwhile, related study on this basis will be widely conducted.

Further, except for the utilization as pure liquid electrode, the liquid metals have also been found as new conceptual electric stimulation modality for tumour therapy through introducing the injectable liquid metal electrode with both extraordinary soft nature and high conductivity together. By means of the unique virtues of such biomedical materials such as being directly injectable, flexible and deformable, it enables the electrodes to realize various desirable configurations, two or even three dimensions, which will help them to conformably attach to the irregular tumor surfaces or any shapes of cavity like stomach, colon or rectum. This would help administrate a highly efficient electric stimulation and adjust expected electric distribution. Aided with the current platform, the liquid metal electrodes have been demonstrated to achieve enhanced tumor destruction effect compared to traditional platinum electrodes. It also clarified via a quantitative way that anode and cathode of the liquid metal electrodes produced more electrochemical products to tumors which is beneficial for treatment purpose. The recorded current from liquid metal group is almost twice as that with platinum under the same voltage. Further, one can attribute the promising performance of the liquid metal to its unique interaction with the external electric field in which such material works as a highly conductive electrode over the electrochemical reaction. Through changing shapes of the liquid metal, the new therapy can easily obtain better output than that with three electrodes, indicating the possibility of decreasing electrode number with liquid metal. Moreover, obvious tumor growth regressions and life spans prolongation were achieved in vivo with liquid metal electrode which promises the future of the present strategy. Without any doubt, the injectable liquid metal electrodes enabled conformable electrochemical treatment of tumor is expected to play an ever important role for better relieving of patients' pain in the coming time.

References

1. Kim DH, Viventi J, Amsden JJ et al (2010) Dissolvable films of silk fibroin for ultrathin conformal bio-integrated electronics. Nat Mater 9(6):511–517
2. Jiang G, Zhou DD (2010) Technology advances and challenges in hermetic packaging for implantable medical devices. In: Implantable neural prostheses 2: techniques and engineering approaches. Springer, Berlin, pp 28–61
3. Bazaka K, Jacob MV (2013) Implantable devices: issues and challenges. Electronics 2(1):1–34
4. ISO 13485 (2003) Medical devices-quality management systems-requirements for regulatory purposes. Geneva, Switzerland. http://www.iso.org/iso/catalogue_detail?csnumber=36786
5. Viventi J, Kim DH, Moss JD et al (2010) A conformal, bio-interfaced class of silicon electronics for mapping cardiac electrophysiology. Sci Transl Med 2(24):24ra22
6. Kim DH, Ahn JH, Choi WM et al (2008) Strechable and foldable silicon integrated circuits. Science 320(5875):507–511

7. Irnich W (2002) Electronic security systems and active implantable medical devices. Pacing Clin Electrophysiol Pace 25(8):1235–1258
8. Adunka O, Kiefer J, Unkelbach MH et al (2010) Development and evaluation of an improved cochlear implant electrode design for electric acoustic stimulation. Laryngoscope 114 (114):1237–1241
9. Halperin D, Heydt-Benjamin TS, Fu K et al (2008) Security and privacy for implantable medical devices. Pervasive Comput 7:30–39
10. Grill WM, Norman SE, Bellamkonda RV (2009) Implanted neural interfaces: biochallenges and engineered solutions. Annu Rev Biomed Eng 11(11):1–24
11. Fountas KN, Kapsalaki E, Hadjigeorgiou G (2010) Cerebellar stimulation in the management of medically intractable epilepsy: a systematic and critical review. Neurosurg Focus 29(2):E8
12. Zrenner E (2002) Will retinal implants restore vision? Science 295(5557):1022–1025
13. Magjarević R, Ferekpetrić B (2010) Implantable cardiac pacemakers-50 years from the first implantation. Zdravniški Vestnik 79(1):55–67
14. Gelinck GH, Huitema HEA, Veenendaal EV et al (2004) Flexible active-matrix displays and shift registers based on solution-processed organic transistors. Nat Mat 3(2):106–110
15. Onuki Y, Bhardwaj U, Papadimitrakopoulos F et al (2008) A review of the biocompatibility of implantable devices: current challenges to overcome foreign body response. J Diab Sci Technol 2(6):1003–1015
16. Cameron T, Liinamaa TL, Loeb GE et al (1998) Long-term biocompatibility of a miniature stimulator implanted in feline hind limb muscles. IEEE Trans Biomed Eng 45(8):1024–1035
17. Williams DF (2008) On the mechanisms of biocompatibility. Biomaterials 29(20):2941–2953
18. International Organization for Standardization ISO 10993. Biological evaluation of medical devices. Part 1: evaluation and testing within a risk management process. Geneva: ISO, 2009
19. Joung YH (2013) Development of implantable medical devices: from an engineering perspective. Int Neurourol J 17(3):98–106
20. Thomas RW (1976) Moisture, myths, and microcircuits. IEEE Trans Parts Hybrids Packag 12 (3):167–171
21. Chlebowski AL, Chow EY, Ellison C et al (2012) Integrated LTCC packaging for use in biomedical devices. Biomed Mater Eng 22(6):361–372
22. Kim SJ, Lee DS, Kim IG et al (2012) Evaluation of the biocompatibility of a coating material for an implantable bladder volume sensor. Kaohsiung J Med Sci 28(3):123–129
23. Chen GQ (2011) Biofunctionalization of polymers and their applications. Adv Biochem Eng Biotechnol 125(125):29–45
24. Guenther T, Dodds CWD, Lovell NH et al. (2011) Chip-scale hermetic feedthroughs for implantable bionics. In: International Conference of the IEEE Engineering in Medicine and Biology Society. IEEE, pp 6717–6720
25. Qin Y, Howlader MMR, Deen MJ et al (2014) Polymer integration for packaging of implantable sensors. Sens Actuators B Chem 202(10):758–778
26. Hwang GT, Im D, Lee SE et al (2013) In vivo silicon-based flexible radio frequency integrated circuits monolithically encapsulated with biocompatible liquid crystal polymers. ACS Nano 7(5):4545–4553
27. Ha D, Kim BG, Lin TY et al. (2010) 3D packaging technique on liquid crystal polymer (LCP) for miniature wireless biomedical sensor. In: Microwave Symposium Digest. IEEE, pp 612–615
28. White TJ, Broer DJ (2015) Programmable and adaptive mechanics with liquid crystal polymer networks and elastomers. Nat Mater 14(11):1087
29. Kim S, Bhandari R, Klein M et al (2009) Integrated wireless neural interface based on the Utah electrode array. Biomed Microdevice 11(2):453–466
30. Ryu SI, Shenoy KV (2009) Human cortical prostheses: lost in translation? Neurosurg Focus 27(1):E5
31. Schalk G, Miller KJ, Anderson NR et al (2008) Two-dimensional movement control using electrocorticographic signals in humans. J Neural Eng 5(1):75

32. So JH, Thelen J, Qusba A et al (2009) Reversibly deformable and mechanically tunable fluidic antennas. Adv Func Mater 19(22):3632–3637
33. Zhang Q, Zheng Y, Liu J (2012) Direct writing of electronics based on alloy and metal (DREAM) ink: a newly emerging area and its impact on energy, environment and health sciences. Front Energy 6(4):311–340
34. Zheng Y, He Z, Gao Y et al (2013) Direct desktop printedcircuits—on-paper flexible electronics. Sci Rep 3(5):759–762
35. Wang L, Liu J (2014) Compatible hybrid 3D printing of metal and nonmetal inks for direct manufacture of end functional devices. Sci China Technol Sci 57(11):2089–2095
36. Jin C, Zhang J, Li X et al (2013) Injectable 3-D fabrication of medical electronics at the target biological tissues. Sci Rep 3:3342
37. Butson CR, Maks CB, Mcintyre CC (2006) Sources and effects of electrode impedance during deep brain stimulation. Clin Neurophysiol 117(2):447
38. Chu V, Otero JM, Lopez O et al (2001) Method for non-invasively recording electrocardiograms in conscious mice. BMC Physiol 1(1):6
39. Salama G, London B (2007) Mouse models of long QT syndrome. J Physiol 578(1):43–53
40. Sun X, Yuan B, Rao W, Liu J (2017) Amorphous liquid metal electrodes enabled conformable electrochemical therapy of tumors. Biomaterials 146:156–167
41. Cabrales LB, Ciria HC, Bruzón RP et al (2001) Electrochemical treatment of mouse Ehrlich tumor with direct electric current. Bioelectromagnetics 22:316–322
42. Wemyss-Holden SA, Robertson GS, Dennison AR et al (2000) Electrochemical lesions in the rat liver support its potential for treatment of liver tumors. J Surg Res 93:55–62
43. Czymek R, Nassrallah J, Gebhard M et al (2012) Intrahepatic radiofrequency ablation versus electrochemical treatment in vivo. Surg Oncol 21:79–86
44. Keisari Y, Hochman I, Confino H, Korenstein R, Kelson I (2014) Activation of local and systemic anti-tumor immune responses by ablation of solid tumors with intratumoral electrochemical or alpha radiation treatments. Cancer Immunol Immunother 63:1–9
45. Nilsson E, von Euler H, Berendson J et al (2000) Electrochemical treatment of tumours. Bioelectrochemistry 51:1–11
46. Li K, Xin Y, Gu Y, Xu B, Fan D, Ni B (1997) Effects of direct current on dog liver: possible mechanisms for tumor electrochemical treatment. Bioelectromagnetics 18:2–7
47. Xin Y, Xue F, Ge B, Zhao F, Shi B, Zhang W (1997) Electrochemical treatment of lung cancer. Bioelectromagnetics 18:8–13
48. Li J, Xin Y, Fan X, Chen J, Wang J, Zhou J (2013) Effect of electrochemotherapy in treating patients with venous malformations. Chinese J integr Med 19:387–393
49. Yen Y, Li J, Zhou B, Rojas F, Yu J, Chou C (1999) Electrochemical treatment of human KB cells in vitro. Bioelectromagnetics 20:34–41
50. Nilsson E, Fontes E (2001) Mathematical modelling of physicochemical reactions and transport processes occurring around a platinum cathode during the electrochemical treatment of tumours. Bioelectrochemistry 53:213–224
51. Cury FL, Bhindi B, Rocha J et al (2015) Electrochemical red-ox therapy of prostate cancer in nude mice. Bioelectrochemistry 104:1–9
52. Belyy Y, Tereshchenko A, Shatskih A (2012) Electrochemical lysis of an intraocular tumour using a combination of electrode placements. Ecancermedicalscience 6:272
53. Czymek R, Dinter D, Löffler S et al (2011) Electrochemical treatment: An investigation of dose-response relationships using an isolated liver perfusion model. Saudi J Gastroenterol 17:335
54. Ren RL, Vora N, Yang F et al (2001) Variations of dose and electrode spacing for rat breast cancer electrochemical treatment. Bioelectromagnetics 22:205–211
55. von Euler H, Nilsson E, Olsson JM, Lagerstedt AS (2001) Electrochemical treatment (EChT) effects in rat mammary and liver tissue. In vivo optimizing of a dose-planning model for EChT of tumours. Bioelectrochemistry 54:117–124
56. Jin C, Zhang J, Li X, Yang X, Li J, Liu J (2013) Injectable 3-D fabrication of medical electronics at the target biological tissues. Sci Rep 3(6163):3442

57. Liu J, Fu TM, Cheng Z et al (2015) Syringe-injectable electronics. Nat Nanotechnol 10:629–636
58. Hong G, Fu TM, Zhou T, Schuhmann TG, Huang J, Lieber CM (2015) Syringe injectable electronics: Precise targeted delivery with quantitative input/output connectivity. Nano Lett 15:6979–6984
59. Kim DH, Lee Y (2015) Bioelectronics: injection and unfolding. Nat Nanotechnol 10:570–571
60. Sheng L, Zhang J, Liu J (2014) Diverse transformations of liquid metals between different morphologies. Adv Mater 26:6036–6042
61. Zhang J, Sheng L, Liu J (2014) Synthetically chemical-electrical mechanism for controlling large scale reversible deformation of liquid metal objects. Sci Rep 4:7116
62. Liu T, Sen P, Kim CJ (2012) Characterization of nontoxic liquid-metal alloy galinstan for applications in microdevices. J Microelectromech Syst 21:443–450
63. Saiz E, Tomsia AP (2004) Atomic dynamics and Marangoni films during liquid-metal spreading. Nat Mater 3:903–909
64. Zavabeti A, Daeneke T, Chrimes AF et al (2016) Ionic imbalance induced self-propulsion of liquid metals. Nat Commun 7:12402
65. Wójcicki M, Drozdzik M, Olewniczak S et al (2000) Antitumor effect of electrochemical therapy on transplantable mouse cancers. Med Sci Monit 6:498–502
66. Turk B, Bieth JG, Björk I et al (1995) Regulation of the activity of lysosomal cysteine proteinases by pH-induced inactivation and/or endogenous protein inhibitors, cystatins. Bio Chem Hoppe-Seyler 376:225–230
67. Kroemer G, Jäättelä M (2005) Lysosomes and autophagy in cell death control. Nat Rev Cancer 5:886
68. von Euler H, Olsson JM, Hultenby K, Thörne A, Lagerstedt AS (2003) Animal models for treatment of unresectable liver tumours: a histopathologic and ultra-structural study of cellular toxic changes after electrochemical treatment in rat and dog liver. Bioelectrochemistry 59:89–98
69. von Euler H, Stråhle K, Thörne A, Yongqing G (2004) Cell proliferation and apoptosis in rat mammary cancer after electrochemical treatment (EChT). Bioelectrochemistry 62:57–65
70. Ikada Y, Tabata Y (1998) Protein release from gelatin matrices. Adv Drug Deliv Rev 31 (3):287–301
71. Azab AK, Doviner V, Orkin B et al (2007) Biocompatibility evaluation of crosslinked chitosan hydrogels after subcutaneous and intraperitoneal implantation in the rat. J Biomed Mater Res, Part A 83(2):414–422
72. Muzzarelli RAA (2009) Genipin-crosslinked chitosan hydrogels as biomedical and pharmaceutical aids. Carbohyd Polym 77(1):1–9
73. Tan H, Li H, Rubin JP et al (2011) Controlled gelation and degradation rates of injectable hyaluronic acid-based hydrogels through a double crosslinking strategy. J Tissue Eng Regenerative Med 5(10):790–797
74. Wang X, Ren Y, Liu J (2018) Liquid metal enabled electrobiology: A generalized easy going way to tackle disease challenges. arXiv:1805.04002

Chapter 9
Liquid Metal as Electronic Medium to Recover Damaged Nerves' Function

Abstract Based on the favourable fluidity, super compliance and high electrical conductivity, liquid metal has been developed for nerve reconnection and repairing due to its owned similar electrical properties to nerve. This chapter explains the basic principle to mold liquid metal as an unconventional medium to help the injured nerve recover the ability to conduct electroneurographic signals. Conceptual experiments on both in vitro and in vivo transected sciatic nerves were given to illustrate the feasibility of liquid-metal based reconnection of damaged nerves.

Keywords Injectable electronics · Implantable medical electronics
Liquid metal · Nerve science

9.1 Introduction

The nervous system can be divided into central and peripheral nervous systems. Its basic functional and structural unit is neuron that plays a key role in message conduction. A neuron is composed of cell body, dendrites and axon (axon is also referred to as a nerve fibre). The nervous system is of great importance in sensing, such as visualizing, hearing, tasting, touching and sensing temperature and pressure. The complete nervous system guarantees the success of signal transmission and controls the activity and function of peripheral tissues and organs. For instance, sciatic nerves are responsible for the hamstring muscle group. The complete transection of such nerve would lead to loss of withdrawal reflex and complete paralysis below the stifle apart from certain sensation in the medial digit [1].

Nerves are subjected to various mechanical stresses all the time. Generally, these stresses cannot cause the nerve injury, unless their intensities exceed the maintenance stress range [2, 3]. Moreover, other factors such as gene mutation can affect the normal function of nerves as well. However, peripheral nerve injuries mainly result from accidents and surgery [4]. Such disease is the main reason contributing to the movement disorders, muscle atrophy, sensation damaged and neuropathic pain, thus life-long disability [5]. Conventional cases of peripheral nerve injury can

J. Liu and L. Yi, *Liquid Metal Biomaterials*,
Springer Series in Biomaterials Science and Engineering10,
https://doi.org/10.1007/978-981-10-5607-9_9

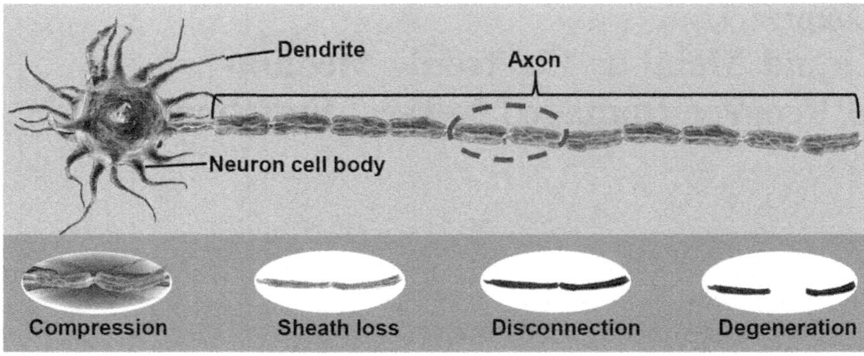

Fig. 9.1 A schematic description of different PNI cases. Nerve compression syndrome (compression neuropathy, entrapment neuropathy) is caused by direct pressure on a single nerve, producing symptoms such as pain, tingling, numbness, and muscle weakness; the process of sheath loss insulating nerves is demyelination, as the hallmark of some neurodegenerative autoimmune diseases; the disconnection refers to the blocking of neural signal circuit, with or without the physical cutting off; axons regenerating grows through an extracellular environment elaborated by glia cells and other nonneuronal cells of the nerve stump, along with Schwann cells proliferated [6]. Picture reproduced with permission

progress into four grades according to the severity of resulted functional loss, which are shown in Fig. 9.1 [6]. Similarly, many factors can cause sciatic nerve injuries including injections, femoral shaft fractures, hip fractures/dislocations, hip arthroplasty, contusions, gunshot wounds, lacerations, and compressions, and iatrogenic causes [7]. Some of the injured nerves are commonly unable to recover when they are completely severed. The extent of nerve injury and prognosis relies on the source of injury. In essence, nerve injuries were classified by Seddon into three categories, i.e. neurapraxia, axonotomesis, and neurotomesis based on the severity of the injury [8]. Thereinto, neurontmesis is the most severe peripheral nerve injury that describes the complete disruption status of nerve and connective tissue [9]. In this situation, surgery is required in an attempt to re-establish the continuity of the peripheral nerve due to the impossibility of nerve regeneration [10]. In the past, nerve repair is difficult to realize due to the deficient knowledge and technology. With the development of sciences and bioengineering, the management of these serious nerve injuries has been greatly improved.

9.2 General Principles

Tremendous efforts have been conducted to treat nervous diseases for decades. Rapid advances in the cognition on anatomy and pathophysiology of the peripheral nerve system, as well as innovations in microsurgical techniques and materials have greatly improved the patients' situation. So far, there are various methods investigated for repairing the transacted peripheral nerve. Typically, neurorrhaphy is a method commonly employed for suturing small nerve gap (less than 20 mm) [11]. Meanwhile, the injured nerve should be hardly contaminated and timely treated. However, for large defects, neurorrhaphy appears inadequate that excessive tension emerges over the repaired nerve resulting in neuralgia and neuroma [12, 13]. The infection and retraction of transected peripheral nerve stumps are main reasons for the increase of gap length. Under this situation, nerve transfer and nerve graft are utilized to solve the problem of longer gap in neurosurgery [14, 15]. Nerve autografting has been recognized as a current gold standard technology for repairing peripheral nerve injury [16]. Although in most clinical cases, nerve autografting is effective, its popularity is restricted by the limited donor graft, a secondary surgery to harvest graft tissue, significant donor site morbidity and short length of available graft resource [17]. Additionally, as an alternative, allograft technology makes use of cadaveric or donor nerve tissues to bridge larger nerve defects [18]. In general, patients treated with such surgery suffer systemic immunosuppression for more than 18 months and have risk of infections and tumor formation [19]. Moreover, nerve transfer operation is a graft-free intervention that connects the proximal nerve stump directly to target muscle belly [20, 21]. In comparison with neurorrhaphy and nerve graft, nerve transfer method shows poorer effects. Besides, nerve entubulation is a method implemented by inserting the nerve stumps into two ends of nerve guidance conduit full of protein-rich fluid and neurotrophic factors for nerve regeneration [22, 23]. There are several commercially available synthetic nerve conduits which have been approved by the U.S. FDA [24, 25]. Nevertheless, nerve disease remains a big challenge for both clinical practice and basic research so far. The effective method for repairing long gap cases is rather lacking, which should be developed with tremendous efforts.

9.3 Liquid Metal Materials as Nerve Signal Conduits

It is well known that the nervous system works depending on the transmission of electric current. The electrical signal alters through changing the concentration of ions including K^+, Na^+ and Ca^{2+}, which further causes the polarization or depolarization of the nerve axon, producing sudden and rapid sequence of induced voltage changes (action potential) [26]. For transected nerve, it loses the function of signal transmission. Thus, the gap should be bridged with electrically conductive material for the recovery of function.

As shown in the above chapters, liquid metal has been introduced with characteristics of outstanding electrical conductivity, excellent flexibility, good chemical stability and biocompatibility, which suggests its potential application in reconnection of transected nerve. For instance, GaInSn alloy composed of 67% Ga, 20.5% In, and 12.5% Sn (mass ratio) has low melting point of 10.5 °C. Thus, such alloy can keep liquid state in a broad temperature range, such as room temperature and body temperature. By virtue of this advantage, liquid metal presents good flexibility and stretchability, which probably display super compliant feature in vivo. Importantly, the electrical conductivity of GaInSn is 3.1×10^6 Sm^{-1} which is much higher than those of electrolyte solutions and non-metallic materials [27]. The high electrical conductivity may enable the conduction of weak electroneurographic signal. Meanwhile, the study has proven that the liquid metal can be directly printed on various materials by tuning its wettability, providing the basis for harmonious cooperation with nerve conduits [28]. In total, the application of liquid metal in nerve repair is valuable to be investigated.

9.4 Preparation of Liquid Metal for Nerve Medicine

With the gradual awareness of the importance of liquid metals, related studies have been rapidly developed in treatment of nerve diseases. Currently, liquid metals have been introduced by the present lab to repair the nerve neurotmesis of bullfrog [29] and mouse [6], which has attracted tremendous attentions throughout the world.

The physical properties of liquid metal are essential for the effect of nerve reconnection. Before the application in function recovery, the electrical characteristics of liquid metal were studied in comparison with Riger's solution [29]. The liquid metal employed was $Ga_{67}In_{20.5}Sn_{12.5}$ alloy. Due to the low melting point, such metal with low viscosity (2.98×10^{-7} m^2/s) displays good fluidity comparable to that of solution at body temperature. The resistance of the liquid metal and Riger's solution was measured by micro-ohmmeter at room temperature. The test samples of two materials were both prepared by being encapsulated in a glass capillary pipette with the length of 10 cm and diameter of 0.5 mm. Based on the measured data and the dimension of samples, the resistance of GaInSn is 4.396×10^{-8} Ω m which is several orders lower than that of Riger's solution (0.8709 Ω m). It demonstrates that GaInSn with low resistivity can perform well in electric conductivity.

Furthermore, the impedance was determined by the SRS Model SR780 2-Channel Network Signal Analyzer from 1 Hz to 1 kHz. The samples were encapsulated in a plastic tube with the length of 40 cm and diameter of 1 mm. Figure 9.2 shows that both the resistance and the reactance of the GaInSn alloy were much lower than those of Riger's solution. Generally, the frequencies of most

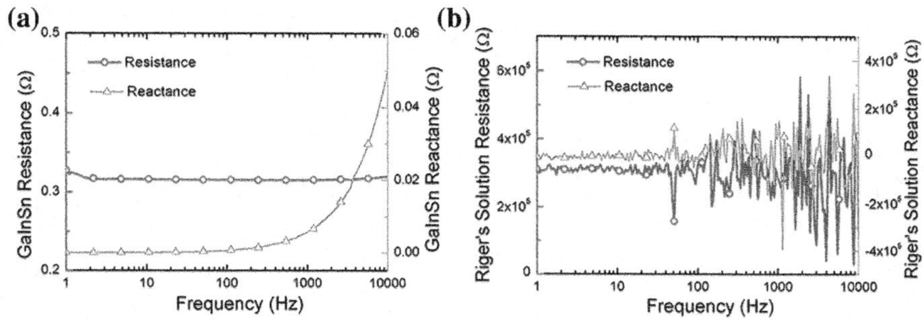

Fig. 9.2 The impedance of the applied liquid metal GaInSn alloy and Riger's Solution [29]. The resistance and reactance curve of the liquid metal (**a**) and Riger's Solution (**b**). All pictures reproduced with permission

electroneurographic signals are below 10 kHz. Thus, the impedance of GaInSn mainly depends on the resistance rather than reactance. According to the curves, the resistance of the GaInSn alloy (Fig. 9.2a) was relatively stable from 1 Hz to 10 kHz, which is obviously distinctive from that of Riger's solution (Fig. 9.2b). It implies that GaInSn alloy is capable of conducting dynamics signals stably compared with Riger's solution. As a kind of liquid metal, GaInSn alloy has embodied advantages in conducting electroneurographic signals, laying foundation for transmission of weak electroneurographic signals.

Moreover, gallium is another commonly used pure liquid metal which has been studied as efficient neural reconnection material. To validate the stability, its electrical properties were measured by micro-ohmmeter under different frequencies and temperatures (Fig. 9.3). It shows that the resistance of gallium sample is stabilized around 5.92 Ω at the frequency range from 1 Hz to 100 kHz (Fig. 9.3a). Meanwhile, its reactance is less than 0.1 Ω when the frequency is lower than 10 kHz, after that, its value increases to 0.84 Ω as the frequency arrives to 100 kHz. No matter resistance or reactance, both of them can remain stable during the frequency below 10 kHz within the working range of neural signals. In addition, Fig. 9.3b displays the performance of resistance of gallium under different temperatures within the range of human's activities. In the given temperature range from −16 °C up to 50 °C, the resistance of gallium samples maintained at 0.51 Ω. These results indicate that the electrical characteristics of gallium are stable which cannot be influenced by change of frequency and temperature in working range.

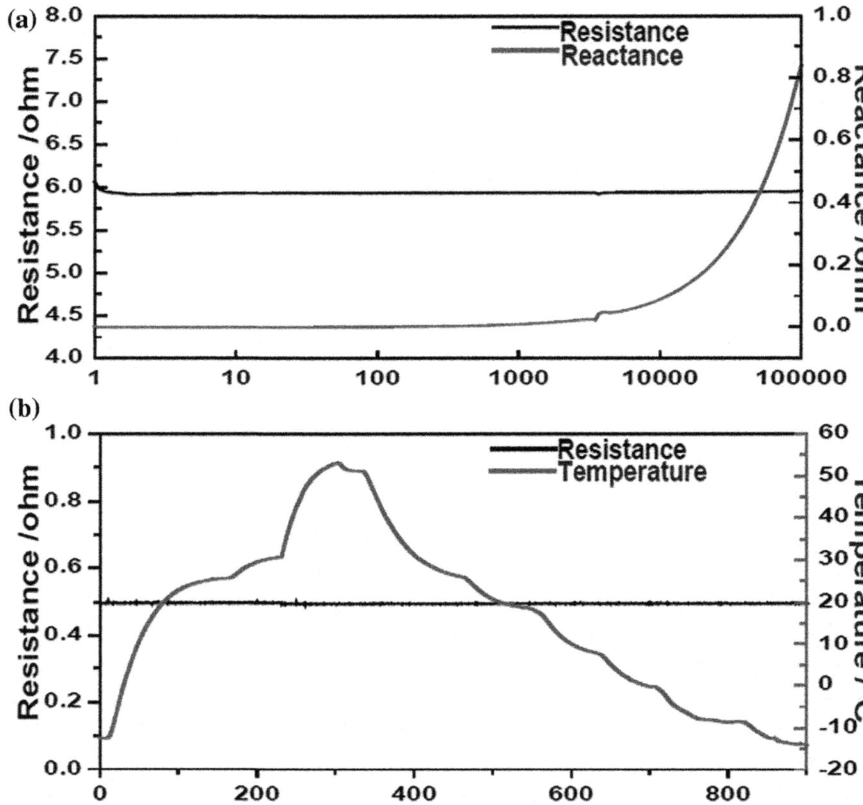

Fig. 9.3 Electrical properties of gallium [6]. **a** The impedance of gallium for signals at different frequencies. **b** The impedance of gallium under different temperatures. All pictures reproduced with permission

9.5 Electrical Reconnection of Bullfrog's Sciatic Nerve

9.5.1 Experimental Animal Model

The bullfrogs are common animal models for studying the function of sciatic nerve, due to their simple nervous structure and being easily available. Hence, GaInSn alloy and Riger's solution were utilized to test the reconnection effect of bullfrogs' sciatic nerve [29]. To expose the intact sciatic nerve with gastrocnemius attached, the double pithing method was carried out. Meanwhile, the extracted proximal sciatic nerve and gastrocnemius with distal sciatic nerve were immersed into Riger's solution to maintain activity (Fig. 9.4). For operation and observation convenience, the transected nerve covered with Riger's solution was placed on the glass slide. Then the nerve was totally transected by ophthalmic scissors. GaInSn alloy and Riger's solution filled in rectangular groove and glass capillary pipette

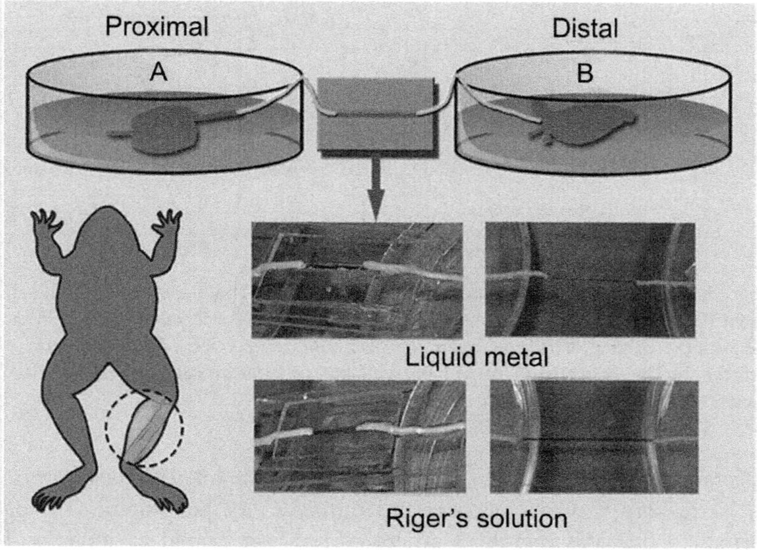

Fig. 9.4 The experimental setup of the transected sciatic nerve reconnected by liquid metal and Riger's Solution, respectively [29]. To improve the visualization, Riger's solution was dyed using red ink. All pictures reproduced with permission

were used to reconnect such transected sciatic nerve, respectively (Fig. 9.4). The dimensions of the transparent plastic groove were 10 mm (length) × 1 mm 0.5 mm. The length and diameter of capillary pipette were 3 cm and 0.5 mm, respectively. This experimental setup was established for the following electrophysiological stimulation.

9.5.2 *Electroneurographic Signal*

In neuroscience research, the electrophysiological stimulation is a typical method to study the nervous structure and function. On the basis of the prepared bullfrog's sciatic nerve, the voltage signal (wave form: square-wave, voltage amplitude: 0.2 V, frequency: 0.5 Hz, duty cycle: 20%) was applied to stimulate the proximal nerve [29]. For the sake of contrastive analysis, the experimental samples were divided into three groups: the intact nerve, the transected nerve reconnected by GaInSn alloy and Riger's solution filled in plastic groove. During the simulation, the innervated gastrocnemius was contracted in these situations. Meanwhile, the output results measured from the distal nerve by data acquisition device are shown in Fig. 9.5. The obtained electroneurographic signals reflected the compound nerve action potentials of various nerve fibers, which are different from that on the single nerve fiber. Therefore, the waveform was biphasic and displayed a positive phase

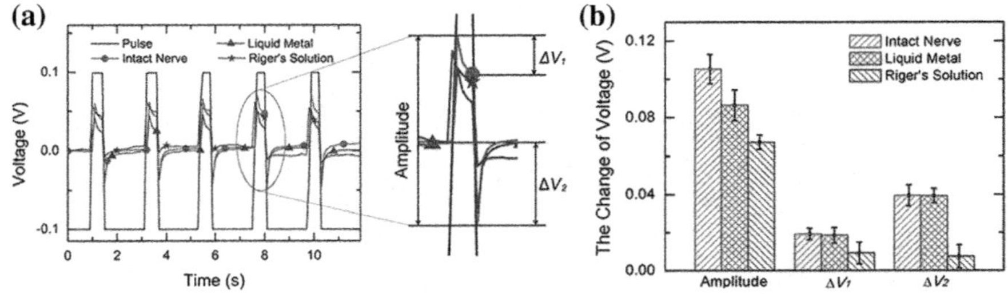

Fig. 9.5 The detection of electroneurographic signal [29]. **a** The electric-stimuli signal and the excitement signal from the intact nerve, the transected nerve reconnected by GaInSn or Riger's Solution with the volume of 10 mm × 1 mm × 0.5 mm, respectively. Amplified detail of partial view (right). **b** The comparison of voltage changes after electrical stimulation. All pictures reproduced with permission

and a negative phase. As shown in Fig. 9.5a, the stimulated signals in these three groups all display similar characteristics during every periodicity. The cause of similar parts is probably that these groups all use background solution, i.e. Riger's solution for maintaining the neuronal activity, whose signals may reflect the electric leakage of solution. Nevertheless, these curves were subtly different at the strategic locations. Obviously, such differences mainly focus on the amplitudes of the electroneurographic signals at peak (ΔV_1) and trough (ΔV_2) position. The differences could denote the action potentials of compound nerve which have been separated from the curves in Fig. 9.5a, see Fig. 9.5b. By contrast, electroneurographic signals of the nerve reconnected by liquid metal were more similar to those of intact nerve. In addition, the same performance was obtained when the liquid metal or Riger's Solution was encapsulated in a glass capillary pipette.

9.5.3 Radiograph of Liquid Metal Reconnection

Due to the high density of metal materials, liquid metals display excellent capabilities in radiological imaging. Thus, liquid metal within biological tissue can be clearly figured out, which have been applied as an efficient vascular contrast agent [30]. On this basis, GaInSn alloy has also been proven with favorable visibility in bullfrog under X-ray irradiation. From this point of view, liquid metal can be aspirated when cooperating with the biodegradable nerve conduits according to needs under the imaging guidance. Such operation can be minimally invasive which prevents the secondary surgery.

9.6 Reconnection of Mouse's Sciatic Nerve

Based on the study of nerve reconnection of bullfrog, another work has employed liquid metal to treat the transected nerve in mouse in vivo [6]. Such investigation on mammalian model would promote further research and application of liquid-metal-based neural reconnection technique in human body.

9.6.1 *Liquid Metal Based Reconnection*

To encapsulate the liquid metal for neural reconnection, gallium was injected into a silicone rubber tube (outer diameter of 1 mm, wall thickness of 0.3 mm and length of 1 cm) by a syringe. Then both ends in the tube were plugged up with 0.8 mm $25^{\#}$ stainless steel wire (diameter of 0.5 mm), preventing the leakage of liquid metal. Such liquid-metal-based tube was already prepared for treating the transaction of sciatic nerve in 8-week-old mouse. Specifically, the epineuriums of two exposed nerve stumps were sutured to each end of the prepared tube using 10-0 prolene suture line, thus the nerve defect was reconnected by gallium.

9.6.2 *Neurological Electrophysiology*

The reconnection effect was evaluated through the measurement of extracellular neural discharges. To achieve this goal, the stimulus signals (wave form: pulse wave; voltage amplitude: low 0 V and high 4 V; frequency: 1 Hz; duty cycle: 10%) were generated using an arbitrary function generator (Tektronix AFG3051C). The relevant electrodes were connected to the skin over gastrocnemius and the muscle dominated by the operated sciatic nerve. On the other hand, the signals from test sciatic nerve were transmitted by using silver-coated copper electrodes and recorded by data acquisition system (PowerLab). Figure 9.6 shows the recorded signals from sciatic nerve in several different situations. The mouse with intact nerve was set as control group. Figure 9.6a, b demonstrate the signal change of intact nerve without and with stimulus, respectively. Obviously, the neural signals in the resting state remained steady at 0 V. When a pulse stimulus was loaded, action potentials with same frequency in pacemaker fashion were induced. It can be explained that the stimulus produced a receptor potential in the specialized receptors (muscle spindles), which triggered an action potential propagating along the axon to the terminal. Such action potential causes the release of neural transmitters where the axon terminal met with muscle fibers.

Then, the signals of nerves in transection and reconnection were compared. There were three methods to detect the output signals of transected nerves: attaching two electrodes onto the proximal stump (Fig. 9.6c), one electrode on the

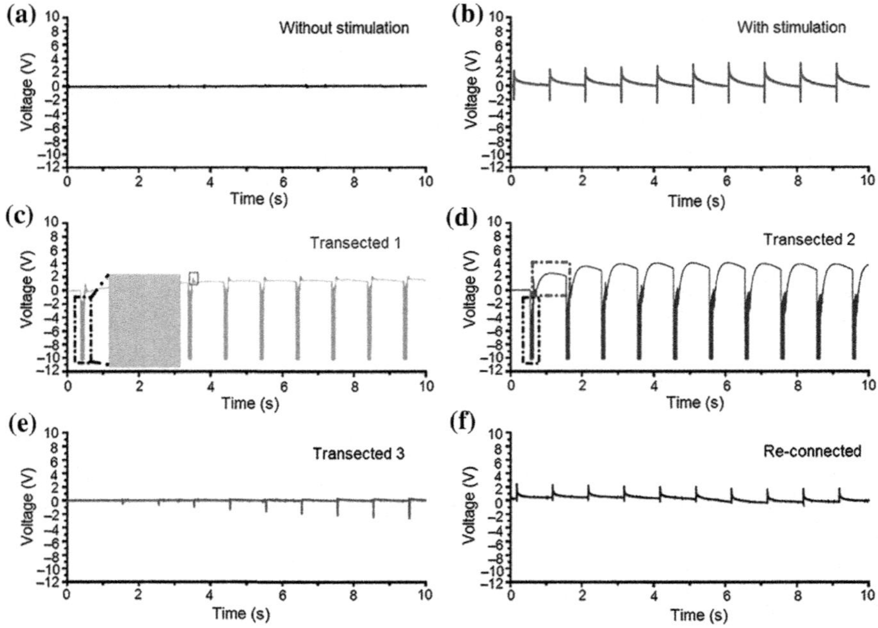

Fig. 9.6 Neurological electrophysiology study on the reconnected sciatic nerve [6]. **a** and **b** The complete nerve without and with stimulus, respectively. **c**, **d**, **e** Transected nerve, with both of two electrodes attached onto the proximal nerve stump in (**c**), one on the proximal stump and another on the distal stump in (**d**), and both on the distal stump in (**e**). The insert with blue background in (**c**) was the expansion of the burst firing. **f** The state of sciatic nerve after reconnection operation. All pictures reproduced with permission

proximal stump and another on the distal stump (Fig. 9.6d), and two electrodes onto the distal stump (Fig. 9.6e). It was found that the voltage signal immediately presented negative bursting firing in the situations of at least one electrode attaching proximal stump (Fig. 9.6c, d). These results are consistent with the view that the presence of burst firing indicates the interruption of nerve signal transduction [31]. In these cases, the stimulus changes the concentration of Ca^{2+} ion, which generates sufficient depolarization and initiates a brief burst of Na^{+}-dependent action potentials. Thus, negative bursting firing is spontaneously triggered in the proximal segment. Moreover, there was an obvious difference between these two situations that the small positive peak (the solid line frame in Fig. 9.6c) was stretched into a positive broadening peak (the dashed box in Fig. 9.6d). Such situation was similar to that of previous study that the probe position can cause the small positive peaks broader [32].

By the contrary, in the case of two electrodes attaching the distal stump, the signal demonstrated only negative tonic firing (Fig. 9.6e) which was assumed to be the antidromic motor signal or the receptor potential. In total, the transaction interrupts the normal neuro-electrophysiological circle, thus the transmission of signal induced from receptor potential is hindered. That is the reason why the receptor potential could be detected only on distal nerve segment, not proximal segment.

Remarkably, the output signal was also obtained from the nerve reconnected by gallium, see Fig. 9.6f. The curve presents virtually similar shape to that of intact nerve, but with smaller amplitude. It should be noted that action potentials in normal nerve transmit without intensity loss rely on the influence on voltage-gated Ca^{2+} channel by hyperpolarization. For gallium-based nerve reconnection, the current conducts by both ion-pumps and the directional migration of free electrons in gallium. Therefore, the decrease of action potential amplitude may result from the resistance of gallium. Nevertheless, the reconnected nerve can transmit the neural signal effectively to a great extent, which proved the validity of gallium.

Additionally, the injured nerves can affect the normal function of relevant muscles. To detect this influence, the common method is to measure the charge of fibrillation potential (Fib). Fibrillation potential is an accepted electrical marker of muscle denervation that occurs in axonal nerve injury [33]. The amplitude of Fib reflects the situation of muscle atrophy. Therefore, the Fib of transected nerves with and without reconnection was also recorded weekly for 3 months. It is preferentially generated in the former end-plate region of a denervated muscle fiber [34, 35]. Therefore, a concentric needle electrode (diameter of 0.3 mm) and earthing electrode were inserted perpendicularly in the gastrocnemius belly and the heel, respectively. The result shows that the Fib curve of denervation case quickly appeared and reached 1.1371 V at the third week, as illustrated in Fig. 9.7. In contrast, the increase of Fib curve of the nerve reconnected by gallium was delayed to the eighth week, indicating the efficiency of executed nerve reconnection surgery

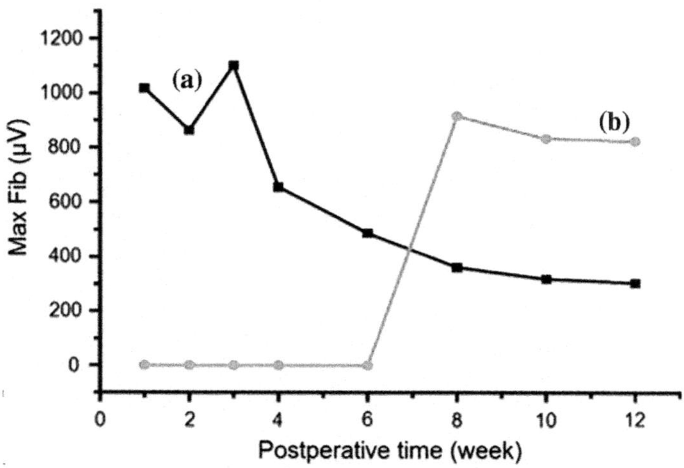

Fig. 9.7 Fib measurements for mice with different treatments [6]: denervation without (**a**) and with (**b**) reconnection. Picture reproduced with permission

in functional recovery and preventing muscle atrophy. However, liquid metal can only reconnect neural signal pathways but not prompt the regeneration of transected nerve, so Fib still appeared and kept at a stable level two months after surgery.

9.6.3 *Histological Analysis*

The histological analysis was carried out to investigate the biological effect of liquid-metal based reconnection. The gastrocnemius muscle was collected and examined for biopsy every week. After three months, the weight maintenance rates (defined as ratio of weight before and after treatment) of muscle with and without nerve repair were 82 and 17% by average, respectively. The biopsies show that gastrocnemius exhibited pathological atrophied muscle fibers in both group. However, the atrophy tendency was distinctly reduced in mice received the nerve reconnection by gallium compared to those with the nerve injury untreated. Such result further supports the conclusion that the transected nerve reconnected by gallium can relieve the muscle atrophy.

9.7 Implantable Liquid Metal Soft Neural Microelectrode Array

9.7.1 *Liquid Metal in Recovering Animal Locomotion Function*

With significant advantages in rapidly restoring the nerve function, electrical stimulation of nervous tissue is a crucial treatment of peripheral nerve injuries leading to common movement disorder. However, the currently available stimulating electrodes are generally based on rigid conductive materials which would cause potential mechanical mismatch with soft neural tissues and thus reduce long-term effects of electrical stimulation. From an alternative, Guo and Liu [36] proposed and demonstrated a flexible neural microelectrode array system via printing approach based on the liquid metal GaIn alloy (75.5% Ga and 24.5% In by weight). Such alloy with unique low melting point (10.35 °C) owns excellent electrical conductivity and high compliance, which are beneficial to serve as soft implantable neural electrodes. The flexible neural microelectrode array embeds four liquid metal electrodes and stretchable interconnects in a PDMS membrane (500 μm in thickness) that possess a lower elastic modulus (1.055-MPa), which is similar to neural tissues with elastic moduli in the 0.1–1.5-MPa range. The electrical experiments indicate that the liquid metal interconnects could sustain over 7000 mechanical stretch cycles with resistance approximately staying at 4 Ω. Over the conceptual experiments on animal sciatic nerve electrical stimulation, the dead bullfrog implanted with flexible neural microelectrode array could even rhythmically contract and move its lower limbs under the electrical stimulations from the implant. This demonstrates a highly efficient way for quickly recovering biological nerve functions. Further, the good biocompatibility of the liquid metal material was justified via a series of biological experiments. Such liquid metal modality for neural stimulation is expected to play important roles as biologic electrodes to overcome the fundamental mismatch in mechanics between biological tissues and electronic devices in the coming time.

9.7.2 Neural Implants and Liquid Metal Electronic Stimulation

Implantable electrical stimulation of nervous tissues engineered to treat the peripheral nerve injuries, which caused the movement disorders or paralysis worldwide in the last few decades [5, 37], has been a unique effective technique to rapidly restore the nerve function compared with the traditional repairs of fracture nerve [38]. The past decade has witnessed the rapid development of the neural implants in both clinic and basic research, such as the deep brain stimulation applied to treat Parkinson's disease, essential tremor, depression, and chronic pain [39]. As one of the most successful clinical application of implantable electrical stimulation of nervous tissue, cochlear implants have been the core effective technique to improve hearing in deaf children [40]. The implantable neural electrodes are also an indispensable apparatus to measure the neural electrical activities of brain in the neuroscience research. For example, some neuroscientists demonstrated that microelectrode sensors close to individual neurons are desirable to monitor their activity in vivo [41, 42]. The implantable electroencephalogram (EEG) recording electrodes are one of the most widely adopted tools of brain-computer interface and have been extensively used for the control of intelligent prosthetic limbs, which both are engineered and designed to improve the movement ability of people with dyspraxia [43]. Recent developments in the field of implantable electrical stimulation of nervous tissue have led to a renewed interest in the peripheral nerve electrical stimulation, which owns the potential to restore the limb locomotor function and body sensory of paralysed and limb disabled patients through directly stimulate the residual peripheral nerve [44, 45]. Current implantable neural electrodes such as micro-wires [46] and micro-electrode arrays [47] are mostly fabricated with inert metal materials, which have excellent electrical conductivity and appropriate biocompatibility, because of their chemical stability. Studies over the past two decades have indicated important information on the challenge of the rigid metal materials restricting long-term bio-integration, which is caused by the cellular reactive responses due to insertion trauma and the chronic foreign body reaction [48]. The mechanical mismatch between implantable electrodes and neural tissues is also regarded as a recurring limitation of the biocompatibility, which increases the electrode–tissue impedance and invalidates the electrodes after long-term implantation [49, 50]. The past decade has seen the rapid development of flexible electronics in many research fields, such as wearable devices [51] and tactile sensors of robots [52]. For example, a recent research on the stretchable conductive polymer realized with a range of enhancers provides a new avenue toward bioelectronics [53]. Studies of the flexible electronics show the application prospect of the flexible neural electrodes and some researches demonstrate that the soft neural implants with the similar mechanical properties of biological tissues display better long-term biointegration and functionality compared with the rigid plastic implants [54].

Recently, the eutectic GaIn alloy has been found to own several intrinsic merits, such as good electrical conductivity, thermal performance [55] and radiation imaging capability [30] (metal features); liquidity and compliance (liquid properties). With a broad temperature range of liquid phase, the room temperature liquid metal GaIn alloy (75.5% Ga, 24.5% In by weight) displays zero stiffness and almost infinite stretchability due to its fluidity, which is super compliant in vivo. Besides, the electrical conductivity of such material is several orders higher than those of non-metallic materials. The liquid metal, with the highly stretchable and conductive features, own the both advantages of inorganic and organic electronic materials. Besides, the fabrication methods of the liquid metal conductors are cheap and simple using the micro channel preparation techniques [56] and spray-printing method [57, 58]. Liquid metal with these unique properties has a broad application prospect in stretchable and wearable electronics [59, 60], such as stretchable interconnections, stretchable pressure sensors [61], dielectric elastomer actuators, and stretchable loudspeaker [62]. More importantly, the biosafety of the liquid metal has been discussed thoroughly in some former researches. For example, the liquid-solid phase transition alloy was demonstrated as reversible and rapid molding bone cement [63], and the liquid metal tested as reconnection agent for peripheral nerve injury [6].

In a latest study, the indium gallium alloy was adopted by Guo and Liu [36] as electrode materials, with polydimethylsiloxane (PDMS) flexible polymer to encapsulate it inside. A straightforward method, the liquid metal spraying printing technology, was adopted to design the shape of liquid metal electrode. In addition to the preparation of liquid metal electrodes, the mechanical properties, electrical characteristics and biocompatibility of such flexible neural microelectrode array were comprehensively evaluated. The results reveal that the liquid metal electrodes have similar mechanical properties with biological tissue, good tensile properties, and maintain electrical stability under tensile state. The related biological experiments demonstrated that a liquid metal displays rather good biocompatibility which promises the practical value of current technology.

9.8 Liquid Metal for Bullfrog Sciatic Nerve Electrical Stimulation

Guo and Liu carried out a series of conceptual experiments to explain their method [36]. The gastrocnemius with sciatic nerve was extracted with the double pithing method. The Riger's Solution was prepared and applied to infiltrate the sciatic nerve and gastrocnemius in order to maintain active state. First of all, the physiological signal amplifiers were connected to the computer. Then, the sciatic nerve was placed in the specimens shielding groove. Two electrodes joints of function signal generator were connected with liquid metal interconnects and electrodes placed on the surface of sciatic nerve. For the control group, two electrodes joints of function signal generator were connected with specimens shielding groove C+ and C− electrode terminals. The measuring electrodes of physiological signal amplifier were connected with specimens shielding groove S2+ and S2− electrode terminals. The sampling rate of the physiological signal amplifier electrode was 40 kHz. The electrical stimulation function signal generator was single phase voltage square wave pulse (amplitude of 1 V, wave width of 10 ms). The in vitro animal tests were approved by the Ethics Committee of Tsinghua University, Beijing, China under contract (SYXK (Jing) 2009-0022).

9.8.1 Electrode Shape and Stability

The liquid metal nerve electrodes (Fig. 9.8a, b, c, d) designed by Guo and Liu [36] integrated the PDMS films (0.5 mm in thickness, 5 mm in width) and included four liquid metal GaIn alloy (75.5% Ga, 24.5% In by volume) interconnects (width of 0.5 mm, wire spacing of 0.5 mm, and the PDMS films were 5 mm in width). One end of the interconnects has four rectangular terminals (points spacing of 1 mm), which are used to connect with other parts of the electrode system, and the other end of the interconnects have 4 holes, which fill liquid metal as the electrode dots (The PDMS films on the two ends were 10 mm in width). Because of the very high surface tension ($\approx$0.6 N/m) of liquid metal [35], the liquid metal at the electrode point will not leak from the holes. This interconnects and electrodes transmit electrical excitation and transfer electrophysiological signals. The packaging material has good biocompatibility and stretchability.

Because of the fluidity of liquid metal, most former works adopted optical mask technology to manufacture micro-channels on the PDMS substrates, then inject liquid metal. However, such method requires a series of complex procedures, leading to a long processing cycle and higher production costs. From an alternative, Guo and Liu [36] adopted the liquid metal spraying technology, with quick fabrication cycle, low costs and simple technology advantages, for patterning the liquid metal electrodes. A detailed fabrication scheme can be found in Fig. 9.9 [36].

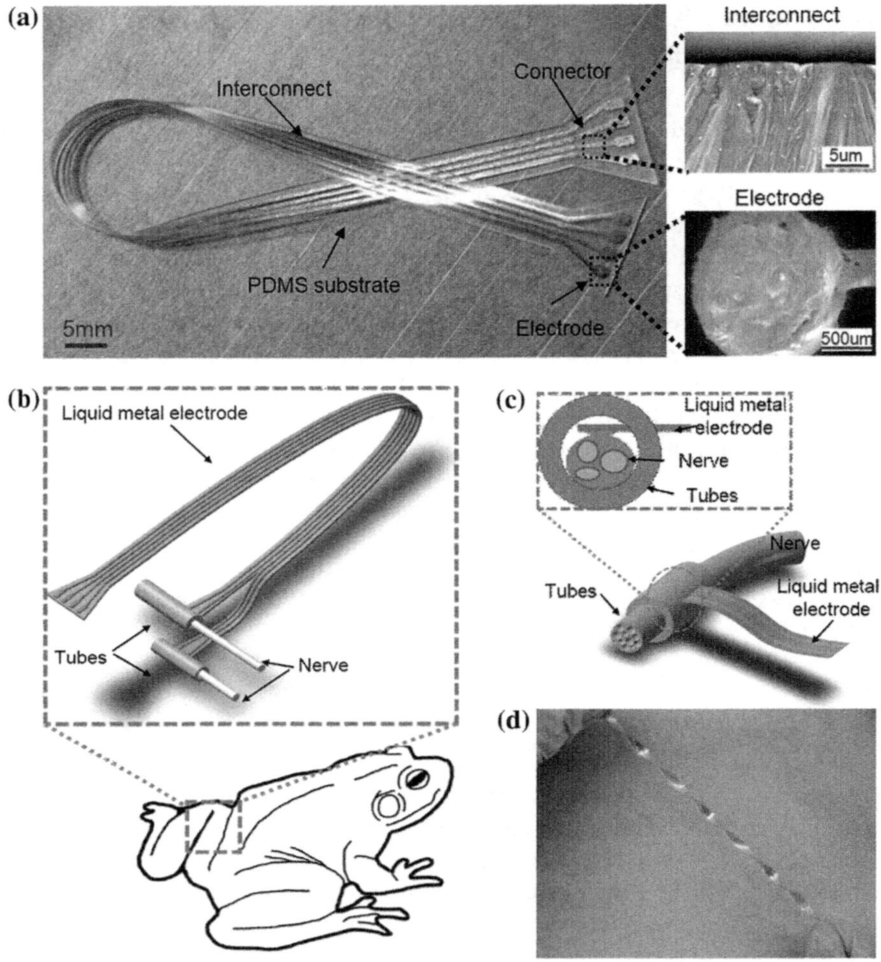

Fig. 9.8 The liquid metal nerve electrodes and the machining process [36]. **a** Optical image of the liquid metal electrodes, and scanning electron micrographs of the electrode and the interconnect. **b** The schematic diagram of the liquid metal nerve electrodes in vivo. **c** A silicone tube was used to fix the electrodes on the nerve. **d** The pictures of the liquid metal nerve electrodes. All pictures reproduced with permission

9.8.2 Mechanical Properties of Liquid Metal Electrodes

In the tensile experiments, four liquid metal electrodes were selected to measure the elastic modulus [36]. The green line in Fig. 9.10a was the stress strain curve of liquid metal electrodes. The elastic modulus of liquid metal electrodes was 1.055-MPa. In addition, compared the elastic modulus with other metal electrodes

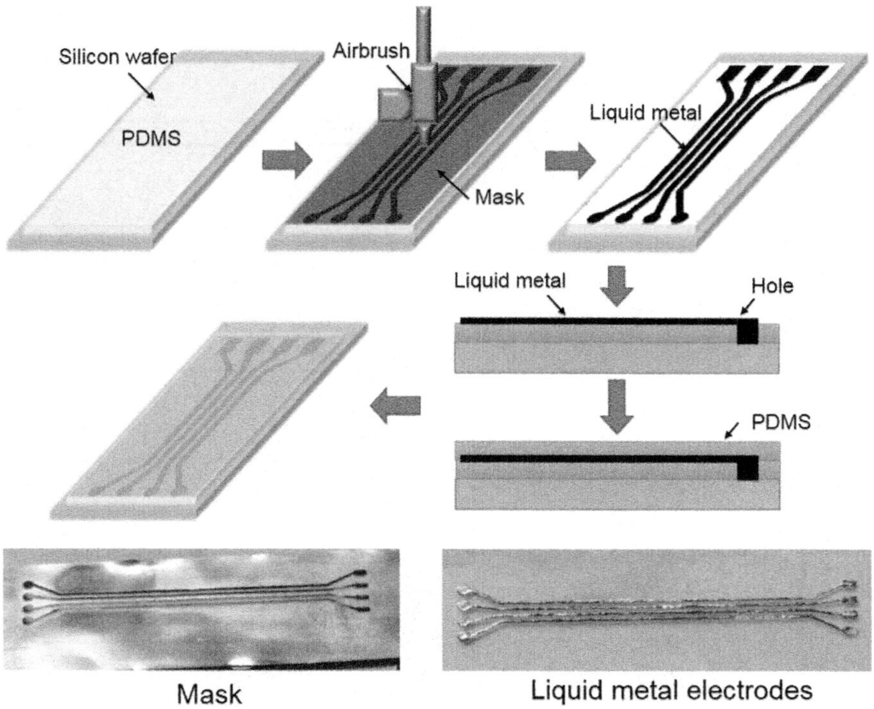

Fig. 9.9 Scheme for patterning and fabricating liquid metal nerve array electrodes [36]. All pictures reproduced with permission

and biological tissues, the liquid metal flexible electrodes had very similar mechanical properties with biological tissues, as shown in Fig. 9.10a.

9.8.3 Electrochemical Characterization of Interconnects

The resistance of the fabricated liquid metal interconnects was approximately 4 Ω, and increased gradually with the extent of stretching. In this experiment, the original length of the liquid metal interconnects was 8 cm, and the maximum tensile rate was 17.5%. Five tensile lengths (original length, uniaxial stretching of 5%, uniaxial stretching of 10%, uniaxial stretching of 15% and uniaxial stretching of 17.5%) were selected to make the AC impedance tests. The impedance modulus and phase spectrum of the liquid metal interconnects under different tensile states were shown in Fig. 9.10b. The DC resistance of the liquid metal electrodes under the applied strain in the uniaxial direction was measured in order to clarify the relationship between electrode elongation and electrical properties (Fig. 9.10c).

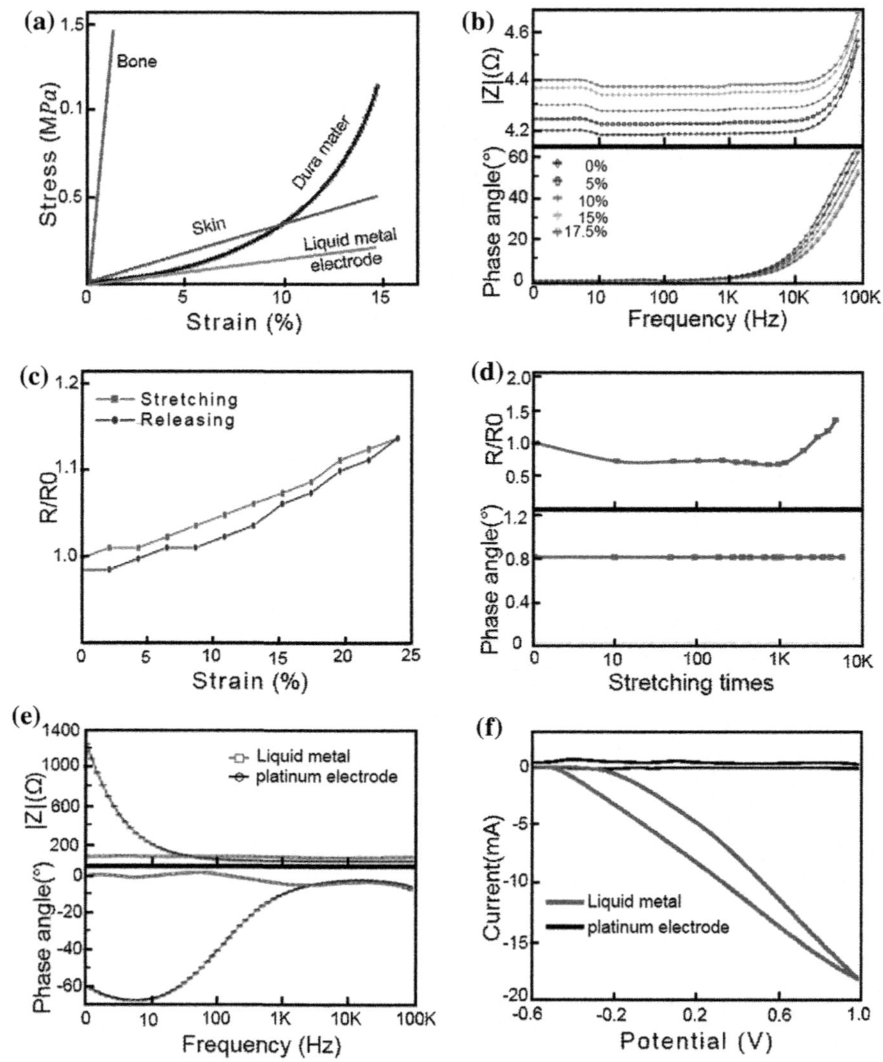

Fig. 9.10 The electrochemical characterization of interconnects [36]. **a** Strain-stress curves of liquid metal electrodes, other metal electrodes and biological tissues. **b** The impedance modulus and phase spectrum of liquid metal interconnects under different tensile states. **c** The DC resistance of the liquid metal electrodes under the applied strain in the uniaxial direction. **d** The relation curve of the drawing times with electrical impedance modulus and phase at 100 Hz. **e** The electrical impedance modulus and phase spectrums of the liquid metal electrode and a platinum electrode. **f** The cyclic voltammograms curve of liquid metal electrode and a platinum electrode. All pictures reproduced with permission

The figures showed that the resistance of the liquid metal interconnects display almost no change (the value of low frequency impedance modulus remained 4.25–4.42 Ω, phases kept at 0°) in mild tensile state (The tensile rate was below 20%). Biological bodies have a large number of repetitive movements every day (such as running), so the liquid metal interconnects should have good fatigue resistance characteristics to meet the long-term implantation in vivo. In the fatigue test, the liquid metal interconnects were stretched to 15% strain over 7000 cycles. Figure 9.10d plotted the relation curve of the drawing times with electrical impedance modulus and phase at 100 Hz. The fatigue tests showed that the resistance of the liquid interconnects did not change much in R/R0 up to 2000 cycles, but it had a ~10% increase upon 4000 cycles of stretching. This is because the length of the liquid metal interconnects increases gradually with the stretching cycles.

9.8.4 Electrochemical Characterization of Liquid Metal Electrodes

The electrochemical characterization of the liquid metal electrodes compared to platinum electrodes (the same length with liquid metal electrodes, the diameter of 1 mm) was measured using AC Impedance tests [36]. To demonstrate the electrochemical stability of the liquid metal electrodes, both cyclic voltammograms (CV) and AC Impedance curves of the liquid metal electrodes and platinum electrodes were recorded in 0.9% saline solution.

The impedance modulus and phase spectrums of the liquid metal electrodes and the platinum electrode were shown in Fig. 9.10e [36]. The liquid metal electrodes had lower resistance compared with the platinum electrode, and its resistance variation was far less than the platinum electrode with the increase of frequency. The result suggested that the liquid metal electrodes display more stable impedance characteristics compared with the traditional platinum electrode.

The CV curves of liquid metal electrodes and the platinum electrode were shown in Fig. 9.10f. The cathodic current of the platinum electrode remained stable with the change of voltage. Electric double layer theory analysis showed that the platinum electrode can be used as an ideal polarization electrode, and the electrode–electrolyte interface had pure capacitance characteristics. Although the electrochemical stability of the platinum electrode was excellent, the interface charge storage capacity was very low. Liquid metal electrode interface, by comparison, currently had a wide change range with the change of voltage, and no obvious REDOX peak appeared in the CV curve, so the electrode–electrolyte interface of liquid metal electrode could be equivalent to a leakage capacitor. The electrodes not only had certain capacitive property, but could also display reversible REDOX reaction. Such electrodes were conducive to the protection of the electrodes and tissues, increasing the cathode electric charge storage capacity.

9.8.5 Biocompatibility of Liquid Metal

Liquid metal could contact with biological tissues directly, so it was necessary to perform a GaIn alloy corrosion test in simulated body fluid environment, and cultured the fibroblast with liquid metal. Physiological saline did not contain the alloy elements of gallium and indium, therefore in the soaking experiment, the content of alloy elements as detected in the solution was the amount of ions, its liquid metal releasing in the solution [36]. Average concentration of gallium and indium elements was shown in Fig. 9.11a. After 48 h of immersion experiment, one could not detect the alloy elements of indium. However, the average concentration of gallium gradually increased with the time, and the maximum concentration of gallium would reach 1.5 ug/ml. It was necessary to test the cytotoxicity of the gallium, even though the concentration of gallium was microcrystalline. The solution pH value decreased with the increase of the immersion time, as shown in Fig. 9.11b. The main reason was that the cultivation environment contained 5% of carbon dioxide, and carbon dioxide dissolved in solution.

The growth situation of the mouse fibroblast was shown in Fig. 9.12a. The green points in the fluorescence micrographs were the living cells, and the red points were

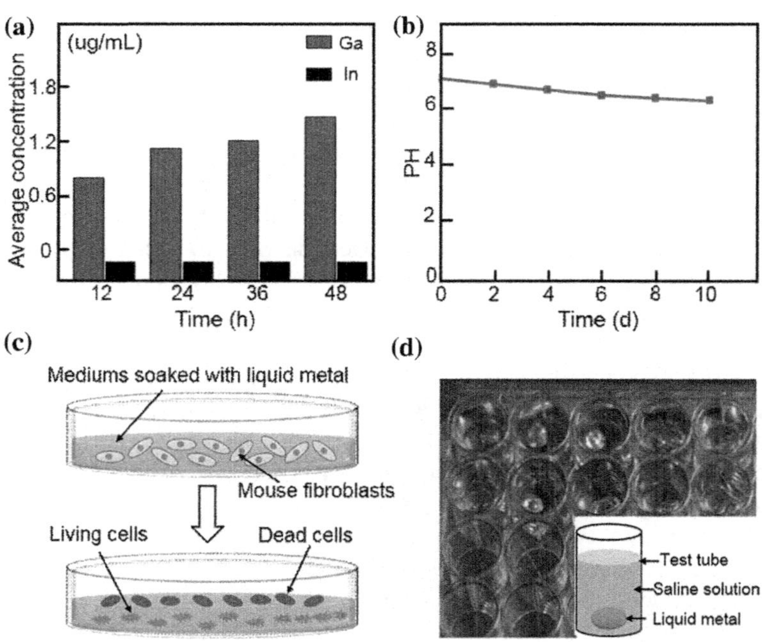

Fig. 9.11 The biocompatibility tests of liquid metal [36]. **a** Average concentration of gallium and indium elements. **b** The pH of physiological saline solution. **c** The schematic diagram of the mouse fibroblasts cultured with the mediums, which soaked the liquid metal for different times. The green points were the living cells, and the red points were the dead cells. **d** The test tube containing the physiological saline solution. All pictures reproduced with permission

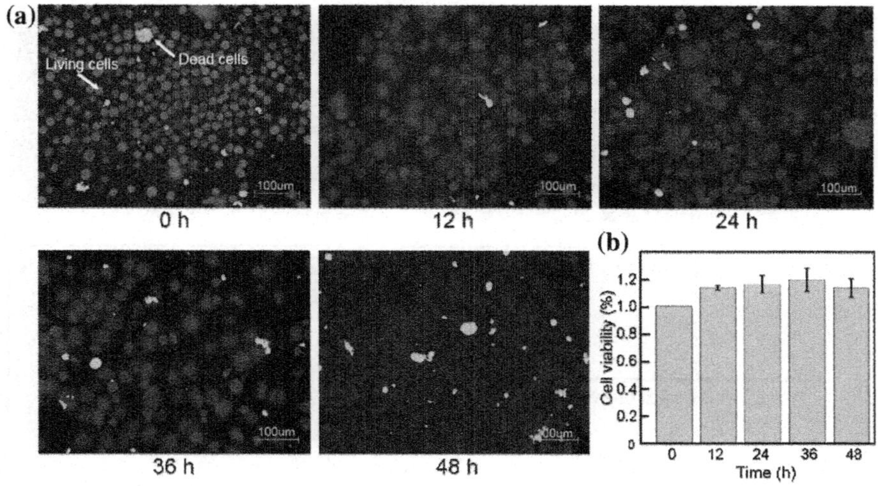

Fig. 9.12 The cytotoxicity tests of liquid metal [36]. **a** The fluorescence micrographs of mouse fibroblasts cultured with the five cell culture mediums. **b** The cell viability of the mouse fibroblasts (n = 4). All pictures reproduced with permission

the dead cells. The living cells grew well in the five kinds of petri dishes and the amount of the dead cells was limited. Figure 9.12b showed the average cell viability of the mouse fibroblasts, which were cultured in five different mediums (soaking the liquid metal for 0, 12, 24, 36 and 48 h, respectively) for 24 h. The cell viability test was repeated four times, and the results showed that the existence of gallium in the mediums was beneficial to the mouse fibroblasts growth and the cell viability of the mouse fibroblasts with the liquid metal elements surpassed this without the liquid metal elements.

9.9 Electrical Stimulation Experiments on Bullfrog Sciatic Nerve

In this conceptual experiment, the adult bullfrog sciatic nerve was selected as the test object (Fig. 9.13), which was one of the most classical biological samples for neuroscience experiments, and easily available. The sciatic nerve was stimulated with liquid metal electrodes and a platinum electrode (Fig. 9.13a), respectively. The effects of liquid metal electrodes were also investigated by comparing these bipolar waveform characteristics of the action potential [36].

Figure 9.13b, c showed the monophasic action potential of sciatic nerve under the stimulus of platinum electrode and liquid metal electrode, respectively. Under the stimulus of two electrodes, the time characteristics of monophasic action potential of sciatic nerve were the same, but the amplitude characteristics were

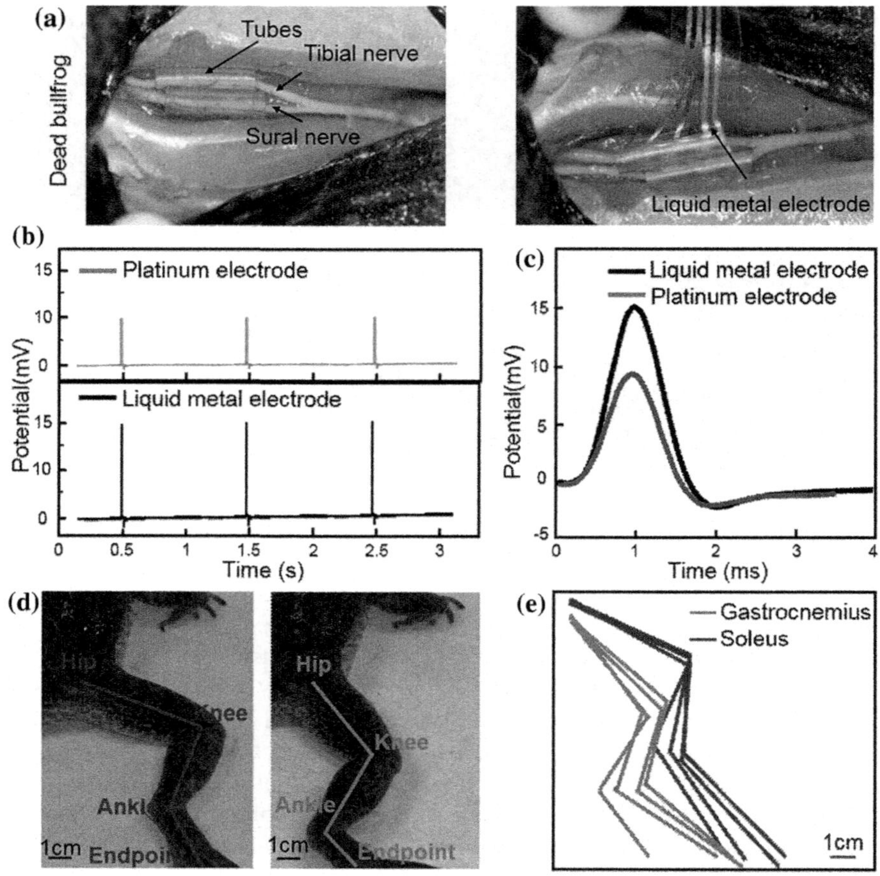

Fig. 9.13 Bullfrog sciatic nerve electrical stimulation experiments [36]. **a** The pictures of the implanted liquid metal electrodes for the bullfrog sural nerve and tibial nerve. **b** The bipolar action potential of sciatic nerve under the stimulus of platinum electrode; the bipolar action potential of sciatic nerve under the stimulus of liquid metal electrode. **c** The amplitudes of bipolar action potential of sciatic nerve under the stimulus of platinum electrode and liquid metal electrode. **d** The hind limb kinematics of a dead bullfrog after implantation. All pictures reproduced with permission

different. In order to further analyze the differences of amplitude characteristics, Guo and Liu [36] selected 4 groups of monophasic nerve action potential under the stimulus of platinum electrodes and liquid metal electrodes, respectively, to compare the amplitudes, as shown in Fig. 9.13c. The result showed that the amplitude of action potential under the stimulus of liquid metal electrode was higher than the platinum electrode (the potential of sciatic nerve under the stimulus of platinum electrode was 10 mV, and the potential of sciatic nerve under the stimulus of liquid metal electrode was 15 mV), and the conductive performance of liquid metal was better than platinum.

The liquid metal electrodes were applied to stimulate the sural nerve and the tibial nerve of a dead bullfrog. In addition, in order to fix the electrodes on the nerves, two silicone tubes were attached to the liquid metal electrodes for sural nerve and tibial nerve, respectively. When the sural nerve was stimulated to control the gastrocnemius, the leg of the dead bullfrog would lift up. When the tibial nerve was stimulated to control the soleus, the leg of the dead bullfrog would lift down (Fig. 9.13d, e). All these first ever conceptual experiments demonstrated the validity of the present technology [36].

In the above study, the liquid metal was packaged in a 500 um thick PDMS membrane using liquid metal spraying technology. Such preparation technology is very simple, which can reduce the manufacturing cost of biological electrodes, and fabricate different patterns of electrodes easily. It is worth noting that the liquid metal in the holes as a stimulating electrode point contacts with nerve tissues. This part of the liquid metal is not fully encapsulated, and there are some potential threats of liquid metal leaking in the holes. However, the tests of the electrode shape and stability showed that the surface tension of the liquid metal was very high, and would not fell off from the electrode points in the physiological saline. PDMS, a kind of common flexible polymer materials and widely used in biological chips and tissue engineering, has similar mechanical properties with biological tissue and good biocompatibility. Theoretically, such liquid metal is zero stiffness and has almost infinite stretchability due to its complete fluidity. The PDMS membrane owns good flexibility and tensile property, and the liquid metal can also compliantly follow the deformation of PDMS membranes.

To investigate the mechanical and electrical stability of the fabricated liquid metal electrodes, the resistance of the liquid metal electrodes was measured according to the applied strain in the uniaxial direction. The results showed that the electrode interconnect in mild tensile state (tensile rate below 20%) could keep stable electrical impedance characteristics. In the experiment of the electrochemical characterization of electrode–electrolyte interface, the liquid metal electrodes had higher charge storage capacity compared with the platinum electrodes and did not display obvious REDOX reaction in aqueous solution. However, the electrochemical characteristic of the surface of liquid metal is not ideal, so in the coming time, further additional researches are needed on the surface modification of the liquid metal electrodes. In the above work, the liquid metal was soaked in the physiological saline for 48 h, and the ion concentration tests found that there was no indium in the physiological saline and the ion concentration of gallium was microcrystalline. This suggests that the indium gallium alloy has good corrosion resistance characteristics in physiological saline. In addition, in the cell viability experiments of the mouse fibroblasts, the existence of gallium in the mediums was beneficial to the mouse fibroblasts growth, so we believed that the liquid metal electrodes will not affect the normal growth of the surrounding tissue. To further test the liquid metal electrodes' stimulation effect of nerve tissue, the liquid metal electrodes were used to stimulate the bullfrog sciatic nerve in vitro, and record the action potential of the nerve fibers. The results showed that the liquid metal electrodes were able to cause gastrocnemius muscle contraction just like the platinum wire electrodes. However, the REDOX reaction on the surface of liquid metal changed the shape of liquid metal drops, and resulted in the deformation of action potential.

Although there are a variety of tests on the performance of the liquid metal electrodes about the mechanical properties, electrical properties and biocompatibility and the experimental results also confirm that the liquid metal electrodes meet some basic requirements of biological electrodes and own a number of advantages over the traditional rigid electrodes. Anyway, in the near future, the long term effects of electrodes still need additional in vivo animal experiments.

9.10 Conclusion

Until now, various trials have been made to employ liquid metal by virtue of its certain characteristics for specific biomedical applications. Based on the favourable fluidity, super compliance and high electrical conductivity, liquid metal has been developed for nerve reconnection due to these similar electrical properties to nerve. This connection serves as not only physical contact, but also an electrical pathway. Liquid metal has been proven with the high stability of electrical resistance under working frequency and temperature. It has demonstrated that the liquid metal as an unconventional medium can help the injured nerve recover the ability to conduct electroneurographic signals. Moreover, the graft of liquid metal tube can effectively delay the muscle atrophy rather than prevention, according to the study of Fib and biopsies of gastrocnemius. Currently, experiments of transected sciatic nerve in vitro and in vivo both proved the feasibility of liquid-metal based reconnection. The application of liquid metal might play a significant role of the functional recovery channel cooperating with nerve conduits during regeneration.

So far, several liquid metals, i.e. $Ga_{67}In_{20.5}Sn_{12.5}$ alloy, $Ga_{75.5}In_{24.5}$ alloy and gallium etc. have been investigated for nerve electrical reconnection or stimulation. There are many other liquid metals composed of different elements in various ratios. Thus, great efforts should be made for comprehensive analysis to achieve optimized results. Furthermore, liquid metal based nerve conduits can be designed with multiple configurations through coupling with advanced technologies and methods. For example, taking advantage of the conventional nerve conduits with microchannels [64], liquid metal can be filled in the peripheral thicker channels. And the paracentral thinner microchannels can be filled with growth factors, Schwann cell or insoluble extracellular matrices to promote the regeneration.

Further, the liquid metal nerve electrode arrays were fabricated via spraying technology and demonstrated to own super compliant merit in vivo, because of its combination of liquid metal and PDMS. Over the experiments, the liquid metal electrodes showed good conductivity and electronic stability in the tensile state. Liquid metal electrode owns lower resistance properties compared with platinum electrode, and its resistance value range is far less than the range of the platinum electrode and the electrodes are conducive to the protection of the electrodes and tissues, and thus increased the cathode electric charge storage capacity. The experiments of biocompatibility and bullfrog sciatic nerve electrical stimulation showed that the liquid metal is avirulent to cells and has similar effects with platinum electrodes. This new conceptual soft liquid metal electrode is expected to play promising role for future implantable prosthesis practices.

In the coming time, one needs to move on to the clinical functional recovery and regeneration of transected nerve with the aid of liquid metal electronic medium. The liquid metal material would benefit the injured peripheral nerve and the optimization of neurosurgery. It is expected that such promising materials provide a game changing way to accelerate the research and clinical applications of nerve reconnection which will contribute a lot for people suffering serious neural diseases.

References

1. Denny HR, Butterworth SJ (2008) A guide to canine and feline orthopaedic surgery, 4th edn. Blackwell Science Ltd, Oxford, UK
2. Shacklock M (1995) Neurodynamics. Physiotherapy 81:9–16
3. Mueller MJ, Maluf KS (2002) Tissue adaptation to physical stress: a proposed "physical stress theory" to guide physical therapist practice, education, and research. Phys Ther 82(4):383–403
4. Liu SQ (2006) Bioregenerative engineering: principles and applications. Wiley, US
5. Widgerow AD, Salibian AA, Kohan E, Sartiniferreira T, Afzel H, Tham T, Evans GR (2014) "Strategic sequences" in adipose-derived stem cell nerve regeneration. Microsurgery 34 (4):324–330
6. Liu FJ, Yu YZ, Yi LT, Liu J (2016) Liquid metal as reconnection agent for peripheral nerve injury. Sci Bull 61(12):939–947
7. Kline DG, Kim D, Midha R et al (1998) Management and results of sciatic nerve injuries: a 24-year experience. J Neurosurg 89(1):13–23
8. Seddon HJ (1943) Three types of nerve injuries. Brain 66(4):238–288
9. Campbell WW (2008) Evaluation and management of peripheral nerve injury. Clin Neurophysiol 119(9):1951–1965
10. Perlmutter GS, Apruzzese W (1998) Axillary nerve injuries in contact sports: recommendations for treatment and rehabilitation. Sports Med 26(5):351–361
11. Yannas IV, Zhang M, Spilker MH (2007) Standardized criterion to analyze and directly compare various materials and models for peripheral nerve regeneration. J Biomater Sci Polym Ed 18(8):943–966
12. Yoleri L, Songür E, Mavioğlu H et al (2001) Cross-facial nerve grafting as an adjunct to hypoglossal-facial nerve crossover in reanimation of early facial paralysis: clinical and electrophysiological evaluation. Ann Plast Surg 46(3):301–307
13. Al-Qattan MM (2000) Prevention and treatment of painful neuromas of the superficial radial nerve by the end-to-side nerve repair concept: an experimental study and preliminary clinical experience. Microsurgery 20(3):99–104
14. Tang X, Xue C, Wang Y et al (2012) Bridging peripheral nerve defects with a tissue engineered nerve graft composed of an in vitro cultured nerve equivalent and a silk fibroin-based scaffold. Biomaterials 33(15):3860–3867
15. Giusti G, Willems WF, Kremer T, Friedrich PF, Bishop AT, Shin AY (2012) Return of motor function after segmental nerve loss in a rat model: a comparison of autogenous nerve graft, collagen conduit and processed nerve allograft (Axogen). J Bone Jt Surg 94(5):410–417

16. Millesi H (1981) Reappraisal of nerve repair. Surg Clin North Am 61(2):321–340
17. Gordon T, Sulaiman O, Boyd JG (2003) Experimental strategies to promote functional recovery after peripheral nerve injuries. J Peripher Nerv Syst 8(4):236–250
18. Evans GR (2001) Peripheral nerve injury: a review and approach to tissue engineered constructs. Anat Rec 263(4):396–404
19. Pabari A, Yang SY, Seifalian AM et al (2010) Modern surgical management of peripheral nerve gap. J Plast Reconstr Aesthet Surg 63(12):1941–1948
20. Moore AM, Novak CB (2014) Advances in nerve transfer surgery. J Hand Ther 27(2):96–105
21. Barbour J, Yee A, Kahn LC et al (2012) Supercharged end-to-side anterior interosseous to ulnar motor nerve transfer for intrinsic musculature reinnervation. J Hand Surg 37(10):2150–2159
22. de Ruiter GC, Malessy MJ, Yaszemski MJ et al (2009) Designing ideal conduits for peripheral nerve repair. Neurosurg Focus 26(2):E5
23. Pfister LA, Papaloïzos M, Merkle HP et al (2007) Nerve conduits and growth factor delivery in peripheral nerve repair. J Peripher Nerv Syst 12(12):65–82
24. Kehoe S, Zhang XF, Boyd D (2012) FDA approved guidance conduits and wraps for peripheral nerve injury: a review of materials and efficacy. Inj Int J Care Inj 43(5):553–572
25. Meek MF, Coert JH (2008) US food and drug administration/conformit Europe-approved absorbable nerve conduits for clinical repair of peripheral and cranial nerves. Ann Plast Surg 60(4):466–472
26. Bean BP (2007) The action potential in mammalian central neurons. Nat Rev Neurosci 8 (6):451–465
27. Liu Y, Gao M, Mei S et al (2013) Ultra-compliant liquid metal electrodes with in-plane self-healing capability for dielectric elastomer actuators. Appl Phys Lett 103(6):064101
28. Gao Y, Li H, Liu J (2012) Direct writing of flexible electronics through room temperature liquid metal ink. PLoS ONE 7(9):e45485
29. Zhang J, Sheng L, Jin C, et al. (2014) Liquid metal as connecting or functional recovery channel for the transected sciatic nerve. arXiv:1404.5931
30. Wang Q, Yu Y, Pan K et al (2014) Liquid metal angiography for mega contrast x-ray visualization of vascular network in reconstructing in-vitro organ anatomy. IEEE Trans Biomed Eng 61(7):2161–2166
31. Johnson SW, Seutin V, North RA (1992) Burst firing in dopamine neurons induced by N-methyl-D-aspartate: role of electrogenic sodium pump. Science 258(5082):665–667
32. Steriade M, Mccormick DA, Sejnowski TJ (1993) Thalamocortical oscillations in the sleeping and aroused brain. Science 262(5134):679–685
33. Willmott AD, White C, Dukelow SP (2012) Fibrillation potential onset in peripheral nerve injury. Muscle Nerve 46(3):332
34. Pisters R, Nieuwlaat R, Lane DA et al (2013) Potential net clinical benefit of population-wide implementation of apixaban and dabigatran among European patients with atrial fibrillation. Thromb Haemost 109(2):328–336
35. Harada M, Luo X, Xiao YQ et al (2012) Transient receptor potential canonical-3 channel-dependent fibroblast regulation in atrial fibrillation. Circulation 126(17):2051–2064
36. Guo R, Liu J (2017) Implantable liquid metal-based flexible neural microelectrode array and its application in recovering animal locomotion functions. J Micromech Microeng 27:104002
37. Noble J, Munro CA, Prasad VS, Midha R (1998) Analysis of upper and lower extremity peripheral nerve injuries in a population of patients with multiple injuries. J Trauma Acute Care Surg 45(1):116–122
38. Scheib J, Höke A (2013) Advances in peripheral nerve regeneration. Nat Rev Neurol 9 (12):668–676
39. Anderson WS, Lenz FA (2006) Surgery insight: deep brain stimulation for movement disorders. Nat Clin Pract Neurol 2(6):310–320

40. Fallon JB, Ryugo DK, Shepherd RK (2014) Consequences of deafness and electrical stimulation on the peripheral and central auditory system. Cochlear Implant, 19–37
41. Lopez CM, Andrei A, Mitra S et al (2014) An implantable 455-active-electrode 52-channel CMOS neural probe. IEEE J Solid-State Circuits 49(1):248–261
42. Borna A, Najafi K (2014) A low power light weight wireless multichannel microsystem for reliable neural recording. IEEE J Solid-State Circuits 49(2):439–451
43. Brandman DM, Cash SS, Hochberg LR (2017) Human intracortical recording and neural decoding for brain-computer interfaces. IEEE Trans Neural Syst Rehabil Eng
44. Tan DW, Schiefer MA, Keith MW, Anderson JR, Tyler J, Tyler DJ (2014) A neural interface provides long-term stable natural touch perception. Sci Transl Med 6(257):257ra138–257ra138
45. Lahiri A, Delgado IM, Sheshadri S, Ng KA, Nag S, Yen SC, Thakor NV (2016) Self-organization of "fibro-axonal" composite tissue around unmodified metallic micro-electrodes can form a functioning interface with a peripheral nerve: a new direction for creating long-term neural interfaces. Muscle Nerve 53(5):789–796
46. Sankar V, Patrick E, Dieme R, Sanchez JC, Prasad A, Nishida T (2014) Electrode impedance analysis of chronic tungsten microwire neural implants: understanding abiotic vs. biotic contributions. Front Neuroeng 7(6):13
47. Williams JC, Rennaker RL, Kipke DR (1999) Long-term neural recording characteristics of wire microelectrode arrays implanted in cerebral cortex. Brain Res Protoc 4(3):303–313
48. Szarowski DH, Andersen MD, Retterer S, Spence AJ, Isaacson M, Craighead HG, Turner JN, Shain W (2003) Brain responses to micro-machined silicon devices. Brain Res 983(1):23–35
49. Barrese JC, Rao N, Paroo K, Triebwasser C, Vargas-Irwin C, Franquemont L, Donoghue JP (2013) Failure mode analysis of silicon-based intracortical microelectrode arrays in non-human primates. J Neural Eng 10(6):066014
50. Potter KA, Jorfi M, Householder KT, Foster EJ, Weder C, Capadona JR (2014) Curcumin-releasing mechanically adaptive intracortical implants improve the proximal neuronal density and blood-brain barrier stability. Actabiomaterialia 10(5):2209–2222
51. Rogers JA, Someya T, Huang Y (2010) Materials and mechanics for stretchable electronics. Science 327(5973):1603–1607
52. Kim J, Lee M, Shim HJ et al (2014) Stretchable silicon nanoribbon electronics for skin prosthesis. Nat Commun 5(5):5747
53. Wang Y, Zhu C, Pfattner R et al (2017) A highly stretchable, transparent, and conductive polymer. Sci Adv 3(3):e1602076
54. Minev IR, Musienko P, Hirsch A et al (2015) Electronic dura mater for long-term multimodal neural interfaces. Science 347(6218):159–163
55. Li HY, Liu J (2011) Revolutionizing heat transport enhancement with liquid metals: proposal of a new industry of water-free heat exchangers. Front Energ 5:20–42
56. Cheng S, Wu Z (2012) Microfluidic electronics. Lab Chip 12:2782–2791
57. Guo C, Yu Y, Liu J (2014) Rapidly patterning conductive components on skin substrates as physiological testing devices via liquid metal spraying and pre-designed mask. J Mater Chem B 2(35):5739–5745
58. Zhang Q, Gao YX, Liu J (2014) Atomized spraying of liquid metal droplets on desired substrate surfaces as a generalized way for ubiquitous printed electronics. Appl Phys A 116:1091–1097
59. Zheng Y, He Z, Gao Y, Liu J (2013) Direct desktop printed-circuits-on-paper flexible electronics. Sci Rep 3(5):1786
60. Wu ZG, Hjort K, Jeong SH (2015) Microfluidic stretchable radio frequency devices. Proc IEEE 103:1211–1225
61. Park YL, Majidi C, Kramer R, Bérard P, Wood RJ (2010) Hyperelastic pressure sensing with a liquid-embedded elastomer. J Micromech Microeng 20(12):125029

62. Jin SW, Park J, Hong SY, Park H, Jeong YR, Park J, Lee SS, Ha JS (2015) Stretchable loudspeaker using liquid metal microchannel. Sci Rep 5:11695
63. Yi L, Jin C, Wang L, Liu J (2014) Liquid-solid phase transition alloy as reversible and rapid molding bone cement. Biomaterials 35:9789–9801
64. Lacour SP, Atta R, Fitzgerald JJ et al (2008) Polyimide micro-channel arrays for peripheral nerve regenerative implants. Sens Actuators A Phys 147(2):456–463

Chapter 10
Phase Changeable Liquid Metal as Injectable and Reversible Bone Cement

Abstract This chapter illustrates the basic principle to adopt the injectable alloy as bone cement through introducing its unique liquid-solid phase transition mechanism. The fundamental characteristics including the mechanical strength, biocompatibility and phase transition-induced thermal effects of such unconventional alloy cement were provided. Prospects for employing the injectable alloy materials as reversible bone cement to fulfill diverse clinical needs were outlined.

Keywords Injectable metal bone · Reversible bone cement · Liquid metal

10.1 Bone Disease

As is well known, diseases in human bone are common that may result in the impairment of bone, including structural deterioration and functional disorders. Generally, bones are capable of repairing themselves [1]. However, for many cases, some severely damaged bones have been clinically verified to be irreparable [2]. Serious bone diseases, such as osteoporosis, arthritis and malignancy, frequently occur among the elderly all over the world. Meanwhile, the fast increase of ageing population has been a global problem which aggravates the resulting severity. Meanwhile, these bone diseases have similar characteristic in affecting bones. In this situation, bones probably display physically weaker or suffer a typical symptom fracture. Patients encountered with bone diseases are threatened by disability and death [3–5]. Moreover, these health issues not only cost individual person and government much, but also bring about social issue, such as unemployment [6].

J. Liu and L. Yi, *Liquid Metal Biomaterials*,
Springer Series in Biomaterials Science and Engineering10,
https://doi.org/10.1007/978-981-10-5607-9_10

10.2 Treatment of Bone Diseases

To improve the life quality of patients with serious bone diseases, bone repair is generally employed in clinics. Here, hip and knee replacements, vertebroplasty and kyphoplasty are introduced as typical treatments of bone damage as follows.

10.2.1 *Hip and Knee Replacements*

For the therapy of bone diseases, total joint replacement (hip and knee replacements) is a particularly common and effective method whose success has caused an increasing demand from an ageing population. Total joint replacement (TJR) has been proven to be a safe operation with high success rate in relieving pain and recovering function. Such method should take into account three main factors: design, materials and surgical technique. With respect to the design and materials, their characteristics should be comparable to those of original joint. In addition, the surgery includes exposure of cancellous bone, pulse lavage, drying, containment, insertion of component.

Clearly, there are two ways to achieve TJR according to the usage of cement, i.e. cemented and uncemented fixation. In a number of total joint replacements, the implant is generally cemented in bone using acrylic bone cement (ABC). Although it was revealed that cementless fixation has become widely used in total joint replacements, especially in total hip joint replacement (THJR) [7], cemented fixation remains the gold standard in total knee arthroplasty (TKA) [8, 9] and the rate of cemented THJR can achieve 90% in some countries [10]. Taking advantages of biostability, good mechanical properties, accurate implantation, low cost [11] and other comparable properties to those of uncemented replacement, cemented arthroplasties are always arousing great attention among the worldwide researchers.

10.2.2 *Vertebroplasty and Kyphoplasty*

The vertebral body consists of a outer cortical bone and an inner cancellous bone. The cancellous bone structure has two horizontal and vertical connecting trabeculaes. In some situations, osteoporosis and tumor invasion, injury by accident usually induce the weak and less stiff of horizontal trabeculae, which may further lead to the compression fracture of vertebral body. It has been familiar that spinal fracture causes pain and deformity of body posture. Traditional open spinal surgery requires long recovery period and patients in appropriate physiological conditions. Therefore, invasive alternatives are urgently needed to improve the surgical experience. In recent decades, vertebroplasty and kyphoplasty have been introduced in solving this issue successfully [12–14]. These methods employ minimally invasive technology to augment fractured vertebral bodies with the aid of X-ray imaging in clinical practice. In vertebroplasty, the augmentation materials like bone cement can be injected into the compressed vertebral body via cannulae. Although the pain can be relieved to a great extent, the vertebral body remains collapsed. By contrast, kyphoplasty imports balloons to restore height of the collapsed vertebroplasty body by inflating the balloons with bone cement [15]. These two methods are promising and increasingly being used in stabilization of the spinal fractures using injectable bone cements.

10.3 Bone Cements

As mentioned above, bone cement has been widely used in treatment of bone diseases. At present, bone repair materials mainly include autogenous bone graft, allograft bone and artificial synthetic biomaterials. However, the limited source of native bones restricts their wide use, mean while, the allograft may cause immunological rejection of transplant recipients with high risk. Therefore, artificial materials, taking advantages of their high stability, good biocompatibility, remarkable availability and low cost have attracted tremendous interests in biomedical area for bone repairment. With the advance of materials and technology, bone cement materials have been developed as critical biomedical materials, thus play a significant role in orthopedic and dental surgery [16], especially being used as the fixing agent in cemented total joint arthroplasty. Notably, bone cement locating between bone and implant transfers stress from the implant to the bone and increases the load-carrying capacity of the system.

10.3.1 Calcium Phosphate Cements and Acrylic Bone Cements

So far, there are two main sorts of bone cements being commonly utilized in clinics, acrylic and calcium phosphate cements (CPCs). PMMA (polymethylmethacrylate) is a typical acrylic cement which was first introduced as bone cement in the early of 1960s [17]. It has two components, solid and liquid phase. Such two parts are separated before use. The working principle of bone cement depends on the polymerization reaction of MMA (methylmethacrylate) by mixing liquid and solid components in situ (Fig. 10.1). During this exothermic reaction, an increase in temperature is induced and a paste is formed in minutes. The paste is capable of conforming the shape of its container. With the completion of reaction, bone cement changes into solid with high mechanical strength, allowing even distribution of implant loads. Commercially available bone cements are various in the market, such as CMW® 1, Palacos® R, Simplex® P and Zimmer® D. Basic characteristics of these

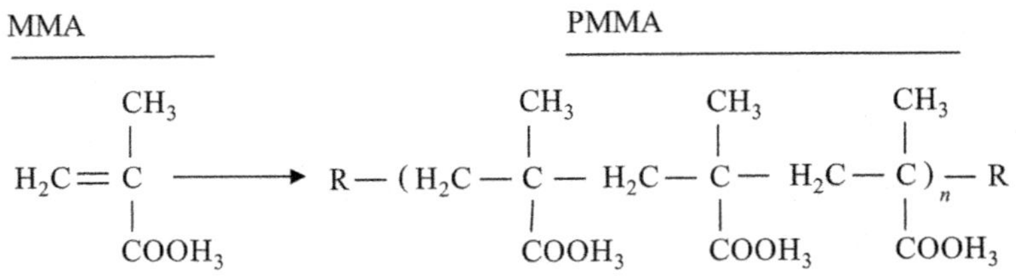

Fig. 10.1 Polymerization reaction of MMA

Table 10.1 Characteristics of typical bone cements [18]

Vacuum mixing	CMW® 1	Palacos® R	Simplex® P	Zimmer® D
Exothermic temperature (°C)	88 ± 1.5	84 ± 0.5	91 ± 1.5	78 ± 1.0
Setting time (min)	11.3 ± 0.5	13.3 ± 0.4	16.2 ± 0.5	13.1 ± 0.2
Flexural modulus (Gpa)	2.51 ± 0.05	2.51 ± 0.16	2.59 ± 0.10	2.21 ± 0.09
Compression strength (MPa)	96 ± 3	97 ± 2	96 ± 2	82 ± 1
Bending strength (MPa)	67 ± 2	72 ± 3	72 ± 2	51 ± 2
Tensile strength (MPa)	47 ± 8	40 ± 8	46 ± 14	46 ± 4
Shear strength (MPa)	63 ± 1	50 ± 12	69 ± 3	60 ± 4
Fracture toughness ($MPam^{1/2}$)	1.75 ± 0.07	1.73 ± 0.17	1.77 ± 0.07	1.56 ± 0.19

bone cements are shown in Table 10.1 [18]. The other essential bone cements, CPCs were discovered in 1980s later than acrylic cements. Such cements also involve two components in liquid and solid phases. Different from the polymerization reaction, their hardening is based on a dissolution and precipitation process. The set cement is similar to hydroxyapatite in both structure and composition. Thus, CPCs are brittle and their poor mechanical strength limits the use in non-load-bearing applications, such as treatment of maxillofacial defects and wrist fractures. Generally, acrylic cements support the bone and prevent further damage, remaining for the rest of the patient's life. Calcium phosphate cements have good bioactivity, degradability and osteoconductivity which promote the surrounding bone to repair itself.

10.3.2 Challenges of Traditional Bone Cements

It is well recognized that bone cements are widely employed in clinical practices. However, the polymerization of acrylic cement is a time-consuming and highly exothermic reaction [19]. The overheat and unreacted monomer released can cause thermal and chemical necrosis of surrounding tissue, coupled with shrinkage of the cement during polymerization [20–22]. This may further contribute to the failures in joint replacements due to aseptic loosening [23–29]. In addition, barium sulphate or zirconium dioxide is often adopted as radiopacifier in most commercial bone cements to facilitate the operation and monitor under radiological imaging [30]. Although these contrast agents have served as an efficient tool in healing process after surgery, their addition would result in the heterogeneity of cement due to the incompatibility between metal salt and acrylic material [31]. Hence, it was suggested that these inorganic particles can cause mechanical weakness [32, 33] and even become fatigue crack initiation sites in the cement [34].

Moreover, failures among bone cements and prothesis occasionally occur as time goes on. The revision is required to fix this problem. Although the revision rate with cement is low, revision of cemented fixation remains a significant concern worth of emphasizing since its appearance over ten years before [8]. Normally, revision is related to some specialized manual instruments and sophisticated technical skills for surgeons. For instance, the sliding trochanteric osteotomy, the extended trochanteric osteotomy (ETO), the extended proximal femur and the cortical windows are conventional methods to remove failed prosthesis and cement [35–37]. These operations require the removal of remaining bones, which not only weaken the remaining bone but also accompanied with complications [35, 36]. On the basis of the above challenges, bone cement should be further improved to settle these problems.

10.4 Bone Cement Based on Liquid-Solid Phase Transition Alloy

With rather easy phase change capability between liquid and solid state, the low melting point metal or alloy was recently found very unique as a kind of injectable bone cement. So far, nearly all the available bone cements are generally non-metallic materials. In fact, metal materials as an important kind of biomaterials have been widely used in orthopedics, such as stainless steel, cobalt alloy, titanium and titanium alloy [38–40]. However, all the commonly used metal materials have high melting points above 1000 °C and their low plasticity makes them difficult in forming various shapes in situ. In the industry, there is a kind of eutectic alloys composed of Bi, In, Sn and Zn that have been supplied as lead-free solder materials. And the melting points for specific alloys vary with different proportion of metal compositions. Moelans et al. have investigated the thermal properties of ternary and quaternary alloy system with these four elements [41]. It was found that the melting point of quaternary system is lower than that of ternary alloy. Moreover, BiInSnZn alloy composed of bismuth (Bi), indium (In), tin (Sn) and zinc (Zn) metals with a corresponding weight ratio of 35, 48.6, 16 and 0.4%, respectively, owns perhaps the lowest melting point among BiInSnZn alloys with other proportions. All these characteristics provide the potential and basis for such eutectic alloy being utilized by direct injection into human body. This alloy can be manipulated with an ordinary medical syringe without needle.

Fig. 10.2 Schematic diagrams of welding and joint replacement

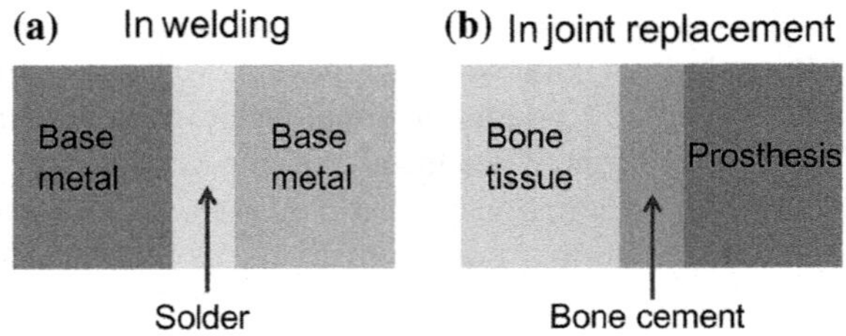

Remarkably, the low-melting-point alloy behaves like acrylic cement in many aspects. The low-melting-point alloys are common lead-free solder in welding. They are widely used to join the dissimilar metals together through melting and solidification process (Fig. 10.2a). Coincidentally, bone cements play a key role in connecting prosthesis and bone tissue (Fig. 10.2b). From this view of point, eutectic alloys have comparable function with bone cement but in different areas. In principle, appropriate bone cement is generally characterized by proper injectability, rapid setting, adequate stiffness, bioactivity, low setting temperature, and radiopacity [42] etc. A generalized way should be developed to simultaneously achieve the above goals. Consequently, a series of tests are required to be implemented to demonstrate the capability of low-melting alloy as bone cement with multi-functions. On this basis, researchers realized the potential of low-melting-point alloys in bone cement materials and made great efforts to investigate the feasibility. With the progress of research in low melting point metal recently [43, 44], it has been reported that 35.0Bi–48.6In–16.0Sn–0.4Zn with melting point less than 60 °C was investigated as bone cement [45]. The comprehensive capabilities of such alloy serving as bone cement are introduced below.

10.5 Flow Characteristics of Alloy Cement

The flow performance of BiInSnZn alloy is one of the most important factors which can affect the filling effect of bone cement. Good fluidity can improve the operability during the injection process. On the other hand, bone cement can suitably fill the target bone cavity with such advantage. Taking into account the flow characteristics, the injectability of cement was firstly demonstrated via droplet experiments. The alloy cement was prepared by heating until melted. Then the droplet was produced by using a medical syringe. With the departure from syringe, the droplet fell vertically to the platform at room temperature. The high speed camera has recorded this dropping process at 500 fps (frames per second), see Fig. 10.3. It was found that the droplet gradually formed into the liquid film when it fell to the ground. This process appears somewhat similar to that of water. Differently, the liquid alloy film solidified ultimately. If the time for the droplet to start contacting with the ground was set as 0 ms. The liquid alloy fully spread on the plane in 8 ms, and completed the fluctuation and solidification in 28 ms.

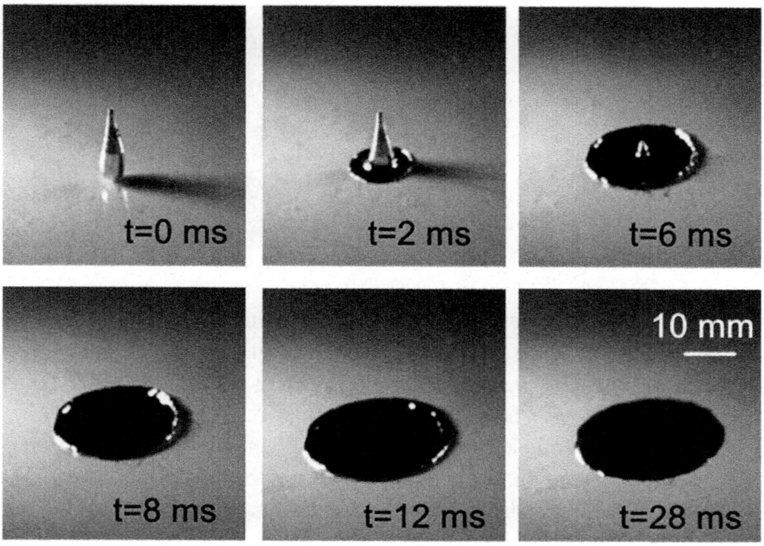

Fig. 10.3 The transient liquid-solid phase transition process of liquid alloy droplet captured by the high-speed camera [45]. Picture reproduced with permission

To quantitatively evaluate the fluidity of alloy cement, the viscosity of alloy cement was measured by using RHEOTRONI C VIII torsional oscillation viscometer. The test results show that the viscosity of BiInSnZn alloy at 74, 95, 150, 203 and 295 °C are 4.0424 ± 0.0459 mPa s, 3.5485 ± 0.0092 mPa s, 2.8599 ± 0.0778 mPa s, 2.3928 ± 0.0345 mPa s and 2.0127 ± 0.0649 mPa s, respectively (Fig. 10.4). The well-known water has excellent fluidity and its viscosity is 1.0025 ± 0.0005 mPa s at 20 °C [46]. Moreover, the viscosity of PMMA paste is relatively constant which is larger than 20 Pa s [47]. In comparison, alloy cement

Fig. 10.4 The viscosity of water and BiInSnZn alloy at different temperatures

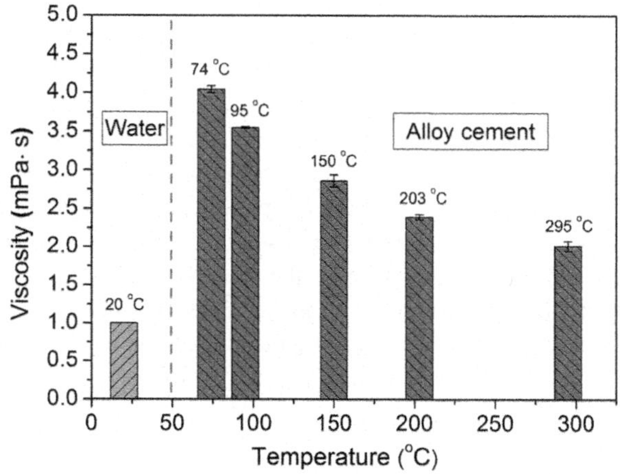

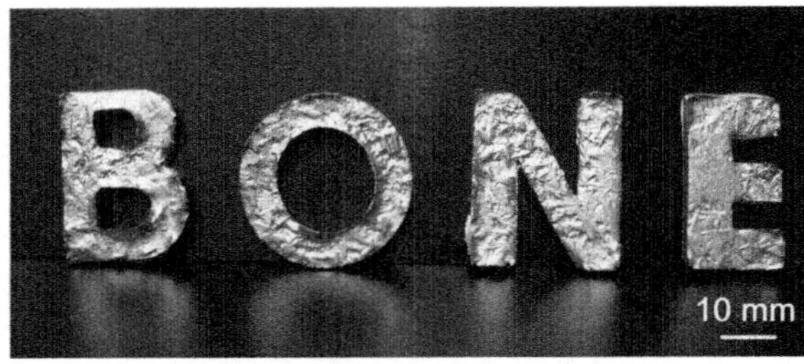

Fig. 10.5 A demonstrated molding of alloy cement in a shape of “BONE” [45]. Picture reproduced with permission

has more superiority on injectability than PMMA cement and this property would allow the alloy cement to be readily administrated in a surgery.

Moreover, the plasticity was evaluated by injecting the melting alloy cement into designed letter molds with height of 3.5 cm. The result shows that the word of “BONE” consisting of four letters made of alloy cement was clearly formed (see Fig. 10.5). It demonstrates that the alloy cement can be easily fabricated in various forms with the aid of injectability and rapid solidification.

10.6 Thermal Physical Properties of Alloy Cement

Thermal physical properties are of great importance for the in vivo applications of bone cements, which have been prescribed in product standard [48]. To validate the thermal characteristics of BiInSnZn alloy, several critical thermal parameters were determined, including DSC curve, peak temperature, setting time, thermal expansion coefficient, thermal necrosis evaluation and reversible capabilities in revision.

10.6.1 DSC Measurement

There are various methods to obtain the melting point of metals. Among them, DSC (differential scanning calorimetry) is a common means by virtue of its high accuracy, low cost and fast speed. Therefore, the fundamental thermal property of BiInSnZn was measured by DSC. In the experiment, alloy cement samples were placed into Al_2O_3 crucible. The predetermined dynamic program was executed in the following process: the temperature first increased to 100 °C at 10 °C/min, then maintained at isothermal phase for 5 min, finally decreased to −20 °C at 10 °C/min. The result shows that the melting point of BiInSnZn alloy is 57.5 °C and the peak rate of heat release is 0.75365 mW/mg. Clearly, the measured value is in accordance with the data reported previously [41].

10.6.2 Peak Temperature

With respect to a new cement, it is significant to clarify the peak temperature thus induced (maximum temperature during the exothermic process, obtained from the maximum of the exotherm curve). The peak temperature of BiInSnZn alloy cement was determined over the liquid-solid transition process. The alloy cement was preheated to melting state at 65 °C for injection. Then the molten alloy was put into PP (Propene Polymer) cylindrical molds (5 mm in diameter of inner bore). A thermocouple was inserted into the center of the mold to measure the temperature at 1 s intervals. The temperature was recorded until it dropped down to the environmental temperature. The change in temperature was shown in Fig. 10.6a. It was found that the central temperature rose sharply to the peak (61.9 °C) when the molten alloy was injected into the mold (T_0 = 1.25 min). Gradually, the temperature decreased under ambient condition. This peak temperature differs from the melting point of alloy, which is related to the preheating temperature. Consequently, the peak temperature would become a little higher than the melting point and approach to the heating temperature to maintain the liquid state of cement. Meanwhile, the peak temperature can be controlled by adjusting the heating temperature which can be close to the melting point. However, it is still a much lower temperature compared to some traditional cements [20].

10.6.3 Setting Time

For acrylic cement, setting time is another important parameter which can be reflected in the liquid-solid transition process together with peak temperature. Setting time (t_{set}) is defined as the period between the start of mixing and the time when the temperature has reached midway from the ambient (20 °C) to peak

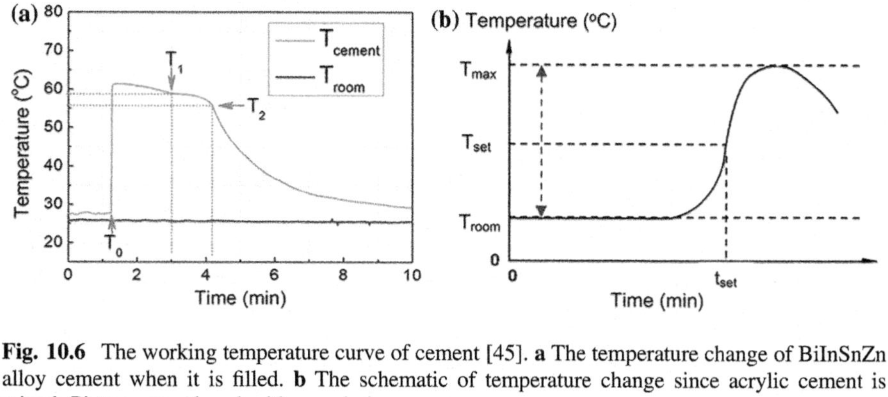

Fig. 10.6 The working temperature curve of cement [45]. **a** The temperature change of BiInSnZn alloy cement when it is filled. **b** The schematic of temperature change since acrylic cement is mixed. Picture reproduced with permission

temperature from the recordings (Fig. 10.6b) [49]. Meanwhile, the time between the dough time and setting time defines the working time of PMMA cement [50]. In fact, alloy cement solidifies without mixing and dough state. Due to the different solidification principles, these definitions for acrylic cements are not suitable to that for alloy cement, which should be distinguished clearly. Accordingly, the whole operation process of alloy cement can be divided as follows: when the molten alloy was injected into the mold, the central temperature rose to the peak immediately. With the heat released under ambient temperature, the liquid cement sequentially started to solidify at the turn point of T_1 (3 min) and completed this process at the T_2 (4.18 min) point. It took 2.93 min for the liquid cement to transform into solid phase. Moreover, the definition of working time for characterizing the alloy cement can be given as the time from injection to solidification, i.e. $T_1 - T_0 = 1.75$ min. This period provides the operation time for the prosthesis implantation. And the solidification time can be regarded as the setting time, i.e. $T_2 - T_1 = 1.18$ min. Therefore, the definitions of setting time and working time for alloy cement should be refreshed according to actual situations.

10.6.4 Thermal Expansion Parameters

In most cases, shrinkage always accompanies with the polymerization reaction of monomer. It was found that the shrinkage of acrylic cement occurs after polymerization. The resulted gaps between cement and prosthesis, cement and bone may lead to micro-motion of the implant [23]. Thus, it is necessary to evaluate the shrinkage of BiInSnZn during its solidification process. Firstly, volume variations were measured through the liquid-solid phase transition experiment. The molten alloy was injected into a 10 mL glass graduate cylinder, and then the water with 2.84 mL was also added over the alloy to make the whole volume reach 6 mL. The same graduate cylinder filling with 6 mL water was used as control. The volume of two samples was first measured at 75 °C and then measured while the temperature dropped to the room temperature by natural cooling. The result shows that the volume change of liquid level was visually invisible at 75 and 22 °C.

Furthermore, the thermal expansion coefficient (δ) of BiInSnZn alloy cement was measured from 25 to 50 °C by dilatometer to verify the relaxation situation at physiological temperatures. It indicates that the thermal expansion rate (δ) of solid alloy cement measured in this temperature range was lower than 0.1%. Meanwhile, corresponding thermal expansion coefficient (α) was stable and restricted in the range of 2.8×10^{-5} to 3.1×10^{-5}/°C (Fig. 10.7). Overall, these results demonstrate that the relaxation of this alloy material could hardly happen with changes in thermal condition, even at physiological temperature for a long time. Such characteristics benefit the working performance of cement a lot.

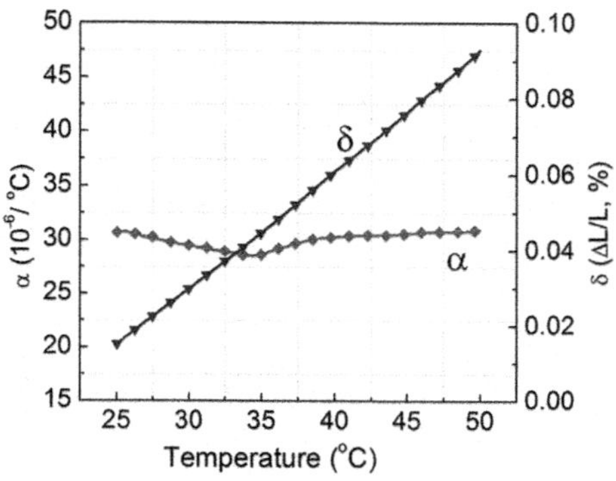

Fig. 10.7 Curves of thermal expansion coefficient (α) and thermal expansion rate (δ) from 25 to 50 °C [45]. Picture reproduced with permission

10.6.5 Thermal Necrosis Evaluation

As mentioned above, the high heat release in the polymerization of PMMA may cause the thermal necrosis of healthy tissue. Therefore, thermal necrosis with adverse effect in vivo is quite worthy of emphasizing. Thermal effect on surrounding tissues was evaluated by the experiments employed with fresh porcine femurs. Femurs were prepared by cutting in half and holes with diameter of 7 mm were drilled on the exposed cancellous bone. Then keep the femurs in 37 °C water bath to simulate the temperature in vivo. Alloy cement was preheated in liquid state at 65 °C and then injected into the holes. At the same time, temperature of bone-cement interface, water bath and ambient temperature were monitored in real-time. When the temperature of bone-cement interface decreased to room temperature, the solidified alloy cement was removed by sawing the bones and the interfacial bone tissue was obtained for histological analysis. Through the change curve of temperature, it can be figured out that the time for the temperature of bone-cement interface standing above 44 °C was 58 s (see Fig. 10.8). This period is less than the 60 s exposure time for acceptable temperature threshold [51]. In

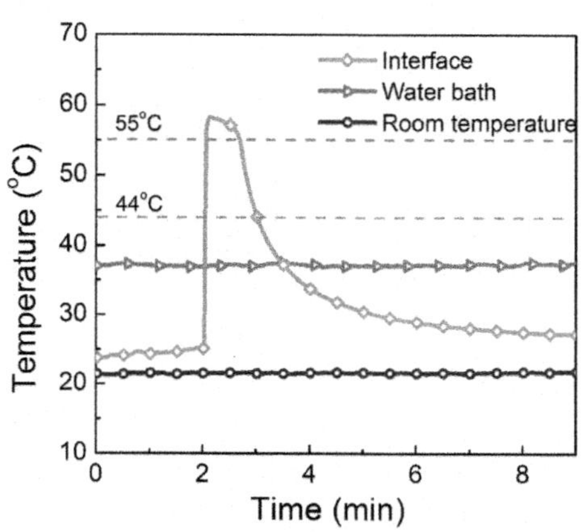

Fig. 10.8 The temperature-time curve of cement injected into porcine bone [45]. Picture reproduced with permission

addition, there was also report that thermal necrosis occurred when bone tissue was exposed to the temperature >55 °C for only 30 s [52]. For alloy cement, the temperature during the solidification between 55 °C and peak temperature (58.3 °C) lasted for 37 s which is a little higher than 30 s. However, HE (hematoxylin eosin) staining shows that the surrounding bone tissue still maintains its structural integrity without any damage after injection of alloy cement.

10.7 Reversible Capabilities of Alloy Bone Cement in Revision

Different from the chemical polymerization of acrylic cement, alloy cement works depending on the physical phase transition. It suggests that the revision of alloy cement may be easy to operate by heating. To verify this, associated experiments were implemented to simulate the revision process intuitively (see Fig. 10.9a). The alloy cement was placed into a PP (Propene Polymer) cylindrical mold (15 mm diameter and 18 mm height) with the thermal couple inserted between the cement and inner wall of mold. The interfacial temperature was recorded with time interval of 1 s. In the revision process, the heating probe was employed to continuously heat the central alloy cement. Along with the alloy melting, the probe was moved down vertically to melt the lower solid alloy. When the specimen became completely melted, remove the heating probe immediately. The working part of the probe used was conical with diameter of 6 mm and height of 12 mm and the heating temperature was 200 °C. The curve of transient temperature profile is shown in Fig. 10.9b. Remarkably, the peripheral temperature was increased to 60 °C within

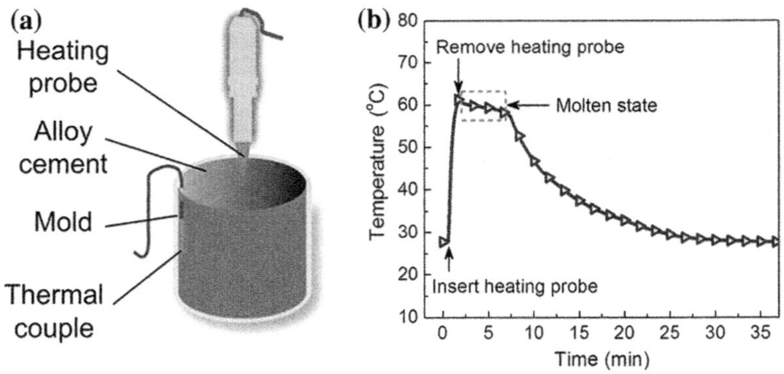

Fig. 10.9 The revision of alloy cement simulated in mold [45]. **a** Schematic of heating solid alloy cement. The heating probe was placed on the center of cement, and the thermal couple was used to monitor the interfacial temperature. **b** The recorded temperature during the operation process which indicates that the cement could be easily removed via syringe when it was melting. Picture reproduced with permission

1 min once the heating probe contacted the alloy cement. That is because the high heat conductivity of BiInSnZn alloy. Meanwhile, the whole cement in the mold have melted completely. By virtue of the temperature recorded in real-time, the heating probe can be timely removed to avoid overheating of surrounding tissue. After the removal of probe, the temperature dropped down slowly in a period of time. This won more time for surgeon to remove the melting cement. In this experiment, operating time was 5 min for aspirating the molten cement. Based on this unique merit, the extraction of prosthesis is also easily accessible.

The experiment has proven the potential of BiInSnZn cement in reversible revision. It is well-known that the melting rate is proportional to the heating temperature. To balance the melting time and minimization of the thermal damage to the peri-prosthetic tissues, a computational model focusing on relationship between heating temperature and thermal distribution was established for further analysis. The heating probe and cement molds were concentric cylinders and detailed dimensions are shown in Fig. 10.10a. In this model, three different heating temperature conditions (T_{heat} = 80, 100 and 120 °C) were investigated respectively, and other parameters were kept constant.

The classical heat transfer equation was utilized to characterize the transient 3D temperature distributions in the alloy cement, i.e.

$$\rho c \frac{\partial T(\mathbf{X}, t)}{\partial t} = \nabla(k \nabla T(\mathbf{X}, t)) \tag{10.1}$$

where, X denotes the three dimensional Cartesian coordinates x, y and z; ρ denotes the density of BiInSnZn alloy, 7.564 g/cm^3; k is the thermal conductivity, 13 W/(m °C); c is the specific heat which transiently varies with the temperature. To implement more accurate simulations, the curve of c was fit by B-spline interpolation function and the estimated result is shown in Fig. 10.10b.

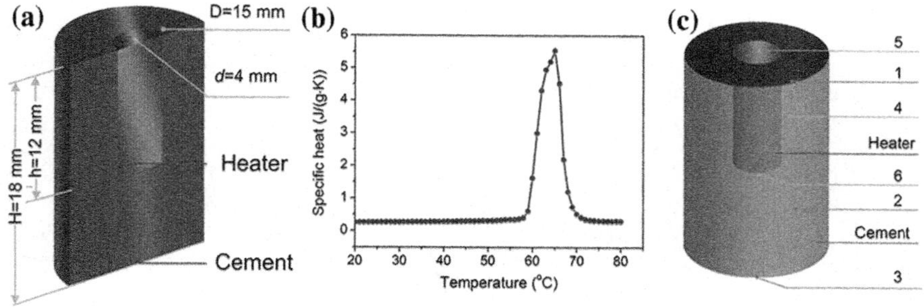

Fig. 10.10 The geometrical model for simulating the thermal effects during the heating [45]. **a** The dimensions of numerical model. **b** The specific heat curve of BiInSnZn alloy via fitting. **c** Geometric theoretical model for thermal distribution. 1–6 are for the boundary conditions of theoretical model. 1–3 denote the upper, profile and bottom surface of the alloy cement. 4–6 denote the profile, upper, and bottom surface of the heating probe. Picture reproduced with permission

The corresponding thermal boundary conditions of 1–3 and 5 (see Fig. 10.10c) are expressed in Eq. (10.2). And the Eq. (10.3) gives the boundary conditions of 4 and 6, i.e.

$$k\frac{\partial T}{\partial n} = 0 \tag{10.2}$$

$$T = T_{heat} \tag{10.3}$$

Through modeling and computational simulation, the temperature distributions of cross-sectional plane are depicted as Fig. 10.11a when peripheric temperature was increased to 60 °C under three heating conditions. Besides, in case of the injury risk resulting from operational errors in delay of removing heating probe, the variation of temperature on the cement edges was simulated when the heating probe kept working for 30 min. As shown in Fig. 10.11b, it took longer time for the whole cement to realize melting at lower heating temperature, whereas such temperature may reduce the risk of thermal injury. Different heating temperatures can be chosen as desired in practical trials. This simulating model has simply given a typical example for revision. Other conditions can also be altered according to actual requirements. For instance, the shape of heating probe can be designed and determined in consideration of different shapes of the filled cements. Thus, the simulating model can be employed to achieve better therapeutic effect through evaluating the effects of practical parameters before revision.

It has been displayed that it is a reversible process for the transitions between liquid and solid alloy cement. Then how to remove the liquid alloy cement from target is also significant that should be paid attention to. With respect to this issue, the experiment has been carried out and proven that the melted metal can be easily removed with medical syringe rather than special and complex device. It not only demonstrates the feasibility of revision using existing instrument but also indicates that the cost caused by the development of new device can be avoided.

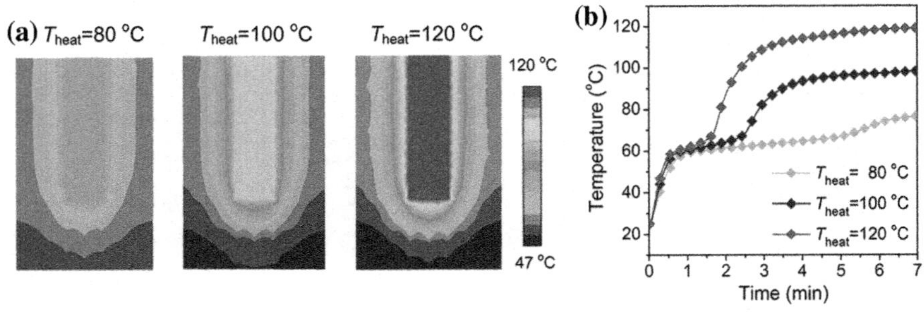

Fig. 10.11 The simulation results of alloy cement revision [45]. **a** The simulated temperature distributions on the cross-sectional plane under conditions of T_{heat} = 80, 100, 120 °C; Here, T_{heat} denotes the heating temperature. **b** The real-time maximum temperature profiles on the sidewalls in three cases of heating conditions. Picture reproduced with permission

10.8 Mechanical Characteristics of Alloy Bone Cement

Proper mechanical characteristics are the basic requirements of bone cement. In Chap. 4, the mechanical properties of BiInSnZn have been introduced and discussed. It has been known that the magnitudes of the compressive strength, bending stress and bending modulus of the alloy cement were 37.6 ± 1.56 MPa, 35.31 ± 1.09 MPa and 6.41 ± 0.81 GPa, respectively. According to the requirements in ISO 5833 standard [48], the mean values of compression strength, bending strength and bending modulus of acrylic cement are larger than 70 MPa, 50 MPa and 1.8 GPa, respectively. Notably, the measured compression and bending strength of alloy cement are lower than the requirements in national standard of acrylic cement. These properties should be further enhanced for the application in THA. In consideration of the current technologies in improvement of mechanical properties of metals, quite a few mature methods can be utilized to modify the behaviors of alloy solder. For instance, it was reported that the methods of regulating the component ratio and (or) adding other components could effectively improve the properties of alloy solder [53]. Additionally, one could attempt to combine the alloy cement with certain nanoparticles as well which have been used to improve the mechanical strength of the materials in future study [22, 54]. On the other hand, the compression and bending strength are comparable with those of CPCs [55, 56]. At this stage, BiInSnZn alloy without more modifications can be rapidly utilized as bone cement in non-load bearing position based on the existing study. Moreover, N_f (number of cycles to failure) results of alloy specimens were 109,373, 106,549, 78,594 and 76,892 with an applied stress of ±15 MPa, at a frequency of 5 Hz. The number of fatigue stress cycles for alloy specimens is close to that of commercial cement such as CMW1, CRX and CXL [57]. Meanwhile, the reported results demonstrated that alloy cement offers better crack resistance compared to acrylic cement in the width control of 32 mm [58]. In total, mechanical characteristics in both short term and long term have revealed the possibility of BiInSnZn alloy serving as bone cement.

10.9 Interaction Between Bone Cement and Multi-factor in Internal Environment

Bone cement is a kind of implantable material. Thus, it should pay great attention to the biocompatibility of novel bone cement, i.e. BiInSnZn alloy. As described in Chap. 4, the interplay between alloy cement and internal environment has been studied in three levels: corrosion, cytotoxicity and animal tests. In the corrosion experiment, alloy samples were immersed into simulating body solution. The result shows that only zinc was slightly increased along with the time and its concentration was 0.8 ± 0.1 μg/mL after 14 days. However, the ratio of zinc in BiInSnZn alloy is very low (0.4%) and the other three metals are nearly insoluble. Generally speaking, BiInSnZn alloy behaves well in static corrosion. In regard to the dissolution problem of zinc, it can be further solved by regulating the ratios of alloy composition and lots of experiments are needed.

On the basis of corrosion behaviour, cytotoxicity of BiInSnZn alloy has been evaluated according to ISO 10993-12 [59]. The cement extract was used to culture BALB/c 3T3 cells. The results indicate that the toxicity of this material is rather low. Furthermore, the alloy cement samples were subcutaneously implanted into the mice. Such in vivo experiment proved that alloy cement takes a good biocompatibility with tissues in a relatively long period of time. The existing literatures also revealed that the elements Bi, In, Sn and Zn are quite safe for human body. Up to the present, all these tests suggest that alloy cement is probably a biocompatible material. The final conclusion can be only obtained by a series experiments, including the cytotoxicity, sensitization, irritation, intracutaneous reactivity, systemic toxicity, subacute and subchronic toxicity, genotoxicity, implantation and haemocompatibility, chronic toxicity, carcinogenicity, reproductive and developmental toxicity and biodegradation [60].

10.10 Contrast Agent for Radiation Imaging

Generally, the radiation imaging is an effective way to monitor and evaluate the status of molding cement in vivo clinically. To achieve this goal, contrast agents are necessary due to the low imaging ability of acrylic cements. On the other hand, BiInSnZn alloy cement is a kind of metal material that may perform well in imaging even without contrast agent added. To investigate the imaging contrast characteristic of the current alloy cement, the radiation images of porcine femurs filling with alloy cement were taken. X-ray photo is the main imaging method in bone diseases, thus X-rays (General Electrics, XR/A) were firstly taken at 50 kV and 4.0 mAs. Under this condition, the radiographs are shown in Fig. 10.12a, b. The alloy cement can be obviously distinguished from surrounding bone through photos, indicating excellent imaging ability of alloy cement. In addition, to quantitatively describe such ability, the grayscale curves of radiographs with and without alloy cement embedded were calculated. The grayscale curves of G1 and G2 lines through bones in Fig. 10.12a, b are shown in Fig. 10.12c. Since the range of gray value is defined as 0–255, gray value of alloy cement with 197 is much higher than that (gray value, 160) of cortical bone (with the highest radiopacity of bone). Such huge difference results in the easy identification of alloy cement. Moreover, gray-level distribution ($F_{contrast}$) was utilized for further characterization. It can be calculated as follows [61]:

$$F_{contrast} = \frac{\sigma}{(\alpha_4)^{0.25}} \tag{10.4}$$

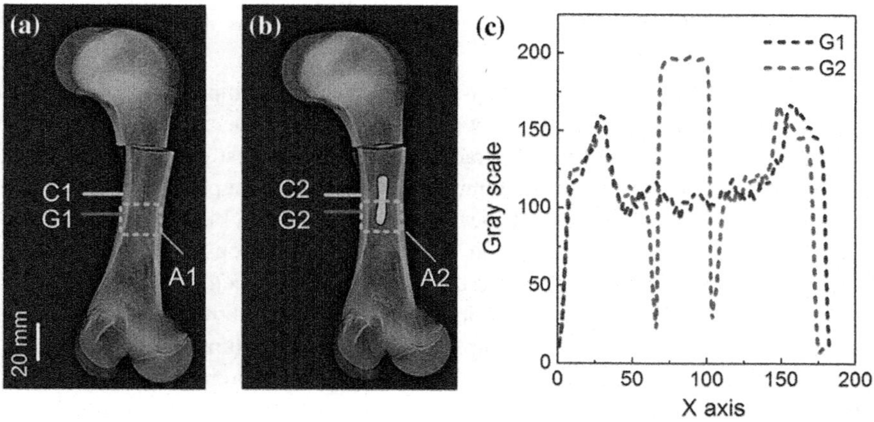

Fig. 10.12 Radiation imaging of porcine femur with alloy cement [45]. **a** X-ray imaging of bone with partial excavation of marrow. **b** X-ray imaging of the bone cavity filled with alloy cement. **c** Grayscale curves of C1 and C2 lines (parts through the bone) in (**a**) and (**b**). Picture reproduced with permission

where, σ and α_4 are standard deviation of mean of the gray-levels probability distribution and kurtosis respectively; The Kurtosis was employed for measuring polarization which is based on the mean μ_4 and the variance σ^2 can be defined as:

$$\alpha_4 = \frac{\mu_4}{(\sigma^2)^2} \tag{10.5}$$

The lines C1 and C2, square A1 and A2 in Fig. 10.12a, b were chosen for comparison. Through calculation using Eqs. (10.4) and (10.5), the contrast value results of C1, C2, A1 and A2 are 16.01, 31.93, 14.76, and 33.1 respectively. Evidently, corresponding numerical values of line and area of alloy cement are much larger, which indicates that alloy cement can dramatically improve the image contrast. In total, alloy cement itself can serve as effective contrast agent in X-ray imaging for convenience of monitoring after surgery.

X-ray imaging provides 2D (dimension) information, which sometimes is insufficient to master the whole structure of the cement filling quality. CT (computed tomography) can solve this problem by 3D imaging. Thus, porcine femurs with alloy cement were scanned by CT (Philips Brilliance 6) at 100 kV and 200 mAs. Although the metal artifacts in CT severely decrease the image quality, alloy cement display clear edges which extends the imaging role for detection. Taking advantage of this, the geometrical model is able to be reconstructed by the CT slices. While using this model, the size of the filling cement can be measured from horizontal or coronal cross section, which is valuable for further medical measurement.

10.11 Conclusion

Conventional cements are general non-metallic materials composed of powder and liquid systems. Prior to use, these two systems have to be mixed in situ at an appropriate ratio. Different from the traditional ones, the latest proposed alloy bone cement has only one system, mitigating the complexity of preparation work. It was found that molten alloy cement performs better fluidity than PMMA paste. A normal syringe would satisfy the required manipulations for alloy cement. Notably, the major difference between the acrylic and alloy cement is their working principle. Rather than the solidification of acrylic cement relying on chemical reaction, alloy cement solidifies simply depending on natural physical process. Thus, the temperature of alloy cement is related to the preheating temperature, which continuously and rapidly decreases from the peak to environmental temperature since it is injected to the target. During the filling process, the released heat is hardly possible to lead the necrosis of surrounding tissues. To further ensure the safety, the preheating temperature could be reduced within a reasonable range. In addition, the reported methods such as pre-chilling prosthesis and bone cavity prior to cement filling [62, 63] are helpful in optimizing the interfacial temperature which can be adopted as well. The resulted advantages include the low incidence of premature failure of the cement mantle and good effects in repairing [64].

Significantly, the revision processes vary with the different working principles of acrylic and alloy cement. Due to the reversible properties in liquid-solid phase transition, alloy cement can not only be performed with traditional method but is also easy to handle by way of simply heating the probe and medical injector. Before practical operation, the calculation model can be constructed for planning the following surgery. The revision methods can be further improved by various attempts as well, such as direct heating on metal prosthesis rather than cement.

Comprehensive mechanical tests carried out had demonstrated that most mechanical properties of solidified alloy cement meet the requirements of acrylic cement based on the measured data. Nevertheless, the compression and bending strength are somewhat lower than those of the national standard of acrylic cement but are comparable with those of CPCs. At present, alloy cements tend to be utilized for non load-bearing position repair. There is a large space to further enhance the material's mechanical strength. Therefore, such deficiency needed to be compensated by advanced technologies and knowledge of materials science. So far, BiInSnZn has been studied as a typical example for cement research. There are still tremendous kinds of low-melting point alloys whose mechanical properties vary with different constituents, waiting for people to test and learn more.

Taken into consideration the biocompatibility, both in vitro and in vivo experiments have displayed consistence in conclusion that the alloy cement is biocompatible to a great extent. However, it is well known that the biocompatibility of implantable material should be rigorous. More investigations are still needed, especially the experiments on human in clinical trials. Besides, by virtue of the intrinsic property of metal, alloy cement itself can serve as image contrast agent which favors the monitoring of the operation. As seen from the radiological imaging data, the gray level and its distribution demonstrate that radiography containing bone and alloy cement together displays high contrast which is hard to realize otherwise by the conventional methods with radiopacifiers added.

Generally speaking, alloy cement consisting of BiInSnZn alloy has shown excellent characteristics including reversible transition, rapid solidification, lower peak temperature, radiopacity, and low cytotoxicity as the bone cement. Moreover, BiInSnZn alloy as a kind of metal performs well in electrical conductivity. It was reported that the electrical stimulation plays a role in controlling bone growth and healing [65, 66], and the electrical polarization of titanium implants may increase the osteoblast differentiation [67]. For traditional non-metallic cements, they are located between metal prosthesis and bone tissue that restrict the transmitting of electrical stimulation due to the poor electrical conductivity. Therefore, the application of alloy cement can contribute a lot in bone healing. In a word, the liquid-solid phase transition alloy cement opens great promise as bone cement with many improved properties which are expected to change the basic concept of current biomedical cement material. Along with the opportunity, these trends suggest that a lot of investigations should be conducted for future enhancement of alloy material performances.

References

1. Taylor D, Hazenberg JG, Lee TC (2007) Living with cracks: damage and repair in human bone. Nat Mater 6(4):263–268
2. Baltzer AW, Lieberman JR (2004) Regional gene therapy to enhance bone repair. Gene Ther 11(11):344–350
3. Johnell O, Kanis J (2005) Epidemiology of osteoporotic fractures. Osteoporos Int 16(Suppl 2):S3–S7
4. Longo V, Brunetti O, D'Oronzo S et al (2012) Therapeutic approaches to myeloma bone disease: an evolving story. Cancer Treat Rev 38(6):787–797
5. Rodan GA, Martin TJ, Rodan GA, Martin TJ (2000) Therapeutic approaches to bone diseases. Science 289(5484):1508–1514
6. Felson DT, Zhang Y (1998) An update on the epidemiology of knee and hip osteoarthritis with a view to prevention. Arthritis Rheum 41(8):1343–1355
7. Berry DJ, Bozic KJ (2010) Current practice patterns in primary hip and knee arthroplasty among members of the American association of hip and knee surgeons. J Arthroplasty 25:2–4
8. Jackson JD, Pagnano MW (2012) Cement fixation for total knee arthroplasty. In: The knee joint. Springer, Paris, pp 759–764
9. Rand JA, Trousdale RT, Ilstrup DM et al (2003) Factors affecting the durability of primary total knee prostheses. J Bone Joint Surg Am 85(2):259–265
10. Garellick G, Rolfson O (2012) The Swedish hip arthroplasty register annual report 2012
11. Dunbar MJ, Richardson G (2012) Cemented femoral fixation: back to the future. Semin Arthroplasty 23(3):155–158
12. Galibert P, Deramond H, Rosat P et al (1987) Preliminary note on the treatment of vertebral angioma by percutaneous acrylic vertebroplasty. Neurochirurgie 33(2):166–168
13. Watts NB, Harris ST, Genant HK (2001) Treatment of painful osteoporotic vertebral fractures with percutaneous vertebroplasty or kyphoplasty. Osteoporos Int 12(6):429–437

14. Hulme PA, Krebs J, Ferguson SJ et al (2006) Vertebroplasty and kyphoplasty: a systematic review of 69 clinical studies. Spine 31(17):1983–2001
15. Eck JC, Nachtigall D, Humphreys SC et al (2008) Comparison of vertebroplasty and balloon kyphoplasty for treatment of vertebral compression fractures: a meta-analysis of the literature. Spine J 8(3):488–497
16. Breusch SJ, Aldinger PR, Thomsen M et al (2000) Anchoring principles in hip endoprostheses. I: prosthesis stem. Der Unfallchirurg 103(11):918–931
17. Charnley J (1960) Anchorage of the femoral head prosthesis to the shaft of the femur. J Bone Joint Surg Br 42B(1):28–30
18. Kindtlarsen T, Smith DB, Jensen JS (1995) Innovations in acrylic bone cement and application equipment. J Appl Biomater 6(1):75–83
19. Cristofolini L, Minari C, Viceconti M (2008) A methodology and criterion for acrylic bone cement fatigue tests. Fatigue Fract Eng Mater Struct 23(11):953–957
20. Ormsby R, Mcnally T, Mitchell C et al (2010) Influence of multiwall carbon nanotube functionality and loading on mechanical properties of PMMA/MWCNT bone cements. J Mater Sci - Mater Med 21(8):2287–2292
21. Stańczyk M, van Rietbergen B (2002) Thermal analysis of bone cement polymerisation at the cement-bone interface. J Biomech 186(2):169–173
22. Yang JM, Lu CS, Hsu YG et al (1997) Mechanical properties of acrylic bone cement containing PMMA-SiO_2 hybrid sol-gel material. J Biomed Mater Res 38(2):143–154
23. Homsy CA, Tullos HS, Anderson MS et al (1972) Some physiological aspects of prosthesis stabilization with acrylic polymer. Clin Orthop Relat Res 83(4):317–328
24. Freeman MA, Bradley GW, Revell PA (1982) Observations upon the interface between bone and polymethylmethacrylate cement. J Bone Joint Surg Br 64(4):489–493
25. Kim YS, Kang YH, Kim JK et al (1994) Effect of bone mineral particles on the porosity of bone cement. Bio-Med Mater Eng 4(1):37–46
26. Dunne NJ, Orr JF, Mushipe MT et al (2003) The relationship between porosity and fatigue characteristics of bone cements. Biomaterials 24(2):239–245
27. Evans SL (2006) Effects of porosity on the fatigue performance of polymethyl methacrylate bone cement: an analytical investigation. Proc Inst Mech Eng Part H 220(1):1–10
28. Gilbert JL, Hasenwinkel JM, Wixson RL et al (2000) A theoretical and experimental analysis of polymerization shrinkage of bone cement: a potential major source of porosity. J Biomed Mater Res 52(1):210–218
29. Kuehn KD, Ege W, Gopp U (2005) Acrylic bone cements: composition and properties. Orthop Clin North Am 36(1):17–28
30. van Hooy-Corstjens CS, Govaert LE, Spoelstra AB et al (2004) Mechanical behaviour of a new acrylic radiopaque iodine-containing bone cement. Biomaterials 25(13):2657–2667
31. Deb S, Vazquez B (2001) The effect of cross-linking agents on acrylic bone cements containing radiopacifiers. Biomaterials 22:2177–2181
32. Artola A, Gurruchaga M, Vazquez B et al (2003) Elimination of barium sulphate from acrylic bone cements. Use of two iodine-containing monomers. Biomaterials 24:4071–4080
33. Manero JM, Ginebra MP, Gil FJ et al (2004) Propagation of fatigue cracks in acrylic bone cements containing different radiopaque agents. Proc Inst Mech Eng [H] 218(3):167–172
34. Bhambri SK, Gilbertson LN (1995) Micromechanisms of fatigue crack initiation and propagation in bone cements. J Biomed Mater Res 29(2):233–237
35. Langlais F, Lambotte JC, Collin P et al (2003) Trochanteric slide osteotomy in revision total hip arthroplasty for loosening. J Bone Joint Surg 85(4):510–516
36. Morshed S, Huffman GR, Ries MD (2005) Extended trochanteric osteotomy for 2-stage revision of infected total hip arthroplasty. J Arthroplasty 20(3):294–301
37. Younger TI, Bradford MS, Magnus RE et al (1995) Extended proximal femoral osteotomy. A new technique for femoral revision arthroplasty. J Arthroplasty 10(3):329–338
38. Li Z, Kawashita M (2011) Current progress in inorganic artificial biomaterials. J Artif Organs 14(3):163–170

39. Long M, Rack HJ (1998) Titanium alloys in total joint replacement—a materials science perspective. Biomaterials 19(18):1621–1639
40. Busscher HJ, Van Der Mei HC, Subbiahdoss G et al (2012) Biomaterial-associated infection: locating the finish line in the race for the surface. Sci Transl Med 4(153):153rv10
41. Moelans N, Kumar KCH, Wollants P (2003) Thermodynamic optimization of the lead-free solder system Bi-In-Sn-Zn. J Alloy Compd 360:98–106
42. Li YW, Leong JC, Lu WW et al (2000) A novel injectable bioactive bone cement for spinal surgery: a developmental and preclinical study. J Biomed Mater Res 52(1):164–170
43. Lei W, Jing L (2014) Liquid phase 3D printing for quickly manufacturing conductive metal objects with low melting point alloy ink. Sci China Technol Sci 57(9):1721–1728
44. Deng Y, Liu J (2014) Flexible mechanical joint as human exoskeleton using low-melting-point alloy. J Med Devices 8(4):044506
45. Yi L, Jin C, Wang L et al (2014) Liquid-solid phase transition alloy as reversible and rapid molding bone cement. Biomaterials 35(37):9789–9801
46. Roscoe R, Bainbridge W (2002) Viscosity determination by the oscillating vessel method II: the viscosity of water at 20 °C. Proc Phys Soc 72(4):585
47. Boger A, Bohner M, Heini P, Verrier S, Schneider E (2008) Properties of an injectable low modulus PMMA bone cement for osteoporotic bone. J Biomed Mater Res B Appl Biomater 86:474–482
48. International Organization for Standardization (2002) ISO 5833: implants for surgery-acrylic resin cements
49. Saito M, Maruoka A, Mori T et al (1994) Experimental studies on a new bioactive bone cement: hydroxyapatite composite resin. Biomaterials 15:156–160
50. Farrar DF, Rose J (2001) Rheological properties of PMMA bone cements during curing. Biomaterials 22:3005–3013
51. Eriksson AR, Albrektsson T (1983) Temperature threshold levels for heat-induced bone tissue injury: a vital-microscopic study in the rabbit. J Prosthet Dent 50(1):101–107
52. Feith R (1975) Side-effects of acrylic cement implanted into bone. A histologicl, (micro) angiographic, fluorescence-microscopic and autoradiog-aphic study in the rabbit femur. Acta Orthop 161(3):163
53. Chang TC, Wang JW, Wang MC et al (2006) Solderability of Sn-9Zn-0.5 Ag-1In lead-free solder on Cu substrate: Part 1. Thermal properties, microstructure, corrosion and oxidation resistance. J Alloy Compd 422:239–243
54. Frogley MD, Ravich D, Wagner HD (2003) Mechanical properties of carbon nanoparticle-reinforced elastomers. Compos Sci Technol 63(11):1647–1654
55. Troczynski T (2004) Bioceramics: a concrete solution. Nat Mater 3(1):13–14
56. Chang CH, Liao TC, Hsu YM et al (2010) A poly (propylene fumarate)-calcium phosphate based angiogenic injectable bone cement for femoral head osteonecrosis. Biomaterials 31:4048–4055
57. Lewis G, Janna S (2003) Effect of test specimen cross-sectional shape on the in vitro fatigue life of acrylic bone cement. Biomaterials 24:4315–4321
58. Lewis G, Mladsi S (2000) Correlation between impact strength and fracture toughness of PMMA-based bone cements. Biomaterials 21:775–7781
59. International Organization for Standardization ISO 10993 (2009) Biological evaluation of medical devices. Part 12: sample preparation and reference materials. Geneva: ISO
60. International Organization for Standardization ISO 10993 (2009) Biological evaluation of medical devices. Part 1: evaluation and testing within a risk management process. ISO, Geneva
61. Tamura H, Mori S, Yamawaki T (1978) Textural features corresponding to visual perception. IEEE Trans Syst Man Cybern 8(6):460–473
62. Toksviglarsen S, Franzen H, Ryd L (1991) Cement interface temperature in hip arthroplasty. Acta Orthop 62(2):102–105
63. Lidgren L, Bodelind B, Möller J (1987) Bone cement improved by vacuum mixing and chilling. Acta Orthop 58:27–32

64. Dunne NJ, Orr JF (2002) Curing characteristics of acrylic bone cement. J Mater Sci - Mater Med 13(1):17–22
65. Lavine LS, Lustrin I, Rinaldi RA et al (1972) Electric enhancement of bone healing. Science 175:1118–11121
66. Luben RA, Cain CD, Chen CY et al (1982) Effects of electromagnetic stimuli on bone and bone cells in vitro: inhibition of responses to parathyroid hormone by low-energy low-frequency fields. Proc Natl Acad Sci 79(13):4180–4184
67. Gittens RA, Olivares-Navarrete R, Rettew R et al (2013) Electrical polarization of titanium surfaces for the enhancement of osteoblast differentiation. Bioelectromagnetics 34:599–612

Chapter 11
Liquid Metal Enabled Flexible Exoskeleton or Artificial Muscle

Abstract This chapter explains the basic concept of a flexible mechanical joint for making human exoskeleton based on a low-melting-point alloy phase change effect. With the liquid-solid phase change capability, this unique joint can easily switch between its flexible and rigid states. In addition, the liquid metal electrode can be an important highly conductive and super compliant electrode for making artificial muscles with the unique capability of two-dimensional in-plane self-healing. Some of such opportunities were discussed.

Keywords Flexible exoskeleton · Artificial muscle · Liquid metal

11.1 Low-Melting-Point Alloy as Human Exoskeleton

The use of a human exoskeleton to strengthen the ability of soldiers and disabled persons has attracted much attention in both academic and industrial circles in recent years [1–6]. The mechanical joint is the core component and plays the important role of supporting the movement and load-bearing functions of the exoskeleton [7–10]. On the one hand, such joint is required to provide appropriate degrees of freedom to enable flexible movement of the body; On the other hand, it should be able to transfer and withstand as much mechanical load as possible to reduce the burden on the human body. Conventional mechanical joints of human exoskeletons generally use bearings and a hydraulic mechanism to achieve flexibility and bear load [11–15]. However, owing to the requirement of pumping machinery, such conventional mechanisms are often characterized by a complicated structure, high cost, and low stability and reliability. Moreover, other advanced mechanical joints such as energy-storing passive joints are incapable of coping with movements of extremely high frequency and intensity [16, 17]. In fact, there has been an urgent need to develop more flexible and powerful mechanical joints with simpler structures, higher degrees of freedom, and more powerful strength and stability for use in human exoskeletons [18, 19]. And a group of important progresses have been made so far (Fig. 11.1).

J. Liu and L. Yi, *Liquid Metal Biomaterials*,
Springer Series in Biomaterials Science and Engineering10,
https://doi.org/10.1007/978-981-10-5607-9_11

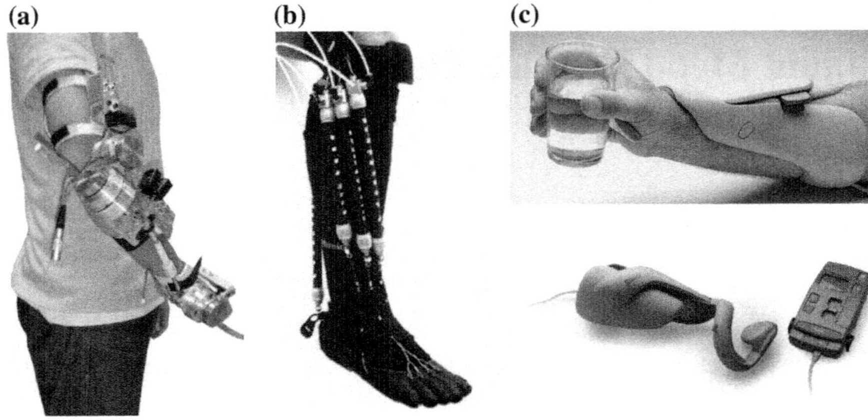

Fig. 11.1 Wearable robotic exoskeleton and powered orthoses for limb rehabilitation: **a** wearable orthosis with electrical actuator [18]. **b** Wearable robotic device with pneumatic actuator [19]. **c** The Bioness H200 based on FES as natural actuator of body muscles (available online: http://www.bioness.com/Products/H200_for_Hand_Paralysis.php; accessed on 7 December 2016). Pictures reproduced with permission

From an alternative, Deng and Liu [20] had ever proposed the concept of a flexible mechanical joint for making human exoskeleton based on a low-melting-point alloy phase change effect. With the liquid-solid phase change capability, this unique joint can easily switch between its flexible and rigid states. The liquid state of the metal ensures excellent moving flexibility, whereas the solid state of the metal allows for extremely high loading capacities. In addition, this flexible and powerful mechanical joint does not require electric motors or pumping machinery, which allows it to be more stable and reliable for use as a practical mechanical joint of a human exoskeleton. Such mechanism allows the fabricated human exoskeleton arm to conveniently and effectively perform the powerful lifting action. This method opens a soft mechanical joint for human exoskeleton in future civilian use. Except for directly applying the low melting point alloy to make exoskeleton, such material can also be adopted as soft electrodes to actuate certain elastomer so as to fabricate artificial muscle. All these efforts suggest that liquid metal offers innovative ways to realize flexible exoskeleton which would significantly expand the category of conventional rigid system. This chapter discusses some of such opportunities.

11.2 Phase Change Properties of Low Melting Point Alloy

Conceptual investigations disclosed that metal-based mechanical joints provided excellent moving flexibility and large loading capacity. Similar to its use as bone cement, the low melting point metal can also be developed as exoskeleton through taking full exploration of its liquid-solid phase changeable capability. Comparative measurements demonstrated that the recently proposed phase change joint responded much faster and could support heavier loads than that of the conventional paraffin-based joint [20].

The key to achieving flexible mechanical joints is to choose a low-melting-point alloy that has a high thermal conductivity, low latent heat, and is nontoxic, stable, and reliable. Until now, there are few alloys with a melting point below 100 °C, primarily gallium-, indium-, and bismuth-based alloys. Table 11.1 lists several typical low-melting-point alloys, for which the melting points were measured and verified in our laboratory. Comprehensively considering the melting point, toxicity, safety, cost, thermal conductivity, and latent heat, the eutectic alloy $Bi_{32.5}In_{51}Sn_{16.5}$ was particularly illustrated here as the phase change material to construct one of the cores of exoskeleton: the mechanical joint. The melting point of such eutectic alloy is 60 °C, with sub-cooling degree always less than 4 °C.

The extremely high thermal conductivity and low latent heat of a low-melting-point alloy ensure that the mechanical joint responds very quickly. Figure 11.2 provides a comparison of the thermal conductivity and latent heat between a low-melting-point alloy and paraffin (conventional phase change material) [20]. It can be seen that the thermal conductivity of the low-melting-point alloy is much higher than that of paraffin; thus, the heat transfer is faster. In addition, the latent heat of the low-melting-point alloy is much smaller than that of paraffin. Furthermore, the low-melting-point alloy has smaller heat capacity. Therefore, the low-melting-point alloy can respond faster and consumes less power under certain heat flux values. This is one of the key advantages of choosing a low-melting-point alloy as the phase change material for making a mechanical joint.

Table 11.1 Melting points of typical low-melting-point alloys

Low-melting-point alloy	Melting point (°C)
$Ga_{61}In_{25}Sn_{13}Zn_1$	8
$Ga_{66}In_{20.5}Sn_{13.5}$	10
$Ga_{75.5}In_{24.5}$	16
Ga	29
$Bi_{32.5}In_{51}Sn_{16.5}$	60
$Bi_{54}In_{30}Sn_{16}$	81

The subscript number represents the mass fraction of each element

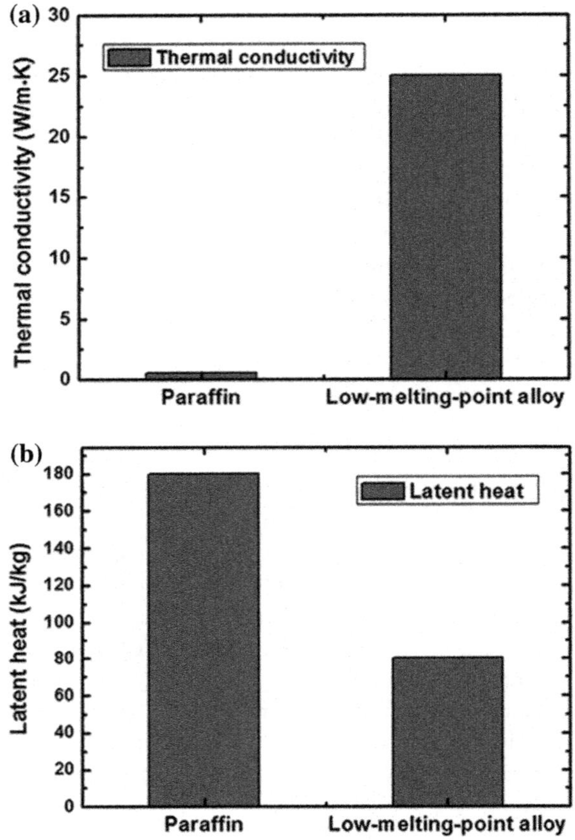

Fig. 11.2 Comparison of the **a** thermal conductivity and **b** latent heat between paraffin and a low-melting-point alloy [20]. All pictures reproduced with permission

11.3 Working of Low-Melting-Point Alloy as Human Exoskeleton

Figure 11.3 presents a working prototype of a flexible mechanical joint using a low-melting-point alloy [20], which is comprised of the forearm, rear arm, metal chamber, thermoelectric device, and sealing ring. In a real application, the forearm and the rear arm of the prototype are connected and fit to the person's upper limb. The thermoelectric device contacts the metal chamber and is responsible for heating and cooling the low-melting-point alloy. At room temperature, the low-melting-point alloy is in a solid state. When the temperature rises to 60 °C, the metal melts into a liquid. Therefore, the mechanical joint can switch between flexible and rigid states. To prevent leakage, the sealing ring was arranged on the top of the low-melting-point alloy chamber. Moreover, a step-like resistance structure was designed in the metal cavity to raise the loading capacity of the joint.

The rigid part of the mechanical joint in Fig. 11.3 is made of $Cr_1Ni_{18}Ti_9$ stainless steel. Its joint chamber is filled with the eutectic alloy $Bi_{32.5}In_{51}Sn_{16.5}$. In

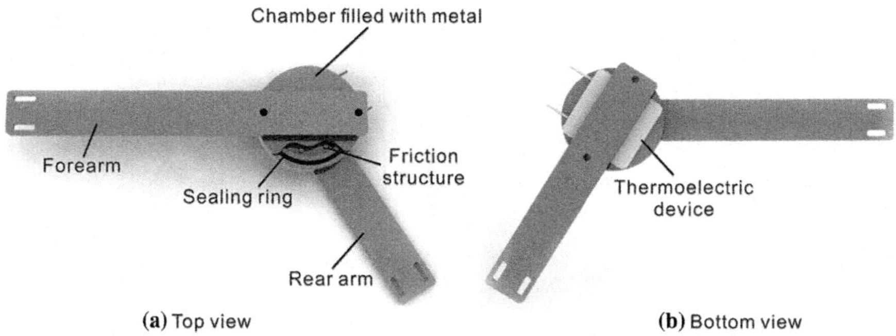

Fig. 11.3 Prototype of flexible mechanical joint based on a low-melting-point alloy [20]. All pictures reproduced with permission

such system, a thermoelectric device was also incorporated for regulating the thermal states of the eutectic alloy. Its heating area is 3 cm × 3 cm, and the maximum heating power is 50 W. Three temperature monitoring points were arranged to measure the temperature of the low-melting-point alloy, metal chamber, and the ambient air, respectively. All the temperature data were collected by Agilent 34970A, and the acquisition interval was 1 s. The power supply is a DC power source, DH1720A, with a maximum output voltage of 20 V and current of 10 A.

Figure 11.4 presents the typical temperature curves of a low-melting-point alloy melting and freezing in a mechanical joint under control of thermoelectric device [18]. The input power of the thermoelectric device is 12 W. Take the melting process for example, in the initial heating stage, the temperature of the low-melting-point alloy rises rapidly. Once the temperature reaches the melting point of the low-melting-point alloy, the alloy begins to melt, and the temperature remains stable. After all of the low-melting-point alloy melts to liquid, the temperature continues to rise again (Fig. 11.4a). A similar however reverse process can be found for the cooling process of such material (Fig. 11.4b). It is evident that the melting point of the eutectic alloy $Bi_{32.5}In_{51}Sn_{16.5}$ is 60 °C with a sub-cooling degree of about 4 °C. Overall, the time for the alloy to complete melting or freezing is about 8 s. Thus, the typical response time of this joint is less than 10 s. If the heating/cooling power is further increased, the joint response time can be significantly shortened. In addition, because the mechanical strength of the low-melting-point alloy is rather high, the amount of filled metal can be optimized and reduced, which will lead to an even shorter response time.

Figure 11.4c, d revealed the relationship between the melting time and heating power as well as the relationship between the freezing time and cooling power of the thermoelectric device, respectively [20]. By analyzing the relationship between the melting/freezing time and power, one can find that the phase transition response time of the mechanical joint is between 5 and 15 s. A higher heating/cooling power produces faster responses of the mechanical joint. In addition, the typical melting time is about 9 s, and the typical freezing time is about 7 s. Environmental heat

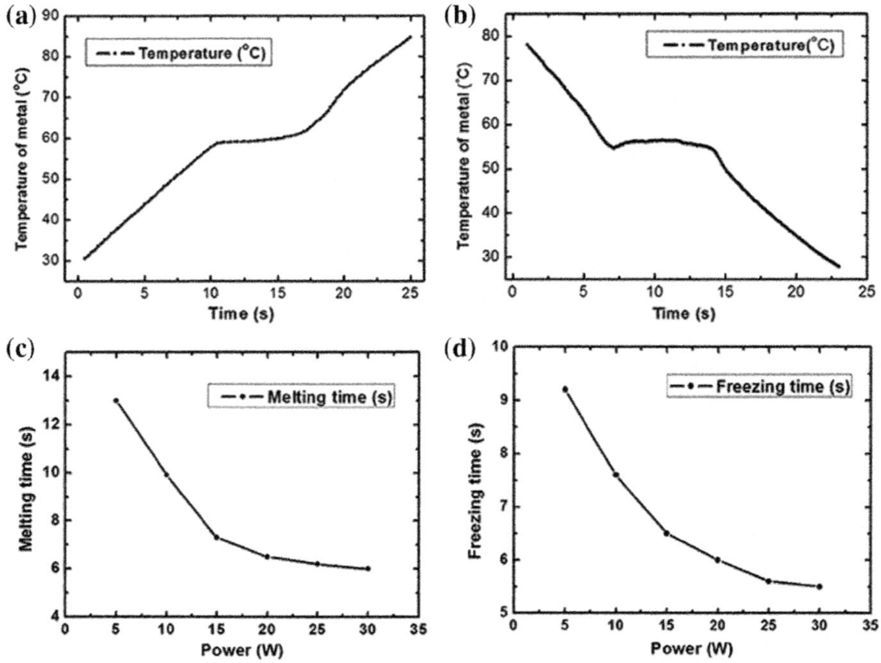

Fig. 11.4 Thermal behaviors of $Bi_{32.5}In_{51}Sn_{16.5}$ in a mechanical joint under heating or freezing [18]. **a** Typical temperature curve during melting; **b** Typical temperature curve during freezing; **c** Melting times under different heating powers; **d** Freezing times under different cooling powers. All pictures reproduced with permission

leakage is the main reason for the shorter freezing time, and it has a negative effect on heating for melting but plays an active role in the cooling stage for freezing.

The thermal conductivity and latent heat of a phase change material are the key factors for determining the response time of the phase transition of the flexible mechanical joint. The higher the thermal conductivity and the smaller the latent heat, the faster the phase change process and shorter the response time. Therefore, the joint is more sensitive to heating power and can quickly switch between rigid and flexible states with lower energy consumption. At present, among all the phase change materials, the low-melting-point alloy has much higher thermal conductivity and much smaller latent heat compared with traditional materials. Thus, it is a great advantage to use a low-melting-point alloy as the phase change material in a solid–liquid phase transition mechanical joint. Under identical experimental platforms but using paraffin instead of the low-melting-point alloy, several shortcomings were found to exist. One is that there was no stable phase transition temperature point. Another is that the response time of the joint was 60 s, which is much higher than that of the low-melting-point alloy. Therefore, for a flexible mechanical human exoskeleton joint, the low-melting-point alloy seems is the best choice for the phase change material.

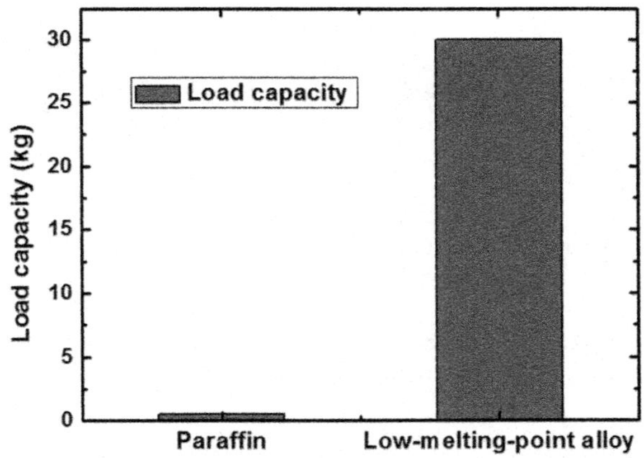

Fig. 11.5 Comparison of mechanical strength between the low-melting-point alloy mechanical joint and that based on conventional paraffin [18]. Picture reproduced with permission

Figure 11.5 compared the mechanical strengths that could offer by the low-melting-point alloy mechanical joint and that of conventional paraffin respectively [20]. In this measurement, the same experimental platform in Fig. 11.3 is used. As seen in Fig. 11.5, the paraffin phase change material can only withstand a load of 0.5 kg, whereas the low-melting-point alloy would sustain more than 30 kg with no sign failure. Therefore, it is obvious that the low-melting-point alloy is more suitable for making powerful mechanical joints. Because the low-melting-point alloy has much better shear strength compared to paraffin, it is able to withstand much larger loads when used for the mechanical joints of a human exoskeleton. This suggests that stronger and more powerful human exoskeletons can be attained and more widely used in the near future.

11.4 Theoretical Evaluation on the Mechanical Joint

Figure 11.6 depicts the application model and stress analysis of a typical low-melting-point alloy mechanical joint [20]. Generally, the joint is under a flexible state and can easily bend which is critical for human wearing comfort. Once the load is put on, the joint rapidly changes to a solid state and can thus withstand enormously heavy loads. With the help of the mechanical joints, the force on the brachialis can be expressed as

$$M = \frac{W \cdot s + G \cdot r - F \cdot m}{l} \tag{11.1}$$

where M is the muscle strength; W the gravity of the forearm; G the gravity of the load; F is the exoskeleton's supporting force; and l, s, r, and m are the lever arms relative to the rotation center. From Eq. (11.1), it can be found that the supporting effect of the mechanical joint can effectively reduce brachialis strength. If the

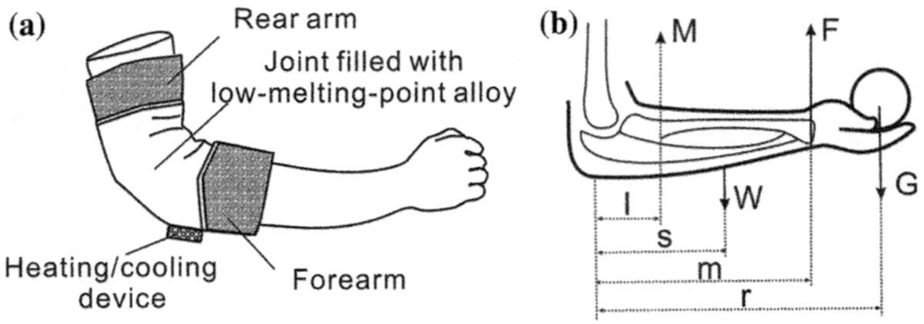

Fig. 11.6 **a** Application model of low-melting-point-alloy-based mechanical joint. **b** Stress analysis model of mechanical joint

mechanical joint is strong enough, the muscle strength equals to zero, which means the user does not feel any pressure during the lifting process.

The response time of the mechanical joint mainly depends on the alloy's solid–liquid phase transition process, which is related to the heating/cooling power and thermophysical property of a low-melting-point alloy. Considering the typical liquid metal in thermal joints in Fig. 11.6, the Biot number can be calculated according to $Bi = hD/K$. Generally, the natural convection coefficient of air is $h = 5$ W/(m^2 °C). The thermal conductivity of the low-melting-point alloy is $k = 25$ W/(m K), and the characteristic length of metal chamber in Fig. 11.6 is $D = 0.05$ m. Thus, the Biot number is calculated as $Bi = 0.01 < 0.1$. Therefore, one can investigate the heat transfer process of a metal-based mechanical joint using the lumped parameter model. In this case for the melting process, the one-dimensional heat transfer model can be described as follows:

$$\begin{cases} \rho CV\frac{\partial T}{\partial t} = hA(T_f - T) + q, & T \neq T_m \\ \rho VQ_L = \left[q - hA(T_m - T_f)\right] \cdot \Delta t & T = T_m \end{cases} \tag{11.2}$$

where ρ, C, V, and T are respectively the density, heat capacity, volume, and temperature, of a low-melting-point alloy. h and A are the air convective heat transfer coefficient and the area, respectively. T_m is the melting point of the metal, T_f is the ambient air temperature, t is the time, q is the electric heating power, Q_L is the latent heat of metal, and Δt is the phase transition time. At the initial stage, $t = 0$, $T = T_0 < T_m$; thus, it can be calculated that (1) the alloy phase transition begins at

$$t_m = \frac{\rho CV}{hA}\ln\left(1 + \frac{T_m - T_0}{T_0 - T_f - q/hA}\right)^{-1}, \tag{11.3}$$

and (2) the total time of phase transition (the joint response time) is

$$\Delta t = \frac{\rho VQ_L}{q - hA(T_m - T_f)}. \tag{11.4}$$

From Eqs. (11.3) and (11.4), one could find that higher initial alloy temperatures with a lower latent heat and higher heating power would result in the shorter joint response time, which means the mechanical joint can respond faster.

11.5 Liquid Metal Enabled Elastomer Actuators as Artificial Muscles

Except for directly using low melting point alloy to make human exoskeleton, liquid metal can also serve as soft electrode to actuate more materials to act which would help mold future soft skeleton. Liu et al. [21] had ever demonstrated a method of directly printing liquid metal films as highly conductive and super compliant electrodes for making dielectric elastomer actuator (DEA). Such soft electrodes enable DE film to approach its maximum strain and stress at relatively low voltages. Its unique capability of achieving two-dimensional in-plane self-healing by merely actuating the DEA would allow actuators more tolerant to fault and resilient to abusive environments. Such high performance actuator has important value in a wide spectrum of situations ranging from artificial muscle, flexible electronics to smart clothing etc.

In the robotics science, human's passion and efforts to mimic nature have never stopped [22, 23]. One of the major challenges in this area lies in the designing of soft linear actuators that could mimic biological muscles [24]. During the past few decades, several dielectric elastomers (DEs) such as 3M VHB 4910 acrylic films which exhibit large actuation strain and effective stress of over 7 MPa have gained ever-increasing interests owing to their potentials as artificial muscles [25, 26]. So far, the performance of dielectric elastomer actuators (DEAs) has been largely dependent on and limited by that of compliant electrodes [27]. Liu et al. [21] described an ultra-compliant liquid metal electrode that could exploit full potentials of DEs with the additional in-plane self-healing capability that would significantly enhance the extreme performance of DEAs as artificial muscles.

In principle, DEAs are capacitors that deform when charged with DC voltages. A basic planar DEA is a sandwich composite with electrodes on both sides and thin DE film in the middle as illustrated in Fig. 11.7a [21]. To achieve electromechanical coupling, when a DC voltage is applied, an electrostatic pressure p is introduced along the thickness direction of the film as $p = \varepsilon_0\varepsilon_r(U/d)^2$, where, ε_0 is the vacuum permittivity, ε_r the relative permittivity of the dielectric film, U the applied voltage and d the resulting film thickness. The pressure compresses the film in the thickness direction and causes it to expand in the plane perpendicular to the direction of compression. The electrodes expand passively as the film expands. As outlined in Fig. 11.7b, an ideal DEA would work under unconfined uniaxial compression when the electrodes do not constrain the planar expansion of the DE film. Clearly, to exploit full potentials of such highly elastic materials, compliant

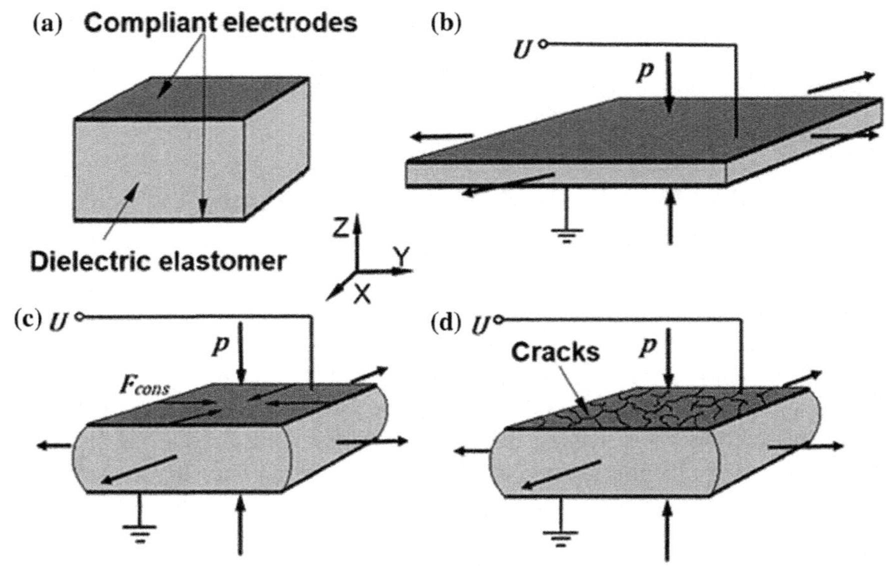

Fig. 11.7 Comprehensive working mechanisms to characterize DEA with or without compliant properties [21]. **a** Operation principle of dielectric elastomer actuation. **b** An ideal DEA working under unconfined uniaxial compression when the electrodes do not constrain the planar expansion of the DE film. **c** Solid electrodes inevitably constrain the planar expansion of the DE film, lowering the actuation strain and rendering actuation hard to model. **d** At high strain (usually larger than 100%), the solid electrodes may be torn apart and thus lose conductivity. Grease electrodes may aggregate and lose conductivity. All pictures reproduced with permission

electrodes should not only be super stretchable with negligible stiffness, but also highly conductive at high strains [28].

Previously, a wide range of DEAs electrodes including solid, semi-solid and liquid electrodes have been developed. The commonly used solid and semi-solid electrodes typically include carbon-based (carbon grease, graphene [29] and single-walled carbon nanotubes (SWNTs) [30]) and metal-based electrodes [31–33]. For carbon-based solid electrodes, a representative type is SWNT which provides a combination of relatively good compliance, conductivity [34] ($\sigma = (2.5–4.0) \times 10^4\ Sm^{-1}$) and self-clearing [30]. For metal-based solid electrodes, a general idea to increase their stretchability is to generate stretchable structures of metals [31]. Various configurations of both in-plane stripes [32] and out-of-plane wavy geometry [33] are thus proposed with strain increase up to 60%. However, when a DEA is actuated, the inherent stiffness of solid electrodes applies constraint force F_{cons} that impedes the expansion of the DEA as reflected in Fig. 11.7c. This may directly restrict the actuation strain or tears the electrodes apart and causes them to lose conductivity. Whichever the case is, the actuation strain is reduced and the actuation becomes hard to model. For solid electrodes, an inevitable problem is the trade-off between stiffness and conductivity. Liquid electrodes like conductive solutions [35], on the other hand, have virtually no stiffness and almost infinite stretchability. However, their poor conductivity and risks of electrolyzation prevent them from being widely used. Semi-solid electrodes, including carbon grease and silver grease, have good conductivity and negligible stiffness. Therefore, they are so far the most widely used electrodes in DEAs [28]. An only pity is that their conductivity is not metallic, and such elements tend to aggregate (Fig. 11.7d) and lose conductivity at high strains, which make them unable to exploit the full potentials of high performance DE materials [28].

11.6 Working Performances of Liquid Metal Elastomer Actuators

To date, few electrodes could simultaneously provide both high conductivity and negligible stiffness at high strain. In Liu et al.'s work [21], their conceptually innovative approach not only combines the superior compliance of liquids and high conductance of metals but also possess in-plane self-healing capabilities with room temperature liquid metals. To demonstrate the working principle, eutectic GaInSn alloy is chosen [36]. Such material has several intrinsic properties that may be advantageous as compliant electrodes: (a) A broad temperature range of liquid phase with a melting point 283.5 K and a boiling point above 1573 K, within which the electrode has, theoretically, zero stiffness and almost infinite stretchability due to its fluidity. The oxide layer significantly reduced the surface tension of liquid metal electrodes, rendering them ultra-stretchable and completely compliant. (b) High electrical conductivity [17] of 3.1×10^6 Sm^{-1}, which is several magnitudes higher than those of non-metallic materials and comparable with many other metallic materials commonly used in electric transmission. Thus, it may minimize ohm loss and increase the overall energy efficiency of DEAs. (c) Chemical compatibility, tunable wettability and the ability to be directly printed on a wide variety of materials such as polymers, clothes, glass and metals [37, 38]. The ease to be applied on various surfaces can largely simplify the manufacturing process and reduce the cost. (d) Good stability. Gallium, as one of the three major components of the liquid metal, is prone to oxidation even exposed to trace amount of oxygen. However, the formation of such oxide layer prevents further oxidation of the underlying material and ensures stability.

In Liu et al.'s experiments [21], gallium, indium and tin with purity of 99.99% used as raw materials were weighted with a weight ratio of 62.1:23.5:14.4. The liquid metal is directly painted on the 300% biaxially prestrained VHB 4905 film to form compliant electrodes. Here, attentions were focused on the one layer DEA case while the practical issues of making stacking multiple layers device were left for future work. The multichannel high voltage power supply used in the tests is

LabSmith HVS448 High Voltage Sequencer. Its voltage output range is −3 to 3 kV. In the test, the specimen is first connected in series with a 10 MΩ current-limiting resistor. Then two channels are connected. For tests of voltages higher than 3 kV, one channel is fixed at 3 kV while the other channel outputs a negative voltage. Over the study, more than 50 samples were tested in total. Generally, the DEAs may experience electric breakdown due to local defects of the DE film or non-uniform prestrain. For illustration purpose, in the depicted curve, only the data of samples that continuously experienced the safe running voltage of 0.5–3.5 kV was presented to explain the most typical performances the current method could offer.

Figure 11.8a, b display the planar DEA before actuation and under actuation at 3.5 kV, respectively [21]. To demonstrate the performances of the liquid metal electrodes, the electrically induced area strain as a function of applied voltage is measured and compared with the control group with silver grease as electrodes. Area expansions of the films were recorded by a digital camera. The area strain was obtained through the calculation $(S_1 - S_0)/S_0 \times 100\%$, where S_1 is the actuated area under high voltage, and S_0 is the area at 0 kV. In this figure, each point on the curve is generated by a total number of at least 9 tests, that is, three samples and three cycles each sample.

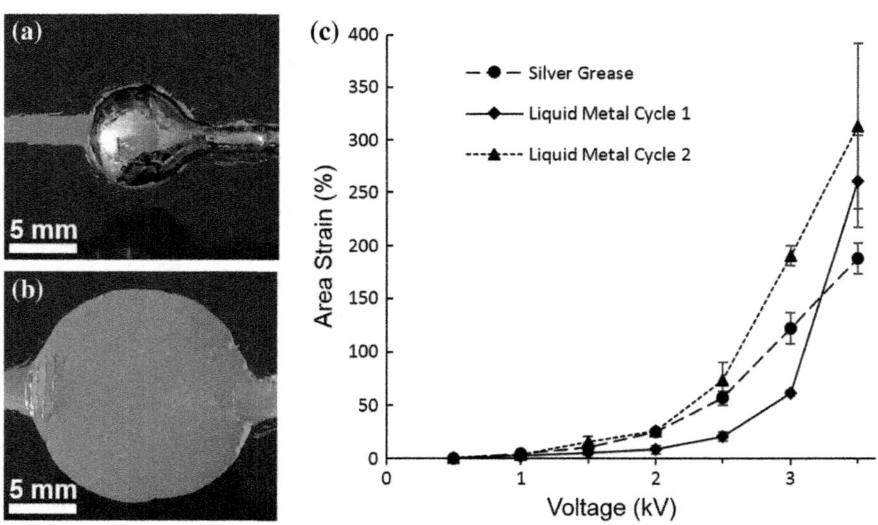

Fig. 11.8 **a** Photo of liquid metal electrodes on 300% biaxially prestrained VHB 4905 acrylic films before actuation. **b** Photo of electrode after applying 3.5 kV DC voltage. The calculated activation strain is 360%. **c** Electrically induced strain as a function of applied voltage on a 300% biaxially prestrained VHB 4905 film with smeared silver grease or liquid metal electrodes on both surfaces. For each point in the curve, at least nine tests (three samples and three cycles per sample) were performed [21]. Error bars indicate standard deviation. All pictures reproduced with permission

In consistence with previous similar standard experiments, the strain-voltage curve in Fig. 11.8c indicates that silver grease electrodes have maintained good performance at area strain lower than 100% and can reach a maximum strain of 190% at 3.5 kV. Due to stiffness of the oxide layer on the interface between liquid metal electrode and the DE film, when actuation voltage is in the range 0.5–3.0 kV, the area strains of the first actuation cycle of the liquid metal group are slightly lower than those of the control group. However, at 3.5 kV, the electrical force breaks the oxide layer and the DEA achieved a strain of over 250%, which is much better than existing approaches. The reason can be explained as follows. After the first cycle, due to the coverage of liquid metal, no new oxide is formed on the electrode-film interface. As a result, area strain performance in the whole voltage range is stable and significantly higher than that of the control group starting from the second cycle throughout the following cyclic actuations. As thin film printed on the DEA, the liquid metal electrode is not prone to inward migration or flow beyond the originally coated area. This guarantees the stable working of the DEA. Overall, the liquid metal group approximates to the maximum area strain of control group ($\sim$200%) at 3.0 kV. It means that with liquid metal electrodes, lower voltage is required to achieve a large area strain. Clearly, liquid metal electrodes exploited more potential of the VHB 4905 film than silver grease electrodes. We have tested the lifetime of the DEAs via actuating them by 3.0 kV at frequency of about 0.5 Hz. Some samples could experience more than 30 cycles of continuous actuation without significant degradation. Besides, some others can even be actuated at 3.5 kV for several cycles without breakdown although it is important to note there is significant deviation at this voltage. These promising features are just enabled by the ultra-compliant liquid metal electrodes, which however are hard to achieve via a conventional rigid electrode. Samples typically fail due to electric breakdown which is more likely caused by defects of the DE films rather than the electrodes. Overall, the experiments indicate that the liquid metal electrode offers a stable option for developing future high performance DEA.

The above performances suggest that the potential of the DE film is being fully exploited. Firstly, the area strain, which could be as large as 360% in some tests at 3.5 kV, is unprecedented in former studies. Considering the initial prestrain, the total area strain of the film is over 7000% and likely to reach the limit of the DE film. Secondly, according to the classic study, the estimated effective compressive stress is 8 MPa for liquid metal electrodes, which slightly eclipses the maximum in previous studies. Thirdly, the area strain at 3.5 kV has large deviation due to the fact that the DE film is less than 8 μm thick and highly prone to electric break down caused by inherent defects. It is reasonable to believe that liquid metal electrode is not only suitable for current DE films but also ready for future DEs with better performances.

11.7 Self-healing Behavior of Liquid Metal Elastomer Actuators

Another important feature that makes liquid metal based DEAs suitable for practical use is the in-plane self-healing capability as revealed below [21]. It has been a major problem that DEAs may experience failure due to loss of electrode conductivity at high strains or when local discontinuity of the electrode is present. In recent studies, by coating stretchable self-healing polymer around liquid metal core, stretchable wires have been made to demonstrate the one dimensional self-healing capability [39]. With nothing but scissors, the self-healing wire can be reconfigured. The above work disclosed the capability of two-dimensional in-plane self-healing in the presence of a macro scale gap without external intervention—the liquid metal electrode heals itself just by actuation.

To simulate a condition when an electrode loses electrical conductivity and severed completely, it can be manually introduced a curved gap of discontinuity with an average width of roughly 1.5 mm on one of the electrodes and completely divided it into two electrically insulated parts (a) and (b) as indicated in Fig. 11.9a. Initially, part (a) is electrically connected to the power source while part (b) is insulated. At resting state, the thin oxide layers on the electrodes prevent the two parts from merging. When a voltage of 3.5 kV is applied, part (a) is actuated while part (b) is only partially actuated as indicated in Fig. 11.9b, indicating that (a) is fully conductive while (b) is partially conductive. When removing and applying voltages for repeated cycles, both part (a) and (b) are electrically connected and achieved a total area strain of more than 210% as indicated in Fig. 11.9c.

The mechanisms of this in-plane auto-healing could be two fold as indicated in Fig. 11.9d. Firstly, once (a) is charged (for example, positively), the boundary of (b) will be negatively charged, creating a capacitor. The opposing charge on both sides of the boundary makes them mutually attractive. At small tips of the two boundaries where charges converge and the distance is shorter and the attraction force is greater, liquid metal is especially prone to break its thin oxide layer film and merge. Consequently, a potential merging site forms. Secondly, actuating the DEA causes expansion of the film, which in turn causes a center-out micro-flow of the liquid metal. Similarly, removing the voltage causes a reverse process. The flow of the liquid metal may facilitate merging of the two parts. The two mechanisms may act independently or cooperatively to count for the self-healing of the electrode. Once the two separated parts are merged, they are electrically connected and new oxide layers form to maintain the connection. The capability of recovering without external interference but just by a few cycles of actuation makes the electrode rather promising as it enhances tolerance to fault and resilience to abusive use.

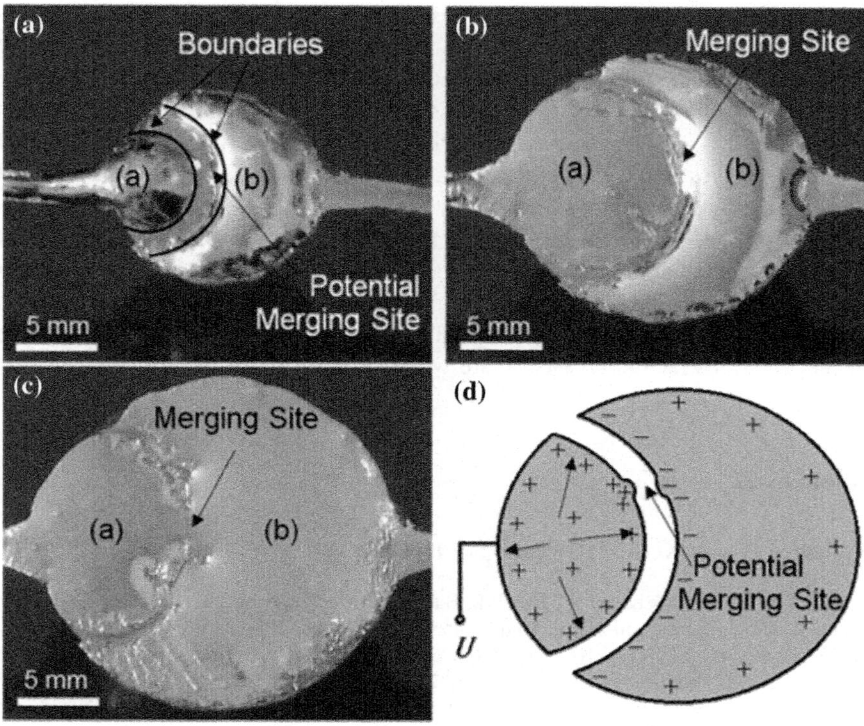

Fig. 11.9 **a** The upper electrode is divided into two mutually insulated parts (*a*) and (*b*) by a curved gap of roughly 1.5 mm. Part (*a*) is connected to the power source. **b** During the first cycle of actuation, part (*a*) is fully actuated at 3.5 kV. The self-healing initiates at the merging site and part (*b*) is partially actuated. **c** Starting from cycle 2, the two parts are connected and fully actuated. **d** The flow of liquid metal and attractive force on the boundaries account for the self-healing effect at the potential merging site [21]. All pictures reproduced with permission

11.8 Conclusion

In summary, the low-melting-point alloy can be directly adopted to make a flexible mechanical joint of a human exoskeleton. Owing to its excellent flexibility and loading capacity, the liquid metal-based mechanical joint technology offers a promising solution for dealing with high-end human exoskeleton applications. In addition, the metal-based mechanical joint responds much faster and would support heavier loads compared to the conventional phase change material. Overall, such low-melting-point-alloy-based mechanical joint opens a feasible and cost-effective technology for future civilian human exoskeletons.

In addition, the liquid metal electrode can be an important highly conductive and super compliant DEAs electrode for making artificial muscles with the unique capability of two-dimensional in-plane self-healing. The negligible stiffness of such electrodes enables DE film to approach its maximum strain and stress at relatively low voltages. The disclosed capabilities of achieving in-plane self-healing by merely actuating the DEA make actuators with liquid metal electrodes more tolerant to fault and resilient to abusive environment in practical usage. In addition, the simple manufacturing procedure and ease to apply on diversified surfaces makes mass production of DEAs more feasible and less expensive. The multitude of advantages makes liquid metal electrodes a type of super compliant electrodes not only suitable for actuators such as DEAs but also a wide spectrum of applications ranging from artificial muscles, flexible electronics to smart clothing. Finally, it should be pointed out that, at this stage, the liquid metal actuator serves primarily as a proof-of-concept. Studies to bring liquid metal electrodes into practical use, such as proper packaging, multi-layer actuator manufacturing and investigation on effects of various factors on DEAs, are worth of pursuing in the coming time.

References

1. Jarrasse N, Morel G (2011) Connecting a human limb to an exoskeleton. IEEE Trans Rob 28 (3):697–709
2. Petrič T, Gams A, Debevec T, Žlajpah L, Babič J (2013) Control approaches for robotic knee exoskeleton and their effects on human motion. Adv Robot 27(13):993–1002
3. Yan L, Wu J, Li YB, Liu JH, Yang F (2013) The design of lower extremity exoskeleton of power assist robot. Mater Sci Eng 278(3):618–621
4. Kao PC, Lewis CL, Ferris DP (2010) Invariant ankle moment patterns when walking with and without a robotic ankle exoskeleton. J Biomech 43(2):203–209
5. Perry JC, Powell JM, Rosen J (2009) Isotropy of an upper limb exoskeleton and the kinematics and dynamics of the human arm. Appl Bion Biomech 6(2):175–191
6. Ferris DP, Sawicki GS, Daley MA (2007) A physiologist's perspective on robotic exoskeletons for human locomotion. Int J Humanoid Rob 4(3):507–528
7. Moreno JC, Brunetti F, Cabello EN, Cordero AF, Pons JL (2009) Analysis of the human interaction with a wearable lower-limb exoskeleton. Appl Bion Biomech 6(2):245–256
8. Kaminaga H, Ono J, Nakashima Y, Nakamura Y (2009) Development of backdrivable hydraulic joint mechanism for knee joint of humanoid robots. In: IEEE International Conference on Robotics and Automation (ICRA 2009), Kobe, 12–17 May 2009, pp 1577–1582
9. Gams A, Petrič T, Debevec T, Babič J (2013) Effects of robotic knee exoskeleton on human energy expenditure. IEEE Trans Biomed Eng 60(6):1636–1644
10. Berring J, Kianfar K, Lira C, Menon C, Scarpa F (2010) A smart hydraulic joint for future implementation in robotic structures. Robotica 28(7):1045–1056
11. Kiguchi K, Iwami K, Yasuda M, Watanabe K, Fukuda T (2003) An exoskeletal robot for human shoulder joint motion assist. IEEE/ASME Trans Mechatron 8(1):125–135
12. Angeles J (2003) Fundamentals of robotic mechanical systems. Springer, Berlin
13. Panich S (2010) Kinematic analysis of exoskeleton suit for human arm. J Comput Sci 6 (11):1272–1275
14. Banala SK, Seok HK, Agrawal SK, Scholz JP (2009) Robot assisted gait training with active leg exoskeleton (ALEX). IEEE Trans Neural Syst Rehabil Eng 17(1):2–8
15. Malcolm P, Derave W, Galle S, De Clercq D (2013) A simple exoskeleton that assists plantarflexion can reduce the metabolic cost of human walking. PLoS ONE 8(2):e56137

16. Wiggin MB, Sawicki GS, Collins SH (2011) An exoskeleton using controlled energy storage and release to aid ankle propulsion. In: IEEE International Conference on Rehabilitation Robotics (ICORR 2011), Zurich, 29 June–1 July 2011, pp 1–5
17. Lee H, Kim W, Han J, Han C (2012) The technical trend of the exoskeleton robot system for human power assistance. Int J Precis Eng Manuf 13(8):1491–1497
18. Rocon E, Belda-Lois JM, Ruiz AF, Manto M, Moreno JC, Pons JL (2007) Design and validation of a rehabilitation robotic exoskeleton for tremor assessment and suppression. IEEE Trans Neural Syst Rehabil Eng 15:367–378
19. Park YL, Chen B, Pérez-Arancibia NO, Stirling L, Wood RJ, Goldfield EC, Nagpal R (2014) Design and control of a bio-inspired soft wearable robotic device for ankle-foot rehabilitation. Bioinspir Biomim 9:016007
20. Deng YG, Liu J (2014) Flexible mechanical joint as human exoskeleton using low-melting-point alloy. ASME J Med Devices 8:044506
21. Liu Y, Gao M, Mei SF, Han YT, Liu J (2013) Ultra-compliant liquid metal electrodes with in-plane self-healing capability for dielectric elastomer actuators. Appl Phys Lett 102:064101
22. Osada Y, Okuzaki H, Hori H (1992) A polymer gel with electrically driven motility. Nature 355:242–244
23. Nawroth JC, Lee H, Feinberg AW, Ripplinger CM, McCain ML, Grosberg A, John OD, Parker KK (2012) A tissue-engineered jellyfish with biomimetic propulsion. Nat Biotechnol 30:792–797
24. Baughman RH (2005) Playing nature's game with artificial muscles. Science 308:63–65
25. Pelrine R, Kornbluh R, Pei Q, Joseph J (2000) High-speed electrically actuated elastomers with over 100% strain. Science 287:836–839
26. Pelrine R, Kornbluh R, Kofod G (2000) High-strain actuator materials based on dielectric elastomers. Adv Mater 12:1223–1225
27. Carpi F, Chiarelli P, Mazzoldi A, Rossi DD (2003) Electromechanical characterisation of dielectric elastomer planar actuators: comparative evaluation of different electrode materials and different counter loads. Sens Actuators A-Phys 107:85–95
28. O'Halloran A, O'Malley F, McHugh P (2008) A review on dielectric elastomer actuators, technology, applications, and challenges. J Appl Phys 104:071101
29. Bae S, Kim H, Lee Y, Xu X, Park JS, Zheng Y, Iijima S (2010) Roll-to-roll production of 30-inch graphene films for transparent electrodes. Nat Nanotechnol 5:574–578
30. Yuan W, Hu LB, Yu ZB et al (2008) Fault-tolerant dielectric elastomer actuators using single-walled carbon nanotube electrodes. Adv Mater 20:621–625
31. Hyun DC, Park M, Park C et al (2011) Ordered zigzag stripes of polymer gel/metal nanoparticle composites for highly stretchable conductive electrodes. Adv Mater 23:2946–2950
32. Gray DS, Tien J, Chen CS (2004) High conductivity elastomeric electronics. Adv Mater 16:393–397
33. Lacour SP, Wagner S, Huang Z, Suo Z (2003) Stretchable gold conductors on elastomeric substrates. Appl Phys Lett 82:2404
34. Bekyarova E, Itkis ME, Cabrera N, Zhao B, Yu A, Gao J, Haddon RC (2005) Electronic properties of single-walled carbon nanotube networks. J Am Chem Soc 127:5990–5995
35. Arora S, Ghosh T, Muth J (2007) Dielectric elastomer based prototype fiber actuators. Sens Actuators A-Phys 136:321–328
36. Morley NB, Burris J, Cadwallader LC, Nornberg MD (2008) GaInSn usage in the research laboratory. Rev Sci Instrum 79(5):112–192
37. Gao Y, Li H, Liu J (2012) Direct writing of flexible electronics through room temperature liquid metal ink. PLoS ONE 7(9):e45485
38. Zheng Y, He Z, Gao Y, Liu J (2013) Direct desktop printed-circuits-on-paper flexible electronics. Sci Rep 3:1786-1-7
39. Palleau E, Reece S, Desai SC, Smith ME, Dickey MD (2013) Self-healing stretchable wires for reconfigurable circuit wiring and 3D microfluidics. Adv Mater 25:1589–1592

Chapter 12
Liquid Metal Enabled Skin Electronics

Abstract This chapter presents the basic principle of the conformal epidermal printed electronics based on the liquid metal to achieve the immediate contact between skin surface and electrode. The remarkable features of the liquid metal skin electronics, such as high conformability, good conductivity, better signal stability and fine biocompatibility were discussed. A series of typical applications on disease therapy or health care were given as examples.

Keywords Skin electronics · Tumor therapy · Health care · Liquid metal

12.1 Introduction

It is well known that skin has the largest flexible and robust surface areas, which covers and protects the biological body from external potential injury, and also serves as an important physiological sensor. This chapter is dedicated to present the basics about the liquid metal skin electronics. Typical routes of directly printing electronics pattern on skin like skin sensors, actuators, skin electrical circuits and so on will be introduced. Typical applications will be illustrated.

Conventional biomedical conductive components generally own advantages of high conductivity and definition process ability. However, they also imply shortcomings requiring complex fabrication conditions. In particular, the classical microelectronics manufacture technologies such as lithography, evaporation, etching, screen printing, micromachining or electroplating etc. heavily rely on special equipments and clean room infrastructure. And most of the existing electrophysiological measurement devices are rigid sensors or circuits, which may encounter troubles such as coupling performance, contact comfortableness, manufacturing complexity and cost etc. Such electrodes may cause discomfort and even hurt to human body due to their mechanically rigid fixing. Recently, the flexible electronics is increasingly investigated and gradually applied to bio-electronic measurement [1–5]. The flexible transistors can be made as electronic skin to mimic the sensitivity of real human skin. Generally, the electronic epidermal devices are integrated

J. Liu and L. Yi, *Liquid Metal Biomaterials*,
Springer Series in Biomaterials Science and Engineering10,
https://doi.org/10.1007/978-981-10-5607-9_12

with a collection of multifunctional sensors, which can be used to detect the temperature or pressure [6], record heartbeats, brain activity and more electrophysiological signals or made as actuators in an array such as micro-heaters [7–10]. So far, most of the skin-electronic devices ever reported are based on solid metals or inorganic semi-conductors. The stretchable skin electronics are usually fabricated on a very thin and flexible substrate, which have intelligent processing capabilities such as sensing and acting. For such an application modality, the electronic devices are isolated from the skin by the substrates. In certain situations, the skin may not be able to directly measure the signal from outside the body. Actually, most of the electrophysiological signals are detected with the electrodes contacting the skin. If the patterned conductive components could be directly printed on the target skin, the interface impedance of the skin and electronic components will be very low. The signal from the human body could thus be well transmitted to the outside for better analysis.

The recently proposed conformal epidermal printed electronics based on the liquid metal offers the way to achieve the immediate contact between skin surface and electrode. This can avoid the skin deformation often caused by the conventional rigid electrode. Through comparing the contact resistances under different working conditions, either ex vivo or in vivo liquid metal electrode-skin model has demonstrated the virtues of direct and immediate contact without deforming the skin surface encountered in traditional rigid electrode strategy. In addition, the electrocardioelectrodes, composed of conformal liquid metal printed epidermal electronics, have been adopted as smart system to monitor the biological electrocardiogram (ECG) signals. The remarkable features of the liquid metal conformal epidermal electrode, such as high conformability, good conductivity, better signal stability and fine biocompatibility, represent a critical step toward accurate medical monitoring and smart treatment.

12.2 Typical Strategy to Print Electronics on Skin

In this section, a pervasive method for printing electronics directly on skin to make conductive patterns via atomized spraying is illustrated [1]. This technology allows manufacturing various more complex components quickly on skin as shown in Fig. 12.1. Considering the requirement at room temperature, most of the existing electronics fabrication methods such as evaporation and sputtering would not work well. In addition, the previously developed functional inks are mainly based on organic substances [11], polymers [12], nano-particles [13] and so on. These electrical inks can be prepared by loading nanoparticles into the base fluids such as silver ink or organic electronic conductive materials such as: poly (3, 4-ethylenedioxythiophene): poly (4-styrenesulfonate) (PEDOT: PSS). However, a big issue exists in such composite inks or organic conductive lines as well as other patterns, because they rely heavily on the high temperature annealing or other more complex process such as evaporation. Besides, these electronic inks' conductive

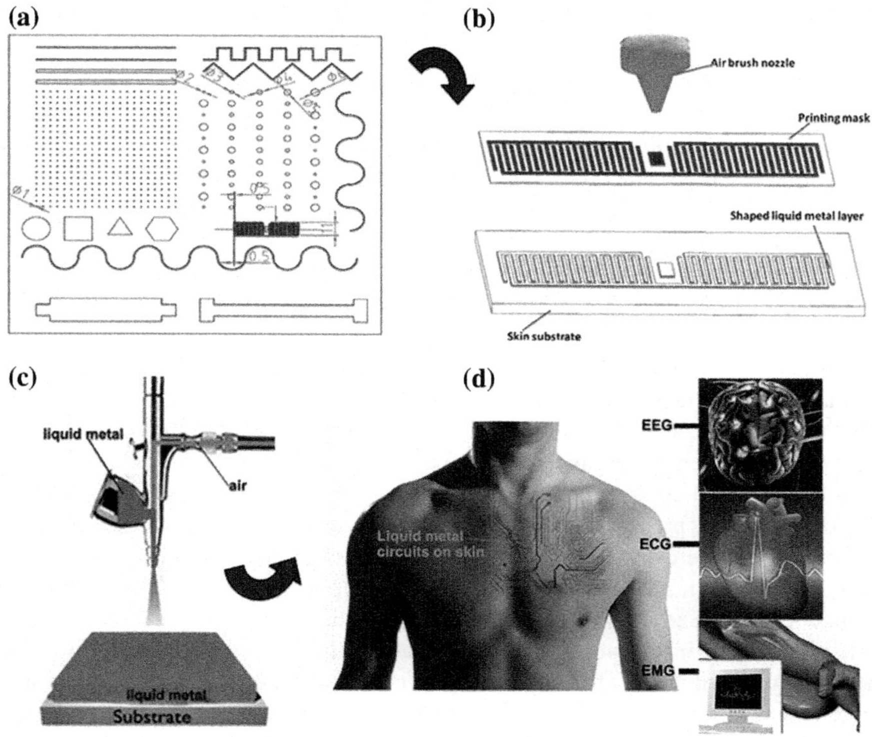

Fig. 12.1 **a** The designed mask for spray-printing. **b** Technical principle of fabricating interdigital electrode on substrate via a mask. **c** The mechanical principle of atomization of liquid metal to form conductive layer by an airbrush and an air pump. **d** The schematic conception of fabricating liquid metal circuits on human skin

performance is not good enough. Until now, there is still no an ideal way of using these materials to fabricate electronics directly on skin. As an alternative, the liquid metal is easy to compose electronics directly on flexible substrates even skin with special convenience at room temperature [14–19]. Such conductive ink owns many unique merits like good electrical conductivity, mechanical flexibility, biocompatibility, low cost and so on, which overcomes in a large extent the shortages facing the conventional materials [14, 15]. This kind of flexible electronics has wide application in making RF electronics [16, 17], injected electrical wire for flexible packaging of solid-state integrated circuit chips [18] and bio-electrodes [19]. The liquid metal ink is increasingly applied to fabricate flexible electronics with the methods to realize direct writing by brush, desktop printing, ball writing [20], injection [18, 21, 22] and stamp [23]. And most of the present printing methods could not fabricate the electrical components on skin, whose geometry is rather irregular and not easy to deposit a circuit. The spray-printing method has been proven to be a very good way to fabricate flexible electronics. It is feasible in fabricating printed circuit board [24]. PEDOT: PSS transparent electrodes are used for solar cells based on the method of spray-printing [25]. The method is also very useful in other situations: ink of copper indium diselenide nanocrystals as the light-absorbing layer for manufacturing photovoltaic devices [26], the printing ink to form metallic silver films [27], the liquid metal to print electronics directly on nearly any desired substrates [28]. This chapter takes the lead in using the atomized spraying technology to directly print the room temperature liquid metal to fabricate electronics on skin in room temperature without requesting a thermal annealing process. The fabricated electronics can be used as testing "Lab on Skin" to form bio-electrodes, sensors, skin circuits and so on. It is expected that such ubiquitous technology will stimulate a series of unconventional application in future bioelectronics.

The chosen printable ink is generally made of gallium-indium alloy [29]. Liquid metal has a high degree of electric conductivity far superior to other flexible conductive materials. For the fabrication, gallium and indium metals with purity of 99.99% were taken as raw materials with a relative weight ratio of 75.5:24.5 in line with the chemical compositions. The detailed procedures were outlined as follows. All beakers were prepared clean with the deionized water. Then the gallium and indium metals were mixed together in the prepared beaker and heated at 100 °C until they were fused completely. The melting point of GaIn24.5 is measured around 15.5 °C (see Table 12.1), which keeps in liquid state at room temperature. When the liquid metal are exposed to the air, GaIn24.5 will quickly form a thin layer of oxide skin, which can help liquid metal maintain the formed shape in a large extent. About 8 mL 30% NaOH solution was added to the metals in order to prevent the configured GaIn24.5 ink from naturally being oxidized. With such low melting point behaviour, all the spraying experiments can be carried out in liquid state at room temperature. Pig skin is chosen as the electronic substrate in the experiments, which is used as the substitute materials for studying human skin due to its similarity in material response to human skin. Fresh pig skin was purchased from a local supermarket. The skin was preserved in 0.9% normal saline solution with a temperature of 4 °C. The lumbar area of the pig skin was cut to make specimens. All of the fat layer, and hairs were removed carefully from the specimens using a surgical scalpel. In this way, the basic behaviours of liquid metal printed skin circuits can be investigated.

Table 12.1 Physical properties for $GaIn_{24.5}$

Material	Melting point (°C)	Density (kg/m^3)	Surface tension (N/m)	Dynamic viscosity (Pa s)
$GaIn_{24.5}$	15.5	6280	0.624	1.6956×10^{-3}

12.3 Principle of Spray Printing Liquid Metal Film on Skin

The basic process for spray-printing liquid metal conductive layer on biological skin is depicted in Fig. 12.1 [1]. The liquid metal was atomized with the equipment of airbrush and the air pump. A stream of liquid metal was disrupted by high-energy gas jets into fine micro-droplets and fell onto the pig skin surface as expected. After atomization, the liquid alloy was broken into micro-droplets, and deposited on the substrate, which finally formed into conductive layer.

Before the printing, one has to make a mask for the replica moulding of liquid metal pattern on skin. Metal chemical etching is used to fabricate the stainless steel mask, which allows any picture, photo, or pattern to be copied onto target substrate. The metal mask is fabricated with a 200 μm thick steel sheet, which is pre-treated to remove the oil on the surface. The metal sheet is washed by de-ionized water. Dry photo-resist membrane layer is heated and attached on metal sheet surface with stress from the hot press roll. The designed picture (see Fig. 12.1a) from the film is transferred to the metal sheet with dry photo-resist membrane layer by exposure and development (Fig. 12.1b). After the dry photo-resist membrane was removed, the next step is chemical etching by following the equations such as:

$$2FeCl_3 + Fe = 3FeCl_2 \tag{12.1}$$

$$2FeCl_3 + Cu = 2FeCl_2 + CuCl_2 \tag{12.2}$$

Here, ferric chloride ($FeCl_3$ solution) has served as the mordant. The mask is fabricated with desired picture designed in advance. Usually the bottom geometries are slightly larger in width than the top geometries so as to compensate for the mask alignment errors. The liquid metal spraying experiments are carried out in a fume hood. The metal mask and the pig skin substrate are cleaned with de-ionized water and dried with N_2. The pig skin substrate is covered by the prepared mask.

The mask must be tightly positioned closely to the substrates to guarantee printed electronics with clear boundaries. Then the electronic components are prepared by the so-called spray-printing method (Fig. 12.1c) until finally deposited on skin surface (Fig. 12.1d).

12.4 Characterizations of Spray Printing of Liquid Metal on Skin

The liquid metal spraying printer has rather diverse capability in manufacturing circuit components on skin [1, 28]. The following is several most typical metal geometric graphics that can be printed to compose complex electrical circuits or devices. In skin electronics, a sensor or antenna is generally composed of various

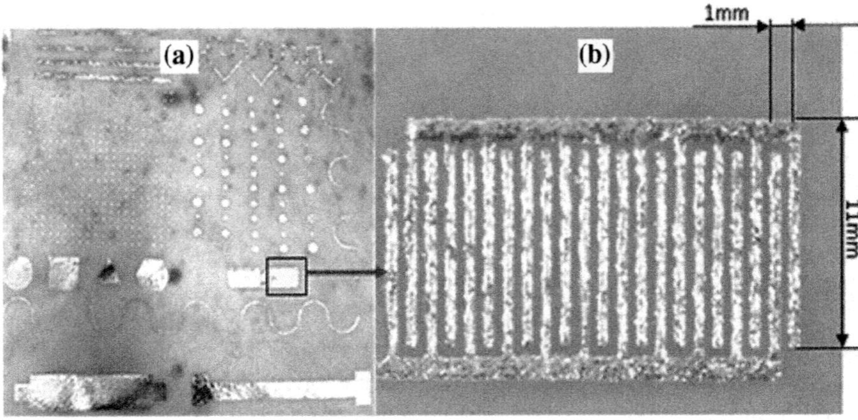

Fig. 12.2 Geometric graphics for liquid metal components on skin using spraying methods [1]. **a** Picture of typical geometric metal graphics of liquid metal on pig skin surface. **b** Inter-digital array microelectrodes (IDAM) of liquid metal on pig skin surface

basic electrical elements such as straight line, circle or complex curve. With a pre-designed stainless mask, the corresponding electronic wires or signs (Fig. 12.2a) can be quickly printed on skin via spray-printing. Traditional inter-digital array (IDA) biosensor is often manufactured with very complex process and equipment. Here, an IDA electrode was fabricated to measure impedance spectroscopy of the pig skin (see Fig. 12.2b). Such biosensor could generate sensitive enough electrochemical signals due to its low ohmic drop, rapid reaction kinetics, and a high signal-to-noise ratio. The quick and straight-forward fabrication of interdigital array microelectrodes (IDAM) is demonstrated. The distance between the two fingers of the IDAM is 0.5 mm and the length of the finger is 11 mm. As shown in Fig. 12.3a–d, the diameter of the micro-droplet which impacted the skin surface was in micro-meter level.

The thickness of the thin film is 2 μm, which is obtained from the SEM image of the thin film's cross section as shown in Fig. 12.3b. The width of the straight line of liquid metal is around 100 μm. Overall, the fabrication accuracy with spray-printing is expected to be around 10 μm. As the SEM figure indicates (Fig. 12.3c, d), the surface tension of the liquid metal micro-droplet is much larger when it is spray-printed on the skin than that on a paper. Therefore, the straight line of liquid metal on the skin is much smoother than on paper. As shown in Fig. 12.4a, the liquid alloy is disrupted into micro-droplet by air-brush with its surface oxidized rapidly in the air. The oxidized liquid metal micro-droplets have polar atoms on the surface, which are somewhat chemically reactive. In addition, the skin surface may also contain certain polar molecules (see Fig. 12.4b). As the micro-droplets of liquid metal impact the skin surface, the atoms or molecules can be firmly adsorbed on the skin surface under the Van der Waals force. After that, the adsorption film of liquid metal conductive layer is formed. For the small size of liquid micro-droplet,

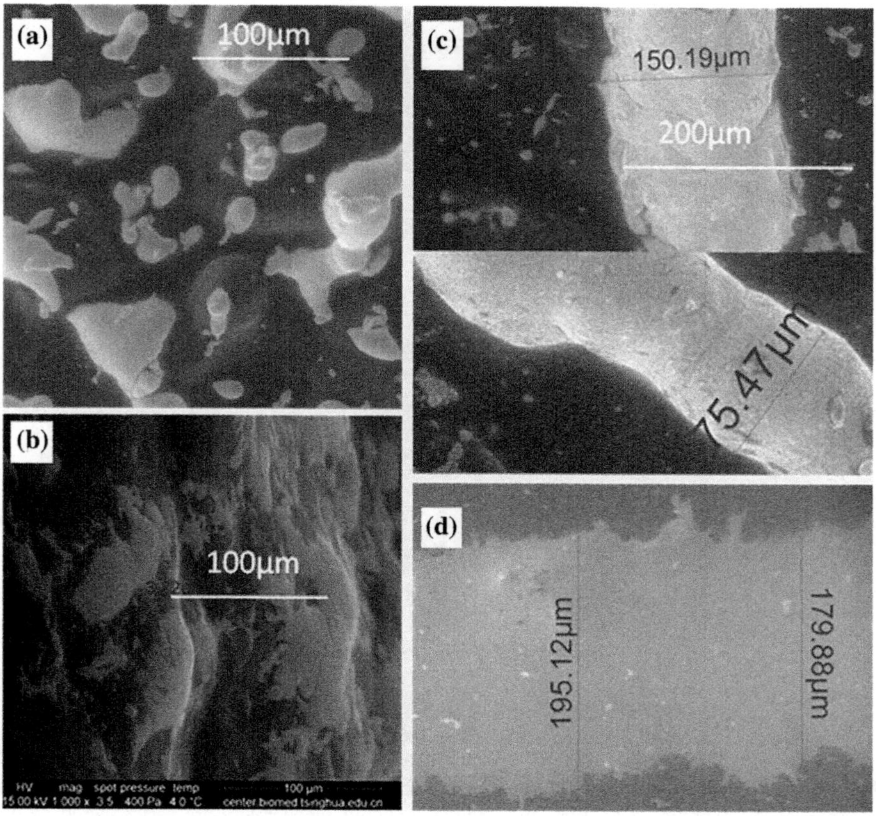

Fig. 12.3 Basic microscopic SEM features of liquid metal spray-printing (LMSP) [1]. **a** SEM of spraying printed liquid metal micro-drops on pig skin under 100 μm scale; **b** vertical direction SEM of spraying printed liquid metal film on pig skin under 100 μm scale to measure the film thickness; **c** SEM image of using LMSP straight line on pig skin; **d** SEM image of using liquid spraying printed straight line on paper

its surface is more active than when it is in normal big size, and the oxidation process as mentioned above become more quick. So it is easier to adhere to the substrates. But the surface oxide would guarantee the purity inside. The liquid metal flow is influenced by the gas flow through the nozzle, so the size of micro-droplet is related to the design of atomization nozzle. Generally, the cohesive strength of the liquid metal and skin surface is described by the work of adhesion [29], i.e.

$$W_d = \gamma_L + \gamma_S - \gamma_{SL} \tag{12.3}$$

where, γ_S, γ_L are the surface tension of the solid and the surface tension of the liquid metal, γ_{SL} the solid-liquid interfacial tension, and the work of adhesion of a liquid metal micro-droplet to a solid surface could be given by Young-Dupre equation as

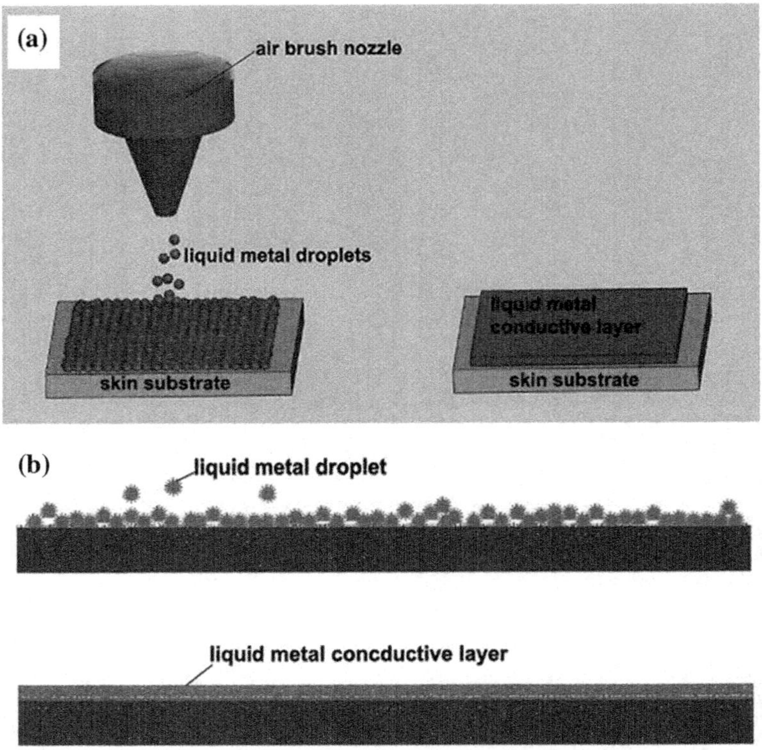

Fig. 12.4 Fundamental process for spraying liquid metal film on substrate [1]. **a** Process of spraying to form liquid metal film. **b** Principle of liquid metal micro-droplets adhered to the substrate and merged film

$$W_d = \gamma_L(1 + \cos\theta) \tag{12.4}$$

where, γ_L is the surface tension of the liquid and θ the contact angle, W_d is the work of adhesion.

Then the adhesion force is:

$$F_a = \frac{dW_d}{dx} \tag{12.5}$$

The contact angle between a liquid metal drop and the skin surface is a measure of the angle to characterize the adhesion strength. In most cases, a larger contact angle means the weaker attraction between the liquid metal and the skin surface. Conversely, a lower contact angle means a stronger attraction. As shown in Fig. 12.5, the static contact angle between a liquid metal drop and the skin surface

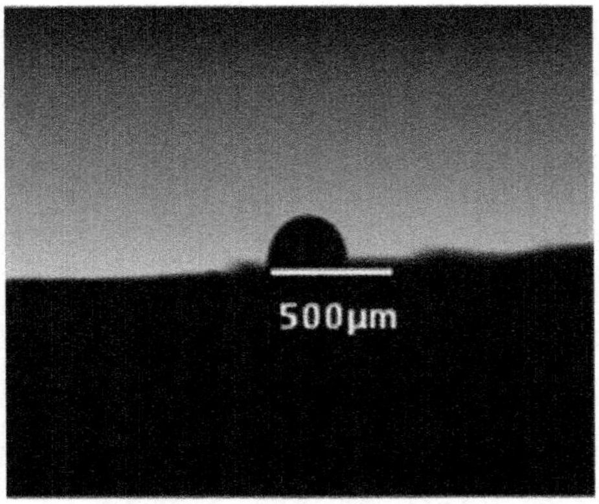

Fig. 12.5 Liquid metal droplet sitting on pig skin surface, 100.5° [1]

is measured as 100.5° by a contact angle meter (JC2000D3, POWEREACH). This is because the micro-droplets are oxidized rapidly in the air with polar atoms on the surface. When the liquid metal drop is placed on skin surface, an attraction develops between the polar molecules in the droplet and the surface. The adhesion strength may be larger than the value which is obtained by only calculating with the static contact angle. The attraction and force of gravity will make the drops to form a thin film. As shown in Fig. 12.6, the experimental results further explain the adhesion principle of spray-printed liquid metal on skin as compared with different methods through depositing GaIn24.5 to the pig skin. Our previous work confirmed that $GaIn_{24.5}$-based liquid metal prepared with oxidation reaction could be directly and easily written on nearly any substrate [29]. It also can be deposited on skin although somewhat difficult to fabricate more complex patterns (see Fig. 12.3c). The surface tension of the skin is much bigger than other substrates such as paper, cloth, polymeric materials and so on. As an alternative, it is easy to quickly make very complex patterns with the methods of spray-printing method [1]. In this way, people can print out various shapes and patterns conveniently on the skin according to demands of the target electrical devices. The energy conservation equation before and after liquid micro-droplet impacts the skin surface can be written as:

$$E_k^i + E_p^i + E_s^i = E_k^f + E_p^f + E_s^f + W_d \tag{12.6}$$

where, E_k^i, E_p^i, E_s^i are the kinetic, potential, surface energies of liquid metal micro-droplet impacting to the skin surface before and E_k^f, E_p^f, E_s^f are the afterwards [30].

The mass of the micro-droplet is not changed after it impacts the skin, for the case, one has:

$$W_d \approx E_k^i + E_p^i + E_s^i \tag{12.7}$$

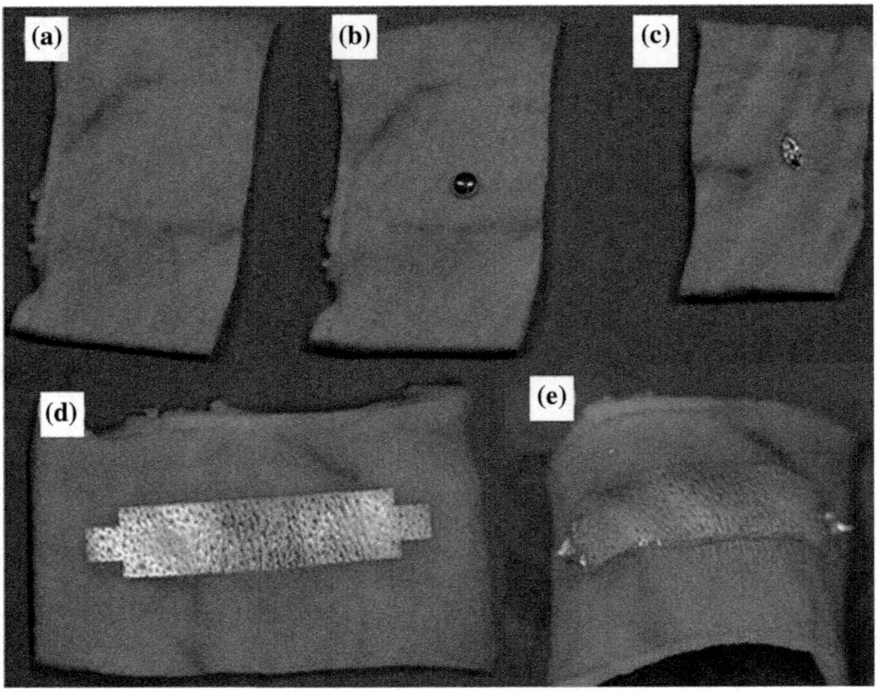

Fig. 12.6 Optical images of comparing GaIn24.5-based liquid metal ink deposited on pig skin under different situations [1]. **a** Optical images of naked pig skin without any GaIn24.5. **b** Optical images of non-oxidized GaIn24.5 injected on pig skin. **c** Optical images of oxidized GaIn24.5 written on pig skin. **d** Optical images of GaIn24.5 spray-printed on pig skin. **e** Optical images of GaIn24.5 spray-printed pig skin in bent states

The kinetic and surface energy before impact can be described as:

$$E_k^i = \frac{1}{2}\rho_L \mathrm{U}_0^2\left(\frac{\pi}{6}d_0^3\right) \tag{12.8}$$

$$E_s^i = \pi d_0^2 \gamma_L \tag{12.9}$$

where, ρ_L, γ_L, d_0 are the liquid metal density, surface tension and diameter of the impacting liquid metal micro-droplet, respectively. U_0 is the velocity of micro-droplet impacting the skin surface. Here, as the liquid metal micro-droplet impacts the solid surface, one has

$$E_p^i \approx 0, \quad E_p^f \approx 0 \tag{12.10}$$

Then one can get:

$$\gamma_L(1+\cos\theta) = \frac{1}{2}\rho_L U_0^2\left(\frac{\pi}{6}d_0^3\right) + \pi d_0^2\gamma_L \tag{12.11}$$

As discussed above, the size of micro-droplets is determined by the physical properties of the main gas-liquid two-phase such as density, viscosity, surface tension, and the velocity of gas flow around the droplet state decisions. The liquid metal micro-droplets in the gas stream are mainly atomized by the influencing factors such as the pressure of the gas, the liquid surface tension and viscous forces.

As the liquid metal micro-droplets impact the surface, a liquid film spreads outwards (see Fig. 12.7a). When the second liquid metal micro-droplet impacts the first micro-droplet, the two liquid micro-droplets will merge (see Fig. 12.7b), and the film will then spread and become thicken (Fig. 12.7c, d). When the second liquid metal micro-droplet impacts the substrate, which is far from the first one, another larger micro-droplet may impact the two micro-droplets which affected the former substrate, and they merged to a film. If the second liquid metal micro-droplet is a larger one it may merge with the first to form a film. According to the SEM measurement on the liquid metal as spray-printed on pig skin, there usually occur six situations of liquid metal micro-droplets impacting on the pig skin substrate (Fig. 12.7a–f). To characterize the electrical properties of the printed electronics on skin, additional experiments were performed as set up in Fig. 12.8a, b. Figure 12.8c shows the resistance results of liquid metal on pig skin according to the measurements. It can be evidently observed that resistances increase with the skin stretched in length. The resistance will increase squarely within the range from 0.4 to 4.1 Ω with the tensile length of the pig skin in a narrow range from 90 to 105 mm.

This stretchable liquid metal pattern has good prospects used as pressure sensor of skin. For impedance measurement, we adopted the SRS Model SR780 2-Channel

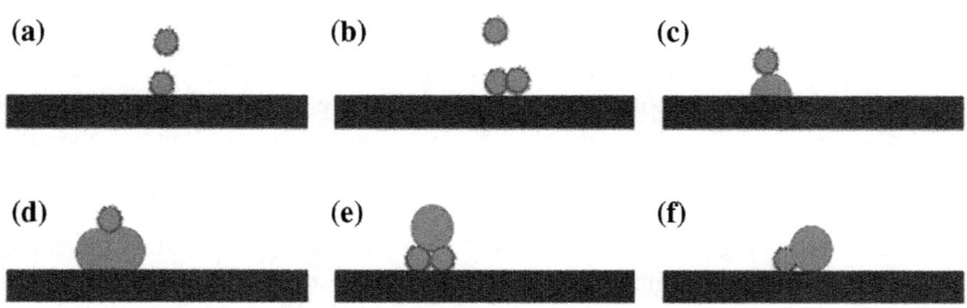

Fig. 12.7 Mechanism of liquid metal micro-droplets impacting the skin substrate [1]. **a** The first micro-droplet impacts the skin surface. **b** The second micro-droplet impacts the skin surface as well as the first micro-droplet. **c** The micro-droplets impact two merged liquid metal. **d** The micro-droplets impact several merged liquid metal micro-droplets. **e** A large micro-droplet impacts two small ones which are not merged yet. **f** A large micro-droplet impacts a small one and then merged subsequently

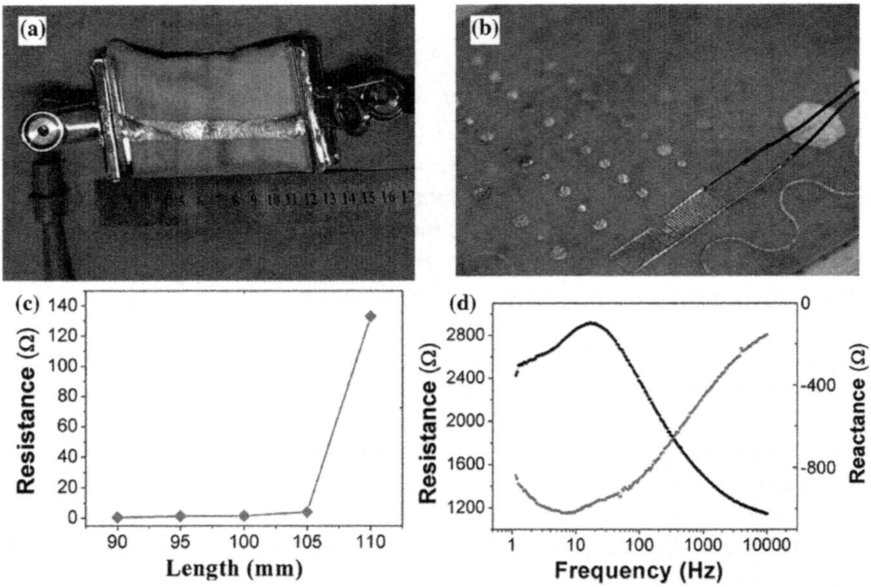

Fig. 12.8 **a** Schematic stretching experiments apparatus of liquid metal on pig skin. **b** Schematic for measurement of impedance spectroscopy of pig skin using IDA. **c** Curve of resistance of the liquid metal line with the length of pig skin. **d** Representative electrical impedance spectroscopy of the IDA electrode. The black line represents resistance of pig skin detected and the red line the reactance [1] (Color figure online)

Network Signal Analyzer to get the data. The impedance spectroscopy of pig skin can be detected with the IDA (see Fig. 12.8d). The impedance of skin reflects the electrical properties of skin, which could be used to evaluate the pathological changes of tissues. The results show that the peak resistance of pig skin is 2900 Ω at the frequency of 20 Hz and the peak reactance of pig skin is 1000 Ω for the frequency of 10 Hz, which provide a very convenient way to measure the physiological parameters of the skin.

Overall, the spray printing has provided a quick forward method to fabricate directly conductive components on skin with spray-printing via pre-designed stainless mask and liquid metal ink. The mask was fabricated using chemical etching method with an accuracy of 100 μm, which serves well to deposit specific conductive patterns. And the liquid metal ink was verified as a perfect material in quite a few emerging skin biomedical practices. According to the SEM images of the liquid metal spray-printing, it was disclosed that the accuracy of the manufactured liquid metal electrical components had reached micro-meter level. Further, it was found that the resistance of the printed film ranging from 0.4 to 4.1 Ω would increase squarely with the tensile length of the pig skin from 90 to 105 mm. An IDAM was fabricated to measure impedance spectroscopy of the pig skin with the distance between the two interdigital fingers as 0.5 mm and the length of the finger as 11 mm, respectively. The impedance spectroscopy of pig skin was detected with the IDAM, which demonstrated its suitability for the on skin physiological measurement. These results promise an important route of quickly and directly making bioelectronics devices as "Lab on Skin" in a variety of practical applications like skin sensors, actuators, and even more complex skin electrical devices in the coming time.

12.5 Drawable Liquid Metal ECG Electrode and Skin Circuit

In biomedical area, electrocardiogram (ECG) was widely known as a reflection of the electrical activity of the heart, which is an essential physiological parameter for both clinical diagnostics and health monitoring. To detect the weak signal of ECG non-invasively, the electrode is usually stuck onto the skin of limbs and chest for better measurement.

So far, there are various ECG electrodes with different materials and shapes, such as flat metal electrodes, suction electrodes and disposable button electrodes etc. However, these conventional electrodes may encounter troubles such as coupling performance, contact comfortableness, manufacturing complexity and cost. The flat metal electrodes are rigid plates that clamp the limbs and the suction electrodes are small evacuated cups that suck tightly to the skin. Both kinds of electrodes are commonly used on the ECG instruments in clinics and hospitals. They usually have poor coupling performance with the skin and high signal noise that has to be overcome with electrolytic gel. And such electrodes may cause discomfort and even hurt to human body due to their mechanically rigid fixing. The disposable button electrodes are mainly used in portable ECG monitor devices with electrolytic gel for conduction enhancement and Ag/AgCl as electrode material to pursue better performance [31]. However, the structure of the button electrodes is quite complicated, including the electrolytic gel, Ag/AgCl disk, steel button cap, adhesive plaster, sealing plastic and paper covers, thus making it more expensive, especially when considering that silver is a noble metal. And the sticking plaster sometimes can take off the hair, causing pain and even inflammation in the hair sac. In order to find out alternative electrodes or ways with better features, various strategies have been investigated. For example, Cauwenberghs' group at UCSD have managed to implement the non-contact electrode to improve comfort degree, which explores a new approach of monitoring ECG and EEG signals wirelessly [32–34]. Another attractive idea is the so-called epidermal electronics, which is developed by Rogers' group [2]. It is a conformal device attached to the skin like a tattoo with stretchable electrical sensors, which could measure physiological variables such as ECG, EEG and EMG. From an alternative, Yu et al. had proposed to use the Ga-based liquid metal ink as skin electrical circuit material [35]. For illustration purpose, the following fundamental measurements of impedance and polarization voltage of the liquid metal ink were adopted to evaluate its basic electrical properties. Conceptual experiments were performed to draw the alloy as bio-electrodes to acquire ECG signals from both rabbit and human via a wireless module developed on the mobile phone. Further, a typical electrical circuit was drawn in the palm with the ink to demonstrate its potential of implementing more sophisticated skin circuits.

With an oxide concentration of 0.34%, the resistivity of the liquid metal ink was measured as 44.1 μΩ cm with quite low reactance in the form of straight line. Its peak polarization voltage with the physiological saline was detected as −0.73 V. The quality of ECG wave detected from the liquid metal electrodes was found as good as that of conventional electrodes, from both rabbit and human experiments. In addition, the circuit drawn with the liquid metal ink in the palm also runs efficiently. When the loop was switched on, all the light emitting diodes (LEDs) were lit and emitted colourful lights.

The liquid metal ink promises unique printable electrical properties as both bio-electrodes and electrical wires. The implemented ECG measurement on biological surface and the successfully run skin circuit demonstrated the conformability and attachment of the liquid metal. Such method is expected to innovate future physiological measurement and biological circuit manufacturing technique in a large extent.

The adopted liquid metal ink is composed of gallium or gallium-indium alloy with oxide. The melting point of gallium is around 30 °C with the nature of supercooling, which keeps it in liquid state at room temperature. By vigorously stirring the liquid metal under strictly controlled conditions, the quantity of oxygen in the material will increase with the stirring time, together with increment of the viscosity and the electrical resistivity of the alloy. Compared with the conventional gallium simple substance, the new material reaches a good balance, which has both good electrical properties and attaching ability.

Through directly printing the liquid metal ink on the skin of either animal or human body with a paintbrush, the alloy layer becomes the simplest electrode and interface for recording electrical signal in human body. Thus, one can measure two basic properties of the liquid metal electrode at room temperature: the impedance and polarization voltage. When the electrode and the electrolyte solution contact, an electrical couple layer is formed at the boundary, causing about the contact voltage and the polarization phenomenon. In Fig. 12.9, the physiological saline was taken as a simulated tissue fluid for the measurement of the voltage with the Ga-based liquid metal at room temperature. Agilent 34970A data acquisition/switch unit was used to record the voltage and the probe material is platinum. For impedance measurement, the liquid metal ink was filled in a 40 cm long plastic tube, which has an inner diameter of 1 mm. And the SRS Model SR780 2-Channel Network Signal Analyzer was adopted for impedance measurement.

To provide practical verification, Yu et al. [35] designed the following conceptual experiments: the liquid metal ink electrode was used for testing the real electrocardiogram of rabbit and human, respectively. The experiments were operated with a miniaturized module (Fig. 12.10a) developed on the mobile phone (Fig. 12.10b) to monitor the ECG wave, which is compatible with both

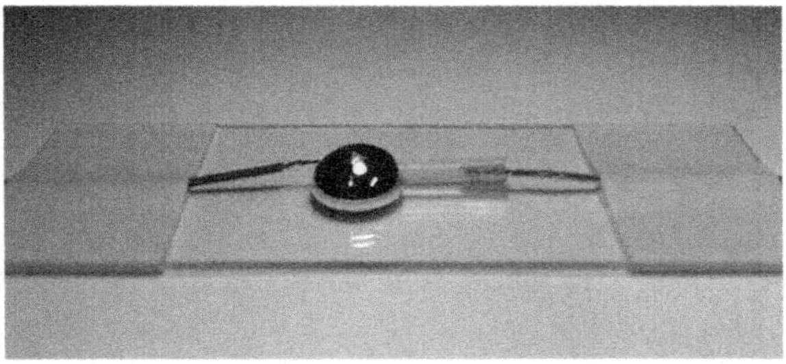

Fig. 12.9 The physiological saline is sealed in a plastic tube [35]. The anode (Pt probe) sticks into the tube and the cathode (Pt probe) into the liquid metal droplet. When the tube and the droplet contact, the polarization voltage emerges and is recorded through the probes

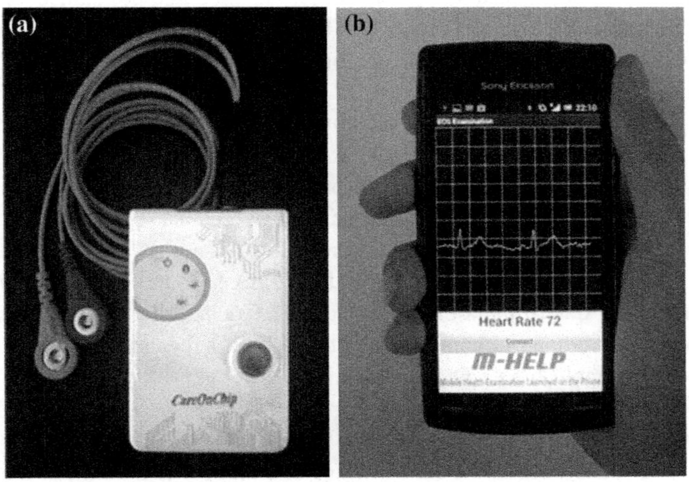

Fig. 12.10 A portable system for ECG monitoring on the mobile phone [35]. **a** The miniaturized wireless ECG module; **b** The ECG monitoring displayed on the mobile phone

conventional Ag/AgCl button electrode and the liquid metal ink. The acquired data can be transmitted to a smart phone (Sony Ericsson lt15i, Android 4.0 OS) via Bluetooth and displayed on the mobile phone screen (Fig. 12.10). The ECG module has two wires for conducting the differential biopotential into the filter circuit. There is a metallic button connector at the end of either wire, which is used for the button electrode to plug in and it can be seen in Fig. 12.10a. The liquid metal ink was printed on the skin surface with a paintbrush, and the button connectors were directly attached to the alloy when using it for acquiring ECG signals. Though it is not a rigid connection, the conformability and wettability of the liquid metal ensures its good contact with both the skin and the metallic button connector, i.e. the module.

In addition, the good wettability and electrical conductivity indicates that the liquid metal ink is not only a favourable bio-electrode, but also an ideal alloy for making conformable circuits on the skin or any other surfaces. Hence, Yu et al. managed to "draw" a basic electrical circuit in the palm using the ink in later section. With batteries hold in hand, the circuit's work status is displayed with four surface mounting LEDs attached in. Such trial can be seen as a symbol of more sophisticated biomedical applications with the material in the near future.

12.6 Implementation of Liquid Metal ECG Electrode

Figure 12.11a shows the resistance and the reactance as a function of frequency from 1 to 10 kHz. The calculation result of the average resistance is 0.225 Ω, representing an electrical resistivity of 44.1 μΩ cm at room temperature. The resistivity of the alloy is higher than common conductive metals such as gold (2.2 μΩ cm), silver (1.6 μΩ cm), copper (1.7 μΩ cm) or pure gallium (25.8 μΩ cm), yet much lower than a more famous liquid metal–mercury (95.8 μΩ cm) [36, 37]. It means while gaining a better wettability, the ink keeps at relatively low resistivity as a liquid conductor. On the other hand, the reactance which is correlated with the shape shows a character of low inductance of about 50 μH in the form of a straight line. Since the frequencies of most biomedical signals are below 10 kHz, the influence of reactance can be negligible and hence the resistance remains the major determinant of the impedance. Considering the liquid state of the metal, the measurement indicates that such ink is a promising choice for constructing conformable biomedical electronics.

The polarization voltage is depicted in Fig. 12.11b. When the metal and the saline contact with each other, the voltage "dives" to −0.73 V. After that, the value goes up slowly according to the time-voltage curve. Yet the magnitude stays higher than 500 mV in a few minutes.

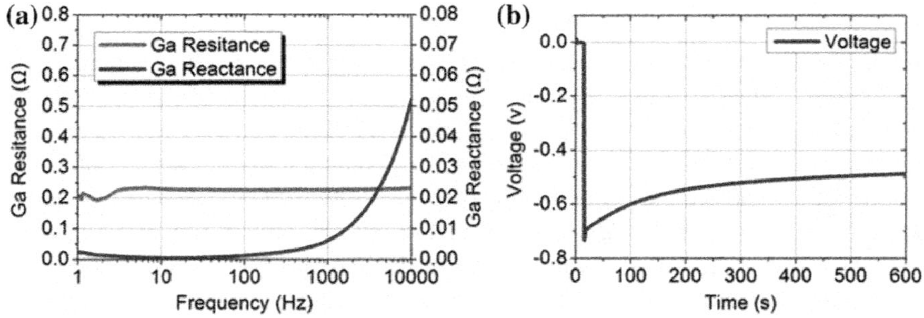

Fig. 12.11 The impedance and polarization voltage of the Ga-based liquid metal ink [35]. **a** The resistance and reactance curve from 1 to 10 kHz for the liquid metal in a 40 cm long tube with a diameter of 1 mm; **b** The polarization voltage curve when the liquid metal contacts with physiological saline

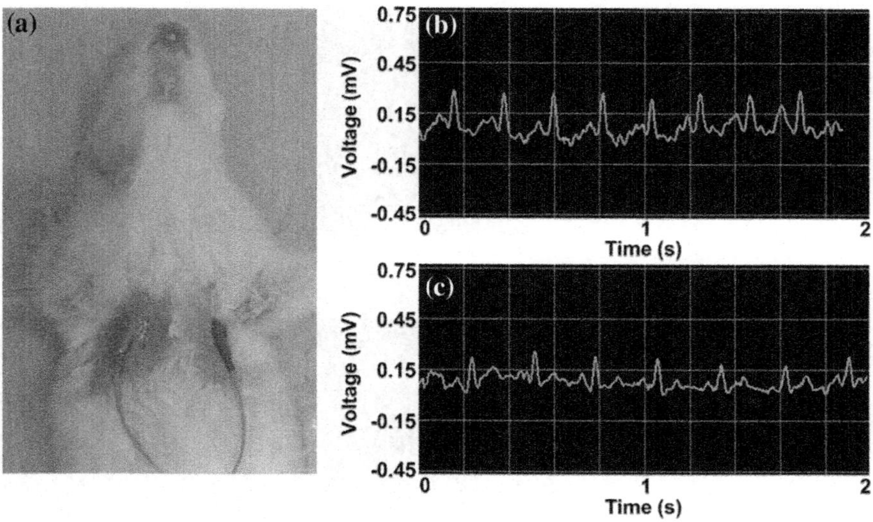

Fig. 12.12 ECG test and results on a rabbit with normal and liquid metal electrode [35]. **a** ECG test on a rabbit; **b** results using button electrode; **c** results using liquid metal electrode

The voltage between different phases is determined by multiple factors, including the metal's inner potential, categories and concentrations of the ions in the electrolyte, the temperature and the electrostatic charge adsorption, respectively. Though some of these factors drift rapidly in the physiological environments and can hardly be accurately measured, the simulation experiments still reveal the trend and scale of its polarization.

The conceptual experiments of measuring ECG with liquid metal ink electrodes were carried out on both rabbit and human respectively, and conventional button electrodes were adopted for a comparison. All the ECG data were acquired by a miniaturized ECG module, which was wirelessly connected to a mobile phone. The ECG waveform can be recorded and displayed in the phone screen in real time. Since the ECG wave amplitude of a rabbit is relatively small, its ECG recording was operated with the lead in the chest, which is displayed in Fig. 12.12a, while the tests on human measured voltage between left hand and right hand (Lead I). Figure 12.12b, c show the consistency of the ECG waveforms that are separately recorded using the button electrodes and the liquid metal ink on the identical rabbit, and Fig. 12.13 displays the similar results with the records of human ECG. Both results have shown that the qualities of the recorded ECG signals were almost the same, which indicates that the liquid metal is competent as a new kind of ECG electrode.

As is well known, it is quite hard to apply ECG test on small animals because of their sizes. The conventional electrodes have to include alligator clips and probes sticking through the skin. This may cause lesions to the animals, while the liquid metal ink overcomes these disadvantages. Thus besides its convenience, the liquid

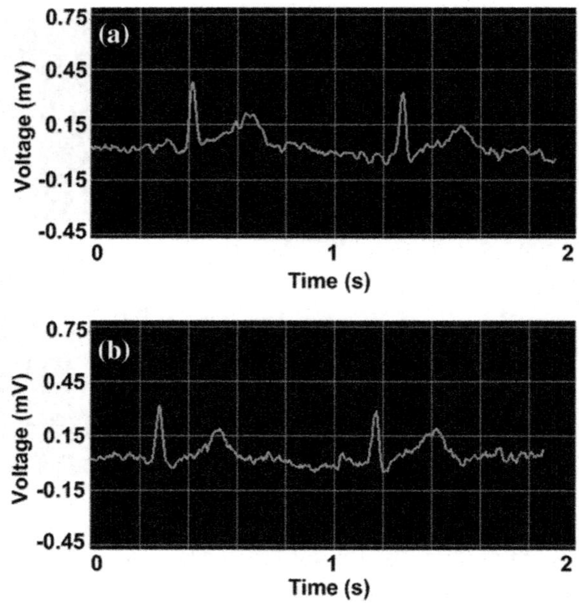

Fig. 12.13 ECG test results on human [35]. **a** Results using button electrode; **b** results using liquid metal electrode

metal ink electrode also brings better humanity, to which the rabbit experiment is a good proof.

It is a basic circuit with battery, resistors and LEDs, except that the wires are made of liquid metal inks, which are simply drawn on the skin with paintbrushes. Either to draw or to modify the circuit is now an easy job because it is just like painting and erasing with normal ink, where the place of canvas has been taken by the palm. Regardless of the veins or the movements, when the batteries are gripped between the thumb and the index finger, the loop closes and everything goes "OK" with the colourful lights, which is presented in Fig. 12.14. While the circuit is working, neither thermal nor electrical stimulation can be sensed from the ink. And though the trace becomes drier and caused a little feeling of discomfort to the skin, yet it can be easily washed off with water and soap, leaving no other perceivable irritation.

Overall, the liquid metal ink shows great virtues that no other conventional material possesses, and the conceptual experiments demonstrate its practical value in biomedical measurement. But before the actual use, there are still many issues need to be clarified.

(a) Safety Issue

The characteristic of the liquid metal ink that people may pay special attention to is about its safety. According to a systematic review on gallium and Galinstan hazards, the metal and its alloy have very low vapor pressures, meaning that a small amount of the material would not evolve any metal vapour [35]. And the gallium and Galinstan do not react with normal electrical insulation, nor do they corrode

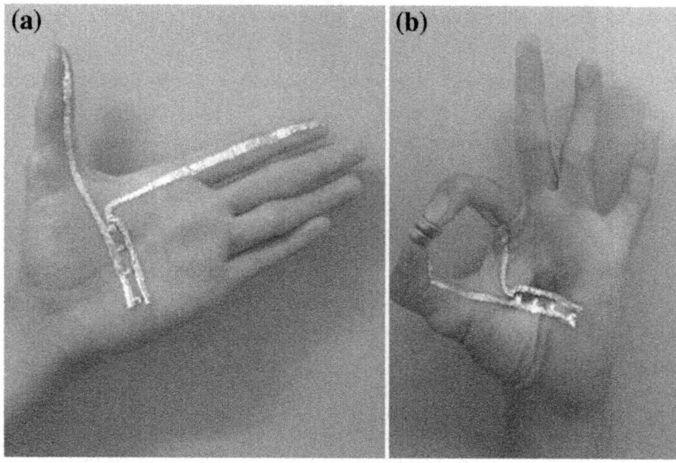

Fig. 12.14 The skin circuit drawn in the palm [35]. **a** The basic circuit drawn in the palm; **b** the circuit works when the batteries are gripped and the hand forms a gesture of "OK"

copper or stainless steel at room temperature. Gallium is insoluble in water and thus can hardly be absorbed through the skin. Long period inhaling of gallium oxide in large quantity may cause lung damage. However, naturally the gallium oxide produced forms a layer instead of becoming dust in the air. There is also report of gallium chloride-containing complexes poisoning, yet case like this is rare even in the laboratory [38]. Only one thing that needs caution is that eye contact or injection through the skin (including contact through wounds) should be avoided. Thus unless contacting the material in long terms or large doses, it is safe for normal use with small amount [39]. There are also other supports on gallium safety: gallium alloy has been used as restorative material in dentistry [40] and Ga-67 scintigraphy is an important body inside medical imaging method [41, 42]. And it is easy to remove the liquid metal by spraying medical alcohol solution, whose evaporation cools the material to solid form and much easier for separation with the substrates.

(b) Electrode Properties of the Ink

The impedance and polarization voltage are among the major concerns when evaluating a material's performance as electrode. The measurements of both parameters illustrate that the liquid metal ink is capable of serving as electrode and circuit material.

Though its resistivity is higher than the normally used metals such as copper or silver, yet it is still acceptable because in most cases this scale of resistance is negligible. But it is obviously not suitable to be an electrical heater unless there are some other energy sources, such as microwave, laser beam and even a contact heater. The reactance varies in different situations such as the change of shape, length and thickness. Thus it is possible to make this use into a sensor of motions, especially in the area of joints and muscles. And the reactance should also be thought about carefully when designing antennas or circuits that involved in high frequency signals.

Though we do not investigate the relative electric potential of the material, the experiment as have been done already reflected the polarization [35]. The magnitude of the contact voltage stays at a high level and it is an unstable but always existing source of noise when recording biopotentials. As a contrast, the polarization magnitude of a button electrode with electrolytic gel is usually smaller than 0.1 V, which means that the ink may not perform as good as an ordinary medical electrode. However, the waveform in both ECG experiments illustrates that the liquid metal is still an acceptable bio-electrode. Thus a device with well designed signal filter and reasonable common mode rejection ration (60–80 dB) is capable to fulfil the request.

(c) Conformable Circuits Technique

The good wettability is another important character the liquid metal ink owns. The skin circuit experiment has verified that it is possible to make an electrical circuit on the rough surface like the skin, which can be easily drawn or erased. As a comparison, it is far more convenient and efficient than the current printed circuit board (PCB) technique, which is rigid and has to make a new one in case of any changes.

This may lead to the unique technique of conformable circuit, which means not only its product is conformable, but also the manufacture of the circuits is adapted to any surface. And the technique can still be divided into two parts: one is electrical circuit drawn by hand or with simple tools, which adequately supports free creation; another is liquid metal printer, which is suitable for precise circuit and industrial production. Both parts can provide supplementary to each other, too. In order to realize multiple functions, it will be valuable to do research in making liquid metal components such as antenna and IC chips, and studies on the embedded batteries or power supply will be important as well. In either case of liquid metal circuit manufacture, the biomedical applications will be an extremely important part of the technique, due to its safety, convenience, low cost and of course flexibility.

(d) Biomedical Application with Liquid Metal

Using the liquid metal as a physiological electrode for ECG detection is a good example of the material's biomedical roles. It is specifically suitable for electrical impedance tomography (EIT) [43–45] due to its electrical property and conformability. Figure 12.15 presents a sketch of a 16-electrode circle array surrounding the breast for EIT. Compared with conventional approaches, the liquid metal ink electrodes provide better contact and more comfortableness with no need of pressing the breast tightly. And similarly, it is a prospective electrode in EIT pulmonary monitoring for the children or the new born. The liquid metal ink electrode is also suitable for various bio-electrical (3D) mapping because the electrodes can be drawn at any area and in any shape, including EIT, ECG and EEG. Clearly, the liquid metal electrode can be extended to defibrillator in emergency first aid, too.

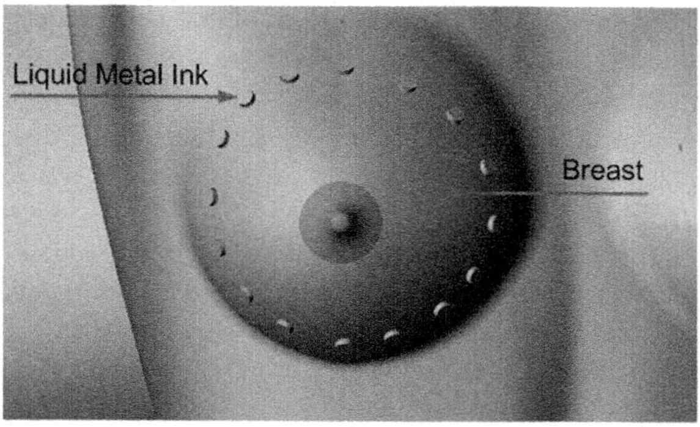

Fig. 12.15 A 3D model of using liquid metal ink as breast EIT electrodes [35]

The contact voltage can be applied in other ways as well. For example, it has been published that using the liquid metal and its matching metal can help make thermal couples, which is a prospective application for body temperature mapping in the future.

Another attractive approach is the functional circuit made by the liquid metal on body surface. For examples, one can use the material to build coils as a signal transmitter for sending out the physiological data acquired in the human body. And the coil can be an energy receiver charged by microwave to realize localized or even whole body heating as well, which is an important method for non-invasive tumor treatment. What's more, one may associate the gallium electrode or circuit with its role in chemical tumor treatment [46] or antimicrobial [47], thus to find its potential value in disease treatment and reasonable ways of releasing it. All of the ideas represent different branches that provide plenty of contents for research, and the liquid metal will make a large difference in biomedical applications.

12.7 Conformal Liquid Metal Printed Epidermal Electronics

12.7.1 Compliance of Biomedical Sensors on Skin

Noninvasion and precision for medical monitoring and treatment indicate the trends for developing advanced health care devices [48]. So far, traditional medical devices for signal measurement or electrical stimulation treatment are often equipped with rigid metallic electrodes such as cooper or platinum which are generally placed on skin directly [49–52]. However, due to non-smoothness of the skin surface and the physiological profile of human body [53], there often exist some air gaps between the rigid metallic electrodes and the skin, which would induce a bad Ohm contact and restrict the accurate monitoring and treatment [54, 55]. According to some researches, it was shown that the poor coupling between metallic electrodes and skin leads to low signal-to-noise ratio (SNR), which causes the degradation of signal performance when measuring the physiological parameters [56]. In addition, the low energy transfer efficiency between metallic electrodes and the target caused by the high resistance of the air gap makes energy mostly deposited on the skin, heating the local surface, which increases the risk of skin injury [57], such as the electronic muscle stimulator (EMS) [58] and defibrillator [59, 60].

In order to overcome the weak coupling of traditional rigid electrodes, some researches impose pressure onto the electrodes to enhance the electrode-skin contact [61]. However, the applied pressure may alter the electrical characteristics of the skin, which results in the deviation from real physiological monitoring. In addition, conductive gel is smeared on the skin surface to facilitate coupling between skin and electrode [62]. However, conductive gel generates additional resistance, and due to the moisture evaporation, it cannot maintain good contact for a long time, which enforces people to reconnect the electrode after monitoring for 24 h.

Since flexible electronic circuits can match the body curve perfectly, they are being increasingly employed to fabricate wearable medical devices for better electrophysiological and biochemical detection [63, 64], such as temperature measurement [65–67], blood flow measurement [66], sweat analysis [68]. Due to good electric coupling with skin, flexible circuits can achieve higher SNR, better security and more robust anti-motion effect [69]. Notably, limited by flexibility, it is only able to keep tight contact with physiological curve, but hard to fit the skin surface microstructure closely. Furthermore, flexible circuits connect to skin indirectly as they need to be printed on some substrates [70].

As it was shown before, with the capability of being printed on skin directly, liquid metal shows a great potential to tackle those technical challenges confronted by the traditional rigid electrodes. Here for the illustration, $GaIn_{24.5}$ (the conductivity: 3.4×10^6 S/m, the polarization voltage dives to −0.73 V) with a mixture of 75.5% gallium (Ga) and 24.5% indium (In) by weight is adopted. Its favourable flexibility enables a direct contact between the electrode and skin via fitting the slightly gully structure of the skin surface, without introducing external mechanical force. In the following, an epidermal liquid metal electrode-skin model [48] was adopted to illustrate the coupling impedance issue of electrode-skin in comparison to rigid electrode.

12.7.2 Coupling Impedance of Ex Vivo Electrode-Skin Model

In the model with rigid electrode, the contact impedance of electrode-skin was affected by the body movement resulted from the transverse tension and longitudinal pressure of the skin. In the model with rigid electrode-gel-skin, the gel reduced the mechanical force caused by the contact between electrode and skin in contrast to the rigid electrode-skin model. Similarly, the liquid metal electrode did not make the skin deformation, which were helpful to reduce the impact of motion and mechanical force as well as keeping the electric potential E_{ep0} stable (Fig. 12.16a). Actually, the electrical resistivity of $GaIn_{24.5}$ (44.1 μΩ cm) was higher than common rigid electrodes, such as copper (1.7 μΩ cm), silver (1.6 μΩ cm) and gold (2.2 μΩ cm). However, the resistance was ignored resulting from the close link of the liquid metal electrode and skin. The liquid metal electrode reduced the contact resistance between the electrode and skin leading to the improved signal to noise ratio of the measured signal. Furthermore, it diminished the impact of skin deformation on the transmission of the electrical signals to

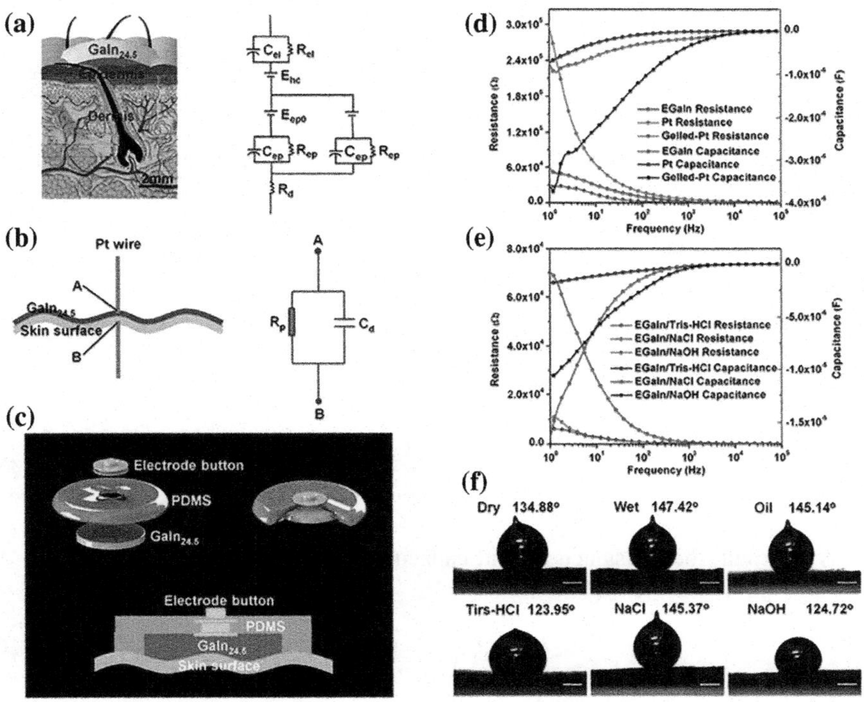

Fig. 12.16 **a** The structural diagram and electronic model of liquid metal soft electrode-skin. **b** The simplified resistance capacitance parallel model of $GaIn_{24.5}$ electrode-skin model. **c** The 3D schematic diagram and its sectional drawing of liquid metal $GaIn_{24.5}$ electrode. **d** Curves of resistance and capacitance of $GaIn_{24.5}$ electrode-skin, Pt electrode-skin and gelled Pt electrode-skin varying with frequency from 1 to 10^5 Hz ('EGaIn Resistance' refers to the resistance of $GaIn_{24.5}$ electrode-skin; 'Pt Resistance' refers to the resistance of Pt electrode-skin; 'Gelled-Pt Resistance' refers to the resistance of gelled Pt electrode-skin; 'EGaIn Capacitance' refers to the capacitance of $GaIn_{24.5}$ electrode-skin; 'Pt Capacitance' refers to the capacitance of Pt electrode-skin; 'Gelled-Pt Capacitance' refers to the capacitance of gelled Pt electrode-skin.). **e** Curves of resistance and capacitance of $GaIn_{24.5}$ electrode-skin under different skin surface treatments (1.0 mol/L Tris-HCl, 1.0 mol/L NaCl, 1.0 mol/L NaOH). **f** The contact angles of liquid metal droplet on the ex vivo skin surface of BALB/c Nude mouse under different treatments (dry, wet, oil, 1.0 mol/L Tris-HCl, 1.0 mol/L NaCl, 1.0 mol/L NaOH). Scale bars: 500 μm [48]

improve the robustness of the motion. In Fig. 12.16a, E_{hc} was half-cell potential; C_{el} and R_{el} were the total capacitance and resistance of the interface of electrode and electrolyte; C_{ep} and R_{ep} were the capacitance and resistance of the epidermis.

The resistance and capacitance of Pt electrode-skin, gelled Pt electrode-skin and $GaIn_{24.5}$ electrode-skin in different frequency were measured by the electrochemical workstation. Due to the limitation of the measurement, the whole electrode-skin model was considered as a simple model consisting of resistance R_p and capacitance C_d (Fig. 12.16b). Consequently, the overall impedance was characterized as

$$Z = \frac{1}{Y} = \frac{R_p}{1 + j\omega C_d R_p} = \frac{R_p(1 - j\omega C_d R_p)}{1 + (\omega C_d R_p)^2} \tag{12.12}$$

$$Z = \frac{R_p}{1 + (\omega C_d R_p)^2} - j\frac{\omega C_d R_p^2}{1 + (\omega C_d R_p)^2} \tag{12.13}$$

Here, Z is the impedance (Z': the real part; Z'': the imaginary part), Y is the admittance (the reciprocal of Z), ω is the angular frequency (unit: rad/s), j is the imaginary number. The real part Z' and imaginary part Z'' of the overall impedance measured from the frequency response analysis could be further described as follows:

$$Z' = \frac{R_p}{1 + (\omega C_d R_p)^2} \tag{12.14}$$

$$Z'' = \frac{\omega C_d R_p^2}{1 + (\omega C_d R_p)^2} \tag{12.15}$$

As a result, the resistance R_p and capacitance C_d can be calculated as:

$$R_p = Z'\left(1 + \left(\frac{Z''}{Z'}\right)^2\right) \tag{12.16}$$

$$C_d = \frac{Z''}{Z'\omega R_p} \tag{12.17}$$

In Fig. 12.16d, the impedance variation tendency under different frequency had apparent distinction among Pt electrode-skin, gelled Pt electrode-skin and $GaIn_{24.5}$ electrode-skin models. Among these three types of electrodes, gelled Pt electrode-skin model had the minimum resistance, while Pt electrode-skin model had the maximum resistance. At frequency of 10 Hz, the EGaIn resistance was $2.93 \times 10^4\ \Omega$, the Pt resistance was $6.53 \times 10^4\ \Omega$ (2.23 times to EGaIn), and the gelled-Pt resistance was $1.57 \times 10^4\ \Omega$ (0.53 times to EGaIn). The capacitance of Pt electrode-skin was the minimum and $GaIn_{24.5}$ electrode-skin was prior to the gelled

Pt electrode-skin model under the whole measured frequency range. At frequency of 10 Hz, the EGaIn capacitance was 5.87×10^{-7} F, the Pt capacitance was 2.9×10^{-7} F (0.49 times to EGaIn), and the gelled-Pt capacitance was 2.24×10^{-6} F (3.82 times to EGaIn). The product of R_p and C_d is the time constant of the resistance—capacitance circuit. Take the frequency of 10 Hz for instance, the $R_p \cdot C_d$ of EGaIn is 1.71991×10^{-2} s, the $R_p \cdot C_d$ of Pt is 1.8937×10^{-2} s and the $R_p \cdot C_d$ of gelled Pt is 3.5168×10^{-2} s. From the above analysis, the time constant of the gelled-Pt electrode is the largest and the charging time that the capacitance C_d requires to reach the steady state is the longest. Attributing to the maximum capacitance, the gelled Pt electrode-skin model caused more oscillation in the circuit than $GaIn_{24.5}$ or Pt electrode-skin model, even though the resistance was the minimum value.

In Fig. 12.16e, the ex vivo skin surface of BALB/c Nude mouse was treated with 1.0 mol/L Tris-HCl, 1.0 mol/L NaCl, 1.0 mol/L NaOH, respectively. Figure 12.16e demonstrated that $GaIn_{24.5}$ electrode-skin model had the maximum resistance and the minimum capacitance with Tris-HCl treating. There were no obvious differences in resistance with NaCl and NaOH treating. At the frequency from 1 to 10 Hz, the capacitance with NaOH treating was lower than that with NaCl treating, but the result was reverse in the frequency from 10 to 10^5 Hz. Figure 12.16f plotted the contact angles (measured by the contact angle instrument JC2000D3, Shanghai) of liquid metal droplet on the ex vivo skin surface of BALB/c Nude mouse with different treatments (dry, wet, oil, 1.0 mol/L Tris-HCl, 1.0 mol/L NaCl, 1.0 mol/L NaOH). The liquid metal droplet fully adapted to the skin surface texture even if it was covered with hair.

Tris-HCl solution and NaOH solution dissolved the thin oxide skin on the surface of liquid metal, which made the liquid metal droplets exhibit approximately the same contact angles. By comparing the resistances and capacitances with Tris-HCl and NaOH treating, there was no distinguishing relationship between the contact resistance and oxide skin. Though the EGaIn/NaCl resistance and EGaIn/NaOH resistance with the same concentration of NaCl and NaOH solution were almost the same values, the contact angles were different. Since Tris-HCl is a kind of buffer solution with incomplete ionization in comparison to NaCl and NaOH, the resistance of 1.0 mol/L Tris-HCl solution (pH = 3.92) was the minimum value. On the whole, comparing the trend of contact angles (under the treatment with 1.0 mol/L Tris-HCl, 1.0 mol/L NaCl, 1.0 mol/L NaOH on skin) with that of the contact resistances, the contact angles of the liquid metal droplet on ex vivo BALB/c Nude mouse skin were not consistent with the contact impedances. Besides, the contact angles of liquid metal droplet on dry skin, wet skin and oil skin (Fig. 12.16f) were not consistent with the contact resistances (Fig. 12.16b).

12.7.3 In Vivo Physiological Monitoring with Liquid Metal Electrode

Figure 12.17 presented the in vivo $GaIn_{24.5}$ electrode-skin contact resistance under different working conditions for the purpose of evaluating the conformability of $GaIn_{24.5}$ electrode. Figure 12.17a demonstrated that the contact resistance of dry skin was higher than that with NaCl solution (0.5, 1.0, 1.5 mol/L) under low frequency. However, the treatment on skin by different concentrations of NaCl solution brought about the same contact resistance. To simulate the skin oil secretion, a thin layer of olive oil was applied on the chest skin, and Fig. 12.17b showed the contact resistances of dry skin, oil skin and normal saline (0.5 mol/L NaCl solution) skin. The contact resistance of oil skin-$GaIn_{24.5}$ was higher than dry skin-$GaIn_{24.5}$ and normal saline skin-$GaIn_{24.5}$, and normal saline skin-$GaIn_{24.5}$ had the lowest contact resistance. Figure 12.17c demonstrated that the contact resistances of skin-$GaIn_{24.5}$ varied under different room temperatures (14, 20, 27 °C). The contact resistance was the largest at 14 °C, the contact resistance was the second at 20 °C, and the contact resistance was the smallest at 27 °C. Figure 12.17d illustrated the contact resistance measurement under different positions (The ear was the largest, the backside was the second, the bosom was the third, and the leg was the last).

By measuring the contact resistance between $GaIn_{24.5}$ bio-electrode and the skin surface under different working conditions, Wang et al. [48] evaluated the conformability of liquid metal electrode. Figure 12.17a inset revealed that positive and negative ions in the NaCl solution enhanced the ion transfer, and increased the current to decrease the resistance. Actually, because of the enough ions in 0.5 mol/L NaCl solution to transfer current, increasing the solution concentration could not reduce the contact resistance obviously. Oil skin increased the contact resistance and the curve fluctuation was quite large in the low frequency region, which showed that the contact resistance was changed largely and signal anti-interference ability was weakened (Fig. 12.17b).

Rabbit was a kind of warm blooded animal. When the external temperature was lower than rabbit body temperature and changed largely, there was much gooseflesh on the rabbit skin surface to adjust the skin temperature. Gooseflesh made the skin so unsmooth that the contact resistance increased when the external temperature was decreased (Fig. 12.17c). At the same time, the reduced temperature transformed the liquid metal from liquid into solid, which also made the $GaIn_{24.5}$ electrode not conformal. Therefore, the $GaIn_{24.5}$ electrode had relatively narrow temperature range for application and should be further designed with a heating system.

At different parts of the rabbit, the skin surface had different shapes and its contact resistance varied greatly, as shown in Fig. 12.17d. When measuring the contact resistance of the ear, it was not shaved and its resistance was the biggest. With regard to the spine existence on the backside, its surface was not flat and its contact resistance was the second. Smooth surfaces at bosom and leg have been

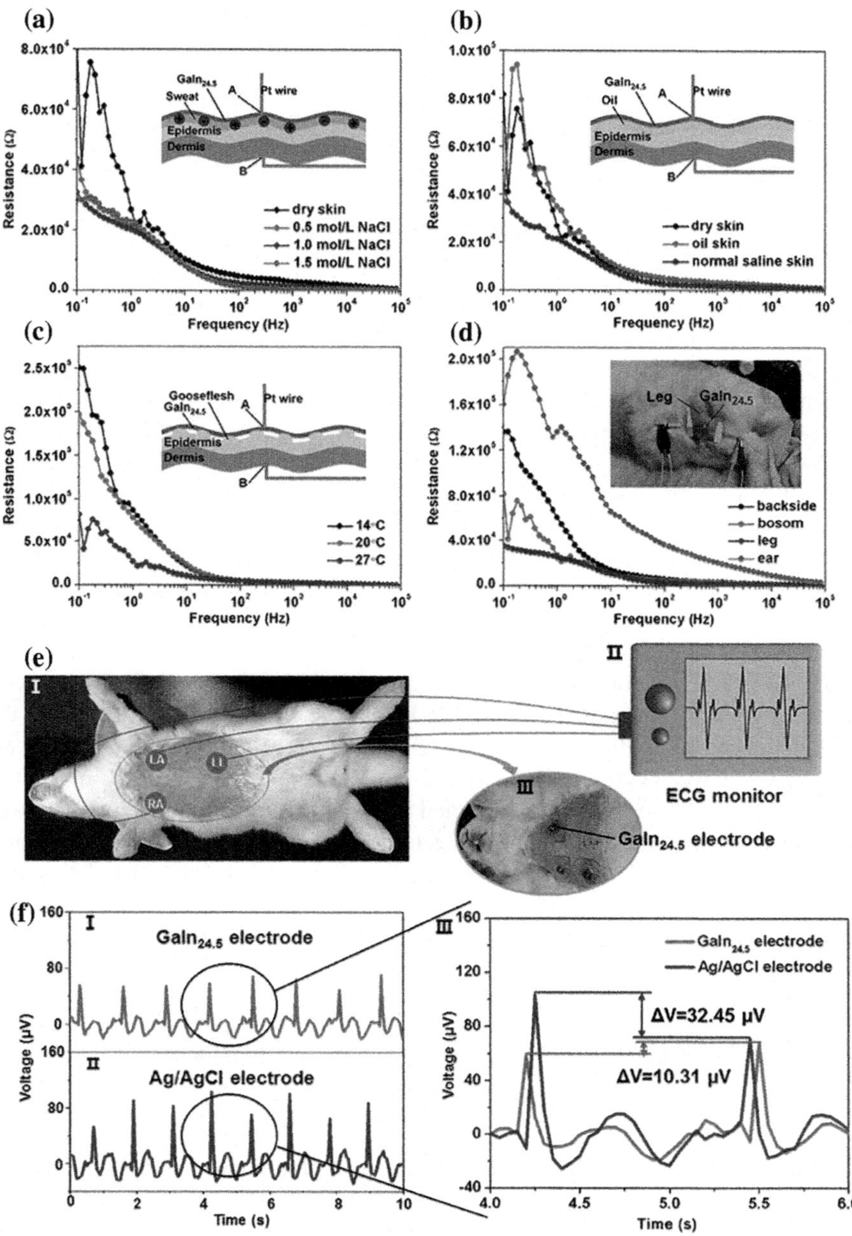
(a)
Galn24.5
Sweat
A
Pt wire
Epidermis
Dermis
B
dry skin
0.5 mol/L NaCl
1.0 mol/L NaCl
1.5 mol/L NaCl
Resistance (Ω)
Frequency (Hz)
(b)
Galn24.5
Oil
A
Pt wire
Epidermis
Dermis
B
dry skin
oil skin
normal saline skin
(c)
Gooseflesh
Galn24.5
Pt wire
Epidermis
Dermis
14°C
20°C
27°C
(d)
Leg
Galn24.5
backside
bosom
leg
ear
(e)
I
LA
LL
RA
II
III
ECG monitor
Galn24.5 electrode
(f)
Galn24.5 electrode
Ag/AgCl electrode
Voltage (μV)
Time (s)
ΔV=32.45 μV
ΔV=10.31 μV

◂**Fig. 12.17** The contact resistance of liquid metal $GaIn_{24.5}$ under different working conditions and the ECG signal measurement of the rabbit [48]. **a** The contact resistance under different NaCl concentrations. **b** The contact resistance under dry skin, oil skin and normal saline skin. **c** The contact resistance under different temperatures. **d** The contact resistance under different measuring positions. **e** The connection of liquid metal $GaIn_{24.5}$ electrodes and ECG monitor, **i** the sketch of three ECG leads on rabbit chest, (II) the ECG monitor measuring ECG signal, (III) the $GaIn_{24.5}$ electrodes on rabbit chest. **f** The ECG signals respectively measured by $GaIn_{24.5}$ electrode and Ag/AgCl electrode, (I) the ECG signal measured by $GaIn_{24.5}$ electrode, (II) the ECG signal measured by Ag/AgCl electrode, (III) the ECG signal comparison between $GaIn_{24.5}$ electrode and Ag/AgCl electrode from 4 to 6 s

chosen, but more subcutaneous fat in the chest leads to larger contact resistance than that in the leg. Hence, the contact resistances were similar in different working conditions in high frequency (up to 10 Hz), which was the frequency range for ECG, EEG (electroencephalogram), PWV (pulse wave) and EMG (electromyographic) detection.

The $GaIn_{24.5}$ bio-electrode was applied to ECG monitoring. By comparing the ECG signals measured by $GaIn_{24.5}$ electrode and Ag/AgCl electrode, we found the similar stable ECG signals between the liquid metal electrode and traditional Ag/AgCl electrode [48]. Figure 12.17e showed the physical map of liquid metal $GaIn_{24.5}$ electrodes according to the theoretical model. The liquid metal electrodes were connected with the ECG monitor through the three leads connections. Figure 12.17f I was the ECG signal measured by the $GaIn_{24.5}$ electrodes with uniformly varying signal and Fig. 12.17f II was the ECG signal measured by the Ag/AgCl electrodes with undulating signal. Figure 12.17f III was the ECG signals comparison between $GaIn_{24.5}$ electrodes and Ag/AgCl electrodes from 4 to 6 s. The variation of peak-to-peak voltage detected by Ag/AgCl electrodes (32.45 μV) was 3.15 times to that tested by $GaIn_{24.5}$ electrodes (10.31 μV). As a result, by comparing Fig. 12.17f I–III, the maximum ECG signal value measured by Ag/AgCl electrodes changed more largely than that of $GaIn_{24.5}$ electrodes, and the $GaIn_{24.5}$ electrodes presented better signal stability and certain reduction of noise.

12.7.4 *Simulation Treatment for Smart Defibrillation of Conformal Liquid Metal Electrode*

To evaluate the treatment for smart defibrillation of the liquid metal electrode, the physical field simulation was carried out to examine the conductivity of liquid metal electrode-skin [48]. The $GaIn_{24.5}$ electrode was closely related to the skin, hence the electric potential distribution along the normal direction of the skin varied evenly. In comparison, the rigid electrode only contacted the convex skin surface and the electric potential distribution in the depression was small (Fig. 12.18). In Fig. 12.18a, b, the electric field distribution of flexible electrode was more uniform compared to that of rigid electrode. Since the directions of the current and electric

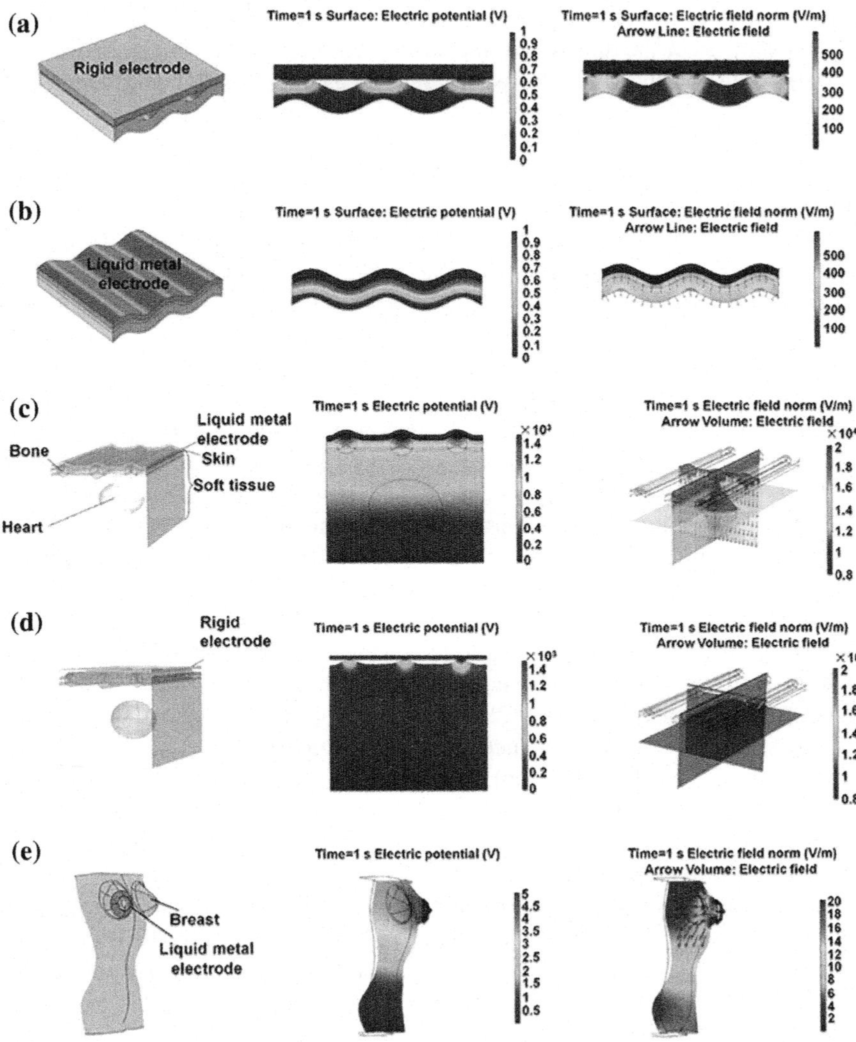

Fig. 12.18 The physical field simulation of rigid bio-electrode and conformal liquid metal bio-electrode on skin surface and human body models, respectively [48]. **a** The electric potential distribution and electric field distribution of skin when applying voltage in the rigid electrode-skin model (the purple area was copper electrode). **b** The electric potential distribution and electric field distribution of skin when applying voltage in the liquid metal electrode-skin model (the purple area was liquid metal $GaIn_{24.5}$ electrode). **c** The defibrillation model of liquid metal flexible electrode covering human body's chest, and the electric potential distribution and electric field distribution of the physical field simulation of the liquid metal flexible electrode model. **d** The defibrillation model of conventional rigid electrode covering human body's chest, and the electric potential distribution and electric field distribution of the physical field simulation of the rigid electrode model. **e** The model of liquid metal ring electrode covering female breast, and the electric potential distribution and electric field distribution of the physical field simulation of the liquid metal ring electrode model (the purple area was liquid metal $GaIn_{24.5}$ electrode)

field were always consistent, flexible electrode was able to generate more uniform effects regardless of the direction of the current. In contrast, the air gap between the rigid electrode and the skin resulted in high impedance, which could damage the skin caused by the generated heat.

Further, based on the electrode-skin models shown formerly, Fig. 12.18c, d exhibited the models of liquid metal flexible electrode and conventional rigid electrode covered on the chest of human body to simulate the treatment for defibrillation via the electrical effect. The simplified chest geometric model was divided into 5 parts, including electrode, skin, bone, soft tissue and heart. In Fig. 12.18c, the liquid metal electrode closely fitted the purple skin surface. On the contrary, there was air void between skin and rigid electrode (Fig. 12.18d). The electrical parameters of the material were shown in Table 12.1. In order to control the variables and compare the difference between the flexible electrode and the rigid electrode, the flexible electrode material here was the liquid metal $GaIn_{24.5}$ and the rigid electrode material was the copper electrode. The upper surface of the liquid metal electrode was provided with a voltage input to simulate the process of defibrillation more realistically. Through the analysis of electrical potential distribution and electric field distribution, the flexible $GaIn_{24.5}$ electrode needed less energy input to realize the same current distribution.

The defibrillation treatment models (Fig. 12.18c, d) revealed that the bone barrier made the rigid electrode hard to pass enough current to the heart especially when the patient was thin. However, the highly conformal bio-electrode had good contact with skin and did not form large surface resistance to accumulate heat and burn skin. Once painting the conductive paste, it completely fitted the electrode and skin (there was usually a small gap). The conductivity of the conductive paste was 1–20 S/m and the $GaIn_{24.5}$ electrode was 3.76×10^6 S/m. Therefore the liquid metal bio-electrode reduced the energy attenuation to reach higher energy at the heart compared to conductive paste.

Additionally, to verify the high conformability of liquid metal electrodes, the liquid metal ring electrode model was built on female breast (Fig. 12.18e). Owing to the fine structure on the contact of the breast and electrodes, there was a high mesh division density. The mesh division density of the electrodes and breast junction region was the highest and the minimum grid density reached 0.1 mm. In the ring electrode model, the human body was assumed as homogeneous soft tissue. The even electric potential and electric field distribution were obtained by the ring electrode tightly fitting the skin curve to highlight the merits of the suitable flexible electrode. To sum up, whether the $GaIn_{24.5}$ electrode was employed in measurement or treatment, it achieved good contact with human body.

12.7.5 Cytotoxicity and Biocompatibility of Liquid Metal

The human melanoma C8161 cells and the human epidermal HaCaT cells were applied to detect the cytotoxicity of liquid metal $GaIn_{24.5}$. Figure 12.19d was the

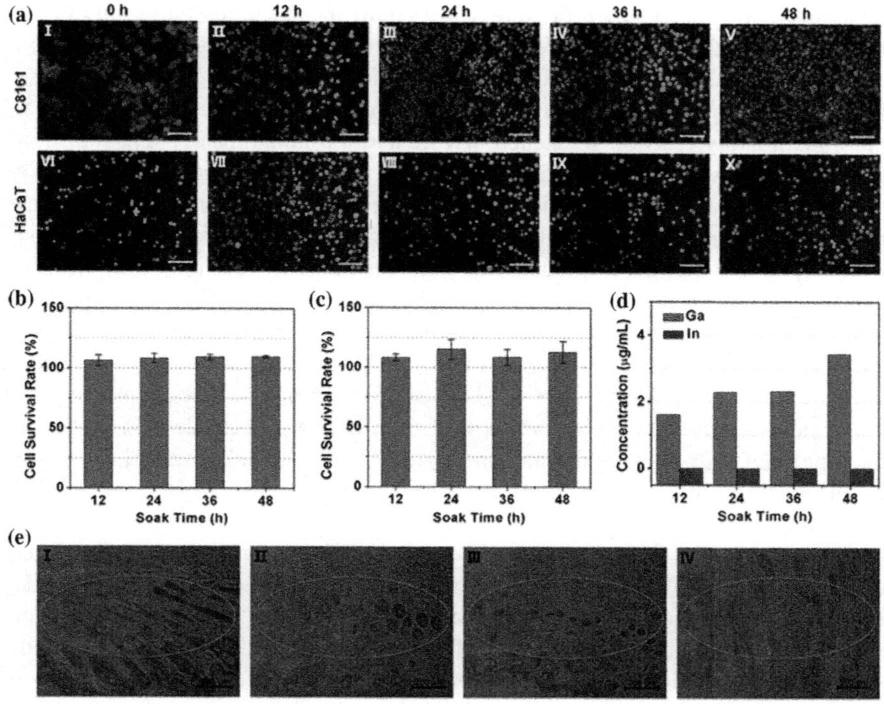

Fig. 12.19 The cytotoxicity and biocompatibility of liquid metal $GaIn_{24.5}$ [48]. **a** Observations of cell live and dead of human melanoma C8161 cells and human epidermal HaCaT cells under fluorescence microscope with cell culture medium immersed by liquid metal $GaIn_{24.5}$ (soak time: 12, 24, 36, 48 h), scale bars: 100 μm. **b** The survival rate of human melanoma C8161 cells by CCK-8 assay with cell culture medium immersed by liquid metal $GaIn_{24.5}$ (soak time: 12, 24, 36, 48 h). **c** The survival rate of human epidermal HaCaT cells by CCK-8 assay with cell culture medium immersed by liquid metal $GaIn_{24.5}$ (soak time: 12, 24, 36, 48 h). **d** Ion concentration in cell culture medium at different soak time (12, 24, 36, 48 h) immersed by liquid metal $GaIn_{24.5}$. **e** Skin biopsies with 0.1 mL liquid metal $GaIn_{24.5}$ injected underneath BALB/c Nude mice skin for different days (0 d, 5 d, 10 d, 15 d), scale bars: 200 μm

ion concentration of gallium and indium in cell culture medium at different soak times (12, 24, 36, 48 h) immersed by liquid metal $GaIn_{24.5}$. Indium was stable and not detected after 48 h immersion [71]. The C8161 cells and the HaCaT cells cultured in the complete medium immersed by liquid metal were almost alive (Fig. 12.19a, green—live, red—dead). The cell survival rate of the C8161 cells and the HaCaT cells (Fig. 12.19b, c) were higher than 100% with different soak times, which demonstrated the nontoxicity of complete medium immersed by liquid metal $GaIn_{24.5}$.

In addition, the liquid metal $GaIn_{24.5}$ was painted on the skin of BALB/c Nude mouse for 30 min and cleaned off the gray residue of liquid metal using the 75% alcohol. The observation of the skin showed that the liquid metal did not cause the skin irritation with skin red or inflamed, and the liquid metal did not block the breaking ability of skin. Furthermore, the liquid metal $GaIn_{24.5}$ (0.1 mL/mouse) was injected underneath BALB/c Nude mice skin for different days (0 d, 5 d, 10 d, 15 d) and the skin biopsies (Fig. 12.19e, in the green circle, circular follicles—inflammatory reaction) indicated that the skin appeared inflammatory reaction at 5d, the inflammatory reaction weakened at 10d, and the inflammatory reaction disappeared at 15d, which manifested its nontoxicity to skin and good biocompatibility.

Overall, the conformal liquid metal electrode shows the merits of small contact resistance, low noise signal acquisition, slow energy diminution and fine biocompatibility. Firstly, its good contact with skin was proven to realize better electrical conduction from physical model and experimental methods. Due to such electrode material's conformal feature, the liquid metal $GaIn_{24.5}$ can not only well adapt to the human body profile, but also fit the subtle gully structure of the skin surface without evident mechanical force to change and deform the electrical properties of electrode-skin. Particularly, according to the liquid metal electrode-skin model and the rigid electrode-skin model and the rigid electrode-gel-skin model, the liquid metal electrode represent the optimal coupling impedance. Besides, the contact resistances of liquid metal $GaIn_{24.5}$ electrode-skin were measured under different working conditions, such as sweat, oil secretion, different temperature and different flatness surface etc. The ECG signal monitored by the liquid metal electrodes had less noise and better signal stability compared with Ag/AgCl electrode. More importantly, the simulation treatment for smart defibrillation of thoracic model electric field distribution achieved the precision therapy by establishing the theory of cardiac defibrillation via the finite element physical field simulation. The conformal liquid metal electrode owns the capability of displaying a more uniform electric potential and electric field distribution with less energy loss compared to the traditional rigid electrode. In addition, the fluorescence imaging of cell live/dead and the survival rate of the C8161 cells and HaCaT cells indicated its nontoxicity, and the weakening of inflammation manifested its excellent biocompatibility. Therefore, the conformal liquid metal electronics offers an excellent way to realize direct and immediate electrode-skin contact with high conformability and good conductivity to improve the stability and precision in physiological monitoring and disease treatment.

12.8 Liquid Metal Printed Skin Electronics as Therapeutic Circuit

12.8.1 About Tumor Treating Field

Liquid metal skin electronics opens significant potential for disease diagnostics and therapy. Li et al. [72] had demonstrated a method of using electrical stimulation for treatment of malignant melanoma through directly spray-printing liquid metal on skin as soft electrodes to deliver low intensity, intermediate frequency electric fields. With patterned conductive liquid metal components on mice skin and under assistance of a signal generator, a sine wave electrical power with voltage of 5 V and 300 kHz could be administrated on treating malignant melanoma tumor. Their experiments demonstrated that tumor volume was significantly reduced compared with that of the control group. Under the designed parameters (signal: sine wave, signal amplitude Vpp: 5 V and Vpp: 4 V, frequency: 300 kHz) of Tumor treating fields (TTFields) with the sprayed liquid metal electrode, four mice tumor groups became diminishing after one week of treatment. The only device-related side effect as seen was a mild to moderate contact dermatitis underneath the field delivering electrodes. The SEM images and pathological analysis demonstrated the targeted treating behaviour of the malignant melanoma tumor. Further, thermal infrared imaging experiments indicated that there occur no evident heating effects in the course of treatment. Besides, the liquid metal is easy to remove through medical alcohol. Overall, TTFields through liquid metal electrode could offer a safe, straightforward and effective treatment modality which evidently slows down tumor growth in vivo. These promising results also raised the possibility of applying spray-printing TTFields as an easy going physical way for future cancer therapy.

12.8.2 Basic Principle of Skin Electronics in Tumor Therapy

As living cells consist of ions, polar or charged molecules, membranes, and organelles, they are responsive to and often generate electric fields and currents. The electric activity of cells plays a key role in many essential biological processes. Low intensity, intermediate frequency, electric fields have been proven to inhibit cancerous cell growth in vitro by an anti-microtubule mechanism of action. However, the classical electrical treatment devices are generally rigid circuit microelectronics which may sometimes encounter troubles such as poor coupling performance and large contact comfortableness etc. Under the huge contact resistance thus induced between circuits and skin, the nearby tissues may easily subject to hurt due to extremely high electrical voltage. On the other hand, such electrodes may cause discomfort and even hurt to human body due to their mechanically rigid fixing property. As an alternative, the recently emerging room temperature liquid metal is easy to manufacture electronics directly on skin with unique convenience which would efficiently help tackle tumor diseases.

12.8.3 Treatment Strategy of Liquid Metal Skin Electronics

According to Fig. 12.20, the current therapy for treating malignant melanoma tumor depends on the soft liquid metal electrodes and electrical fields delivered into

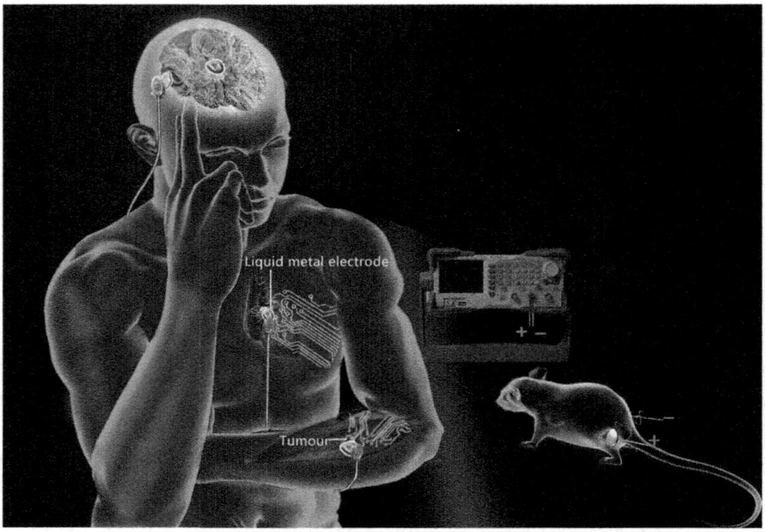

Fig. 12.20 Principle of using liquid metal electrodes to deliver electrical stimulation for tumor therapy [72]

the target site. To test the effectiveness in destroying tumor cells in vivo, an animal tumor model of C57BL/6 mice inoculated intradermally with malignant melanoma cells (B16F10) was adopted. Tumor treating fields (TTField) was administrated by means of 15-mm-long insulated wire needle (outer diameter, 0.3 mm; insulation thickness, 0.1 mm; Tefzel) inserted intradermally on one side of the tumor, then liquid metals were sprayed on the surface of the tumor, leaving only 4 cm^2 normal skin on the other side of the tumor. Another identical wire needle was inserted intradermally into the 4 cm^2 normal skin left on the other side of the tumor. TTFields were generated between liquid metals plus inserted (intradermal) wholly insulated wire needle placed on one side of the tumor and inserted (intradermal) wholly insulated wire needle placed on the other side of the tumor. Mice with inserted electrodes were treated 90 min per day for 6 days beginning 1 week after cell inoculation. The animal study has been approved by the Ethics Committee of Tsinghua University, Beijing, China under contract [SYXK (Jing) 2009-0022].

12.8.4 Animal Tests on Tumor Treatment

Eight healthy C57/BL mice were tested, whose subcutaneous skin were inoculated with melanoma B16 tumor cell lines [72]. After 14 days, the mice were divided into two groups: six mice in the experimental group, and two mice in the control group. The experimental group was divided into three experimental groups with different test conditions: (A) Electrical stimulation parameters of mice model (signal: sine wave, signal amplitude Vpp: 5 V, frequency: 300 kHz); (B) (signal: sine wave, signal amplitude Vpp: 5 V, frequency: 100 kHz) and (C) (signal: sine wave, signal amplitude Vpp: 4 V, frequency: 300 kHz) respectively. Each group has 2 mice. The mice in the control group were sprayed with liquid metal electrodes on the surface of the tumor, leaving only 4 cm^2 normal skin on the other side of the tumor without TTFields. The sine wave signal of TTFields through the electrode was administrated by means of 15-mm-long insulated wire needle. Mice were treated with TTFields 90 min per day for 6 days.

In the control group, the mice were also sprayed with liquid metals electrodes, with the same time length and interval of treatment without TTFields. Percutaneous measurements were made on tumor volume in eight mice, in the treatment of the beginning of the first 1 d, 2 d, 6 d, and 7 d. Tumor volume can be calculated via formula: $V = (a \times b^2)/2$, where a is the longest diameter of the tumor, and b is the longest perpendicular diameter length of a.

After 6 days of complete electrical stimulation treatment, in each group a mouse was sacrificed. The tumor tissues were removed and fixed with 10% formalin for histopathological examination. Magnetic resonance imaging (MRI) examination was performed 24 h after the TTFields treatment with sprayed liquid metals electrodes removed by ethanol.

12.8.5 Performance of the Method

The average volume of the three experimental groups and control group tumor are presented in the following Table 12.2.

Through in vivo treatment of tumors in C57BL/6 (B16F10 syngeneic tumor model), significant slowing of tumor growth and extensive destruction of tumor cells were obtained within 6 days. We found that 300 kHz of TTFields at low intensities of 5 V/cm effectively inhibited malignant melanoma growth compared with other electrical stimulation parameters [72]. Photographs of examples of treated mice models with 300 kHz of TTFields at low intensities of 5 V/cm and other electrical stimulation parameters are given in (Fig. 12.21a–c) for comparison. Clearly, the sizes of the treated tumors were significantly smaller than that of control tumors at the end of treatment. In addition, total process was found to be both safe and effective in slowing tumor progression. These findings demonstrate the potential applicability of the described spray-printing TTFields as a novel therapeutic modality for tackling malignant tumors.

Magnetic resonance imaging (MRI) data from a representative mouse that showed an almost complete response to the spray-printing TTFields treatment is shown in Fig. 12.22. It indicates that, a tumor was visible before TTFields treatment (Fig. 12.22a) while almost no tumor was detected 24 h after treatment (Fig. 12.22b). The tumor volume post-treatment was significantly smaller than that of the pre-treatment (23 mm^3 vs. 197 mm^3) (Fig. 12.22a, b).

Table 12.2 Comparison of tumor volume between experimental group and control group after TTfields was applied (mean value ± standard deviation) [72]

Group	Days after the electric field applies (day)			
(A)	305.92 ± 90.88	98.5 ± 37.12	–[a]	–[a]
(B)	1567.60 ± 595.60	10518.40 ± 8331.8	21445.31 ± 708.51	22,803.63 ± 894.53
(C)	5147.27 ± 2984.07	3515.92 ± 2100.8	–[a]	–[a]
(Control)	1714.78 ± 228.72	6530.90 ± 875.10	7916.85 ± 1145.65	11,512.3 ± 1541.3

[a]Tumor is too small to measure

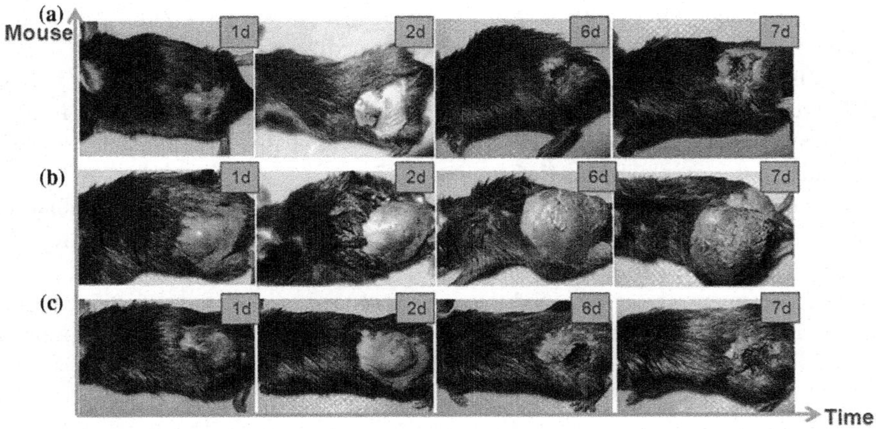

Fig. 12.21 Pictures of electrical stimulation treatment of malignant melanoma tumor on mice model based on liquid metal spray-printing [72]. **a** Electrical stimulation parameters of mice model (signal: sine wave, the voltage is 5 V, the electric field strength of about 2 V/cm, the frequency is 300 kHz). **b** Electrical stimulation parameters of mice model (signal: sine wave, voltage: 5 V, the electric field strength is about 2 V/cm, the frequency is 100 kHz). **c** Electrical stimulation parameters of mice model (signal: sine wave, voltage: 4 V, the electric field strength is about 1.6 V/cm, the frequency is 300 kHz)

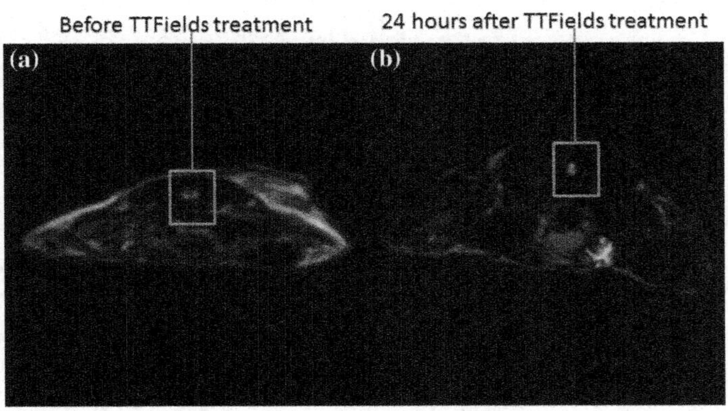

Fig. 12.22 Magnetic resonance imaging (MRI). Exemplary partial radiological response to therapy in a representative mouse [72]. **a** T1-weighted axial MRI images with pre-treatment (left panel). **b** 24 h after treatment (right panel)

Observed by naked eyes, after electrical stimulation therapy, in the experimental group mice (A) and (C), partial tumor becomes necrosis 2–3 days after applied TTFields treatment. And the tumors display central depression, with uneven surface. Then a week later, new tissue was seen around the necrotic tissue. In the (A) group, tumor group of mice after treatment gradually reduced within a week, and finally disappeared. In the (C) group, tumor group was diminishing after one week of treatment, but more slowly. In the (B) group and the control group, the tumor of the mice continues to grow after treatment.

As the MRI image indicates (Fig. 12.22a–b), a tumor was visible before TTFields treatment (Fig. 12.22a) while almost no tumor was detected 24 h after treatment (Fig. 12.22b). The tumor volume post-treatment was significantly smaller than that of the pre-treatment (197 mm^3 vs. 23 mm^3).

In the (A) group, as shown in Fig. 12.23a, c, 24 h pathological examination demonstrated that a carbide changed the tumor tissue on the surface of the skin, and the cancer nests on the integrity of the structure was completely destroyed.

After treatment, the tumors and their adjacent tissues were fixated, stained with H&E, and analyzed histopathologically. Histopathological evaluation of treated

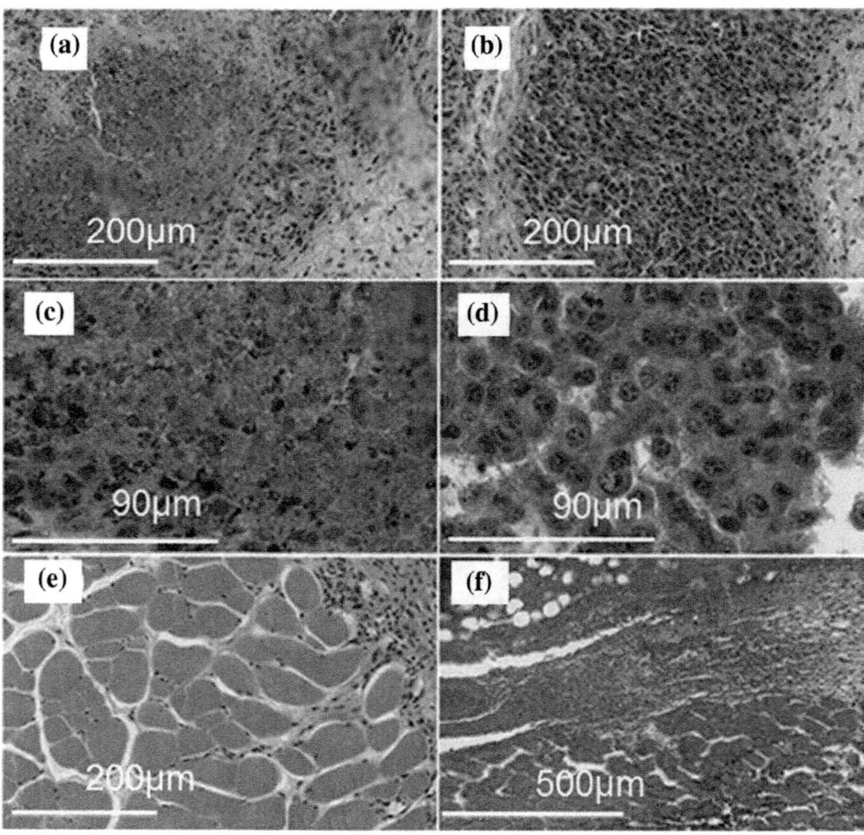

Fig. 12.23 The pathological pictures as the mouse was subjected to electrical treatment 3 times after 72 h [72]. **a** The picture for the case of most of the tumor cells was died. **b** The picture for the case of most of the tumor cells were apoptosis after electrical treatment based on liquid metal spray-printed electrodes. **c** The picture for the case of normal muscle tissues beside the tumor. **d** The enlarged picture where the tumor cells were apoptosis. **e** The enlarged picture of the tumor cells being died. **f** The section picture of tissue without tumor cells

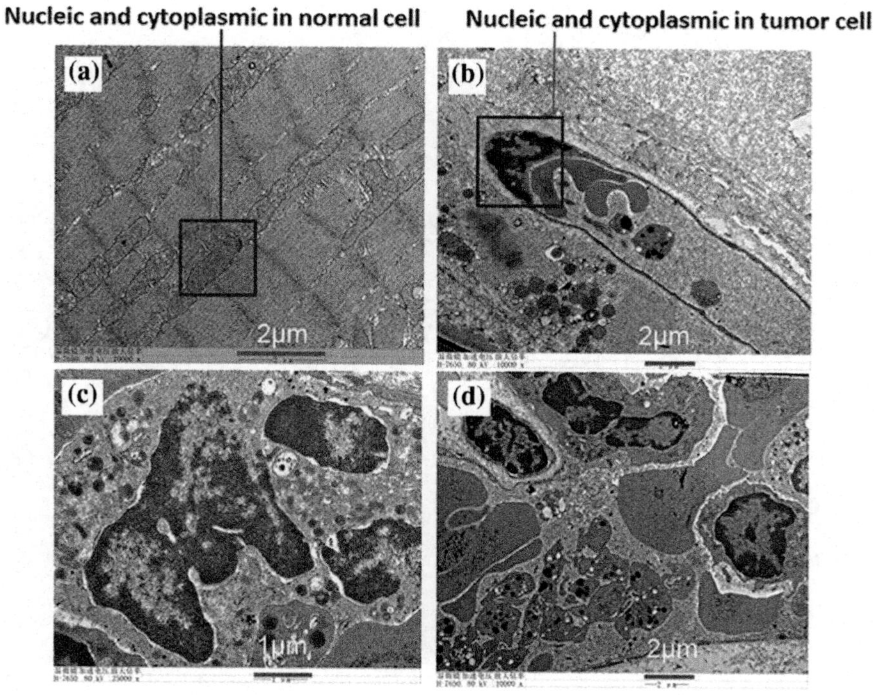

Fig. 12.24 The SEM pictures as the mouse was electrically treated 7 times after 168 h [72]. **a** The picture of normal muscle tissues beside the tumor. **b** The picture where the tumor cell was died. **c** The picture where the nucleus of the tumor cell undergone fragmentation. **d** The picture where the fragmentation of the nucleus is outside of cell

tumors showed extensive necrotic tissues and cellular debris. No damage to the surrounding tissues was detected (Fig. 12.23a–f). As the SEM figure indicates (Fig. 12.24a–d), there were no damage to the nucleus in normal cells, but the nucleic and cytoplasmic contents were losing in tumor cells. It can be explained that this treatment has produced good output regarding targeted therapy.

To confirm the mouse mode of tumor cell death induced by spray-printing TTFields treatment, we performed further transmission electron microscopic tests. Necrotic cell death manifested by rupture of the plasma membrane and loss of nuclear and cytoplasmic contents was readily detected using transmission electron microscopy in post-treatment tumor. In contrast, tissues beside the tumor (muscle) resembled those untreated normal control, displaying intact plasma membrane and preserved nuclear architecture (Fig. 12.24a–d). Thus, spray-printing TTFields treatment induces necrosis in melanoma cells only.

To exclude the temperature effect in the experiments, infrared camera (FLIR, US) was used to monitor the temperature change on the skin surface above the treated tumors in vivo, which showed no significant elevation in temperature during

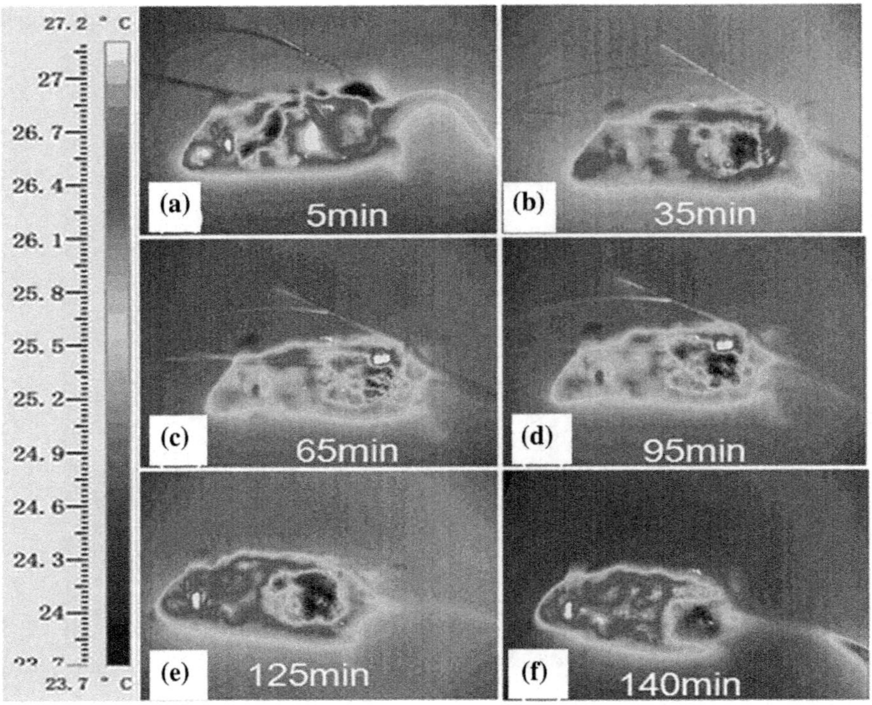

Fig. 12.25 Thermal infrared images as the mouse was electrically treated from 5 to 140 min under anesthesia [72]. **a** It is the 5th min before the spray-printing of liquid metal on the back of mouse with the 5 V voltage, 300 kHz sine wave electrical signal. **b–d** It is the 35th min, 65th min, 95th min after the spray-printing of liquid metal on the back of mouse with the 5 V voltage, 300 kHz sine wave electrical signal respectively. **e–f** It is the 125th min, 140th min, after the end of electrical treatment, and liquid metals were removed by medical alcohol

the period of treatment compared with pre and post-treatment (Fig. 12.25a–f). The results validate the existence of a non-thermal effect during spray-printing TTFields treatment.

12.8.6 Development Prospect

Traditionally, oncology therapy includes chemotherapy, surgery, and radiation, or a combination thereof. More recently, molecularly targeted therapy and vaccines have held great promise for prolonging survival and, in some cases, preventing cancer. Physical modalities, other than ionizing radiation and heating, have been systematically studied as cancer treatment in just the past decade. Electric fields, while being utilized in various fields of medicine, had fallen into this category until very recently. In the past decade, antimitotic, frequency-tuned electric field therapy (low-intensity, intermediate-frequency alternating fields), also referred to as TTFields, has been studied, and represents a promising regional oncology therapy.

TTFields is a noninvasive, regional antimitotic treatment modality that delivers low-intensity (1–3 V/cm), intermediate-frequency (100–300 kHz), and alternating electric fields to the tumor using transducer arrays placed on the skin around the region of the body containing the tumor. TTFields has been approved for the treatment of recurrent glioblastoma by the U.S. FDA and has a CE mark in Europe [73]. TTFields therapy affects metaphase, by disrupting mitotic spindle formation, and anaphase, by dielectrophoretic dislocation of intracellular constituents, resulting in apoptosis. TTFields therapy relies on frequency tuned to specific cancer cell types. The antimitotic effect of TTFields therapy has been demonstrated in multiple cell lines when the appropriate frequency was utilized. Compared with active chemotherapy, TTFields therapy is associated with minimal toxicity, better quality of life, and comparable efficacy in recurrent glioblastoma patients. Preclinical data demonstrated that the antimitotic effect of TTFields is intensity and frequency dependent and has additive or synergistic activity with chemotherapy [74–76]. In addition, TTFields therapy has been shown to inhibit systemic metastases in animal models [77]. Clinical data demonstrate comparable efficacy in recurrent glioblastoma with a more favorable safety profile and better quality of life than chemotherapy (with U.S. Food and Drug Administration (FDA) approval in 2011).

In Guo et al.'s work [72], it was shown that spray-printing TTFields could evidently inhibit the growth of tumors in mice while causing no general side effects or local histopathological damage. This demonstrated the strategy's inhibitory effect in all proliferating cell types as tested, whereas, nonproliferating cells and tissues were unaffected. Temperature measurements on the skin above treated tumors in vivo, showed no significant elevation in temperature. This indicates that this effect is nonthermal.

The method of directly printing electronics pattern TTFields therapy owns the potential to completely change the treatment paradigm for solid tumor oncology, as a regional therapy that can encompass entire body regions, such as brain, lungs, or liver, which are the most common sites of solid tumor metastasis and the most common cause of mortality once involved. Meanwhile, the directly printed electronics pattern TTFields cancer treatment modality avoids the conventional cytotoxic systemic side effects and may enable chronic and continuous cancer therapy. Previous attempts to increase cell killing with chemotherapy through increasing dose density had limited success due to the cumulative toxicities of high-dose chemotherapy, and radiation doses are limited due to potential damage to surrounding normal tissues.

Combination of the directly printing electronics pattern TTFields therapy with chemotherapy (surgery, radiation) may benefit from several ways: (1) Enhanced cell killing by chemotherapy due to a potential synergistic effect; (2) Continuous cytoreductive effect by TTFields therapy in between chemotherapy infusions to minimize tumor regrowth, DNA repair, and emergence of drug resistance; (3) Continuous cytoreductive effect by TTFields therapy in between lines of chemotherapy; (4) Absence of overlapping toxicity; and (5) Inhibiting the metastasis. Together, these may add up to an exponential increase in cell killing, possibly sufficient to result in long-term tumor regression and control.

Compared with the conventional TTFields therapy, the liquid metal electrode increased the contact area with the skin, enhanced therapeutic effects and reduced conventional TTFields adverse effects. The advantages of this liquid metal electrode TTFields therapy is expected to increase acceptability and is easy for patient use in the near future. Optimization of the field-generating device in terms of size, weight, and longer battery life may enable long-term carrying and continuous cancer therapy throughout the day.

12.9 Electrically Induced Reorganization of Liquid Metal Printed on Biological Skin

Although liquid metal has been proven to be directly printed on biological skin as biomedical elements, many fundamental issues remained unclear which may impede further application of the liquid metal skin electronics. Guo et al. had ever disclosed an intriguing phenomenon of electrically induced reorganization of liquid metal [78]. It was found that, when applying an external electric field to liquid metals which were spray printed on biological skin, it induced unexpected transformations of the liquid metals among different morphologies and configurations. These include change from a large liquid metal film into a tiny sphere and contraction of liquid metal pool into spherical shape. The impacts of the size, voltage, orientation were clarified. Furthermore, effects of different substrates like in vitro skin and in vivo skin affecting the liquid metal transformations were investigated. Compared to the intact tissues, the contraction magnitude of liquid metal electrode appears weaker on in vivo skin of nude mice under the same electric field.

In the following, several unusual transformations of the liquid metals between different morphologies and configurations were presented. The experiments were conducted using droplets of $GaIn_{24.5}$ under different arrangements of the electrodes. Fresh pig skin is adopted as one of the substrate materials in the experiments. Another substrate material is skin from eight-week-old male nude mice CD-1 NU. As compared to the in vitro pig skin, one of the experimental mice was sacrificed. The lumbar area of the nude mice skin was cut as specimens. Power supply and camera are also used in the experiments to supply electrical power and record the test videos. The liquid metal was atomized to deposit on the substrate and formed into liquid film [9].

As shown in Fig. 12.26, experiments were carried out under different arrangements of the liquid metal electrodes. Figure 12.26a shows that power supply is to supply electrical power, and Fig. 12.26b shows the camera utilized to record video of experimental results. As is found in Fig. 12.26c, when a non-uniform electric field was applied on $GaIn_{24.5}$ liquid metal electrode, the electrode will contract to center probe. As shown in Fig. 12.26d, the contacting electrode rapidly transform

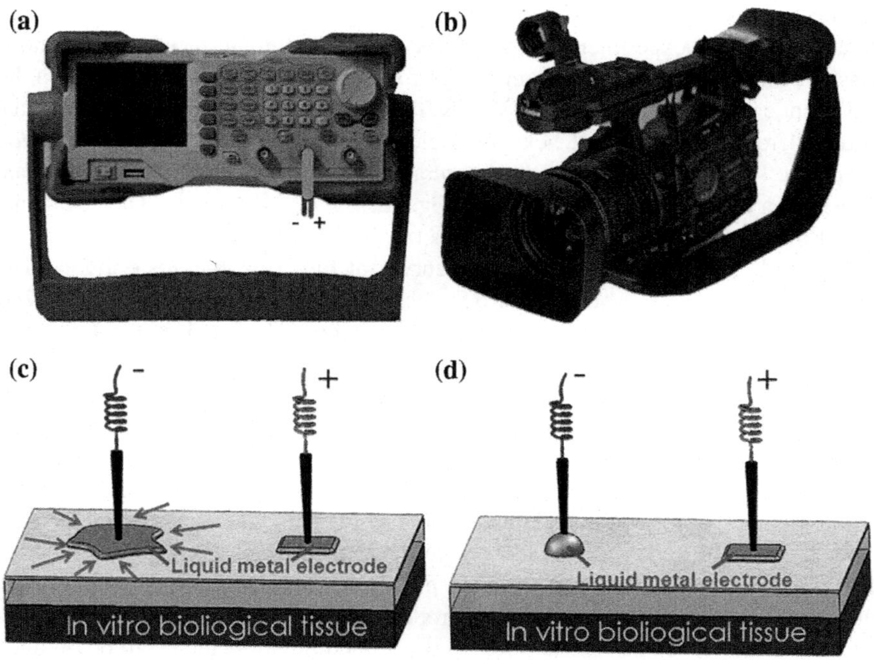

Fig. 12.26 Diagram for the experimental set up. **a** Power supply. **b** Video camera. **c** Schematic of liquid metal transformation on skin with electric leads. **d** Schematic of liquid metal contraction to a sphere on skin with electric leads

into sphere. The observed liquid metals on skin transformations mainly varied in accordance with the shape of the two electrodes, the relative position of the two electrodes and the intensity of the applied electrical field, and different kinds of skins: in vitro pig skin, in vitro nude mice skin, living nude mice skin, and dead nude mice skin etc.

As shown in Fig. 12.27a, sixteen liquid metal flattened electrodes on pig skin was investigated. There were four kinds of shape of liquid flattened electrodes: triangular, round, square, and hexagonal. Every four electrodes are fabricated with each the same shape. Two of them are used to carry out the experiments with electrical field; the other two are used as comparison. As indicated in Fig. 12.27b, the copper-wire anode was attached to the triangular liquid flattened electrode, and the cathode was attached to the other. When the electricity was switched on, it was found that the liquid metal near the cathodic quickly transformed from its original flattened shape into spherical one. Here direct current was supplied by a 5 V voltage. To obtain a visual observation of the electro-induced contraction of liquid drop, after the electricity was applied, the triangle liquid metal electrode transformed from triangular shape into a contraction status at 0, 1, 2, 3, and 4 s, respectively. Surface molecules are under the strain of the liquid surface tension from internal of liquid metal, which results in spontaneous contraction into the smallest surface area trend. The molecular force inside the liquid metal drop is very weak. During the experiments, it was observed that the liquid metal drop at anode was not changed. And the two control electrodes which are used as comparison did not change also. As shown in Fig. 12.27b, the experiments are carried out using the flattened round, square, and hexagonal electrodes. The contraction phenomenon keeps the same as before. But their contraction time are 10, 12, 16 s, which are longer than the triangle one as shown in Fig. 12.27c, d, respectively. The hexagonal liquid metal electrode contraction process displays the longest time.

Figure 12.27g–j are the area change curves of Fig. 12.27b–e respectively. The speed of contraction of square electrode decreases in whole process (Fig. 12.27g). And the speed of contraction of triangular electrode decreased in the first three seconds but increased in the last second; the round electrode increased in the first six seconds but decreased in the 6–9 s, then increased in the 9–12 s again. The square electrode decreased in all the 10 s. The speed contraction of the hexagonal electrodes alternatively grew or reduced (Fig. 12.28).

In order to clarify the difference regarding the contraction phenomena between liquid metal on in vivo skin and that on in vitro pig skin when subject to electrical field, the skin of nude mice is adopted in the experiments. The liquid metal was atomized by airbrush and deposited on nude mice skin with prepared mask. As shown in Fig. 12.29, liquid metal electrodes are spray printed on nude mouse's lumbar area. 5 V voltage was applied on the printed liquid metal electrode on nude skin and lasted for 30 s as shown in Fig. 12.29a. It is surprised to find that the contraction phenomenon of liquid metal was not obvious. But when 10 V voltage was applied, phenomenon of liquid metal contraction happened as shown in Fig. 12.29b–l. However, the liquid metal was moving much slower than that on in vitro pig skin.

As shown in Fig. 12.30a, experiments are carried out to research the relationship of relative position of liquid metal electrodes on pig skin and the contraction time. Figure 12.30b shows that after applying the electric field, the liquid metal transformations occurred. It was found that the contraction time was roughly an inverse proportion function with relative position of liquid metal electrodes (Fig. 12.30c). Figure 12.30d shows that the higher the voltage applied on the two electrodes, the faster the liquid metal cathode contracted to a sphere.

Skin conductivity is mainly contributed by various ions. The volume of ion is usually much larger than that of electron. However, the conductive process is generally blocked by the biological membranes. The barrier layer and the base layer prevent ions from transferring across the membrane. So ions with different polarities will attract each other and result in ions accumulation. These anions make the $GaIn_{24.5}$ liquid metal surface negatively charged and result in an accumulation of positively charged ions in a diffuse layer of electric double layer (EDL) behind cathode electrode. So the skin with charge storage capacity plays the role of capacitance. The film will also make some ion "leakage" in the passage, like a poor quality of the electrolytic capacitor, film capacitor and resistor conductive available parallel to the equivalent as shown in Fig. 12.31. The EDL can be modeled as a charged capacitor. Due to the high conductivity of the liquid metal, the potential

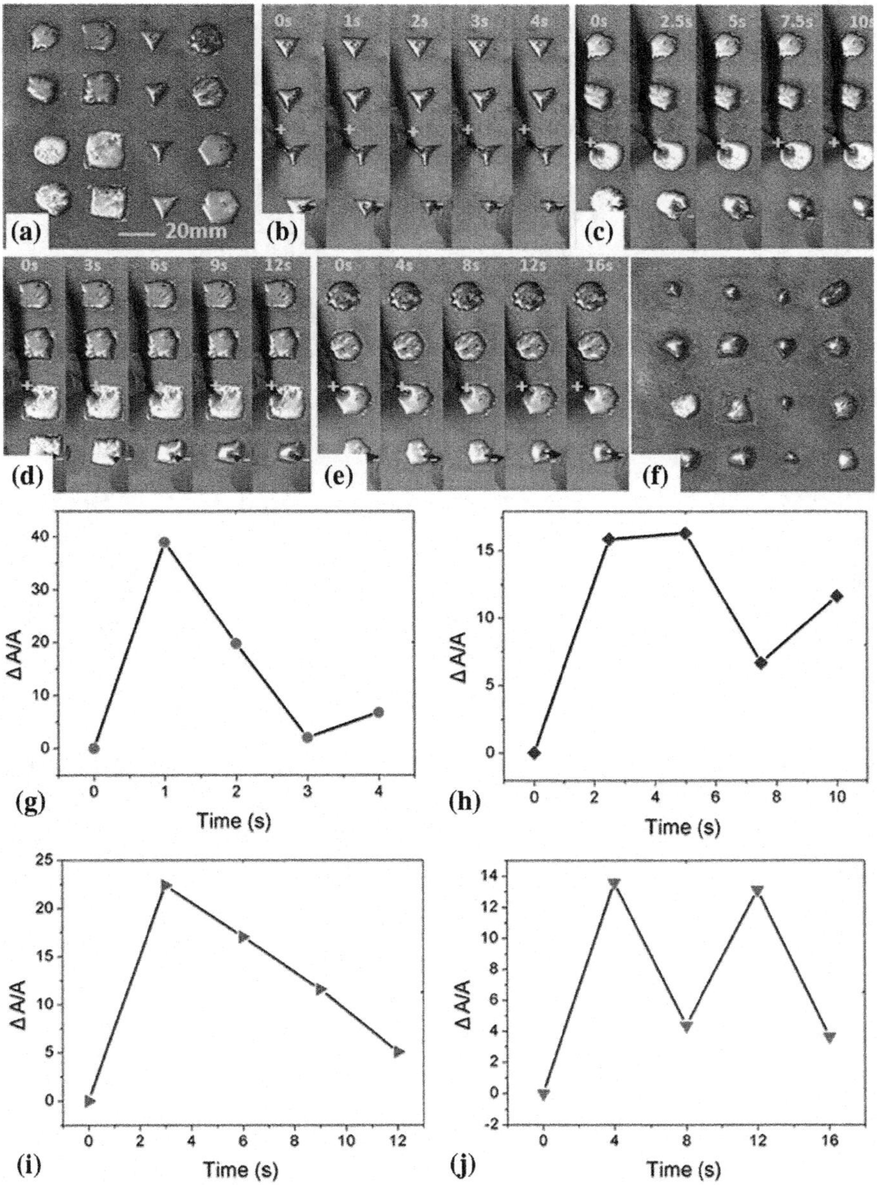

Fig. 12.27 Experimental results of liquid metal moving on pig skin surface [78]. **a** Sixteen liquid metal flattened electrodes with four kinds of shape: triangular, round, square, and hexagonal. **b–e** The process as electrodes were contracting on pig skin with triangular, round, square, hexagonal shape respectively. **f** The picture of last situation of contracted liquid metal flattened electrode on pig skin. **g–h** The relative change of the cross sectional area along with the time of **b–e** respectively. The symbols ΔA and A respectively refer to the change of the cross sectional area and the original cross sectional area of round, square, hexagonal electrodes are upon 0.4 mL liquid GaIn24.5 respectively, and triangle electrode is 0.2 mL

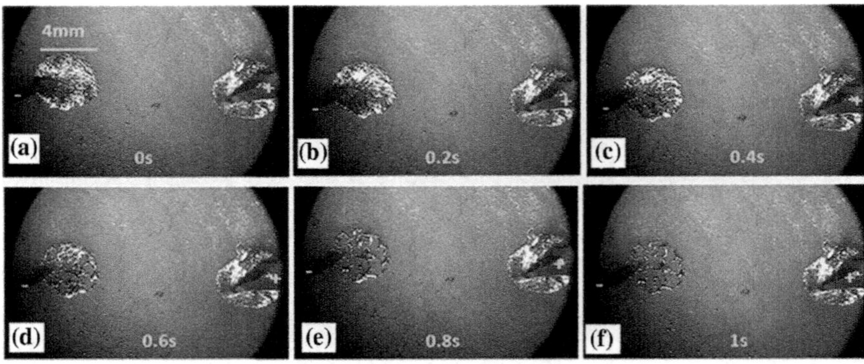

Fig. 12.28 **a–f** are pictures of contracting liquid metal film electrode on pig skin at 0, 0.2, 0.4, 0.6, 0.8, 1 s, respectively [78]

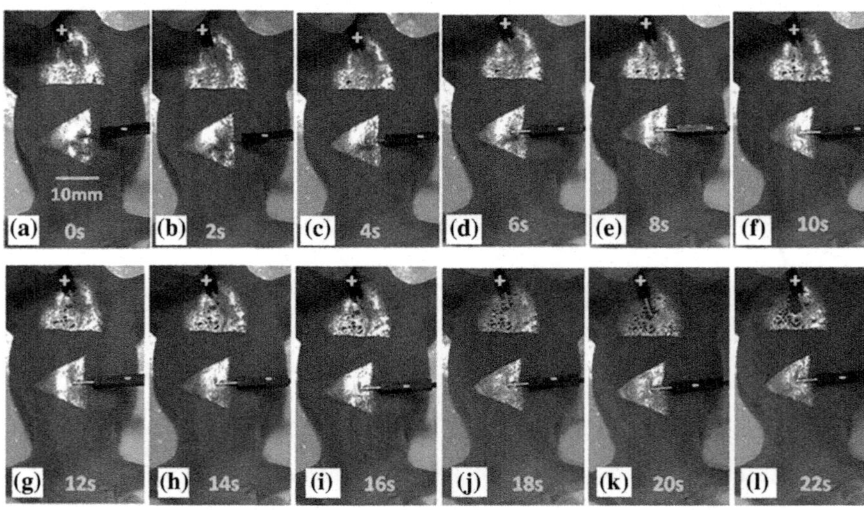

Fig. 12.29 **a–l** Experimental pictures of electrically induced liquid metal contraction on nude mice skin with 10 V voltage applied on spray printed liquid metal electrode from 0 to 22 s [78]

must be approximately uniform throughout the liquid metal electrode. Conversely, the skin has a finite conductivity. When the electrical field was applied on liquid metal electrode on skin, electro-chemical reduction reaction can occur in gallium (the more dominant metal) of the cathode electrode, whose oxidation occurs on the anodic electrode. This induces liquid metal electrode surface negative charge accumulated. The surface tension of liquid metal and skin are very different from each other. This process indicates significant variations of the interfacial tension on the liquid metal. In theory, surface tension of liquid is related to its density. The internal molecular distance is small in liquid when the density is large. Then

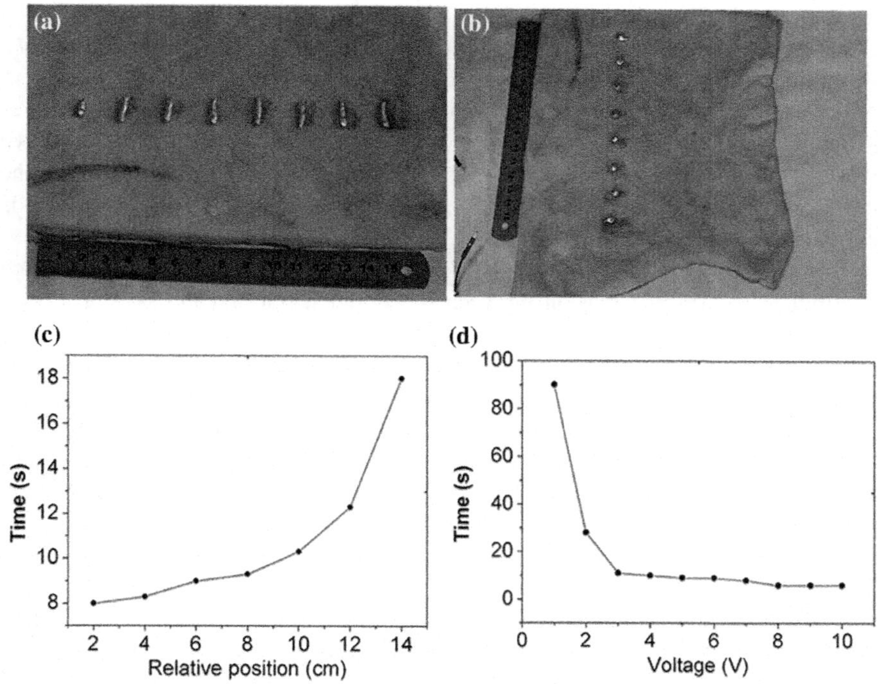

Fig. 12.30 **a** Experiments regarding the relationship of relative position of liquid metal electrode on pig skin and the contraction time. **b** Test results of (**a**). **c** Curve of relative position of the liquid metal electrode with the contraction time. **d** Curve of the voltage applied on the liquid metal electrode with the contraction time [78]

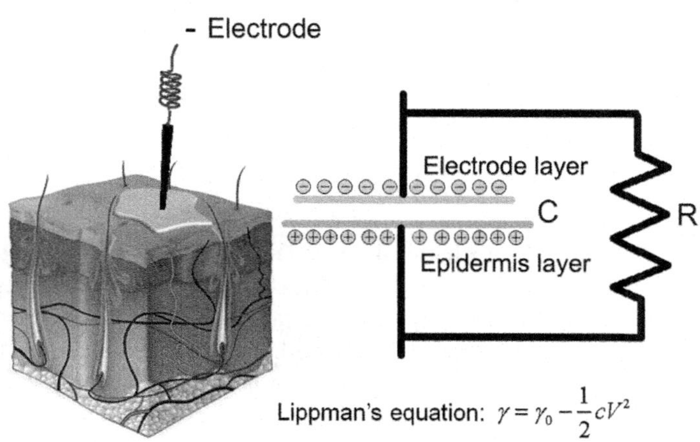

Fig. 12.31 Schematic of liquid metal electrode contraction on skin

attractive forces between molecules in liquid metal are greater than in skin. As a result, the surface tension of the liquid metal is much larger than skin. For example, the surface tension of a liquid metal such as gallium alloy is over ten times that of water. The density of skin is similar to water, the surface tension of liquid metal is also much larger than skin. As shown in Fig. 12.31, equivalent circuit is shown adjacent to the liquid metal electrode–skin interface. The resistance R is now the effective resistance associated with interface effects of the gel between the electrode and the skin.

The capacitance C and potential difference V are the major parameters which determinate the surface tension between the liquid metal and the skin. The skin consists of three principal layers that surround the body and they also serve as appropriate interfaces. The outer most layer or epidermis, affects most to the resistance in the electrode-skin interface. The nude mouse skin surface attracts positively charged ions, forming an ionic double layer. The fluid flow drives the ions in the double layer along the surface till a counterbalancing electronics. Biological skin can be equivalent to electrochemical electrolyte. The equivalent circuit is shown in Fig. 12.31. According to Lippman's equation, the surface tension is determined by capacitance C and potential difference voltage. In vivo nude skin must have different capacitance from in vitro pig skin. To confirm this conjecture, electrochemical impendence spectra (EIS) of four kinds of skin with liquid metal spray printed liquid metal electrodes are measured. The electrochemical impendence spectra were performed on CHI 660D potentiostat-galvanostat (CHI instruments Inc.) in the frequency range of 0.01–90,000 Hz. The four kinds of skin are in vitro pig skin, living nude mouse skin, dead nude mouse skin, and in vitro mouse skin, respectively. As shown in Fig. 12.29, the impedance is composed by resistor and capacitor in parallel form. And the impedance can be described by the function as follows:

$$\frac{1}{Z} = \frac{1}{Z_R} - \frac{1}{Z_C} = \frac{1}{R} + jwC \tag{12.18}$$

$$Z = \frac{1}{\frac{1}{R} + jwC} = \frac{\frac{1}{R} - jwC}{\frac{1}{R^2} + (wC)^2} \tag{12.19}$$

Figure 12.32a, b are electrochemical impendence spectra of in vitro pig skin and in vitro mouse skin respectively. The electrochemical impendence spectrum of in vitro pig skin displays more capacitance characteristics, and nude mouse performs more resistance characteristics. This explains that when higher voltage was applied, phenomenon of liquid metal contraction happened on living nude mouse. Overall, such findings have both fundamental and practical values, which remind further technical strategies in developing future electronically controlled liquid metal electronics on skin.

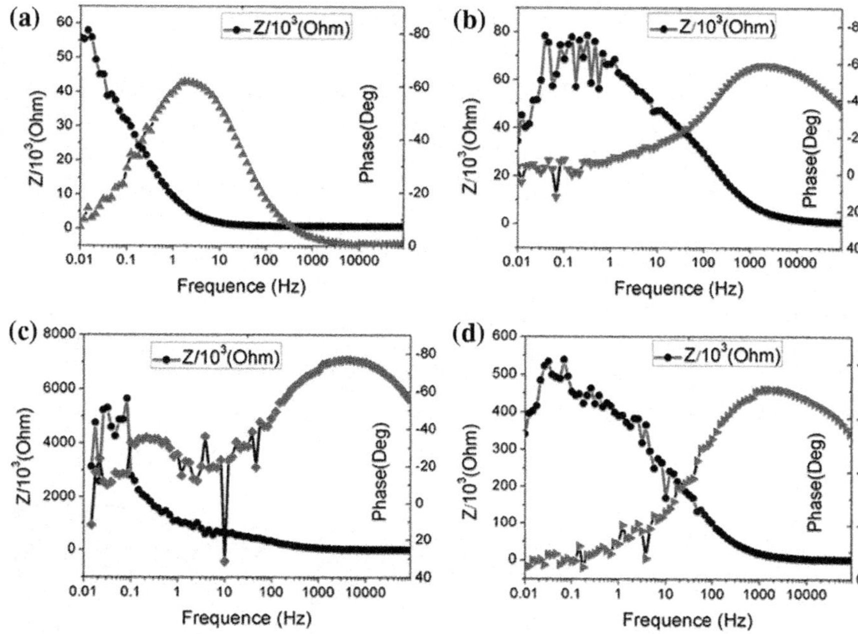

Fig. 12.32 EIS spectra recorded for the different kinds of skin using electrodes which are fabricated by liquid metal [78]. **a** EIS spectra recorded on in vitro pig skin. **b** EIS spectra recorded on in vitro nude mouse skin. **c** EIS spectra recorded on living nude mouse skin. **d** EIS spectra recorded on dead nude mouse skin

12.10 Stretchable Wearable Liquid Metal Electronic Skin

Conventional rigid electronics are usually unconformable with soft skins and tend to fail in accurate physiological monitoring and precise treatment. Electronic skins (e-Skins) made by conductive and stretchable materials offer mechanical compliance for fabricating flexible and conformable wearables. Compared to common organic or inorganic conductive materials, gallium-based liquid metals alone own superior conductivity and compliance. Guo et al. demonstrated a highly conductive and stretchable electronic skin with liquid metal circuits (LMCs) embedded in silicone rubber film, which are functionalized for physiological signals monitoring [79]. It was found that, LMCs maintained good electrical conductivity and functionality under over 100% strain. Also, a wearable electrocardiogram (ECG) recording device was fabricated and tested. The device was able to acquire steady state signals during real-time measurement of physical activities. The proposed liquid metal e-Skin can be further extended to conformable bio-integrated healthcare devices and intelligent health monitoring networks.

12.10.1 Fabrication of Stretchable Liquid Metal Circuits

In Guo et al.'s work [79], RTLM is made of gallium–indium alloy (EGaIn) with a relative weight ratio of 75.5:24.5. The platinum-catalyzed two-part silicone rubber Ecoflex 00-30 (Smooth-On, PA, USA, mixed at 1:(1) was used to fabricate elastomer substrates and encapsulate LM, because of its stretchability and easy preparation. The RTV silicone adhesive/sealant was chosen as the fixed glue to fix the connectors between the rigid components and LM wires.

Figure 12.33 showed the schematic diagrams about the preparation process of LMCs. First, a layer of Ecoflex membrane (500 μm in thickness) was even spun on the smooth silicon wafer, and cured at room temperature for 15 min. Then, a stainless steel mask, which was fabricated by the metal chemical etching, was tightly positioned closely to the Ecoflex substrate. EGaIn was atomized to fall onto

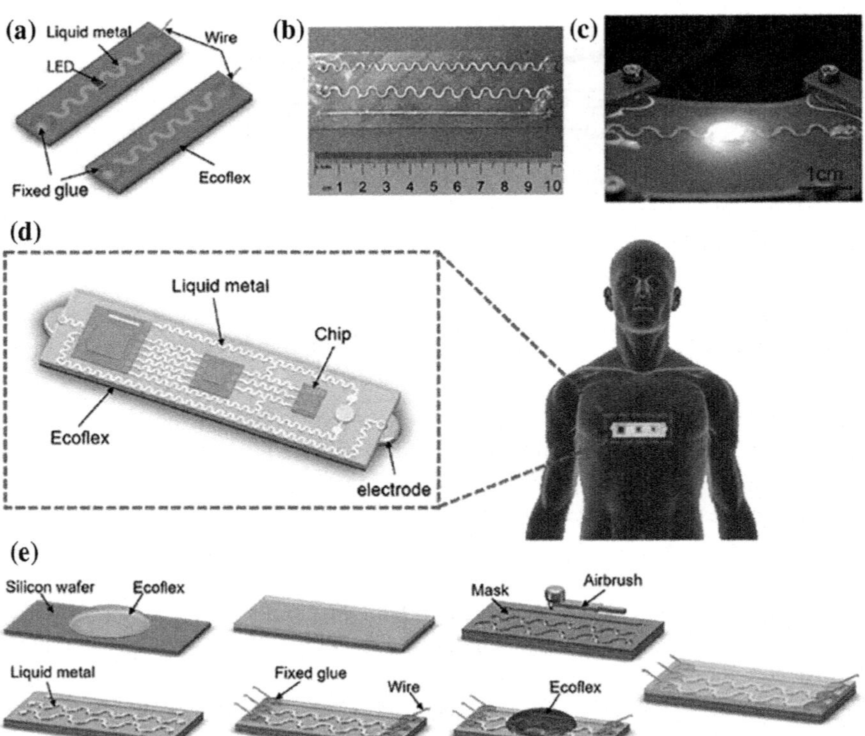

Fig. 12.33 **a** The structures of the LMCs (without and with LED) [79]. **b** Three kinds of LMCs (Linear, r = 1.5 mm and r = 2 mm). **c** The photograph of the conductor with rigid active component (a LED). **d** The functional LM e-Skin for ECG measurement. **e** The LMCs preparation process

the Ecoflex substrate to obtain certain shape after removing the stainless steel mask. One end of the iron wires (0.1 mm in diameter) were welded in the connectors of rigid components, and the other end were inserted in LM. Later, e RTV silicone adhesive/sealant was painted on the connectors between EGaIn wires and rigid components to fix the iron wires. Finally, other layer of Ecoflex membrane (500 μm in thickness) was spun on LM layer.

To demonstrate the application of LM as interconnects, ECG monitoring device was designed with LMCs connected rigid sensors and chips. The device included four parts: electrodes, ECG sensor, A/D conversion chip and Bluetooth chip. Here, two silver chloride electrodes were selected as measurement electrodes, which connected the ECG sensor by two LMCs (r = 1.5 mm). ECG sensor (IN AMP chip AD620) could magnify physiological signal 500 times, and transferred the expanded ECG signal to A/D conversion chip. MSP430 microcontroller, a kind of low cost A/D conversion chip, was chose to record the expanded ECG signal, and linked the Bluetooth chip by some LMCs (r = 1.5 mm). The Bluetooth chip transmits the ECG signal to a computer, and display-related software rendered a near real-time graphical representation on screen. In addition, the ECG device was powered by a button battery with diameter 10 mm, and its output voltage was 3 V. The schematic diagrams of the functional LM e-Skin were shown in Fig. 12.33d.

LM was sprayed on elastomeric substrates and encapsulated in Ecoflex membranes, as shown in Fig. 12.33a. When fabricating the LMCs, a large number of EGaIn droplets sprayed from an airbrush, and gathered on the smooth surface of Ecoflex membranes (Fig. 12.33e). Figure 12.33b, c presented liquid metal wires and the connection with rigid active component (a LED). It was apparent from these photographs that LM droplets fused into LM layers, which adhered to the surface of elastomeric substrates and connected the LED. Figure 12.34a showed some scanning electron microscope (SEM) images about the surface of LMCs. The surface of LM layer was covered with a layer of oxide skin to preserve its shape. The schematic diagrams and optical images of LED pins in the ends of LMCs and the iron wires inserted in LM assessed the connection between LMCs and rigid components (Fig. 12.34b). The pins and iron wires were dipped into EGaIn, and fixed glue was used to improve the stability of the structure. In Fig. 12.34c, three groups of LM wires (linear (defined as Liner), curved with radius of 1.5 mm (defined as r = 1.5 mm) and curved with radius of 2 mm (defined as r = 2 mm) deformed under different tensile strain in the axial direction (0% strain, 50% strain and 100% strain). There were significant elongations of linear LMCs in the direction straining, and the width decreased when stretching length increased. However, LMCs of r = 1.5 mm and r = 2 mm had an obvious increase in line width. Because of the liquidity of LM, there was no breakage of the three kinds of LMCs in different strain conditions, while the shape shifting could result in resistance variation.

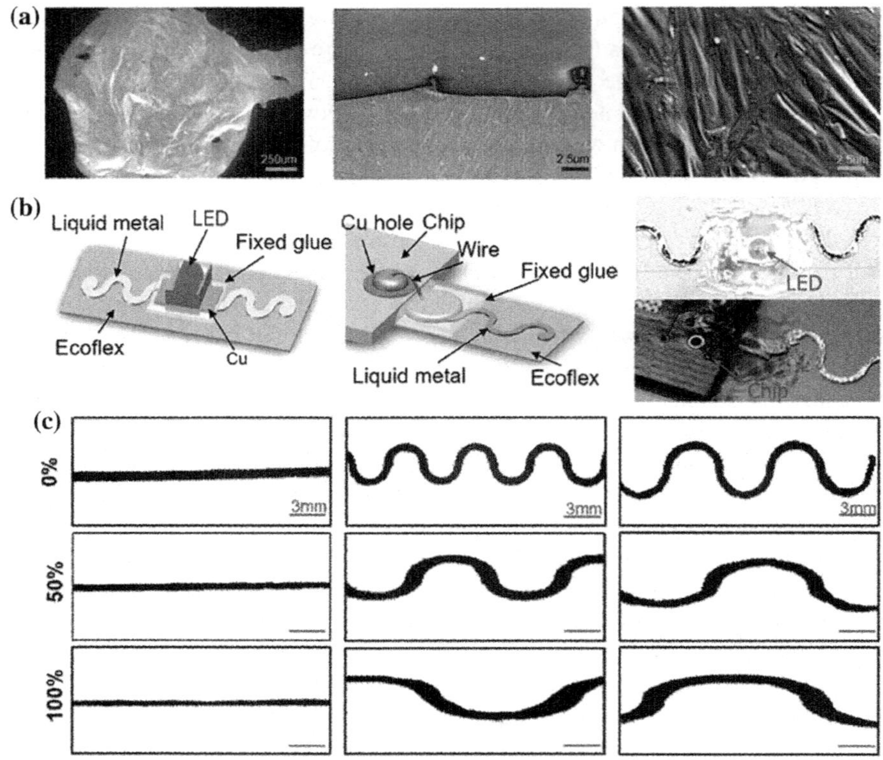

Fig. 12.34 The morphological characterization of LMCs [79]. **a** SEM images of LMC surface. **b** The schematic diagrams and optical images of LED pins in the ends of LMCs (the left image and the top of the right image) and the iron wires inserted in liquid metal (the main image and the lower of the right image). **c** The deformation of three groups of LMCs (left images: Linear, middle images: r = 1.5 mm, right images: r = 2 mm) under different tensile strain in the axial direction (0% strain, 50% strain and 100% strain)

12.10.2 Physical Properties of Stretchable Liquid Metal Circuits

In tensile test, four groups of LMCs (Ecoflex without liquid metal (defined as Ecoflex), linear, r = 1.5 mm and r = 2 mm) were stretched to the same length (175% strain), and the measurements of stress were carried out to get the stress-strain curve [79]. Figure 12.35a showed the stress-strain curves of the four groups of LMCs. In addition, we calculated the elastic modulus of the four kinds of LMCs (Ecoflex: 0.069 MPa, Linear: 0.041 MPa, r = 1.5 mm: 0.050 Mpa, r = 2 mm: 0.055 MPa). Compared to conventional rigid metal conductors, LMC elastic modulus was several orders lower.

When measuring its resistance, the original length of LMC was 10 cm, and the maximum tensile rate was 105%. The DC resistance of three groups of LMCs under

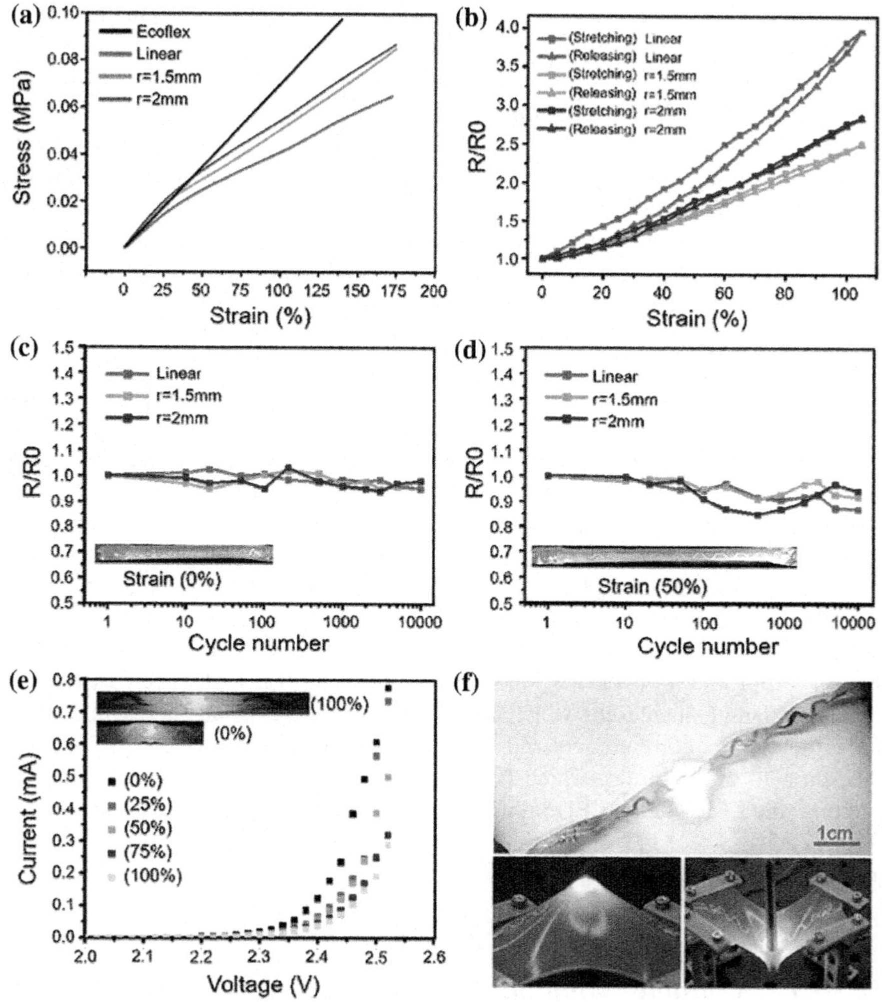

Fig. 12.35 The mechanical and electrical properties of LMCs [79]. **a** The stress-strain curves of four groups of LMCs. **b** The changing curves of electrical resistance of three kinds of LMCs under different tensile states. **c** The relation curve of drawing times with the LMCs resistance at 0% strain. **d** The relation curve of drawing times with the LMCs resistance at 50% strain. **e** I–V curves of LMCs with a rigid LED light under different strain conditions (from 0% strain to 100% strain). **f** LMCs with a rigid LED lights were twisted (the top picture) and compressed with a sharp object (the lower two pictures)

the applied strain in the force direction was measured to demonstrate the relationship between conductor elongation and electrical properties. Under original length condition, the resistance of Linear was 2.3 Ω, the resistance of r = 1.5 mm was 3.5 Ω, and the resistance of r = 2 mm was 3.9 Ω. The resistance difference was mainly caused by the length change of three shapes of LMCs. In fact, the lengths of r = 1.5 mm and r = 2 mm were the same, and longer than Linear, so the resistance of curviform was higher than linear.

The changing curves of three kinds resistance under different tensile states were shown in the Fig. 12.35b. The impedances increased gradually with the extent of stretching, while under the same tensile state, the resistance had almost no change in stretching and releasing process. Comparing the three kinds of LMCs, the resistance variation of r = 1.5 mm was lowest, thus this kind of LMCs were selected to connect rigid sensors and chips. There was a significant change of LMCs resistance in stretching process, and the maximum resistance ratio (defined as R/R0) was about 2.5. But the maximum resistance variation of LMCs (approximately 5 Ω) was slight compared with the resistance of functional components, such as the LED (above 3 kΩ).

In fatigue test, Guo et al. [79] stretched LMCs to 50% strain over 10,000 cycles, and plotted the relation curves about resistance variations and cycle numbers (Fig. 12.35c, d). The fatigue tests showed that LMCs resistances did not change significantly along with 10,000 cycles at the 0% strain and 50% strain. The test results suggested that flexible printed circuits based on LM had excellent electrical stability.

In order to assess the effects of resistance variation of LMCs on component function, a LED was connected. Figure 12.35e showed the I–V (Current–Voltage) curves of LMCs with LED under different strain conditions (0% strain to 100% strain). From the I–V curves, the current through the LED decreased when stretching length increased, which resulted in the increase of LMCs resistance. Nevertheless, the current decreased 0.4 mA at the working voltage of 2.5 V from 0% strain to 100% strain, which had slight effects to electronic components. In addition, the LMC with a LED light was warped and compressed by a sharp object (Fig. 12.35f). The LED could maintain normal brightness, even though LMCs occurred serious deformation.

12.10.3 Wearable Liquid Metal E-Skin with ECG Measurement Circuit

Figure 12.36a presented an overview of wearable LM e-Skin with ECG measurement circuit. The Ecoflex band was about 10 cm long and 4 cm wide, on which LMCs and some rigid functional components were packaged. LMCs curved with radius of 1.5 mm were selected to connect rigid functional components, which were fixed on the surface of the lower Ecoflex layer by fixed glue and covered with the upper Ecoflex layer. Owing to its fluidity and conductivity, LM was able to maintain the connection of the conductors, when the flexible circuit board was stretched to 33% strain and bent arbitrarily (Fig. 12.36b, c).

To measure physiological signals, two silver chloride electrodes were directly attached to the chest, with stuck on the lower surface of flexible circuit board via the

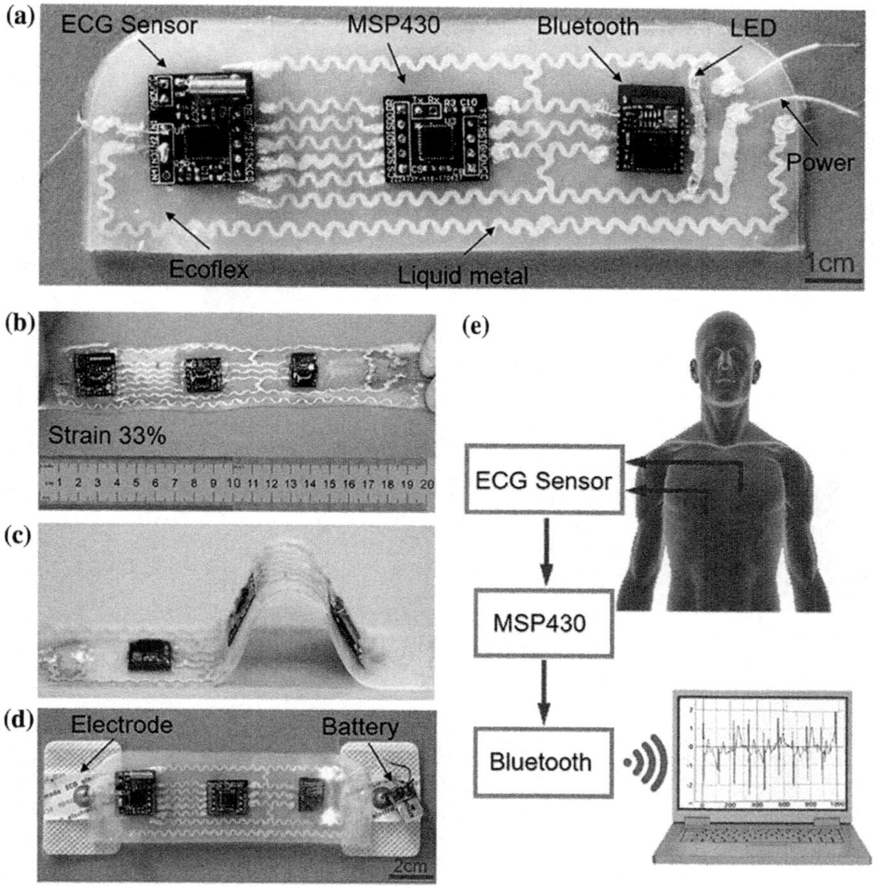

Fig. 12.36 The working process of wearable LM e-Skin with ECG measurement circuit [79]. **a** LM e-Skin ECG device. **b** The flexible circuit board was stretched to 33% strain. **c** The flexible circuit board was bent arbitrarily. **d** The connection between flexible circuit board and silver chloride electrodes. **e** Working process of LM e-Skin ECG device

fixed glue (Figs. 12.36d and 12.37a). The metal caps of silver chloride electrodes were stuck on both edges of the board, and weld with the iron wires (0.1 mm in diameter) together, which were inserted in LMCs encapsulated in elastomer substrates.

In Fig. 12.36e, the ECG signal, collected from human body by silver chloride electrodes, was enlarged about 500 times by ECG sensor (ADS620). Controlled by computer software, MSP430 read out the voltage signal from the sensor, and sent the data to Bluetooth via a two-wired digital communication protocol immediately. After receiving Bluetooth-transmitted data packages, the computer software interpreted the ECG value and the real-time curve was drawn on the screen.

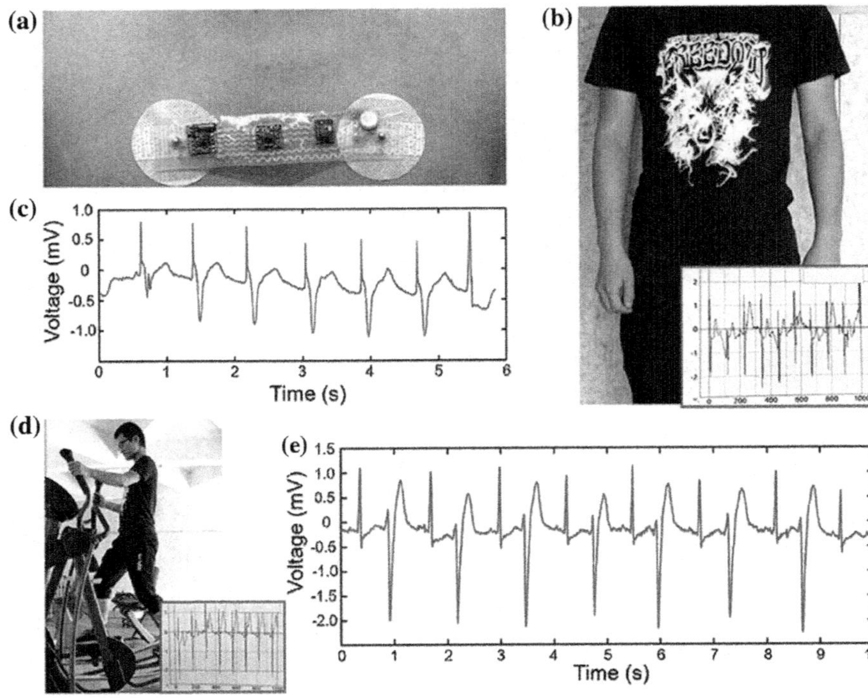

Fig. 12.37 **a** The photo of LM e-Skin ECG device attached on the upper chest of a human body. **b** The LM e-Skin collected the signal and showed it on the computer screen, when the body was in still. **c** The processed ECG data in still by MATLAB software. **d** The LM e-Skin collected the signal and showed it on the computer screen, when the body was in motion. **e** The processed ECG data in motion by MATLAB software [79]

When the body was in still, LM electronic skin collected the ECG signal and showed it on computer screen (Fig. 12.37b). Later, the recorded data was processed by MATLAB software, and Fig. 12.37c showed the correct time and signal amplitude. In order to demonstrate the functional stability of the LM e-Skin, ECG signals in body movement state were detected (Fig. 12.37d, e).

12.10.4 Future Outlook

LMCs presented high stretchability and conductivity compared with traditional rigid conductive materials. Meanwhile, silicone rubber Ecoflex 00-30 was easy to process and had excellent stretchability with the maximum elongation of 300%. Under the microscope, LM layer was encapsulated in soft film steadily under different tensile strain. A series of experiments were carried out to assess the mechanical and electrical properties of LMCs. According to these data, one can infer that LMCs did not significantly impact the elasticity of silicone rubber Ecoflex, and electrical connections were kept stable, even if they were stretched over 100%. Although LMCs resistance gradually increased in stretching process, the resistance variation was limited and did not impact the function of rigid components. Besides, fatigue test suggested that LMCs could be used long-termly with flexible circuit board attached to skin in the daily life.

Wearable LM e-Skin with ECG measurement circuit could monitor physiological signals in different states. Even in body movement, the output signals were still clear and effective. Due to high flexibility, LMCs could also assemble other kinds of functional circuits, such as temperature measurement circuit, sweat analysis circuit, pulse signals detecting device, gait analysis device and the Electroencephalography (EEG) measurement device, to integrate intelligent e-Skin monitoring network. Of course, there also existed certain limitations that should be noticed. For example, the width of LM wires was greater than the wires in conventional rigid circuit boards. The thickness of LM e-Skin device was several times larger than the wearable and stretchable electronics made by other inorganic and organic materials. In future research, one could design finer LMCs, which are thinner, smaller and more precise. Besides, the functionality of LM e-Skin is frail, and some other sensors will be added in flexible circuit board. With high strechability and conductivity, liquid metal circuits form wearable electronical skin. Attaching the functional flexible device onto soft skin, stable physiological signals are detected even in human activities.

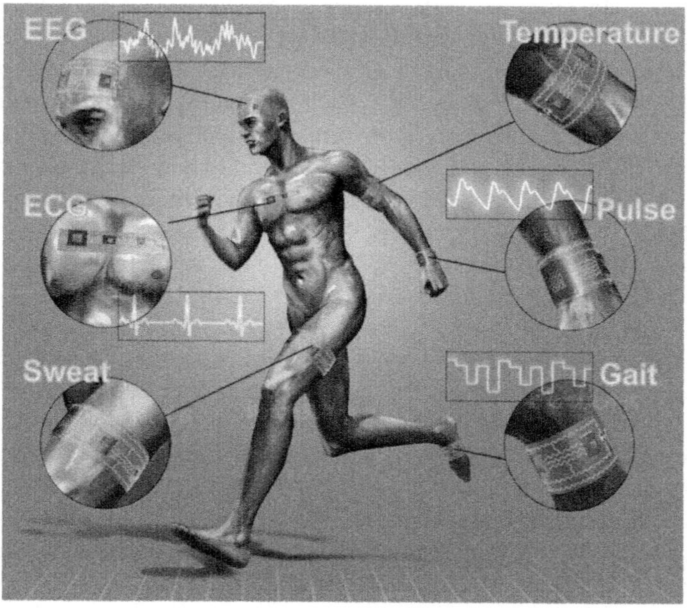

Fig. 12.38 The intelligent electronic skin network based on the liquid metal electronic skin [79]

Intelligent electronic skin network (Fig. 12.38) based on liquid metal flexible electronics is expected to come true in the future.

12.11 Ni-GaIn Amalgams Enabled Wearable and Wireless Healthcare Electronics

The commonly used liquid metal sometimes may not be easily printed on target substrate. Therefore, Guo et al. [80] developed a kind of directly-printed Ni-GaIn functional amalgams which can efficiently construct wearable healthcare monitors. Unlike EGaIn, Ni-GaIn amalgam owns a tunable and enhanced adhesion, which makes it easy to directly paint on various substrate for customized circuits.

In Guo et al.'s work, EGaIn was mixed with different Ni particles (φ = 0–30%) and the electro-conductivity and adhesion force of the amalgams was measured to determine the suitable doping ratio for fabrication of flexible electronics. Straining, bending or compressing the Ni-GaIn circuits tested the electrical properties of the flexible coils to demonstrate the advantages of printable Ni-GaIn amalgam for the fabrication of flexible electronics. Combining the wireless power transfer, a wearable LED array wireless power circuit and pulse wave monitor device were designed respectively, which could be attached to skin. The pulse wave monitor device was utilized to collect pulse wave signal from the wrist for providing body realtime health conditions. It was expected that the printable Ni-GaIn mixture had more functional applications in individualized wearable electronics.

Mixed in GaIn alloy (EGaIn), metal particles were covered with a layer of oxidized EGaIn (Fig. 12.39a), and the mixing process could accelerate the oxidation of EGaIn. The oxidized EGaIn had lower surface tension and could be painted on any soft substrate surface directly. With the increase of doping ratios, more EGaIn was oxidized and its surface performance was changed. However, because the oxidized EGaIn resulted in a decrease of fluidity and electro-conductivity of LM, the curve in Fig. 12.39c indicated that the conductivity of Ni-GaIn amalgam decreased gradually with φ increasing. Besides, its adhesion force increased when φ increased (Fig. 12.39d). In order to find the most appropriate φ with adequate electrical conductivity and adhesion force, Guo et al. [80] printed six Ni-GaIn wires (φ from 5 to 30%) on Ecoflex substrate (Fig. 12.39e). Finally, the wire with φ = 15% was demonstrated that it could be printed on Ecoflex substrate easily, and its conductivity was able to meet the requirements to be a conductor.

Figure 12.40c has presented the fine connection between Ni-GaIn LM and the components LED in the circuit. From the image, Cu wire was entirely covered with Ni-GaIn. More importantly, the fabrication of flexible circuit based on printable Ni-GaIn amalgam could be customizable. Various shapes of flexible Ni-GaIn circuits could be printed by designing various shapes of stainless steel masks, such as circle, square and triangle (Fig. 12.40d).

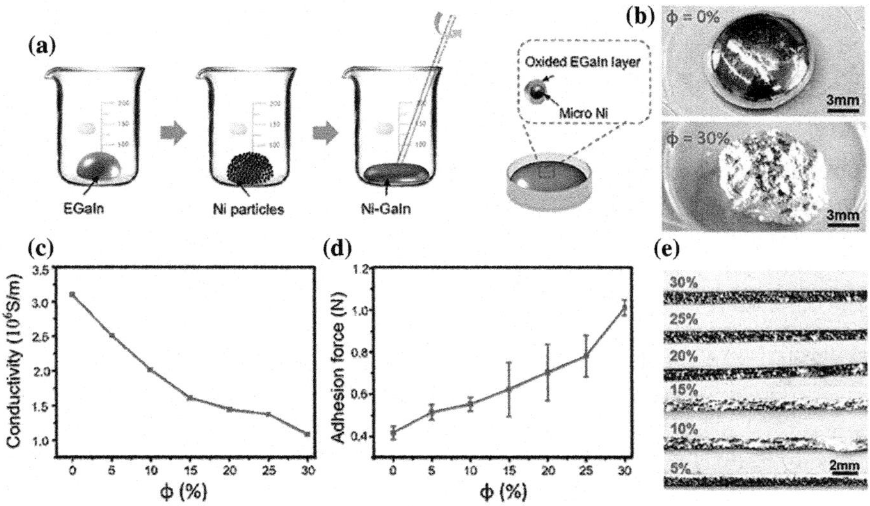

Fig. 12.39 The properties of Ni-GaIn amalgams [80]. **a** The preparation process of Ni-GaIn amalgam. **b** Upper picture: EGaIn ($\varphi = 0\%$), bottom picture: Ni-GaIn ($\varphi = 30\%$). **c** Electro-conductivity of Ni-GaIn. **d** Adhesion force of Ni-GaIn. **e** Directly-painted Ni-GaIn wires on Ecoflex substrate with different doping ratios (from 5 to 30%)

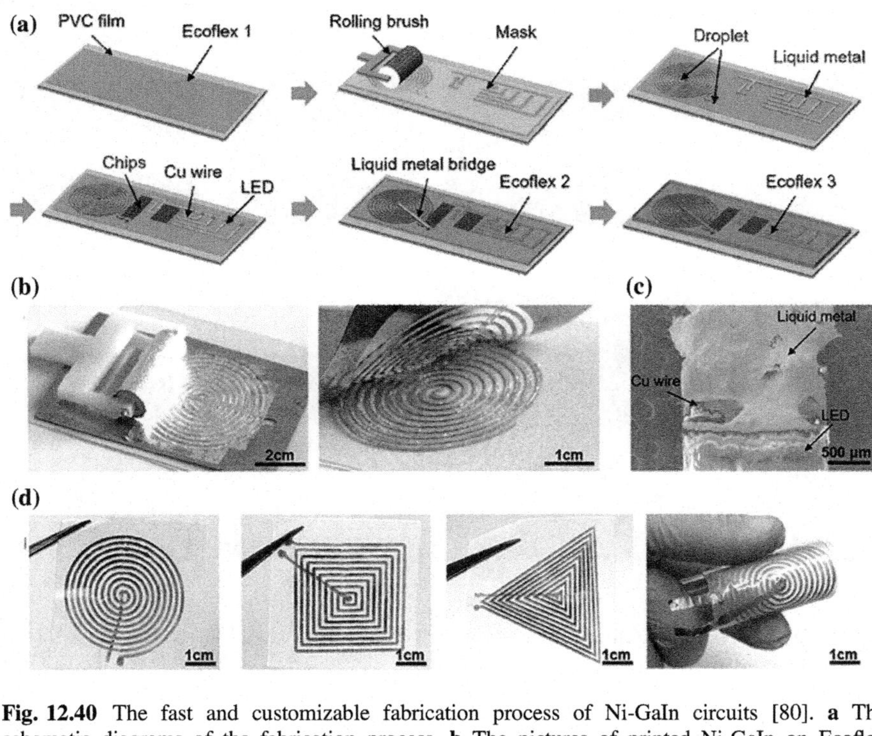

Fig. 12.40 The fast and customizable fabrication process of Ni-GaIn circuits [80]. **a** The schematic diagrams of the fabrication process. **b** The pictures of printed Ni-GaIn on Ecoflex substrate via a rolling brush. **c** The SEM image of the junction of LED and Ni-GaIn wire in the circuit. **d** Three different shapes of flexible Ni-GaIn coils

Ni-GaIn amalgam was printed on Ecoflex substrate directly by a rolling brush and encapsulated by Ecoflex membranes (Fig. 12.40a). The left image of Fig. 12.41a showed that the surface of Ni-GaIn wires were covered with a layer of its oxide. From the right image of Fig. 12.41a, there were some agglomerates of Ni micro-particles mixed in EGaIn. Besides, Fig. 12.41b, c showcased the uniform distribution of elements (Ni, Ga, In and O) into the Ni-GaIn amalgam. The results indicated that there were tiny micro Ni particles on the Ni-GaIn surface, which suggested that most micro Ni particles were covered with the EGaIn. In addition, the printed Ni-GaIn wires appeared serious deformation under different tensile strain in the axial direction (0% strain and 200% strain) (Fig. 12.41d). There were dramatical elongations, and its width decreased significantly with the increase of stretching length. Under assistance of the optical profiler, the Ni-GaIn wire surface appeared relatively rough, while the contact area between Ecoflex substrate and the Ni-GaIn was much larger, and the layer thickness was enough, thus it ensured good connectivity for the Ni-GaIn wire (Fig. 12.41e).

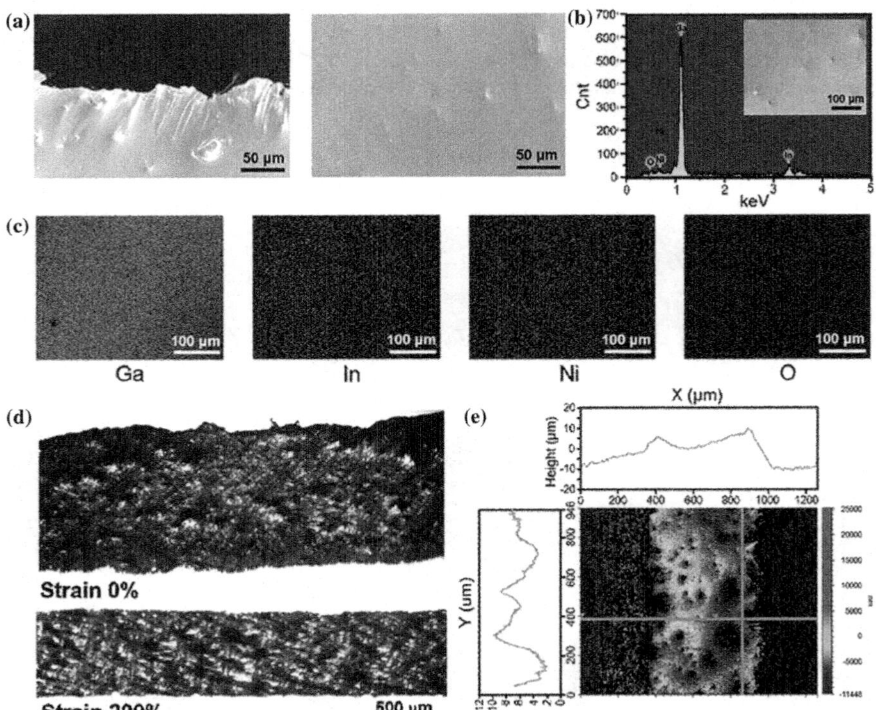

Fig. 12.41 Morphological characterizations of printed Ni-GaIn wires [80]. **a** The surface SEM images of the printed Ni-GaIn wires. **b** The content of elements (Ni, Ga, In and O) on the Ni-GaIn surface. **c** Its elements distribution (Ni, Ga, In and O). **d** The optical photographs of the printed Ni-GaIn wires under different tensile strain in the axial direction (0% strain and 200% strain). **e** The topography of the Ni-GaIn wire surface with the assistance of the optical profiler

The flexible Ni-GaIn coils were prepared as the wireless power transfer, which was able to be used in wearable electronics [80]. In the resistance measurement experiments, the original diameter of the flexible coils was 4 cm, and the maximum strain rate was 70%. The DC resistance of the original flexible coils was about 21.3 Ω, and the maximum resistance ratio was about 1.9. The resistance of the flexible coils increased gradually with the strain rate increasing in the stretching process, and there was a slight resistance variation in the releasing process (Fig. 12.42a). The increase of resistance was related to the decrease of power efficiency at applied strain (Fig. 12.42a, blue line). There was a significant drop (drop to 11 from 19%) in the power efficiency between transmitting coil and receiving coil with the increase of strain rate. Because the flexible coil should keep good electrical stability when it was attached to the skin (Fig. 12.43 showed that the flexible coils was attached to an artificial caoutchouc hand to simulate human skin), one can test the dc resistance of flexible coil when it was bent and compressed with a sharp object (Fig. 12.42b, c, red lines). Different from the stretching process, there was only a slight increase in the DC resistance of flexible coils, and the maximum resistance ratio was about 1.004 in the bending process. While, in the bending process, there was a significant drop (drop to 13.3 from 17.8%) in the power efficiency of the flexible coil (Fig. 12.42b, black line). Similarly, there was also a significant drop (drop to 2 from 17.8%) in the power efficiency of the flexible coil, when it was compressed with a sharp object (Fig. 12.42c, black line).

In the fatigue test, one could stretch the flexible coils to 50% strain over 1000 cycles, and plotted the relation curve of the drawing times with the resistance (Fig. 12.42d). The fatigue tests showed that the resistance of the flexible coils did not change much in R/R0 up to 1000 cycles. In addition, the power efficiency was measured when the receiving coil was moving out of the coaxial position (Fig. 12.42e). It can be seen from the curve that the transferred power was diminished gradually with the moving of the coil. More importantly, the output voltage of the flexible coils decreased as the power transmission distance increased (Fig. 12.42f). Specially, when the power transmission distance was no more than 5 mm, the voltage chip could provide a DC voltage of 3.3 V for the circuit.

Figure 12.44a presented an overview of the LED array flexible circuit with wireless power transfer, and the pulse wave measurement circuit was shown in Fig. 12.44d. In order to demonstrate the stretchability of the LED array flexible circuit, one could stretch the Ecoflex substrate over 30% strain and folded it to different shapes. The results showed that all the components could keep in working status and the LEDs were able to light normally (Figs. 12.44b and 12.45). In addition, the LED array flexible circuit could be wrapped around the wrist and attached to the skin (Fig. 12.44c).

As shown in Fig. 12.44e, the pulse wave measurement circuit was flexible and wearable, which was applied to the skin easily. The pulse wave sensor was put onto the wrist and recorded the pulse wave signals then the signals were processed by MATLAB software (Fig. 12.44f). In addition, the pulse wave measurement circuit was stretchable, and even could keep good working status under 25% strain (Fig. 12.44g).

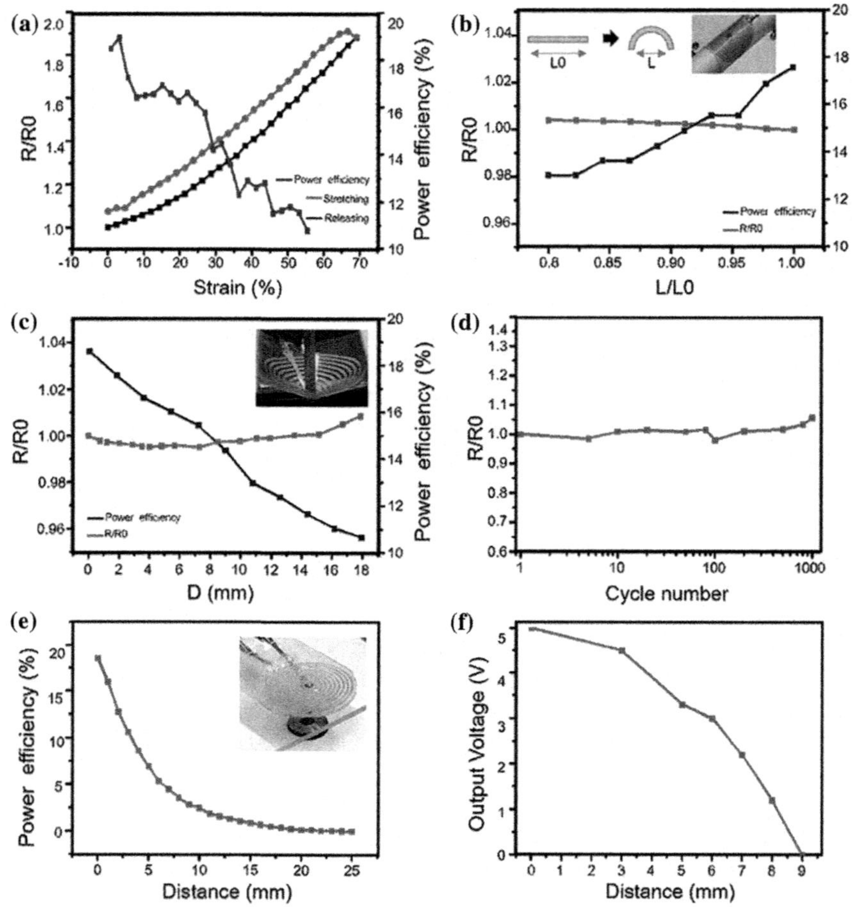

Fig. 12.42 Electrical properties of flexible Ni-GaIn coils [80]. **a** The changing curves of resistances (the red and black lines) and the power efficiency (the blue line) of the flexible coil under different tensile states. **b** The changing curves of resistances (the red line) and the power efficiency (the black line) of the flexible coil when it was bended. **c** The changing curves of resistances (the red line) and the power efficiency (the black line) of the flexible coil when it was compressed with a sharp object. **d** The relationship between drawing times and the resistances of the flexible coil. **e** The changes of power efficiency under different distance between the transmitting coil and receiving coil. **f** The changes of output voltage under different power transmission distance (Color figure online)

Different from previous LM printing technologies, this fabrication of flexible electronics based on printable Ni-GaIn amalgam is efficient and customizable. Because of the presence of oxidized EGaIn, the printable Ni-GaIn amalgam has lower surface tension and higher adhesion force compared with pure EGaIn. However, the doping ratio of Ni particles is limited due to the decrease of electrical conductivity of Ni-GaIn amalgam. Overall, the printable Ni-GaIn amalgam has a

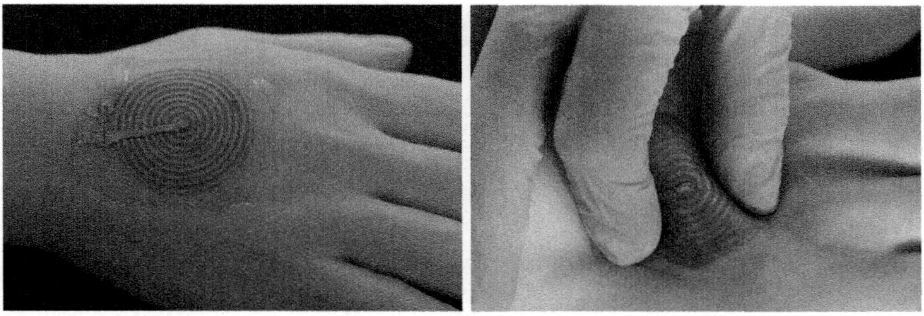

Fig. 12.43 The flexible coils were attached to a caoutchouc artificial hand to simulate the human skin [80]

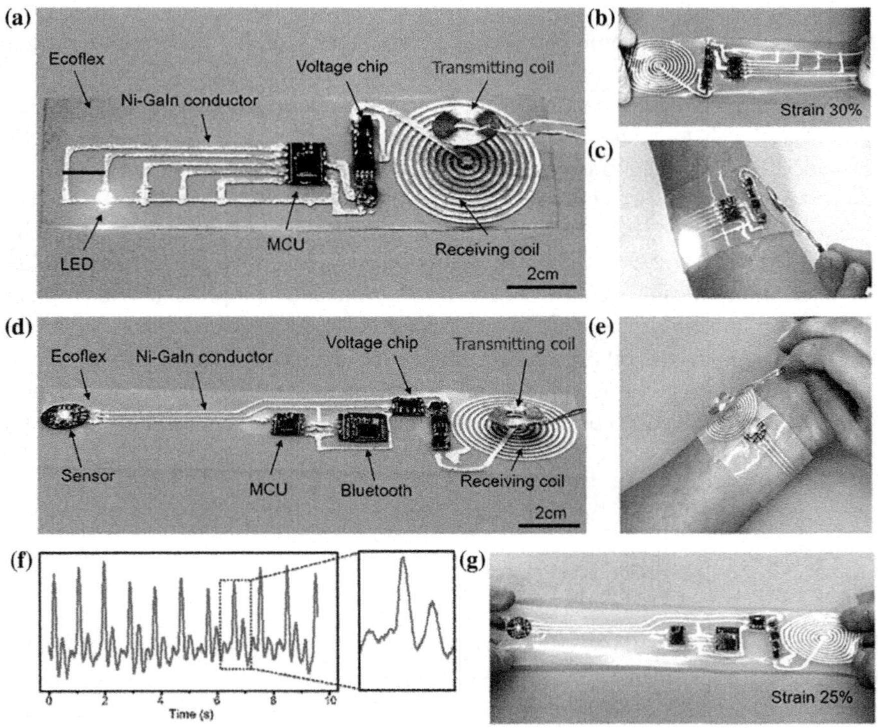

Fig. 12.44 The wearable healthcare device with wireless power transfer based on printable Ni-GaIn amalgam [80]. **a** An overview of the LED array flexible circuit with wireless power transfer. **b** The flexible circuit board was stretched to 30%. **c** The LED array flexible circuit was wrapped around the wrist and attached to the skin. **d** An overview of the pulse wave measurement circuit. **e** The pulse wave sensor was put on the wrist. **f** The pulse wave signals recorded by the wearable device and processed by the MATLAB software. **g** The flexible circuit board was stretched to 25%

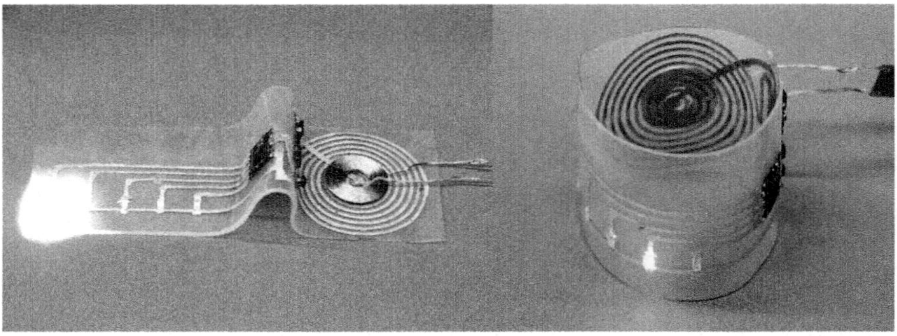

Fig. 12.45 The pictures of the LED array flexible circuit when it was folded to different shapes [80]

degree of liquidity and compliance, which can be stretched in the stretching process of Ecoflex substrate.

The results of these electrical properties tests indicate that the printed Ni-GaIn flexible coil can maintain low resistance. There is a remarkable increase of the resistance in stretching process, which can reduce the power efficiency of the receiving coil, but the maximal resistance variation (approximately 19 Ω) was quite slighter compared with the resistance of functional components, such as the resistance of LED light (above 3 kΩ). In addition, the resistance of the flexible coil does not have a significant increase when it was bent and compressed with a sharp object, and the power efficiency loss is mainly due to the shifted center alignment between the receiving coil and transmitting coil. The distance between the receiving coil and transmitting coil is limited, and the effective transmission distance is about 5 mm. Thus, one needs to put the transmitting coil near the receiving coil within the distance of 5 mm.

12.12 Conclusion

This chapter illustrated the feasibility and advantages of printing liquid metal alloy as electronic components. Overall, the alloy contacts the skin well and has relatively low polarization voltage, which ensures the good signal quality. The results indicated that the liquid metal could serve as a favourable electrode material for detecting physiological signal such as ECG. Though still in its primary stage, the liquid metal skin electronics opens a wide area of new applications on human healthcare.

It is also noteworthy that, the adopted liquid metal ink is safe, inexpensive and easy to use. Hence the alloy, as a new form of bio-electrical sensor and printable skin circuit material, is fully compliant with pervasive healthcare. It can be printed and erased easily, making it much easier to realize the self-service of bio-electrical detections, mapping and treatment. With good wetting ability, the liquid metal ink enables to make the biomedical system on the skin, which may significantly shape the conventional technology in the near future.

One thing needing to be cautious is that, electric-field may induce reorganizations of spray printed liquid metal electronics on skin with different configurations and on different electrochemical environments such as dead skin or living skin, in vitro skin or in vivo skin, pig skin or mice skin have been discovered. These include transformation from a large liquid metal film into a tiny sphere, contraction of several shapes of liquid metal objects to sphere. Various effects will be caused under different size, voltage, orientation. Further, various substrates like in vitro skin and in vivo skin would lead to different liquid metal transformations. The experiments revealed that the phenomena of reorganization of liquid metal electrode related to types of skin and intensity of electrical field. These findings have both fundamental and practical significances for developing future liquid metal skin electronics.

For those substrates or skin where liquid metal inks can not be printed, further modifications on the inks will help resolve the difficulty. For such examples, the Ni-GaIn amalgam as described in this chapter offers direct printing ability which could help fabricate a customized wearable device for healthcare with wireless power transfer. Such Ni-GaIn amalgam contains a certain amount of oxidized EGaIn and can be printed on Ecoflex substrate easily. With different mask, various soft circuits can be printed to realize their rapid customization. Moreover, Ni-GaIn owns a good connection with rigid pins for fabricating hybrid flexible electronics. In the coming future, the skin electronics based on functional liquid metal materials can be pervasively applied in various biomedical scenes.

References

1. Guo C, Yu Y, Liu J (2014) Rapidly patterning conductive components on skin substrates as physiological testing devices via liquid metal spraying and pre-designed mask. J Mater Chem B 2:5739–5745
2. Kim DH, Lu NS, Ma R et al (2011) Epidermal electronics. Science 333:838–843
3. Takei K, Takahashi T, Ho JC, Ko H, Gillies AG, Javey A (2010) Nanowire active-matrix circuitry for low-voltage macroscale artificial skin. Nat Mater 9:821–826
4. Maheshwari V, Saraf RF (2006) High-resolution thin film device to sense texture by touch. Science 312:1501–1504
5. Tee BC, Wang C, Allen R, Bao Z (2012) An electrically and mechanically self-healing composite with pressure- and flexion-sensitive properties for electronic skin applications. Nat Nanotechnol 7:825–832
6. Schwartz G, Tee BC, Mei J, Appleton AL, Kim DH, Bao ZN (1859) Flexible polymer transistors with high pressure sensitivity for application in electronic skin and health monitoring. Nat Commun 2013:4
7. Webb RC, Bonifas AP, Behnaz A, Zhang YH, Yu KJ, Rogers JA (2013) Ultrathin conformal devices for precise and continuous thermal characterization of human skin. Nat Mater 12:938–944

8. Lin P, Yan F (2012) Organic thin film transistors for chemical and biological sensing. Adv Mater 24:34–51
9. Lumelsky VJ, Shur MS, Wagner S (2001) Sensitive skin. IEEE Sens J 1(1):41–51
10. Jeong GS, Baek DH, Jung HC et al (2012) Solderable and electroplatable flexible electronic circuit on a porous stretchable elastomer. Nat Commun 3:977
11. Forrest SR (2004) The path to ubiquitous and low-cost organic electronic appliances on plastic. Nature 428:911
12. Yoshioka Y, Jabbour GE (2006) Desktop inkjet printer as a tool to print conducting polymers. Synth Met 156:779–783
13. Yu RM, Lin D, Pan CF, Niu SM, Liu HF, Wang ZL (2012) Effect on the transport properties of GaN nanobelts for active flexible electronics. Adv Mater 24:3532–3537
14. Gao YX, Li HY, Liu J (2013) Biomedical implementation of liquid metal ink as drawable ECG electrode and skin circuit. PLoS ONE 8(3):e58771-1–e58771-6
15. Zheng Y, He ZZ, Gao YX, Liu J (2013) Direct desktop printed-circuits-on-paper flexible electronics. Sci Rep 3:1786-1–1786-7
16. Cheng S, Wu ZG (2010) Microfluidic stretchable RF electronics. Lab Chip 10:3227–3244
17. Kong TF, Peng WK, Luong TD, Nguyen NT, Han J (2012) Adhesive-based liquid metal radio-frequency microcoil for magnetic resonance relaxometry measurement. Lab Chip 12:287–294
18. Zhang B, Dong Q, Korman CE, Li ZY, Zaghloul ME (1098) Flexible packaging of solid-state integrated circuit chips with elastomeric microfluidics. Sci Rep 2013:3
19. Yu Y, Zhang J, Liu J (2013) Biomedical implementation of liquid metal ink as drawable ECG electrode and skin circuit. PLoS ONE 8(3):e58771-1–e58771–16
20. Zheng Y, Zhang Q, Liu J (2013) Pervasive liquid metal based direct writing electronics with roller-ball pen. AIP Adv 3:112117-1–112117-6
21. Jin C., Zhang J., Li X. K., Yang X. Y., Li J. J., Liu J. Injectable 3-D fabrication of medical electronics at the target biological tissues. Scientific Reports, 2013, 3: 3442-1-7
22. Kaydanova T, Miedaner A, Perkins JD, Curtis C, Alleman JL, Ginley DS (2007) Direct-write inkjet printing for fabrication of barium strontium titanate-based tunable circuits. Thin Solid Films 515:820–3824
23. Hansen TS, West K, Hassager O, Larsen NB (2007) Direct fast patterning of conductive polymers using agarose stamping. Adv Mater 19:3261
24. Siegel AC, Phillips ST, Dickey MD, Lu N, Suo Z, Whitesides GM (2010) Foldable printed circuit boards on paper substrates. Adv Func Mater 20:28–35
25. Tait JG, Worfolk BJ, Maloney SA, Hauger TC, Elias AL, Buriak JM, Harris KD (2013) Spray coated high-conductivity PEDOT:PSS transparent electrodes for stretchable and mechanically-robust organic solar cells. Sol Energy Mater Sol Cells 110:98–106
26. Akhavan VA, Goodfellow BW, Panthani MG, Reid DK, Hellebusch DJ, Adachi T, Korgel BA (2010) Spray-deposited $CuInSe_2$ nanocrystal photovoltaics. Energy Environ Sci 3:1600–1606
27. Dong TY, Chen WT, Wang CW et al (2009) One-step synthesis of uniform silver nanoparticles capped by saturated decanoate: direct spray printing ink to form metallic silver films. Phys Chem Chem Phys 11:6269–6275
28. Zhang Q, Gao YX, Liu J (2013) Atomized spraying of liquid metal droplets on desired substrate surfaces as a generalized way for ubiquitous printed electronics. Appl Phys A 116:1091–1097
29. Zhang Q, Zheng Y, Liu J (2012) Direct writing of electronics based on alloy and metal ink (DREAM Ink): a newly emerging area and its impact on energy, environment and health sciences. Front Energy 6(4):311–340
30. Mundo C, Sommerfeld M, Tropea C (1995) Droplet-wall collisions: experimental studies of the deformation and breakup process. Int J Multiph Flow 21:151–173
31. Thaker NV (1999) Biopotentials and electrophysiology measurement. In: Webster JG (ed) The measurement, instrumentation and sensors handbook. CRC Press, Boca Raton, pp 74-1–74-19

32. Chi YM, Wang YT, Wang Y et al (2012) Dry and noncontact EEG sensors for mobile brain-computer interfaces. IEEE Trans Neural Syst Rehabil Eng 20:228–235
33. Chi YM, Cauwenberghs G (2010) Wireless non-contact EEG/ECG electrodes for body sensor networks. In: International conference on body sensor networks (BSN). IEEE Press, Singapore, pp 297–301
34. Chi YM, Deiss SR, Cauwenberghs G. Non-contact low power EEG/ECG electrode for high density wearable biopotential sensor networks. In: Sixth international workshop on wearable and implantable body sensor networks (BSN 2009). IEEE Press, Berkeley, pp 246–250
35. Yu Y, Zhang J, Liu J (2013) Biomedical implementation of liquid metal ink as drawable ECG electrode and skin circuit. PLoS ONE 8(3):e58771-1–e58771-16
36. Matula RA (1979) Electrical resistivity of copper, gold, palladium and silver. J Phys Chem Ref Data 8:1147–1298
37. Dean JA (1999) Lange's handbook of chemistry. McGraw-Hill Inc., New York, p 1291
38. Ivanoff CS, Ivanoff AE, Hottel TL (2012) Gallium poisoning: a rare case report. Food Chem Toxicol 50:212–215
39. Cadwallader LC (2003) Gallium safety in the laboratory. Energy Facility Contractors Group (EFCOG) Safety Analysis Working Group (SAWG) 2003 Annual Meeting, INEEL/CON-03-00078 Preprint
40. Dunne SM, Abraham R (2000) Dental post-operative sensitivity associated with a gallium-based restorative material. Br Dent J 189:310–313
41. Chen WC, Tsai KD, Chen CH et al (2012) Role of Gallium-67 scintigraphy in the evaluation of occult sepsis in the medical ICU. Intern Emerg Med 7:53–58
42. Hagemeister FB, Fesus SM, Lamki LM, Haynie TP (1990) Role of the gallium scan in Hodgkin's disease. Cancer 65:1090–1096
43. Brown BH (2003) Electrical impedance tomography (EIT): a review. J Med Eng Technol 27:97–108
44. Cherepenin VA, Karpov AY, Korjenevsky AV et al (2002) Three-dimensional EIT imaging of breast tissues: system design and clinical testing. IEEE Trans Med Imaging 21:602–607
45. Cherepenin VA, Karpov AY, Korjenevsky AV et al (2001) A 3D electrical impedance tomography (EIT) system for breast cancer detection. Physiol Meas 22:9–18
46. Seligman PA, Moran PL, Schleicher RB, Crawford ED (1992) Treatment with gallium nitrate: evidence for interference with iron metabolism in vivo. Am J Hematol 41:232–240
47. Martens RJ, Harrington JR, Cohen ND et al (2006) Gallium therapy: a novel metal-based antimicrobial strategy for potential control of Rhodococcus equi foal pneumonia. AAEP Proc 52:219–221
48. Wang X, Zhang Y, Guo R, Wang H, Yuan B, Liu J (2018) Conformable liquid metal printed epidermal electronics for smart physiological monitoring and simulation treatment. J Micromech Microeng 28:034003
49. Shimizu H (2007) Shimizu's textbook of dermatology, 1st edn. (Chap. 1). Nakakyama Shoten, Hokkaido University Press, Sapporo City, Japan
50. Kletenik YB, Aleksandrova TP (1997) Submicron regeneration of the working surface of indicator electrodes: regeneration of metal electrodes. J Anal Chem 52(7):680–682
51. Lehew G, Nicolelis MAL (2008) State-of-the-art microwire array design for chronic neural recordings in behaving animals. In: Methods for neural ensemble recordings, 2nd edn., pp 361–371
52. Lee H, Kim HB, Im TG, Jeong JI, Ahn S (2003) Characterization of platinum electrode using unbalanced magnetic field sputter for implantable biomedical applications. Plasma Science. In: The 30th International Conference on IEEE Conference Record-Abstracts. ICOPS 2003. IEEE. doi: 10.1109 (2003)
53. Wu F, Wang L, Zou J, Huang X, Yuan X (2012) Clinical features, mutation of the GNAS1 and pathogenesis of progressive osseous heteroplasia. Chin J Pediatr 50(1):10–14
54. Cömert A, Honkala M, Hyttinen J (2013) Effect of pressure and padding on motion artifact of textile electrodes. Biomed Eng Online 12:26

55. He L, Lin D, Wang Y, Xiao Y, Che J (2011) Electroactive SWNT/PEGDA hybrid hydrogel coating for bio-electrode interface. Colloids Surf B 87:273–279
56. Bera SC, Chattopadhyay S, Chakraborty B (2004) An experimental analysis of the non-linear behaviour of a bio-electrode polarisation impedance with excitation frequency. Measurement 35:363–370
57. Plam U, Keeser D, Schiller C, Fintescu Z, Nitsche M, Reisinger E, Padberg F (2008) Skin lesions after treatment with transcranial direct current stimulation (tDCS). Brain Stimul 1:386–387
58. Ahadian S, Ramón-Azcón J, Ostrovidov S et al (2013) A contactless electrical stimulator: application to fabricate functional skeletal muscle tissue. Biomed Microdevice 15:109–115
59. Esibov A, Chapman FW, Melnick SB, Sullivan JL, Walcott GP (2015) Minor variations in electrode pad placement impact defibrillation success. Prehospital Emerg Care 20:292–298
60. Killingsworth CR, Melnick SB, Litovsky SH, Ideker RE, Walcott GP (2013) Evaluation of acute cardiac and chest wall damage after shocks with a subcutaneous implantable cardioverter defibrillator in Swine. Pacing Clin Electrophysiol 36(10):1265–1272
61. Martins AC, Moreira A, Machado AV, Vaz F, Fonseca C, Nóbrega JM (2015) Development of polymer wicks for the fabrication of bio-medical sensors. Mater Sci Eng C 49:356–363
62. Xu S, Dai M, Xu C, Chen C, Tang M, Shi X, Dong X (2011) Performance evaluation of five types of Ag/AgCl bio-electrodes for cerebral electrical impedance tomography. Ann Biomed Eng 39:2059–2067
63. Abellán-Llobregat A, Jeerapan I, Bandodkar A, Wang J, Morallón E (2017) A stretchable and screen-printed electrochemical sensor for glucose determination in human perspiration. Biosens Bioelectron 91:885–891
64. Mishra RK, Hubble LJ, Martín A, Kumar R, Wang J (2017) Wearable flexible and stretchable glove biosensor for on-site detection of organophosphorus chemical threats. ACS Sens 2:553–561
65. Zhang Y, Webb RC, Luo H et al (2016) Theoretical and experimental studies of epidermal heat flux sensors for measurements of core body temperature. Adv Healthcare Mater 5: 119–127
66. Webb RC, Ma Y, Krishnan S, Li Y, Yoon S, Guo X, Feng X, Rogers JA (2015) Epidermal devices for noninvasive, precise, and continuous mapping of macrovascular and microvascular blood flow. Sci Adv 1(9):e1500701
67. Gao L, Zhang Y, Malyarchuk V, Jia L, Jang KI, Webb RC, Rogers JA (2014) Epidermal photonic devices for quantitative imaging of temperature and thermal transport characteristics of the skin. Nat Commun 5. doi:10.1038
68. Huang X, Liu Y, Chen K, Shin WJ, Lu CJ, Kong GW, Rogers JA (2014) Stretchable, wireless sensors and functional substrates for epidermal characterization of sweat. Small 10: 3083–3090
69. Neuman MR (1997) Biopotential electrodes. In: Webster JG (ed) Medical instrumentation: application and design, 3rd edn. Wiley, New York, pp 183–232
70. Kim J, Salvatore GA, Araki H, Chiarelli AM, Xie Z, Banks A, Rogers JA (2016) Battery-free, stretchable optoelectronic systems for wireless optical characterization of the skin. Sci Adv 2 (8):e1600418
71. http://datasheets.scbt.com/sc-257605.pdf
72. Li J, Guo C, Wang Z, Gao K, Shi X, Liu J (2016) Electrical stimulation towards melanoma therapy via liquid metal printed electronics on skin. Clin Transl Med 5(1):1–7
73. Stupp R, Wong ET, Kanner AA et al (2012) NovoTTF-100A versus physician's choice chemotherapy in recurrent glioblastoma: a randomised phase III trial of a novel treatment modality. Eur J Cancer 48:2192–2202
74. Schneiderman RS, Shmueli E, Kirson ED, Palti Y (2010) TTFields alone and in combination with chemotherapeutic agents effectively reduce the viability of MDR cell sub-lines that over-express ABC transporters. BMC Cancer 10:229
75. Kirson ED, Schneiderman RS, Dbalý V et al (2009) Chemotherapeutic treatment efficacy and sensitivity are increased by adjuvant alternating electric fields (TTFields). BMC Med Phys 9:1

76. Kirson ED, Gurvich Z, Schneiderman R et al (2004) Disruption of cancer cell replication by alternating electric fields. Can Res 64:3288–3295
77. Kirson ED, Giladi M, Gurvich Z et al (2009) Alternating electric fields (TTFields) inhibit metastatic spread of solid tumors to the lungs. Clin Exp Metas 26:633–640
78. Guo C, Yi L, Yu Y, Liu J (1070) Electrically induced reorganization phenomena of liquid metal film printed on biological skin. Appl Phys A 2016:122
79. Guo R, Wang X, Yu W, Tang J, Liu J (2018) A highly conductive and stretchable wearable liquid metal electronic skin for long-term conformable health monitoring. Sci China Technol Sci. https://doi.org/10.1007/s11431-018-9253-9
80. Guo R, Wang X, Chang H, Yu W, Liang S, Rao W, Liu J (2018) Ni-GaIn amalgams enabled rapid and customizable fabrication of wearable and wireless healthcare electronics. Adv Eng Mater. https://doi.org/10.1002/adem.201800054

Chapter 13
Liquid Metal Printed Biosensor

Abstract This chapter illustrates a series of liquid metal printed biomedical sensor systems, particularly for quantitative measurement of various physiological signals. By virtue of the low melting point, the introduced liquid metal ink makes it possible for the direct writing or printing of the biomedical circuits in a moment. Unlike the prior art, the current fabrication process appears rather straightforward, labor-saving and cost-effective. This is expected to fulfill certain increasing needs in the coming home or society health care. In some cases, the developed sensors have already displayed rather beneficial properties.

Keywords Biosensor · Direct printing · Liquid metal

13.1 Introduction

As the new generation electronic ink, liquid metal can certainly be directly printed into various sensors for the measurement of specific physiological signals such as electrical, mechanical, thermal, including chemical parameters of human body. Such a role can lead to many practical applications in health care. Previously, conventional fabrication processes are generally time consuming and expensive. From an alternative, liquid metal electronics provides an innovative way to quickly make biosensors. For example, among all biosensors, electrochemical ones are often adopted for health administration purpose. A typical case is pervasive detection of blood glucose which is rather critical for the real-time disease diagnosis and would provide valuable guidance for treatment planning. The present lab had ever established a biomedical platform along this direction through incorporating the glucose detection with liquid metal printed sensor and the smart phone monitoring system together. The liquid metal ink composed of bismuth indium stannic (BIS) alloy was identified as appropriate sensor material to be quickly written or printed on polyvinyl chloride (PVC) substrate at around 59 °C to form desired electrodes. It therefore eliminated the complicated procedures as usually required in conventional sensor fabrication strategies. The alloy electrodes can be characterized

J. Liu and L. Yi, *Liquid Metal Biomaterials*,
Springer Series in Biomaterials Science and Engineering10,
https://doi.org/10.1007/978-981-10-5607-9_13

via cyclic voltammetry to demonstrate their practical functionality. Unlike the commonly adopted glucometer, the smart phone serves as the data acquisition and display center to help improve the portability and ubiquitous virtue of the detection system. Glucose solution in different concentrations can be assayed via this platform. The good linear relationship between the concentration and the integral value of the curve recorded by the mobile phone confirms the feasibility of the new method. Such quantitative point-of-care system has pervasive feature and is expected to be very useful for future low cost electrochemical detection. In fact, except for the electrochemical detection of glucose level in human body, liquid metal was also found critical in more and more biomedical areas. This chapter illustrated several representative applications and fundamental sciences enabled from the liquid metal printed biosensors.

13.2 Blood Glucose Detection in Health Care

In modern medicine, pervasive blood glucose detection has great significance for real-time diagnosis of disease and provides valuable insights associated with treatment evaluations [1]. Over the past few decades, tremendous efforts have been made to find out a sensitive and effective way for the glucose detection. Some studies had ever been focused on the colorimetric measurements [1–3], where assays are based on enzymatic reactions or small molecule dyes. The color intensity would indicate the glucose concentration. Such method presents remarkable advantages, such as visualization and real time. However, an external equipment should always be needed which is usually large and complex to operate. Recently, camera phones or portable scanners were developed and employed to digitize the color intensity [4–10]. An only pity is that, detections from this approach are restricted to the lighting conditions and require assistance in analysis from medical professionals. From an alternative, electrochemical method not only offers a solution with better accuracy and higher sensitivity in many biochemical application cases [11–13], but also plays an increasingly important role in both miniaturization and integration of device design. In a large extent, the portability and point of care are believed to be the way to improve the pervasive value of medical devices in the near future [14–19].

So far, commercial glucometers based on electrochemical principle are the most widely used devices by diabetic patients. Nevertheless, most of them simply display the numerical results and are unable to save the results as records, which may limit their full play of multi-functions. Along with the emerging information and communication technology, the demand towards desirable in-home health monitoring increases rapidly. Cell phone is one of the most widespread consumer electronics. It has become an essential tool in peoples' daily life. For example, 96% of the U.S. population own mobile phones and 35% adults among them use smart phones [20]. Clearly, the universality of such tool makes it possible to meet the need of home health care. More importantly, the computational capability of mobile phones is becoming closer to that of the personal computer. Therefore, if phones can be developed as medical device, the test results could be conveniently saved there and synchronized with PCs. As a result, people could easily check their daily glucose records whenever needed. So far, some studies have investigated the electrochemical method coupled with smart phone [21–23]. The phone could receive the electrical signal from sample reaction. Nevertheless, the detection module has to be plugged directly into the smart phone through the audio jack or USB port. Compared to USB interface, the application of Bluetooth breaks the restriction of space. For example, people can put the detection platform on table, and hold the phone in hand more comfortably. Consequently, one can develop a mobile phone-based platform utilizing Bluetooth to carry out the electrochemical detection.

Another major concern in the glucose monitoring clearly lies in the design of the electrochemical sensor. Despite their success in fabrication, these sensors have also shown limited capability in dealing with the situations like time costing, high temperature treatments and expensive equipment. From an alternative, the present lab had ever demonstrated that GaIn10-based material was capable of being directly written on various substrates such as epoxy resin board, glass, plastic, silica gel, paper, cotton, and fiber etc. [24]. This suggests a unique way for the direct fabrication of electronics. However, due to its lower melting point and liquid state at room temperature, GaIn10 is inappropriate as an electrode material which requires to be inserted into the detection slot. From a different material strategy, we turn to another kind of ink material composed of bismuth indium stannic (BIS) alloy. In regard to the toxicity, BIS alloy has been investigated as a kind of green and clean material and applied in industry to replace the toxic lead [25]. Its melting point is around 59 °C. Taking advantage of its fusible characteristic, prototyping of BIS alloy electrodes is simple and feasible for handwriting. This printing method offers a new way for the rapid manufacture of electrodes. As the 3D printing technology develops, the fabrication of alloy electrode will become quicker and simpler [26]. The electrode material was composed of BIS: Bi (32.5 wt%), In (51 wt%) and Sn (16.5 wt%). The price of the BIS alloy takes the average price of its components according to their proportions. Overall, the price of the BIS alloy is between that of graphite ink and the classical silver Ag/AgCl ink. In addition, the graphite and silver ink have to be provided by producers. The performance of the electrodes may be influenced by ink from different producers. From such comparison, it can be seen that the composition and preparation are relatively simple for BIS alloy. In addition, experiments also demonstrated that BIS alloy owns good performance as printable electrodes which may incubate future pervasive biochemical sensor fabrication technology.

In recent years, paper-based material has aroused tremendous interest for its potential use as substrate in biological and chemical tests. In fact, it has been investigated in the electrochemical detection area [27–30]. Whereas, the results from paper-based substrate are sensitive to the moisture due to that the reaction zone is hydrophilic. Non-reaction area of paper substrate involves hydrophobic treatment to separate the reaction zone. With regard to this, other materials have to be adopted as the substrate of alloy electrode through the contrastive analysis. We have proven that polyvinyl chloride (PVC) could better satisfy the demands in liquid alloy printing with its easy availability and less processing requirement [1]. More importantly, PVC has higher adhesion with BIS alloy when compared to several other candidate materials. Accordingly, PVC material was determined as electrode substrate after comprehensive consideration of multiple factors.

The following section illustrated the method for rapid prototyping of electrochemical sensor system for wireless glucose detection [1].

13.3 Sensor Materials and Printing Methods

The electrode material was composed of Bi (32.5 wt%), In (51 wt%) and Sn (16.5 wt%) (BIS). This alloy was prepared through mixing these metals with weighted ratio. Firstly, they were placed into a beaker and heated at 500 °C for 24 h until melted together completely. Then, the mixtures were stirred magnetically at 80 °C for 4 h to achieve the homogeneity. The melting point of the obtained

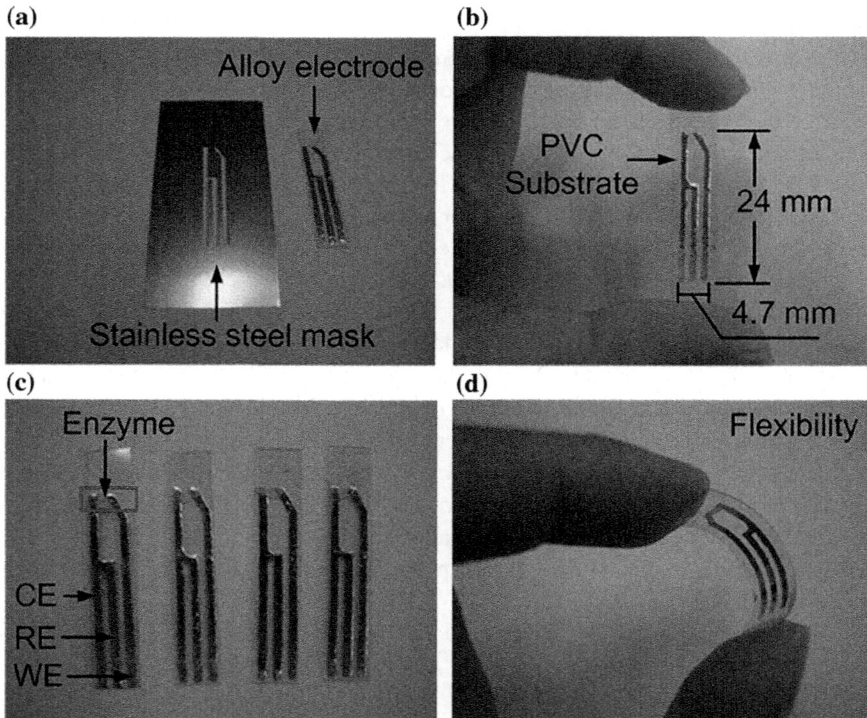

Fig. 13.1 The photos of BIS alloy electrodes [1]. **a** The stainless steel mask for patterning and fabrication of electrode. **b** Dimension of electrodes. **c** The basic design of the alloy electrode. **d** The electrodes attached firmly to the PVC substrate. All pictures reproduced with permission

eutectic alloy is 59 °C [31]. Such metal ink is stable and could be stored at room temperature for quite a long time. In the fabrication of the electrochemical sensor, a mask made of stainless steel as well as a PVC substrate were employed, respectively. To achieve the high adhesion between electrodes and substrates, the BIS alloy was stirred continuously in the air until it was oxidized of 5%.

An overall design of the electrode can be depicted in Fig. 13.1 [1]. The thickness of the stainless steel mask is 50 μm (Fig. 13.1a). In order to provide a good comparison and ensure the matching between electrodes and detecting slot, the alloy electrodes designed were on the same order of commercial electrodes, but with different shapes to simplify the fabrication process (Fig. 13.1b). Alloy electrodes consisting of working electrode (WE), counter electrode (CE) and reference electrode (RE) were fabricated through direct hand printing on the PVC substrate (Fig. 13.1c), and the whole electrode was made of BIS alloy.

Figure 13.2 depicts the detailed procedures for making the present alloy electrodes. Firstly, the BIS alloy was preheated at 70 °C to maintain its molten state [1]. Meanwhile, the mask of electrode was placed over the PVC substrate and they were

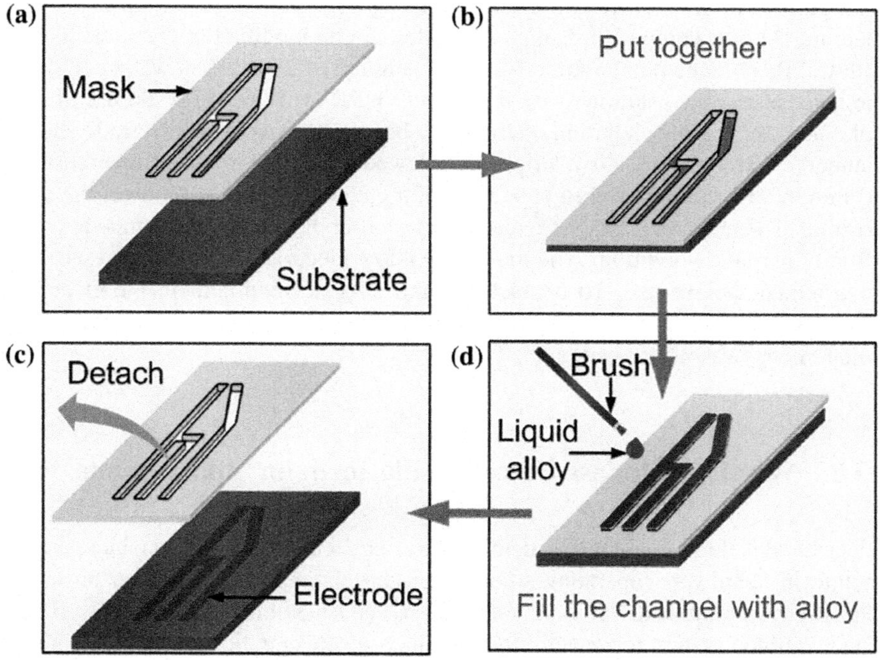

Fig. 13.2 Schematic of the fabrication process of alloy electrodes [1]. **a** The design of the mask and substrate. **b** The mask is placed on the substrate in full contact. **c** The channel is filled with alloy by brushing. The substrate is on the heating platform with the temperature higher than 59 °C to keep the alloy in liquid state. **d** Detach the mask from the substrate, and the alloy electrodes are obtained when the substrate is removed from the platform. All pictures reproduced with permission

held together tightly on the heating platform of 59 °C during the printing procedure. Then dip the liquid alloy with a brush to cover the channels until the mask was fully filled. After that, the mask was detached from the substrate and cooled naturally at room temperature. Since their surfaces were coarse, the achieved electrodes were treated with abrasive paper and then cleaned ultrasonically in distilled water. Before modification, the electrochemical characterization of the alloy electrodes was performed via cyclic voltammetry by dropping 4 μL phosphate buffer solution (PBS) and glucose solution respectively on the zone between counter electrode and working electrode. The measurements were taken using a CHI 660C electrochemical work shop (Shanghai, CN). All cyclic voltammetric tests were operated at 100 mV/s under room temperature.

13.4 Modification of Electrodes as Electro-Chemical Sensors

The commercial glucose testing strips (SANNUO®) employed can be immobilized with glucose oxidase on carbon electrodes using potassium ferricyanide as electron medium [1]. For comparison, alloy electrodes can be modified in the same way as follows: Prepare the potassium ferricyanide solution of 250 mM in water and dilute the glucose oxidase solution to 1000 units/mL in PBS (pH 7.0) [32]. Spot 2 μL of a potassium ferricyanide solution on the space between the working electrode and the counter electrode. The alloy strip was allowed to dry at room temperature for 20 min in dark condition, then spot 2 μL of a glucose oxidase solution at the same position. The reaction zones were ready for test after drying at room temperature for 20 min in dark condition. The modified alloy electrodes were stored at 4 °C environment before use. To characterize the enzyme modified on the electrode, 4 μL of glucose solution was dropped on the reaction area, and the cyclic voltammetry was performed.

13.5 Wireless Glucose Detection Platform on Smart Phone

Yi et al. developed a wireless detection system which includes an independent monitoring hardware, operating software on the phone and PVC-based biosensor [1]. Their communications were established via Bluetooth protocols (Fig. 13.3). The integrated system for quantifying the glucose concentration mainly depends on the specific biochemical reactions between glucose and enzymes with the help of potassium ferricyanide as the electron transfer mediator.

The operating principle of the detection system is shown in Fig. 13.4. A constant excitation voltage was provided by microcontrollers to motivate the free electron produced in the oxidation-reduction reactions. Thus, the dynamic current was

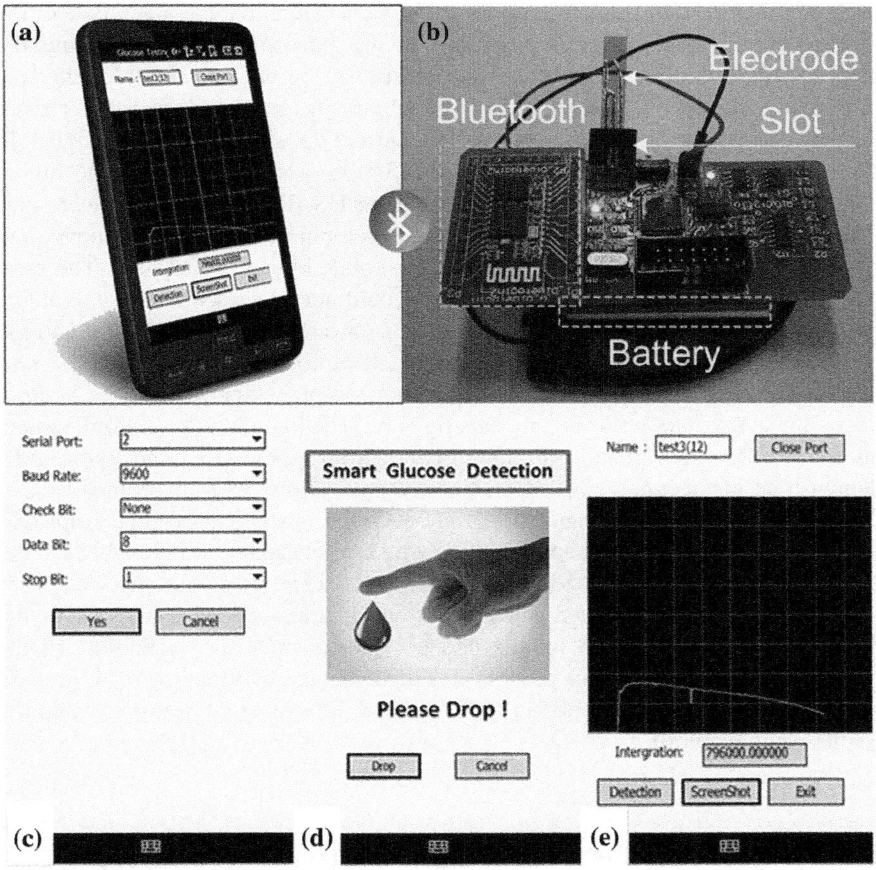

Fig. 13.3 The wireless detection system integrated with smart phone and related hardware [1]. **a** Smart phone interface for operating the glucose detection. **b** The independent detection device communicating with smart phone via Bluetooth. The glucose detection interfaces on smart phone. **c** Screen for parameters setting. **d** The screen reminding user to drop the sample. **e** Screen of glucose reaction. All pictures reproduced with permission

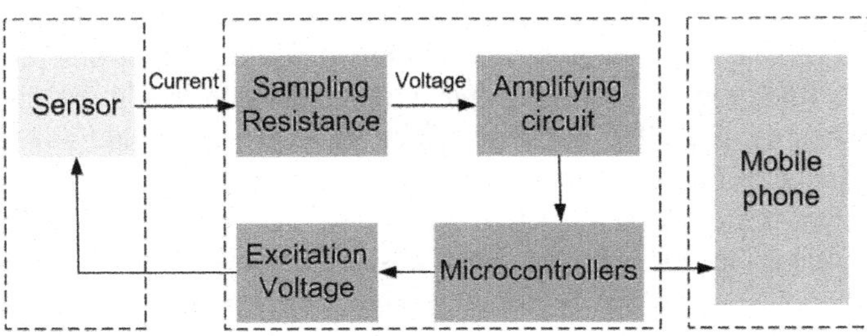

Fig. 13.4 The operating principle of detection system based on mobile phone [1]. Picture reproduced with permission

induced. Theoretically, under the same enzyme concentration, the magnitude of the induced current was strictly in proportion to the glucose concentration. Thus the glucose concentration can be calculated by measuring the magnitude of the corresponding current. To facilitate the measurements, we conducted the current through a sampling resistance to convert the current transferred to voltage signal. In addition, Micro-programmed control unit MSP430 was used as analog to digital converter which meanwhile transmitted data over USART (Universal Synchronous Asynchronous Receiver Transmitter) to the Bluetooth module BC04 (Chongqing, China). After that, the final data was sent to mobile phone in real time. The sampling rate was 512 Hz and data acquisition would not be ceased until data volume reached 10,000. The printed circuit board was power-supplied by a 3.3 V battery, occupying 9.5 cm × 3.5 cm (Fig. 13.3b) which can be easily held in hand.

One can take the multi-functional smart phone as processor, running on Android operating system to perform the experiments. The ubiquitous Android system allows seamless transplant of utility software from laptops to smart phones. To demonstrate the accuracy and effectiveness of the whole platform, comparison of the commercial glucometer and mobile phone system using commercial strips was carried out by testing the glucose solution with concentration of 5, 7.5, 10, 15, and 20 mM, respectively. Each test with different concentration was repeated three times. After that, the printed alloy strips were employed combining with the detection platform based on mobile phone to demonstrate the availability of the whole integrated system. This process was implemented by dropping 4 μL glucose solution with concentration of 5, 10, 20, 30, and 50 mM to the test zones and the results were analyzed.

13.6 Direct Printing of BIS Alloy Electrodes as Glucose Sensor

The BIS eutectic alloy has the melting point of 59 °C. This temperature is much lower than that of most electrode materials. Taking advantage of the low melting point, circuits and electrodes with various shapes and sizes are capable of being "written" or "printed" directly and immediately by a brush on a heating platform [1]. Whereas, due to the surface tension of the alloy material, the adhesion between the liquid alloy and the PVC substrate is limited. To deal with this problem, we managed to find a way of improvement that adhesion could be significantly increased when the BIS alloy was oxidized of 5% in the air. In addition, due to the specific adhesion of this alloy, materials of the mask required to be strictly selected. In fact, a poor adhesion was preferred between the liquid alloy and the mask material to make their detachment much easier. Meanwhile, the mask should be rigid enough so as to repetitively use and protect the fine structure.

Because the mask of electrode and the PVC substrate were both put on the heating platform, and the writing process was carried out there as well, the heating temperature should be controlled higher than 59 °C to prevent the liquid alloy from solidifying immediately at the low environmental temperature. Moreover, the temperature of the heating platform should be set below 80 °C. If exceeding this scale, the PVC substrate will deform. Remarkably, to combine the alloy with the substrate tightly, gentle pressure was required to fill the gap between mask and substrate with liquid alloy while printing. When the mask was detached from the substrate, the initial prototype of the solid electrode was accomplished. Then the substrate already printed with liquid alloy was removed from the heating platform by cooling at room temperature within only one minute, the liquid alloy got solidified rapidly and an electrode was thus made. The BIS alloy electrodes can firmly attach to the PVC substrate, and will not break or peel off from the PVC substrate when subject to bending (Fig. 13.1d). This process was superior to screen printing which requests longer drying process. Moreover, compared to the graphite electrode, the economic efficiency of BIS alloy is higher due to its recyclability. Most importantly, the entire procedure to fabricate alloy electrode does not involve the complicated operation which is rather time and cost saving.

13.7 Cyclic Voltammetric Tests on BIS Alloy Electrode Sensor

Before applied to the measurement of various glucose concentrations, the basic characterization of the BIS alloy electrode should be evaluated using cyclic voltammetry [1]. The electrodes can be modified with potassium ferricyanide solution. After the alloy strip was dried at room temperature, phosphate buffer solution was dropped and cyclic voltammetry was performed at different scanning rates. The results at the scanning rates of 10, 50, 100 and 150 mV/s are shown in Fig. 13.5a. It can be observed that the anodic and cathodic peaks are stable and reversible. The insert in Fig. 13.5a shows that anodic and cathodic peak current have good linear relation with the scanning rate between 10 and 150 mV/s. The cyclic voltammetry of unmodified electrodes in 0.1 M PBS and 20 mM glucose solution and the modified electrodes in 20 mM glucose solution were comparatively studied. As the solution dropped onto the position modified with glucose oxidase (For unmodified electrodes, solution was dropped on the same position corresponding to the modified electrodes.), the cyclic voltammetric curves were obtained. Figure 13.5b demonstrates that the peak current from the reaction on modified electrodes was much larger than the ones happened on the unmodified electrodes, which proves that BIS alloy dose not react with either the composition of PBS or glucose solution. The reaction between glucose and glucose oxidase was the prominent one taken place on alloy electrodes. Therefore, alloy electrodes could truly reflect the signal from the glucose oxidation and it confirms that the BIS alloy electrodes can be well utilized in glucose detection.

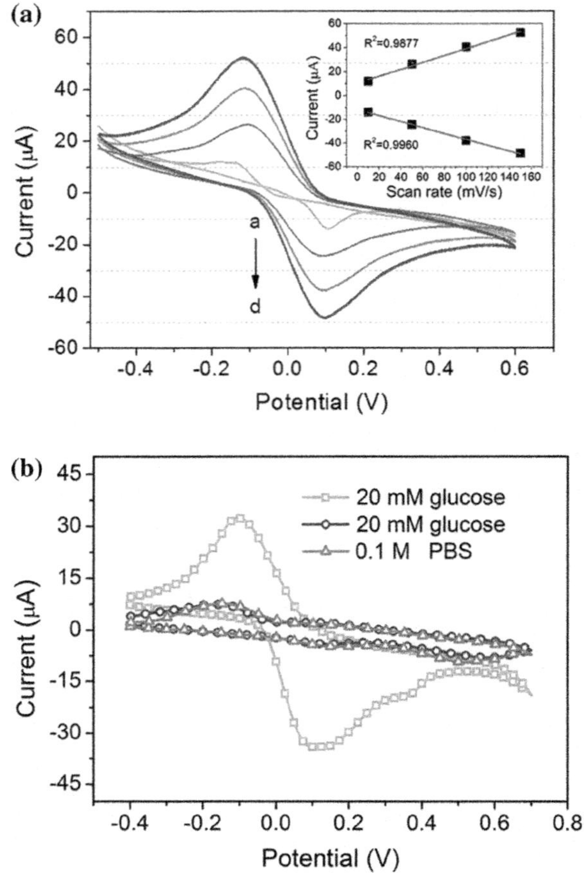

Fig. 13.5 Characterization of alloy electrodes [1]. **a** Cyclic voltammograms of alloy electrodes in PBS at different scanning rates of 10, 50, 100 and 150 mV/s (**a–d**). The insert denotes the relationship between the peak currents with the scanning rates. **b** Cyclic voltammograms of the enzyme-modified BIS alloy electrodes in 20 mM glucose solution, unmodified electrodes in 20 mM glucose and 0.1 M phosphate buffer solution (pH 7.0) at a 100 mV/s scan rate. All pictures reproduced with permission

13.8 Wireless Glucose Detection on Smart Phone

The comparison test implemented between the mobile phone platform and commercial glucometer by employing commercial glucose electrodes, validated the reliability of the wireless detection system [1]. Figure 13.3 shows the interfaces of the glucose detection application. In the screen of the smart phone, the Open/Close Port button provided access to the serial setting interface, where user can select the serial port number, set up transport protocol parameters like baud rate, and connect to the Bluetooth device (Fig. 13.3c). After that, insert the biosensor to the slot, click Drop button (Fig. 13.3d), press Detection to run the program (Fig. 13.3e), and then drop 4 μL glucose solution to the entrance of the commercial strips. At this point, the interface turns to present the dynamic reaction curve (Fig. 13.3e). The reaction signal was transmitted synchronously to the phone via Bluetooth, and the curve displayed in the gridlines reflects the electrochemical response in real time. After receiving the information, we took 1000 data before and 4000 data after the maximum value as the valid data and computed the sum as integral.

The phone gives the curvilinear integral automatically which indicates the glucose concentration indirectly. Besides, through comparison with the conventional glucometer, the screen capture function is added in the phone system and the result can be saved for any late check. By detecting multiple groups of glucose solution with concentration of 5, 7.5, 10, 15, and 20 mM, the result shows that the integral value increased linearly with the increasing concentration and accord well with the relationship between concentration and the measured value from glucometer (Fig. 13.6a). Although the result provided by the phone was integral value, the unknown concentration could be determined through the comparison between the concentration and integral value. It is proven that the mobile phone system is with good performance in detecting the glucose concentration. On this basis, the BIS alloy electrodes were applied in combination with the smart phone to test different glucose concentrations at 5, 10, 20, 30, and 50 mM respectively. The relationship between the obtained integral value and the corresponding concentration was displayed in Fig. 13.6b. The results indicate that there existed a good linear relation between the integral value and the concentration. It suggests that the alloy electrode could be utilized for sensitive electrochemical detection. In addition, the results shown were not fully consistent under the same concentration every time, it is probably due to that the hand-brushing results in the differences in shape of the electrode and the enzyme modified zone. To confine the sample solution, the reservoir with permanent volume or the siphon channel on traditional test strips will be designed and added for the improvement of alloy sensors in batch production. In this regard, the influence brought about by hand would be improved or avoided through simple mechanized equipment, which is worth of pursuing in the near future.

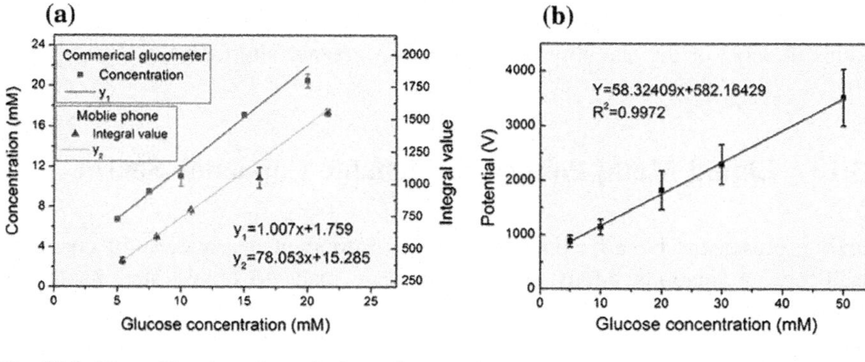

Fig. 13.6 The calibration plots of electrodes based on mobile phone system and commercial glucometer [1]. **a** Glucose solution with concentration of 5, 7.5, 10, 15, and 20 mM was tested using mobile phone system and commercial glucometer. **b** The BIS alloy electrodes were characterized in combination with the smart phone through determination of glucose concentration at 5, 10, 20, 30, and 50 mM, respectively. All pictures reproduced with permission

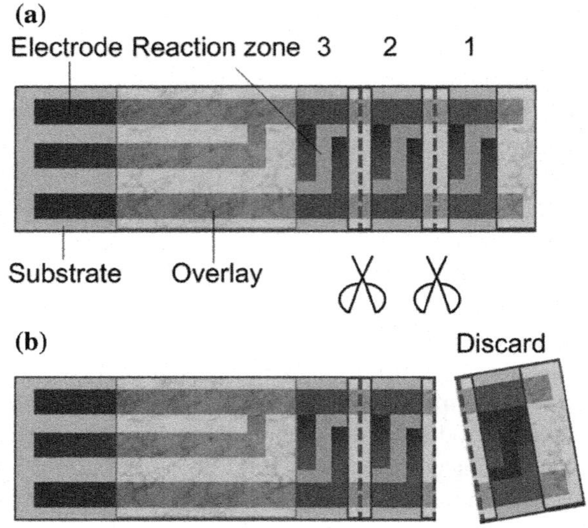

Fig. 13.7 The design of alloy sensor with multi-reaction zones [1]. **a** The designed sensor has three reaction sections. **b** The test could be carried out from the 1st reaction part. The test area would be cut off and discarded when the reaction was accomplished. All pictures reproduced with permission

13.9 Pattern Design of Electrodes for Repetitive Measurements

One advantage of the integrated system is its simplicity. Besides the improvements on materials and device, Yi et al. [1] further proposed a multi-reaction pattern design of alloy sensors which can also be applied in the practical system (Fig. 13.7). Compared to the commercial and traditional test strip, another prominent merit of the sensor are its multiple detection zones. The contact area between enzyme modified zone and electrode is pretty large which improves the sensitivity of the signal response. With the multiple detection zones, one strip can be used for three or more times, depending on the designed number of detection zones. People can cut off the reacted section before a new test begins. This method will not only reduce the cost of the test strip but also offer a greener alternative.

13.10 Liquid Metal Painted Stretchable Capacitor Sensor

Flexible biosensors have become increasingly important in a variety of emerging healthcare applications. Many efforts have been made to obtain stretchable and highly conductive biomaterials, most of which are based on gold or silver nanoparticles. However, such materials have a number of disadvantages. From an alternative, the present lab had ever developed flexible capacitor sensors based on 3M VHB 4905 tape and GaInSn and designs a wearable biosensor monitoring device that uses the CAV444 chip [33]. The system exhibits highly linear response to stretching, rotation, and pressure. The practical applications of these sensors are explored, such as measuring the motion angle of the wrist and finger joint and responses to pressure. The proposed flexible capacitor sensors have many potential biomedical applications, such as parameter measurement, accident alert, electronic skin, motion feedback, and remote control.

13.10.1 Sensor Materials for Motion Measurement

The monitoring of physiological signals such as human motions via biomedical sensors is usually considered effective for health assessment or disease diagnosis. Such sensors are usually fabricated on rigid substrates, which make them not well match human skin. Stretchable electronics, a class of large-area electronics, has potential application in wearable health monitoring and the collection of sensitive tactile information. Conventional production process needs higher requirement on the temperature tolerance of the base film material. For example, plastic materials must be treated under 150 °C [34], and commonly used flexible materials, such as organic film and paper, are often subjected to a high-temperature environment. Therefore, an ideal conductive material for the production of flexible electronic components requires the ability to be manipulated at room temperature. Several conductive materials have potential to overcome these problems, including metal nanoparticles, carbon nanotubes, conductive polymer PEDOT/PSS, polypyrrole, graphene, room-temperature liquid metals such as gallium-indium-tin alloy (GaInSn) [33], PDMS-based conducting composites. These materials have potential applications in flexible displays, solar cells, electronic skin, flexible batteries, and radiofrequency antennas.

Among the above candidate materials, room-temperature liquid metal GaInSn (67% Ga, 20.5% In, and 12.5% Sn, by volume) has a low melting point and simple production process, which are beneficial in the production of flexible electronic components. GaInSn is a non-toxic, low-viscosity fluid. Unlike commonly used metal nanoparticles, whose conductivity heavily depends on the production process, GaInSn is always highly conductive ($\sigma = 3.4 \times 10^6$ S/m) due to its intrinsic properties and simple production process. Some researches used an elastomer embedded with a micro-channel filled with liquid metal or stamp lithography to produce stretchable capacitor sensors. These fabrication methods may not be able to produce complex patterns and are time-consuming. To set up a cost-effective fabrication method to form large-scale and uniform electronic skin, Sheng et al. [33] developed a flexible capacitor sensor that uses GaInSn liquid metal as a conductive material and 3M VHB tape as a dielectric material [33]. The liquid metal was brushed on both sides of the film or packaged into a multilayer structure, which demonstrates the printability of the material and simplifies the production process. The proposed sensor shows some excellent properties, such as stretchability, linear correlation, sensitivity, repeatability, and stable electrical properties. In addition, the flexible capacitor sensor can monitor human physiological signals, such as the motion angle of the wrist or finger joint and the pressure of fingers.

13.10.2 Design of Liquid Metal Capacitor Sensor

The flexible capacitor sensor is based on the 3M VHB 4905 tape [33] as the dielectric elastomer and a liquid-phase GaInSn alloy as the conductive electrode. A schematic diagram of the capacitor sensor is shown in Fig. 13.8a. The capacitor sensor has three layers of 3M VHB tape. The top and bottom layers of the VHB tape were used as packaging, preventing the oxidation of the liquid metal and direct contact with the electrodes. The middle layer of the VHB tape in this sandwich structure worked as a capacitor dielectric. Liquid metal painted on the both surfaces of capacitor dielectric worked as the capacitor electrode. 3M VHB 4905 tape is a clear double-sided pressure-sensitive acrylic tape with a red polyethylene film liner. The general purpose adhesive on both sides is suitable for high-surface-energy substrates. The tape has a thickness of 0.5 mm, a width of 570 mm, and an extension coefficient of 150%. The capacitance of this capacitor sensor can be expressed as:

$$C = \frac{\varepsilon_r \varepsilon_0 A}{d} \tag{13.1}$$

where A represents the area of the liquid metal electrodes, ε_0 is the permittivity of a vacuum, whose value is 8.86×10^{-12} F/m, ε_r represents the relative dielectric constant of the film, and d is the thickness of the capacitor dielectric.

Based on the above design, a multilayer capacitor sensor was developed. Its schematic diagram is shown in Fig. 13.8b. The basic structure is almost the same as that of the single-layer capacitor sensor, but with two additional layers of 3M VHB tape and liquid metal electrodes. The advantages of this design lies in its improved

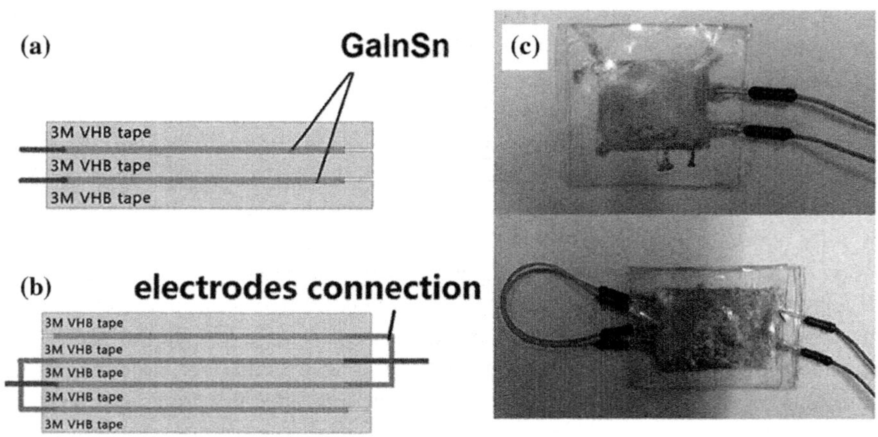

Fig. 13.8 Design of liquid metal capacitor sensor [33]. **a** Single-and **b** multilayer capacitor sensor designs and **c** photographs of their respective experimental samples. All pictures reproduced with permission

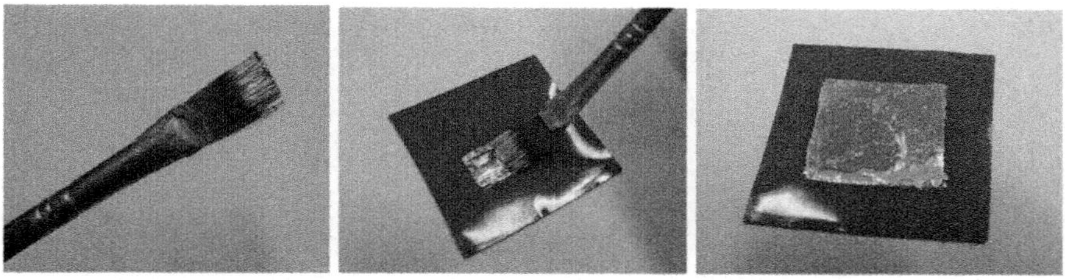

Fig. 13.9 Manufacturing method of capacitor sensor [33]. Liquid metal was directly painted on surface of VHB tape. All pictures reproduced with permission

sensitivity and increased capacitance. The experimental samples of the two designs are shown in Fig. 13.8c. The capacitor sensor is fabricated via the direct printing of liquid metal electrodes onto the surface of 3M VHB tape using a small paint brush, as illustrated in Fig. 13.9. This process is simple and fast.

13.10.3 Design of Sensor Measurement Circuit

To measure the voltage changes in the capacitor sensor, a measurement circuit based on the CAV444 chip was designed. CAV444 is an integrated capacitance-to-voltage transducer. The block diagram of CAV444 is shown in Fig. 13.10a. A schematic diagram of the circuit is shown in Fig. 13.10b. The system transfer function can be expressed by Eq. (13.2), where $\triangle V_{CM}$ = 2.1 V and V_{REF} = 2.5 V. The values of C_W are related to $C_{M,max}$, as expressed in Eq. (13.3).

$$V_{OUT} = \left(\frac{3 \cdot \triangle V_{CM} \cdot R_{CM}}{8 \cdot C_W \cdot R_{CW}}\right) \cdot C_M + V_{REF} \tag{13.2}$$

$$C_W = \frac{C_{M,max}}{1.6} \tag{13.3}$$

The operation principle of the CAV444 sheet can be found in the datasheet by Analog Microelectronics. CAV444 has a wide capacitor measurement range and linear transfer behavior. Changing the *f/V* converter capacitor (CW) alters the measurement range and the resolution of the circuit. The printed circuit board (PCB) design is shown in Fig. 13.10c. The dimensions of the PCB are 4.5 cm 2.3 cm. CW is proportional to the measurement range and inversely proportional to the resolution. Four values (62, 100, 220, and 330 pF) of CW were selected to verify this relationship, and the output responses of the detection circuit were measured. The output characteristics of the circuit with various CWs are shown in Fig. 13.10d. The maximum value of capacitance can be estimated from the saturation voltage of this circuit (4.5 V) and the corresponding values of CWs. The

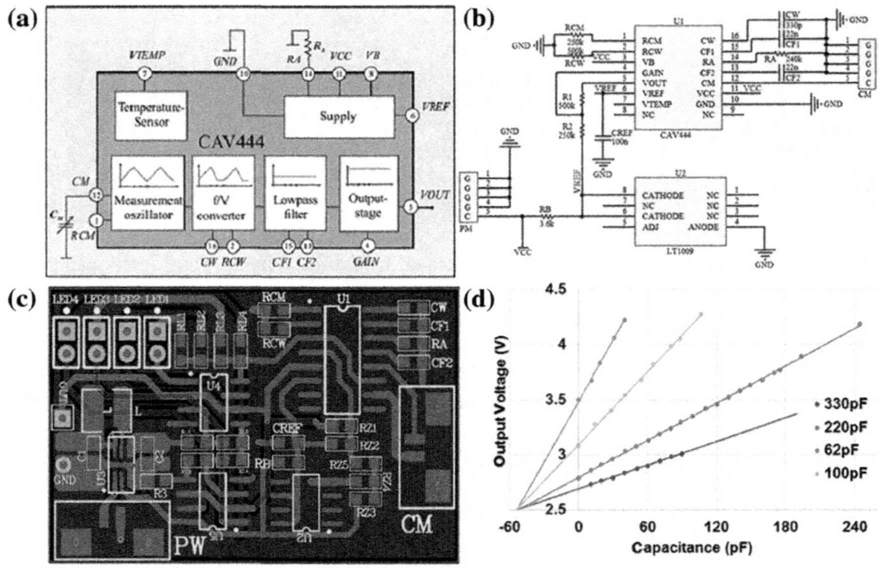

Fig. 13.10 Design of measurement circuit [33]. **a** Block diagram of CAV 444, **b** schematic of circuit, **c** PCB design, and **d** output characteristics of circuit with various *f/V* converter capacitors. Circuit has stray capacitance of 53 pF. All pictures reproduced with permission

empirical equation of the relationship between CW and CM with a correlation coefficient of 0.9978 was obtained as:

$$C_{\mathrm{M,max}} = 1.6442C_{\mathrm{W}} - 44.974 \tag{13.4}$$

The values of stray capacitance of the detection circuit were obtained using Eqs. (13.3) and (13.4). Figure 13.10d shows that the circuit had a stray capacitance of 53 pF, which would affect the measurement range of the circuit.

13.10.4 Performance of Liquid Metal Capacitor Sensors

Equation (13.1) indicates that the capacitance of the sensor is proportional to the area of the electrode. Measurements of eight samples of liquid metal capacitor sensors (each sample was measured five times using a Victor 6013 digital capacitance multimeter) are shown in Table 13.1. The average capacitance per unit area of the capacitor is 0.077 pF/mm^2, with a standard deviation of 0.0017 pF/mm^2. Using Eq. (13.1), the relative dielectric constant of each sample capacitance sensor is about 4.348, which is almost equal to the relative dielectric constant of 3M VHB tape (about 4.35), proving the stability of the capacitor sensor. Five multilayer samples were tested. The capacitance increased three-fold (0.23 pF/mm^2, with a

Table 13.1 Stability test of single-layer capacitor sensor [33]

Sample	Area (mm^2)	Mean of capacitance value (pF)	Standard deviation	Dielectric constant	Average capacitance per unit area (pF/mm^2)
1	392.68	31.48	0.098	4.529	0.080167057
2	526.04	38.94	0.445	4.182	0.074024789
3	465.66	36.26	0.120	4.399	0.077867972
4	463.32	34.14	0.242	4.163	0.073685574
5	591.53	45.56	0.102	4.351	0.077020608
6	1116.58	86.66	0.120	4.385	0.077611994
7	1183.81	92.50	0.141	4.415	0.078137671
8	380.00	29.32	0.744	4.359	0.077157895

standard deviation of 0.007 pF/mm^2) in this design compared to the single-layer design under the same area of electrodes. This was due to the additional two layers of 3M VHB tape, which served as the dielectric material. Sensitivity was improved by the increase in the change of the sensor's capacitance to strain.

Repetitive tests were conducted on the liquid metal capacitor sensor, with results shown in Table 13.2. The capacitance values of eight samples were recorded after stretching various numbers of times. The capacitor sensor was proven to be stretchable. It was stretched over 500 times with little influence on performance. This was due to the liquid form of GaInSn giving the sensor a certain degree of self-healing ability. The frequency response of the stretchable capacitor sensor was characterized. The results show that the capacitor sensor had a quick response (<10 ms) to strain. As shown in Fig. 13.11a, the abscissa represents time and the frequency can be observed by the time, the output voltage showed the corresponding change to the frequency response. The output voltage was measured using the CAV444 measurement circuit and recorded using an Agilent 34970A data acquisition unit.

Table 13.2 Repetitive tests of single-layer capacitor sensor [33]

Sample	Capacitance value after sensor stretched different numbers of times (pF)					
	0	100	200	300	400	500
1	31.3	31.4	31.5	31.5	31.5	31.6
2	39.2	39.0	39.4	38.8	39.4	38.9
3	36.2	36.1	36.2	36.2	36.2	36.5
4	33.7	33.9	34.3	34.1	34.2	34.4
5	45.5	45.5	45.6	45.4	45.6	45.7
6	86.8	86.7	86.6	86.5	86.8	86.6
7	92.6	92.6	92.5	92.7	92.4	92.3
8	29.0	28.7	30.0	29.8	29.8	28.0

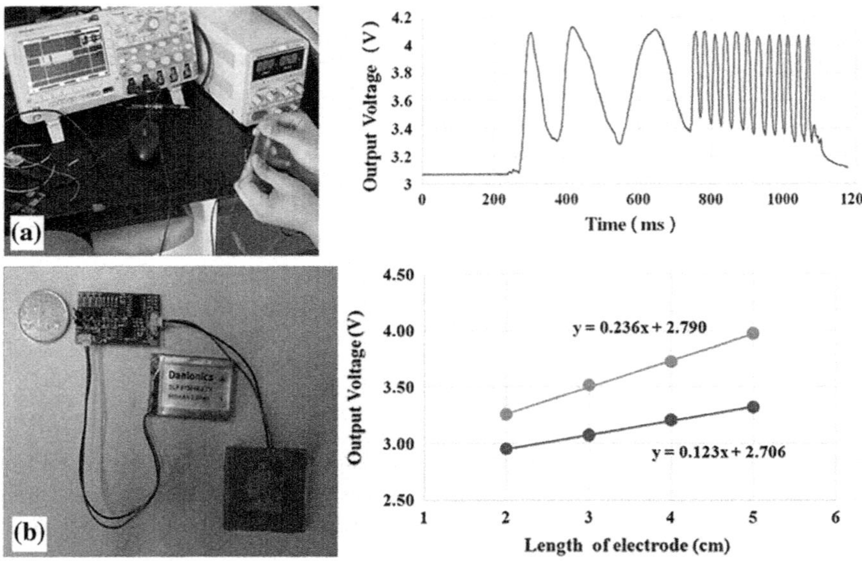

Fig. 13.11 Tests of liquid metal capacitor sensor [33]. **a** Capacitor sensor was under different time and the frequency can then be observed (left), with output voltage showing corresponding change to frequency (right). **b** System used for stretching test of single- and multilayer capacitor sensors (left) and linear correlation of stretch data recorded for these sensors (right). All pictures reproduced with permission

13.10.5 Sensitivity of Liquid Metal Capacitor Sensors

Single-and multilayer capacitor sensors were used in the strain test. They both had square electrodes (2 cm × 2 cm). The output voltages were recorded while the sensors were stretched to 3, 4, and 5 cm in a given direction, respectively. The tests were repeated 10 times. The output voltages were statistically analyzed. Figure 13.11b shows that both sensors had a good linear relationship to stretching and that the multilayer capacitor sensor had twice the sensitivity of the single-layer capacitor sensor. For the single-layer capacitor sensor, the linear regression formula is $V = 0.1235L + 2.7063$, and the correlation coefficient is 0.999, where L is the length of the electrode and V is the voltage. For the multilayer capacitor sensor, the linear regression formula is $V = 0.2365L + 2.7905$, and the correlation coefficient is 0.998.

13.10.6 Typical Applications of Liquid Metal Capacitor Sensors

To further explore the practical use of the liquid metal capacitor sensor for monitoring physiological motion signals, two bending tests (from 0° to 90°) at different parts of the human body were performed 10 times. First, a circular capacitor sensor with a diameter of 30 mm was pasted on the wrist, as shown in Fig. 13.12a. The angle of the wrist is defined in Fig. 13.12b for quantitative analysis of the relationship between a rotating wrist and capacitance value. The relationship between the angle of the wrist and the output voltage of the CAV444 measurement circuit (CW = 220 pF) is shown in Fig. 13.12c. The statistics results show that they had a good linear relationship. The linear regression formula is $y = 0.0012^* \times x + 3.245$, where x is the angle of the wrist and y is the measurement voltage, with a correlation coefficient of 0.996. A smaller capacitor sensor with square electrodes (25 mm × 25 mm) was then pasted on a finger joint, as shown in Fig. 13.12d. The measurement voltage (CW = 100 pF) was recorded while the finger was being bent. The linear regression analysis of the recorded data is shown in Fig. 13.12e. The linear regression formula is $y = 0.0012 \times x + 3.6347$, with a correlation coefficient of 0.986. As it was shown in the experiment, a liquid metal capacitor sensor with an LED was used to demonstrate its tensile properties. The LED lights up successively as the stretching increases. Further, various levels of stress were applied to the sensors. The tests were repeated three times. As shown in Fig. 13.13, there was a very good linear relationship between pressure applied and capacitance value. The linear regression formula is $y = 0.597x + 60.43$, with a correlation

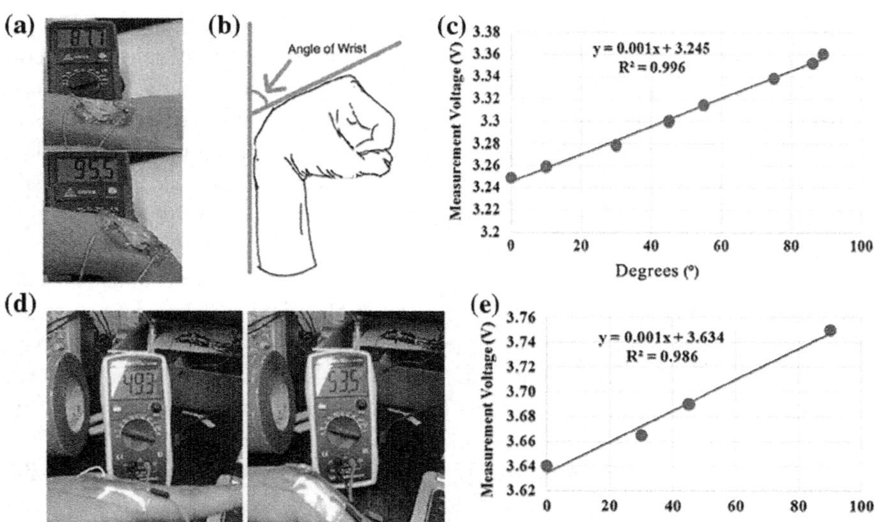

Fig. 13.12 Complete dynamic analysis of wrist and finger joint movement [33]. **a** Capacitance of sensor changed when wrist was rotated. **b** Definition of angle of wrist. **c** Linear correlation of measurement voltage of CAV444 circuit (CW = 220 pF) and angle of wrist, with linear regression formula of $A = 799.8 \times V - 2595.5$. **d** Capacitance changed when finger was bent. **e** Linear correlation of measurement voltage of CAV444 circuit (CW = 100 pF) and angle of finger joint, with linear regression formula of $A = 770.2 \times V - 2794.1$. All pictures reproduced with permission

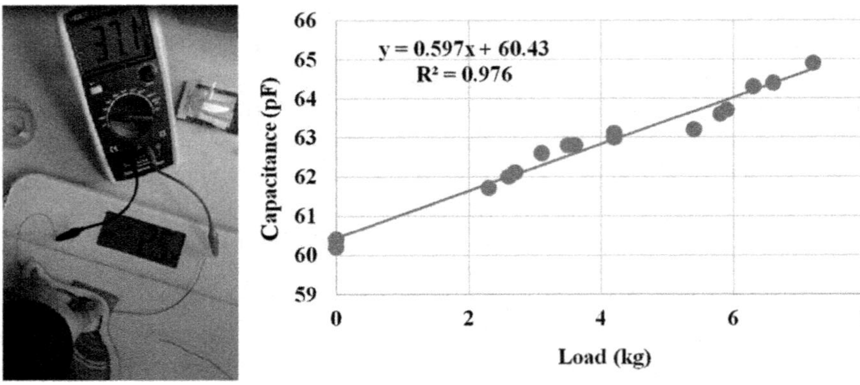

Fig. 13.13 Linear correlation of three sets of data from pressure test, showing good linear relationship between loads applied and capacitance change [33]. All pictures reproduced with permission

coefficient of 0.976. This indicates that the proposed capacitor sensor has potential to be used as a pressure sensor. Further, a liquid metal capacitor sensor with an LED was also used to demonstrate its pressure properties. The LED lights up successively as the pressure increases.

The above study illustrated a capacitor sensor based on the liquid metal. The use of a liquid metal as deformable capacitive plates offers unique benefits over conventional solid components, such as robustness to cracking and fatigue. Such sensor is also easy to fabricate, low-cost, and robust, uses non-toxic components, has a large degree of flexibility, and allows repeatable measurements. The sandwich structure and multilayer design give the sensor stable electrical properties, especially the multilayer design, which triples the performance of the single-layer capacitor sensor design (0.23 pF/mm^2 vs. 0.077 pF/mm^2). This design method and the capacitance values can provide a reference for flexible/stretchable capacitor design. The multilayer design gives good enough electrical properties when circuit noise is large. The stretching sensitivity of different designs was quantitatively analyzed. The multilayer capacitor sensor had twice the sensitivity compared to that of the single-layer capacitor sensor. The multilayer design outperformed the single-layer design and should be preferable for future designs.

Another merit of this work is that it proves the feasibility of fabricating flexible sensors using a very simple method. Because all tests were conducted at room temperature, and the humidity is almost constant, the test results were not influenced by temperature or humidity. Factors such as stain or pressure are two ways to change the capacitance and they do not affect each other for measuring related parameters. After 500 cycles, the baseline capacitance and sensitivity did not drift.

It is also worth mentioning that the packaging of the sensor enables the electrodes to work on the skin without direct contact, thus avoiding the direct effect of the liquid metal on the human body. This is quite beneficial for developing an attachable or wearable biomedical device for physiological tests. The performance of the capacitor sensor can be further improved. For example, the production process can be improved by introducing other technologies, such as mask printing, lithography, micro-channel technology, and 3D printing. The selection of other advanced dielectric materials can also improve sensor performance. The capacitor sensor shape can be changed to adapt to different uses.

13.11 Liquid Metal Based Printable Thermocouple

Temperature measurement is commonly needed in biomedical areas. If fully explored, the liquid metals can also be adopted to make such sensors. Li et al. [35] had ever proposed a way for the direct printing of thermocouples based on liquid metal. Their fabricated temperature sensor composed of gallium and its matching metal exhibited excellent linear dependence between thermoelectric voltage and temperature within the range from 0 to 200 °C. It was disclosed that liquid metals with high purity could be used for high precision thermocouples with tiny size, which were quite convenient for micro channel measurement due to their fluidity in making sensors; while liquid metals with a small amount of oxides were handy for depositing on the substrate by "hand-written" style, with thin film thickness of approximately 50 μm.

Temperature measurement on the micro- or nano- scale has been a challenging but critically important task in many physical, chemical, and material science areas. Among various temperature sensing methods, platinum temperature sensors and thermocouple (especially thin film one) are commonly used. Platinum is a noble metal, temperature sensors made by which have high precision but cost too much. On the other hand, the qualities of the thin film are greatly influenced by the substrates and the fabrication process, which increases the complexity in making thin film thermocouples.

The sensing characteristics of liquid metal materials have important value in many measurement situations. Previously, Ga-filled carbon nanotubes and mercury have been presented as temperature sensors, based on the principle of contact resistance and thermal expansion of a liquid metal with respect to temperature increment, respectively. Both methods are useful. However, fabrication of such tiny thermocouples is rather difficult. A more flexible approach, recurring to which the thermocouples can be fabricated with an extremely simple structure and in very tiny scale, should be developed with the potential for nano- or micro scale measurements.

Based on the concept of directly printing the thermocouple by using the liquid metal ink [35], the fabricated thermocouple offers certain distinctive advantages, such as little contact thermal and electric resistance, no need to weld, easy integration with various substrates without pretreatment, and could function over a wide range of temperature. Such sensors show a potential to be widely adopted in a broad range of applications, especially in nano- or micro scale areas for temperature measurements.

In Li et al.'s study [35], gallium with 99.99% purity (hereinafter referred to Ga for simplicity) and Ga with 0.25 wt% Ga oxides were used as samples, while constantan, two types of tungsten-rhenium alloys (WRe_5 and WRe_{26}), as well as $GaIn_{21.5}$ eutectic alloy (weight percentage, Ga 78.5 wt%, In 21.5 wt%), were chosen as matching metals, respectively. It should be noted that 0.25 wt% is the minimum content of the oxides in liquid metal to warrant that the liquid metal ink can be written directly on the paper continuously. The samples of Ga with 0.25 wt% Ga oxides dispersed uniformly were prepared by a controlled oxidation reaction method, and the corresponding gallium-indium eutectic alloy with 0.25 wt% Ga oxides was prepared in the same way. In this case, all liquid metal samples were encapsulated into the 14# silicone tube with inner diameter of 1.6 mm to prevent further oxidation, and all the tube ends were sealed with 704 silicon rubber.

Figure 13.14 depicts the schematic of the experimental setup, which characterizes a typical thermocouple connection for measuring Seebeck effect [35]. As is well understood in the thermocouple art, when heat is applied to one junction of a thermocouple to bring it to an elevated temperature, while the other junction is kept at a lower temperature, thereby electro-motive force (emf) is generated in the thermoelements and proportional to the temperature difference between the junctions, which can be described in accordance with Kirchhoff's voltage law:

$$S_A \cdot (T_h - T_c) + S_C \cdot (T_c - T_v) + \text{emf} + S_C \cdot (T_v - T_c) + S_B \cdot (T_c - T_h) = 0, \tag{13.5}$$

where, S_A, S_B are the Seebeck coefficients of thermocouple wire materials, S_C is the Seebeck coefficient of the wire used in the voltage measuring circuit, T_h is the temperature at the hot junction, T_c is the temperature at the cold junction (assumed as the same for both wires), T_v is the internal temperature of all the voltmeter circuit elements.

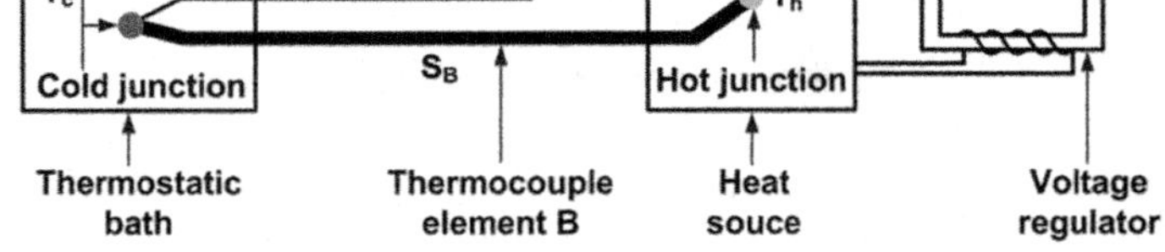

Fig. 13.14 Schematic diagram of the experimental setup [35]. Thermocouple elements refer to liquid Ga and matching metal wires including constantan, WRe_5, WRe_{26}, and $GaIn_{21.5}$. Heating power of heat souce was kept at 50 W. Picture reproduced with permission

Rearranging and simplifying Eq. (13.5), one has:

$$\mathrm{emf} = (S_A - S_B) \cdot (T_h - T_c) \quad (13.6)$$

As is well known, Seebeck effect consists of the basic principle of the thermocouples, which can be explained by theories of electron diffusion within a material's molecular structure due to the temperature gradient in a conductor or a semiconductor. To gauge the magnitude of this effect, Seebeck coefficient (also called thermal power) is introduced. The voltage across each metal element depends on its Seebeck coefficient so that the potential difference between the two wires will depend on $S_A - S_B$ based on Eq. (13.6), and $S_{AB} = S_A - S_B$ is defined as the thermoelectric power for the thermocouple pair A-B.

It can be deduced that the voltage of the two measuring wires (WRe_{26} alloy wires here) is the emf as long as the cold junctions are both at temperature T_c, and the elements in the voltmeter circuit are both at temperature T_v. Here, the heat source consisted of a copper block and a heating rod, which was powered from a voltage regulator. The open ends were connected to voltage measuring wires, with the junctions immersed in a water-bath at 40 °C. Type T thermocouples were used to record the temperatures at the respective locations of the system, whose accuracy of ±0.5 °C primarily determined the precision of the system. The hot and cold junction temperatures, as shown in Fig. 13.14, as well as the generated emf were monitored by an Agilent 34970A. Proper precautions were taken to prevent solidification of liquid Ga. Tests were performed by raising the heat source temperature with the voltage regulator at the constant power of 50 W, and triplicate temperature measurements were made precisely at the same location for each thermocouple pair in ambient air.

Figure 13.15 presents the voltage–temperature difference profiles of the thermocouples consisting of Ga and the matching metal wires. It is apparent that all these thermocouples exhibit nearly linear behavior in the experimented temperature range, but the slopes (S_{AB}) differ greatly due to large distinction of Seebeck coefficients, as shown in Table 13.3. Linear curves fitting to the experimental data show an average slope of 47.64 μV/°C for Ga-constantan thermocouple, which is very similar to conventional wire thermocouples, just a little smaller than that of Type T thermocouple (51 μV/°C) but bigger than that of Type K thermocouple (41 μV/°C). In comparison, S_{AB} of Ga-WRe_{26} and Ga-$GaIn_{21.5}$ thermocouples were considerably smaller (1.27 and 0.11 μV/°C, respectively). Thus, it can be concluded that the thermocouple consisting of Ga and constantan is much more responsive. The main reason can be inferred as that the Seebeck coefficients of Ga and WRe_{26} are closer to each other compared to those of Ga and constantan. As a result, a smaller thermoelectric power is obtained. The case of Ga and liquid $GaIn_{21.5}$ can also be explained in the same way.

As for the cases with Ga oxides, similar situations are demonstrated in the first three cases that contained solid metal wires, and even no obvious discrepancy is exhibited compared to those without Ga oxides. This could be explained by the fact that in the first three cases, the Seebeck coefficient of solid metal is rather larger or

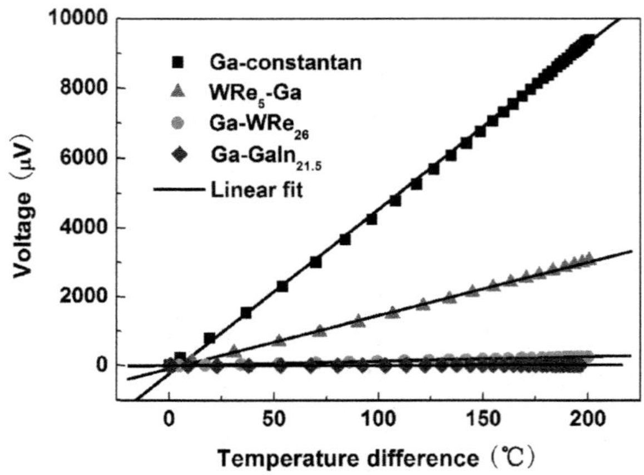

Fig. 13.15 Measured thermoelectric voltage as a function of temperature difference between Ga and constantan, WRe_5, WRe_{26}, and $GaIn_{21.5}$, respectively [35]. The diameters of WRe_5, WRe_{26} and constantan wires were 0.5 mm, while the diameters of Ga and $GaIn_{21.5}$ were 1.6 mm, respectively. The accuracy of thermocouples was ±0.5 °C. Picture reproduced with permission

Table 13.3 Linear fit parameter values for different thermocouple pairs [35]

Parameter	Ga-constantan	WRe_5-Ga	Ga-WRe_{26}	Ga-$GaIn_{21.5}$
S_{AB} (μV/°C)	47.64	15.41	1.27	0.11
R^2	0.9990	0.9985	0.9996	0.9929

smaller than the Seebeck coefficient of gallium, and thus, the former becomes dominating, resulting in an imperceptible nuances of the thermoelectric power when the latter alters slightly with the oxides added in. Figure 13.16a shows the situation adopting WRe_{26}, which could be a representative of these three cases. However, when two liquid metals are used for constituting a thermocouple, as shown in Fig. 13.16b, more complex situation arises. In the case of Ga-$GaIn_{21.5}$ thermocouple, the open circuit may occur during temperature-rise period sometimes, and will restore connectivity during temperature-drop period. This situation is even more frequent when oxides exist in liquid metals. Moreover, the existence of oxides also leads to an increase of average slope by 27%, which was meaningful at the temperature difference range that above 50 °C. The increase could also be explained by the clarification that Seebeck coefficients of gallium and $GaIn_{21.5}$ alloy were all changed when oxides are added and both of them are close to each other, thus, no one can dominate. Consequently, the thermoelectric power was influenced strongly by the addition of the gallium oxides. There still should be mentioned that the slopes of the voltage–temperature curves of these thermocouples are nearly identical after repeated cycling, indicating excellent stability and reproducibility over the course of multiple cycles.

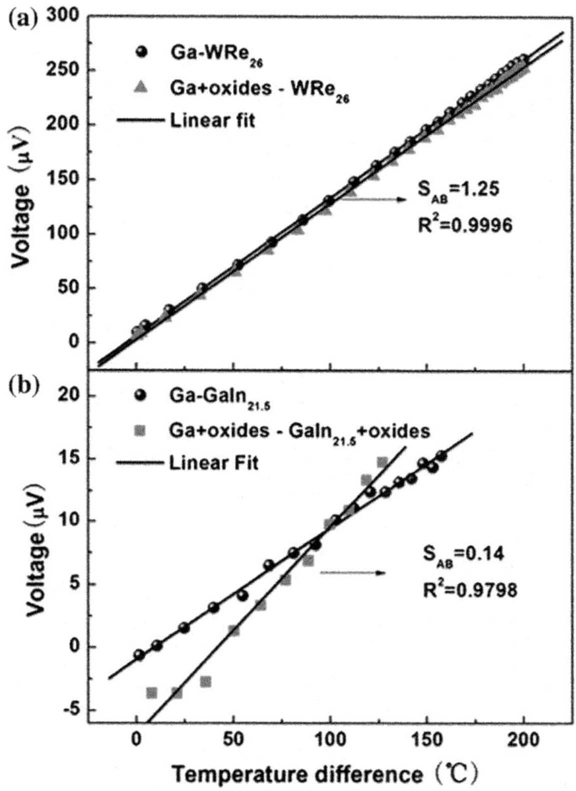

Fig. 13.16 Measured thermoelectric voltage [35] as a function of temperature difference between **a** Ga-WRe_{26} thermocouple and Ga with 0.25 wt% Ga oxides—WRe_{26} thermocouple, as well as **b** Ga-$GaIn_{21.5}$ thermocouple and Ga with 0.25 wt% Ga oxides—$GaIn_{21.5}$ with 0.25 wt% Ga oxides, respectively. The diameters of WRe_{26} wires are 0.5 mm, while the diameters of Ga and $GaIn_{21.5}$ were 1.6 mm, respectively. The accuracy of thermocouples was ±0.5 °C. All pictures reproduced with permission

The thermoelectric response is a complex function of the imposed thermal gradient, the Seebeck coefficient, and the surrounding environment [36]. The Seebeck coefficient of Ga has been discussed half a century ago [37], which stated that Ga had positive Seebeck coefficient which was close to zero in the temperature range from 330 to 660 K. This means that electrons migrate from cold to hot end of the Ga conductor. In the case of commercial WRe_5-WRe_{26} thermocouple pair, WRe_5 is generally taken as positive polarity while WRe_{26} as negative polarity. The difference between WRe_5 and WRe_{26} in the Seebeck coefficient may be explained as follows. If the stoichiometric ratio of rhenium to tungsten is different, it would affect the corresponding thermoelectric properties. But in the case of WRe_5-Ga thermocouple pair, WRe_5 and Ga act as positive and negative polarity, respectively. As for the Ga-WRe_{26} and Ga-constantan thermocouple pair's cases, Ga is proven to be positive polarity. Based on these findings, one could arrange the experimented metals in a thermoelectric series: constantan, WRe_{26}, $GaIn_{21.5}$, Ga, WRe_5. In this series, the two metals forming a thermocouple are apart further, emf of the thermocouple is greater. Also, the direction of the current at the hot junction is from the metal lying in the front of this series to the metal lying in its back. Considering the fact that the position of a metal in this series is dependent upon the temperature and also somewhat upon its purity, the application in the occasion outside the experimental temperature range should be checked carefully. Besides Ga, the Seebeck coefficients of other liquid metals could also be found in [37]. Consequently, the Seebeck coefficients of thermocouples consisting of various liquid metals and corresponding matching metals could be deduced in the same way. It is also well known that the Seebeck coefficient is independent of the shape and size of each thermocouple element, so the liquid metal element could be encapsulated into more tiny tubes, such as carbon nano tube, or directly prints on the substrate with thin film thickness in micro scale (when oxides exists), as illustrated in Fig. 13.17. On the other hand, environmental conditions such as stress, chemical corrosion, radiation, etc. may affect molecular structure anywhere along the length of the thermocouple wire, thus errors can be created. For example, thermocouples with liquid metals are subject to severe oxidation at elevated temperatures, which may cause errors. Therefore, measures such as vacuum casing are necessary at elevated temperature measurement in the near future.

Overall, the thermocouples formed by gallium and matching metal exhibit excellent linear behavior in the temperature difference range from 0 to 200 °C. Owing to its wide temperature range of liquid metals in the liquid state, it could be predicted that the measurable temperature range can be extended to over 2000 °C as long as vacuum casing is equipped to cut off oxygen. The thermocouples based on pure liquid metals have inherent liquidity and excellent linear dependences on temperature with high accuracy, which are appropriate for precision measurement in microfluidic pipeline; while the thermocouples consisting of liquid metals with a small amount of oxides will give rise to "hand-written" thermometric element with accuracy guaranteed by calibration, which will lead to the emergence of a printable temperature sensor. The adhesion of liquid metal ink to various surfaces including

Fig. 13.17 The Ga with 0.25 wt% Ga oxides—$GaIn_{21.5}$ with 0.25 wt% Ga oxides thermocouple printed on the paper by "hand-written" style with thin film thickness of approximately 50 μm [35]. Picture reproduced with permission

ceramics is proportional to the content of oxides in the liquid metal. And it is very convenient to fabricate such liquid metal ink by a simple oxidation reaction within only several minutes. Owing to such flexibility, these thermocouples are relatively easy to fabricate, and are suitable for micro- or nano- measurement in restricted space or temporary condition. Further modifications to the thermocouple elements could result in a larger responsivity so that higher thermoelectric power could be attained. There is one problem which should be noted that excessive oxidation may affect properties of the thermocouples, so special steps are necessary to prevent this situation, such as vacuum casing, just like tungsten-rhenium thermocouple. There still exist some other barriers that hinder the application of thermocouple formed by two liquid metals, such as reversible open circuit, shorter temperature range, etc., which needs additional efforts. Once these thermocouples are put into use, the micro thermopiles based on liquid metals could even be directly printed on target substrate in the near future.

13.12 Fabrication of Flexible Sensor System via Liquid Metal Dual-Trans Printing

Flexible electronics, which allow electronic circuits to respond with elasticity under mechanical deformation while maintaining their normal functions, have kept attracting intensive attentions over the past few years, especially for some newly emerging consumer electronics and biomedical application purposes. To date, the design and fabrication of the flexible electronics have involved many state-of-art innovations on both materials and manufacture strategies, among which two main approaches have been particularly adopted [38]. One most popular way is to uniformly mix tiny conductors such as nano-particles or metal droplets with elastomeric matrices. Another basic solution relies on the use of various wavy structures [39], while the conductive materials could be conventional thin enough copper or gold wires. Such methods significantly enable the flexible circuits with more performances and functions.

As an alternative, the liquid metal such as gallium or its alloy with indium, tin, zinc and so on directly provides a conductive metal ink that could stay in liquid phase under room temperature. Meanwhile, various techniques that targeted for patterning the liquid metal have also been put forward [38]. However, due to the alloy's high surface tension and heavy density, it still remains a challenge to pattern the liquid metal with sufficient time-efficiency, precision and robustness on a soft substrate to fulfill various specific needs, especially for making functional circuits which usually have to deal with plenty of components, arbitrary turns and intersections.

The recently established tapping mode liquid metal delivery technique successfully improves the wettability of liquid metals on the substrates [40], which performs very well on the PVC (polyvinyl chloride) plastic film. As for soft substrate, the PDMS (Polydimethylsiloxane) features better elasticity and bio-compatibility. This makes it rather suitable for realizing flexible and biomedical applications. However, the static contact angle of the liquid metal on the cured PDMS is measured as 150° ± 2° [41], which implies low wettability. As a result, even when using this tapping mode direct printing, the results are still a little far from being favorable. The barely printed or written line turns to break arbitrarily, or deform easily due to the poor wettability.

As a remedy, Wang et al. [38] put forward a fabrication strategy termed as liquid metal dual-trans printing based on the liquid metal transfer printing and the freeze phase transition mechanism. It overcomes the obstacles as explained above and works much simpler and faster to fabricate flexible and functional circuits encased in the elastic substrates. The principle as it was presented shows a promising approach for individualized electronic design and manufacture with high compatibility to classical component and sensor techniques.

13.12.1 Transfer Printing Strategy of Liquid Metal Flexible Circuits

With the aid of the liquid metal printer (see Fig. 13.18), the functional liquid metal circuit can be directly printed on top of the PVC film, which serves as the primary substrate of the alloy ink. Then the circuit is covered with fluidic PDMS solution with various quantities as desired for making either a thin or thick substrate. After the PDMS is cured as the secondary substrate, the multi-layer structure is cooled down below the melting point of the metal, so that for the alloy to freeze and then the PVC film can be easily peeled off. After recovering to normal temperature, the PDMS would firmly hold the original shape of the liquid metal circuit and ensure its flexibility at the same time.

Regarding the flexibility of the PDMS-PVC, a schematic diagram for the analytical model of thermal stress for PDMS-PVC structure is shown in Fig. 13.19.

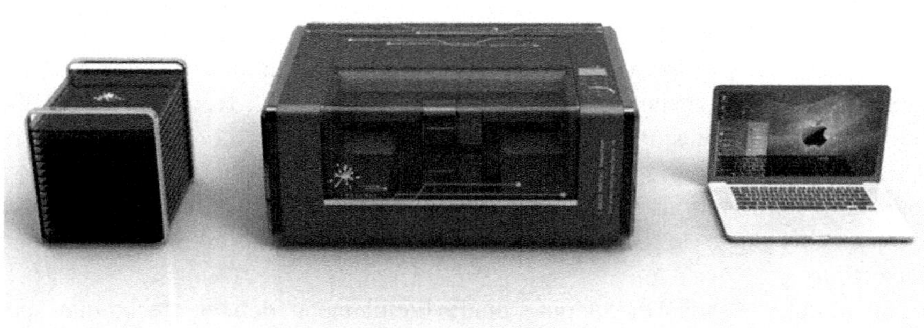

Fig. 13.18 The appearance of the liquid metal printer system, developed in the present lab at Technical Institute of Physics and Chemistry, Chinese Academy of Science

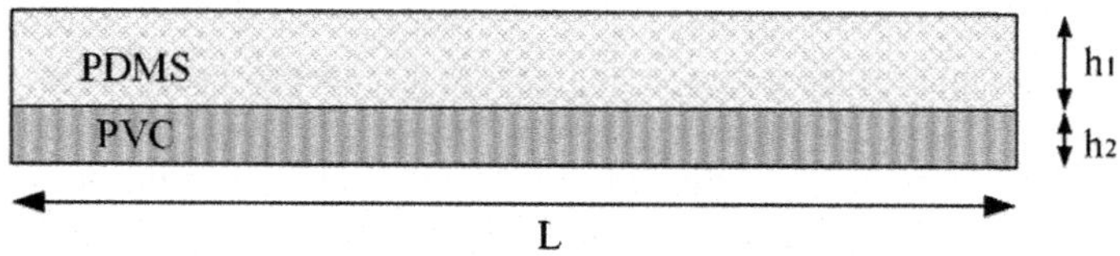

Fig. 13.19 Schematic diagram of PDMS-PVC model for thermal stress analysis

The contraction lengths caused by the temperature change in PDMS and PVC without considering the thermal stress are expressed as

$$\Delta l_1 = \alpha_1 L \Delta T \tag{13.7}$$

$$\Delta l_2 = \alpha_2 L \Delta T \tag{13.8}$$

where, α is the coefficient of thermal expansion, L is the initial length and ΔT is the temperature decrease. Before the separation, the relative position equilibrium gives

$$\Delta l_1 - \sigma_1 L / E_1 = \Delta l_2 + \sigma_2 L / E_2 \tag{13.9}$$

where, σ is the thermal stress and E the elastic modulus. According to force equilibrium, it gives

$$\sigma_1 h_1 = \sigma_2 h_2 \tag{13.10}$$

where, h is the thickness.

Therefore,

$$\sigma_1 = \frac{(\alpha_1 - \alpha_2) E_1 E_2 \Delta T}{(E_2 + E_1 h_1 / h_2)} \tag{13.11}$$

$$\sigma_2 = \frac{(\alpha_1 - \alpha_2) E_1 E_2 \Delta T}{(E_2 h_2 / h_1 + E_1)} \tag{13.12}$$

The typical values for all the parameters are listed as follows:

$$\begin{aligned} \alpha_1 &= 9.07 \times 10^{-4}\ \mathrm{K}^{-1} \\ \alpha_2 &= 2.9 \times 10^{-5}\ \mathrm{K}^{-1} \\ E_1 &= 1.8\ \mathrm{MPa} \\ E_2 &= 2000\ \mathrm{MPa} \\ h_1 &= 300\ \mu\mathrm{m} \\ h_2 &= 175\ \mu\mathrm{m} \\ \Delta T &= 75\ \mathrm{K} \end{aligned}$$

In detail, there are two manipulating sequences for the dual-trans printing according to whether the circuit components are incorporated after or before peeling. Figure 13.20 demonstrates the major steps of both the "after peeling" and "before peeling" approaches with the cross-sections of the multi-layer structure shown at each stage. For the "after peeling" approach (Fig. 13.20a), the liquid metal

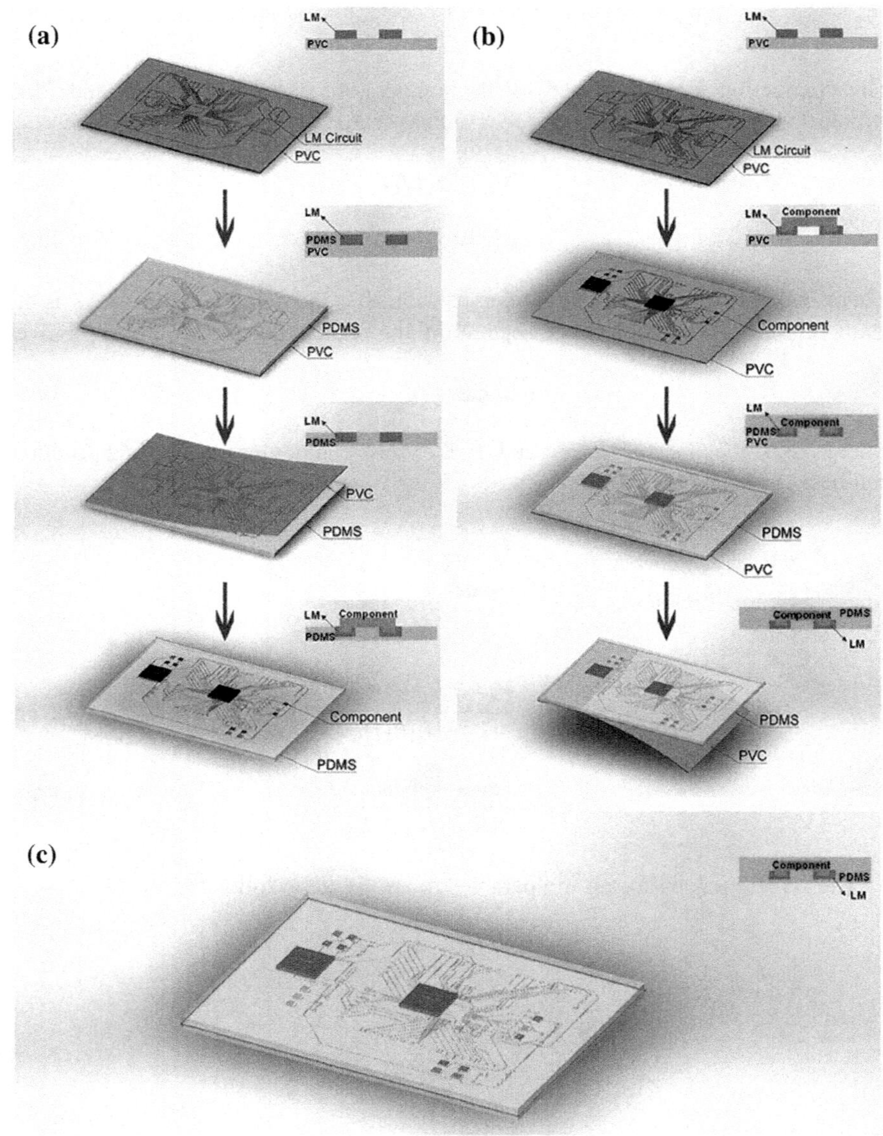

Fig. 13.20 Schematic illustrations of the dual-trans printing fabrication process [38]. The right-hand side corner inset represents the cross-sections of the multi-layer structure at each stage. **a** Steps of "after-peeling" approach. **b** Steps of "before-peeling" approach. **c** Implementation of flexible liquid metal functional circuit encapsulated with PDMS. All pictures reproduced with permission

is printed as mirrored circuit pattern on the top of the PVC film which is then covered with liquid PDMS solution. After the PDMS is solidified, the multi-layer structure is cooled down to freeze the GaIn alloy and the PVC film can be peeled off. Then the liquid metal circuit layout embedded inside the PDMS is prepared, and the electronic components such as micro control units (MCUs), resistors and capacitors can be positioned to the circuit pads according to the layout design. During the manipulation, trace amounts of GaIn alloy can be added to the pins and pads as solder in order to enhance the connection between the components and the pads mechanically and electrically. Here, the role of the liquid metal is similar with the solder paste in the traditional PCB fabrication.

Figure 13.20b illustrates the steps for the "before peeling" approach. A bit different from the "after-peeling", there is no need to mirror the printed circuit pattern, because the electronic components are directly placed on the PVC substrate with the liquid metal layout, which also uses extra liquid metal solder. Then the liquid PDMS solution covers the liquid metal circuits together with the electronic components. When the PDMS is solidified, the liquid metal circuit is frozen to peel the PVC off the secondary substrate, yet with electronic components already inside this time. However, the liquid metal layout below a component sometimes may disconnect because of no PDMS protection, thus the "after peeling" sequence is preferred. Finally, the dual-trans printed electronics in either sequence is encapsulated with additional PDMS, and the flexible liquid metal functional circuit can then be implemented (Fig. 13.20c).

With the dual-trans printing, the liquid metal circuit can be easily embedded into the elastic substrate with good quality. Figure 13.21a shows the liquid metal circuit in the PDMS substrate with thickness of 300 μm fabricated by the dual-trans process. Each line is straight with uniform liquid metal, as displayed in Fig. 13.21b. Figure 13.21c depicts the profile of the liquid metal as printed on the PVC and covered by the PDMS. It can be seen that the liquid metal between the PVC and PDMS substrates is semi-oval, and the interface between the PDMS is cambered. The reason lies in that when the alloy is first printed onto the PVC film, the top of the printed liquid metal is convex due to fluidic surface tension and its good wettability to the PVC. When the covering PDMS is solidified and the PVC is peeled off, the cover naturally forms a channel in reverse, which ensures the robustness of the liquid metal layout in the transferred substrate.

During the transfer process, slight mechanical deformation might occur due to two possible reasons. One is the volume contraction of the PDMS film in the process of solidification, while another lies in the volume variations with the temperature for both the alloy and the substrate. Figure 13.21d, e compares the differences between the liquid metal lines directly printed on the top of the PVC film and those subsequently transferred into the PDMS. The results indicate that there is no evident change for these liquid metal lines printed with various widths and distances during the fabrication. In other words, the dual-trans printing method could ensure the same accuracy and precision with the original printed liquid metal patterns.

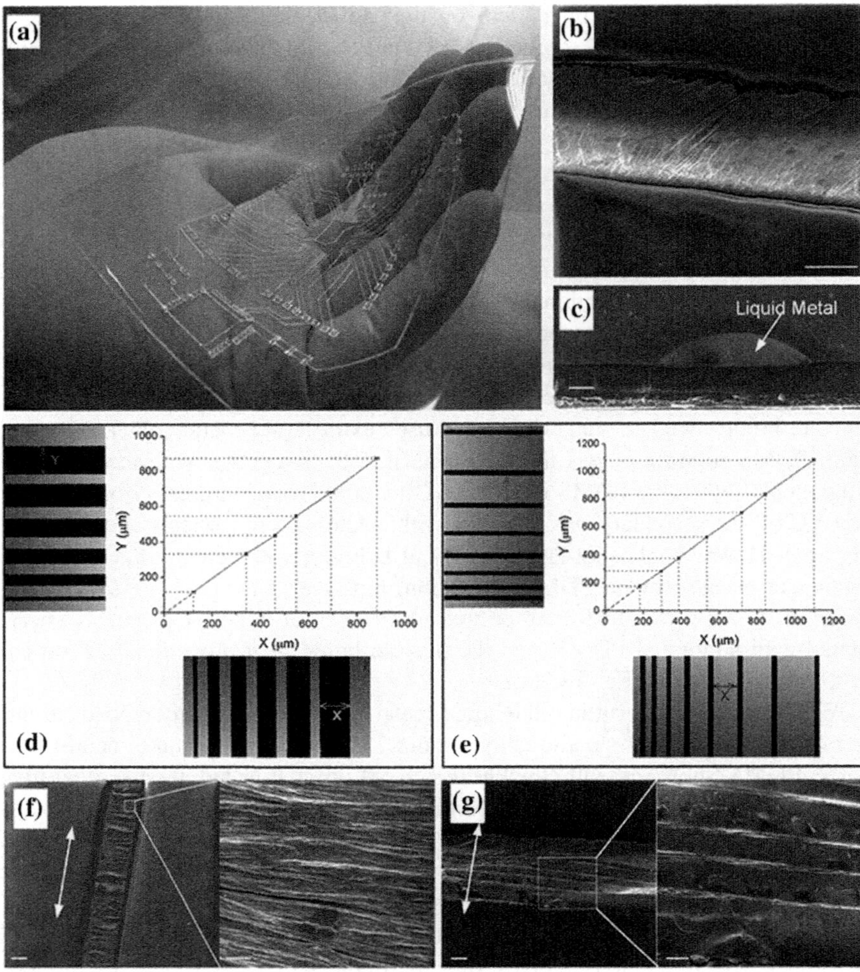

Fig. 13.21 Mechanical properties of the liquid metal lines fabricated by the dual-trans method [38]. **a** The image of the liquid metal circuit embedded in the PDMS substrate fabricated by the dual-trans printing process. **b** The SEM image of the top view of a liquid metal line embedded in the PDMS substrate. Scale bar, 100 μm. **c** The SEM image of transversal surface of a liquid metal line embedded in the PDMS substrate. Scale bar, 100 μm. **d** The widths of the liquid metal lines transferred to the PDMS substrate vs. the widths of the liquid metal lines originally printed on the PVC substrate. **e** The distances of the liquid metal lines transferred to the PDMS substrate versus the distances of the liquid metal lines originally printed on the PVC substrate. **f** The SEM image of the liquid metal line after stretching up to 130% of the original length along the axial direction for 100 times (the arrows represent the direction to stretch), and some wrinkles appear on the surface. Scale bar, 100 μm. The inset: scale bar, 10 μm. **g** The SEM image of the liquid metal line after stretching up to 110% along the radial direction for 100 times (the arrows represent the direction to stretch), and some wrinkles appear on the surface. Scale bar, 100 μm. The inset: scale bar, 25 μm. All pictures reproduced with permission

When the PDMS channel is stretched, the fluidity of the soft alloy allows to guarantee the stability of the flexible circuit connection. To prove that, several unenclosed PDMS films with liquid metal lines embedded are intentionally stretched for 100 times. As characterized by the scanning electron microscope (SEM) images in Fig. 13.21f, g, some wrinkles appear on the surface of the liquid metal perpendicular to the tensile direction after the repeatedly stretching movements. For the convenience to observe SEM, the liquid metal line has to be bared in the air, which will be oxidized on its surface. The wrinkles would form because the oxide layer breaks and regenerates during repeated stretching, which demonstrates that the liquid metal indeed deforms with the stretch of the PDMS channels. However, it ought to be noted that in the fabricated circuits, the alloy is encased in the PDMS substrate, which efficiently avoids the oxidization. Therefore, the encased metal will flow compliantly to the substrate's deformed site in the transferred channels, which also means the wrinkle phenomenon will not appear in that case. In addition, the change of relative resistance as a function of the number of the stretching cycles (Fig. 13.22) displays that the resistance variation is irregular yet within a range of 50%.

Here, the transfer phenomenon and principle are of particular focus. According to the comparative experiments, if the PVC is directly peeled off under normal temperature, the liquid metal could not be transferred to the PDMS substrate thoroughly. It would even spill out of the PDMS channels to destroy the circuit (Fig. 13.23a). While if performing freeze phase transition processing as proposed in

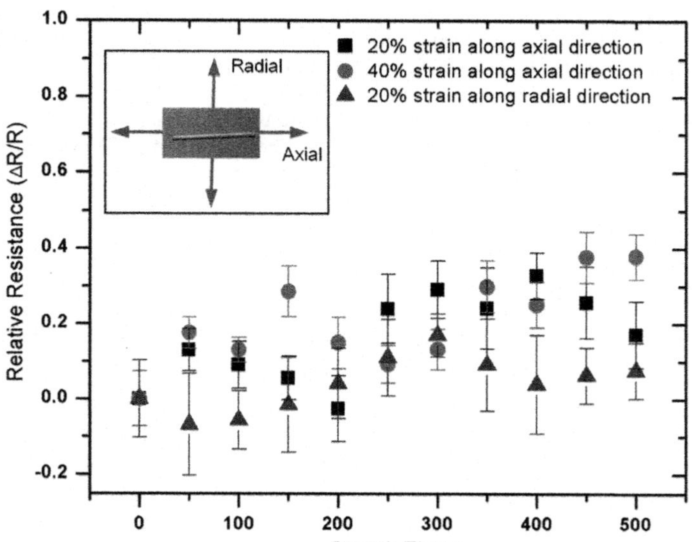

Fig. 13.22 Relative resistance change as a function of stretch times at various elongations [38]. The thickness of the PDMS substrate is 350 μm. The inset: Schematic diagram of the stain direction. Picture reproduced with permission

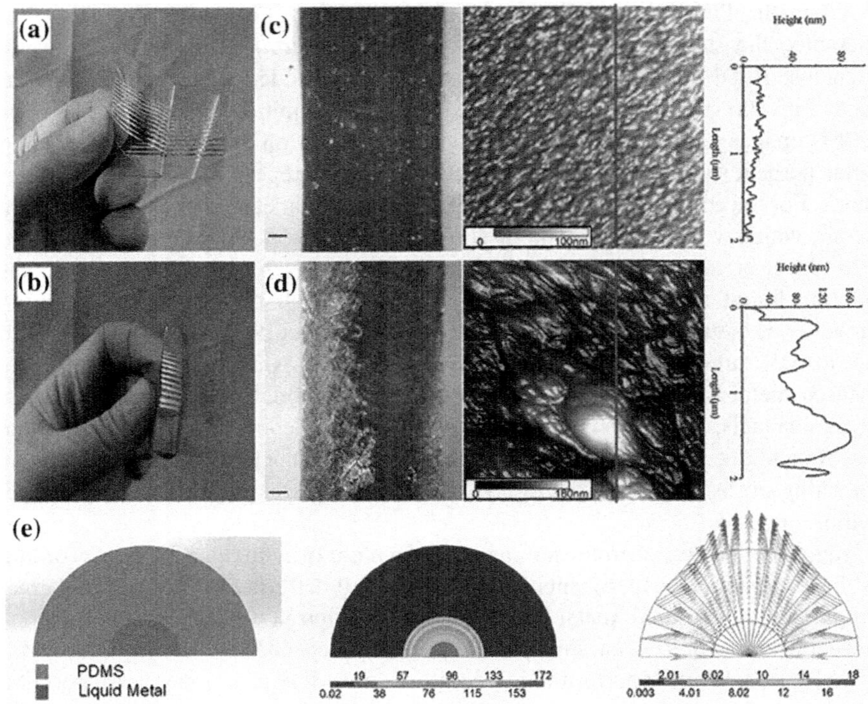

Fig. 13.23 Principle of freeze phase transition separation process in the dual-trans method [38]. **a** Peeling off the PVC substrate under normal temperature. **b** Peeling off the PVC substrate after the metal solidification. **c** Surface topography of interface between the PVC film and the liquid metal line. **d** Surface topography of interface between PDMS film and liquid metal line. In **c**, **d**, the left are the optical images of the contact surfaces of the liquid metal line meeting the PVC and the PDMS under the stereomicroscope, respectively. Scale bar, 100 μm. The middle are the AFM images of a 2 μm × 2 μm area captured by the atomic force microscope. The right curves are the variation in height across line in the middle images. **e** Simulation results of the thermal stress distribution (middle, the unit is MPa) and translation vector (right, the unit is μm) for the model (left), the temperature is decreased from 25 to −50 °C. All pictures reproduced with permission

current method, the PDMS and the whole solidified liquid metal circuit can be easily separated from the PVC substrate (Fig. 13.23b). Figure 13.24 provides a closer look for both cases via the optical microscope. Clearly, it indicates an almost complete removal of the metal without leaving any residue when it is frozen.

The mechanism can be interpreted as follows. Along with the decrease of the temperature, the PDMS and the PVC both contract. Yet, their different contraction coefficients will generate thermal stress on the interface between the two substrates. As a result, when the thermal stress becomes larger than the adhesion force, the two substrates can be separated easily.

Further, a pair of liquid metal patterns that are separately printed on the PVC and transferred to the PDMS in identical shape and size (10 mg, 2.0 mm × 2.0 mm)

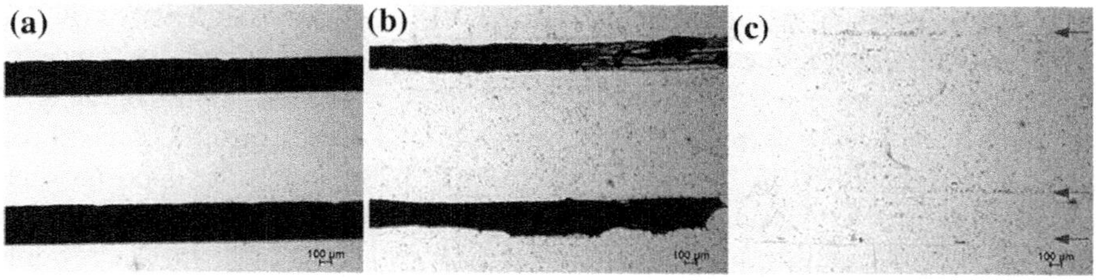

Fig. 13.24 Optical microscope images of the PVC substrate after different manipulations [38]. **a** The PVC substrate printed with liquid metal. **b** The PVC substrate directly peeled when the metal is in liquid phase. **c** The PVC substrate separated when the metal is frozen. The arrows indicate the residual traces of liquid metal lines. All pictures reproduced with permission

have been fabricated to measure the adhesion forces between the frozen alloy and the two substrates (as shown in Fig. 13.25). The results from the samples indicate that the adhesion force between the frozen metal and the flat PVC substrate is 4770 μN, while the frozen metal with similar shape and weight embedded in the PDMS film requires a tension of 0.87 N to be pulled off completely. Though the value and ratio for the adhesion forces in the real liquid metal circuits will be different due to varied specific shape and size of the liquid metal patterns, the results

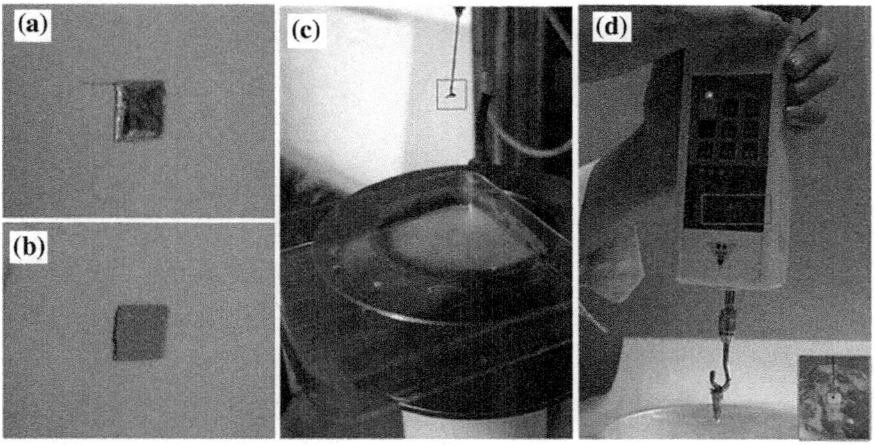

Fig. 13.25 The measurement of adhesion force for samples on different substrates [38]. **a** A liquid metal pattern in the shape of 2.0 mm × 2.0 mm square is printed on the PVC, which is prepared for measuring the adhesion force between frozen liquid metal and PVC substrate. **b** An identical liquid metal pattern in the shape of 2.0 mm × 2.0 mm square is transferred to the PDMS with the PVC off, which is prepared for measuring the adhesion force between frozen liquid metal and PDMS substrate. The 2.0 mm × 2.0 mm liquid metal pattern is transferred to the PDMS. **c** The adhesion force measurement with the dynamic contact angle measuring device and tensiometer. The probe has pulled the liquid metal off from the PVC. **d** The adhesion force measurement with the digital force gauge. The max tension value is displayed as 0.87 N. All pictures reproduced with permission

from the samples have undoubtedly proven the significant differences in the adhesion force magnitude between the two substrates. With the assistance of the stereomicroscope and the atomic force microscope (AFM), the topography of the contact surfaces between the PVC substrate and liquid metal line has been obtained and displayed in Fig. 13.23c. And Fig. 13.23d shows the opposite sides that towards the PDMS substrate. These images indicate that the surface between the PVC substrate and the metal is smooth and flat, while the other surface towards the PDMS substrate appears relatively rough. Besides, the contact area between PDMS substrate and the metal is much larger, which can be inferred from Fig. 13.21c. Thus when applying low temperature to solidify the alloy into a whole entity, it is the differences in shape and roughness of the two interfaces that dominate the significantly varied adhesion ability with the frozen metal. This leads to an easy transfer of the liquid metal.

What's more, without the encasing PDMS substrate, the frozen metal would not spontaneously separate from the PVC, but just keep its adhesion to the substrates (as shown in Fig. 13.26). The reasons of the spontaneous separation as indicated in Fig. 13.23b also include the thermal stress due to the temperature fall. Figure 13.23e depicts the results from a static finite element analysis of the situation between the solidified metal and the PDMS. After decreasing to a low temperature,

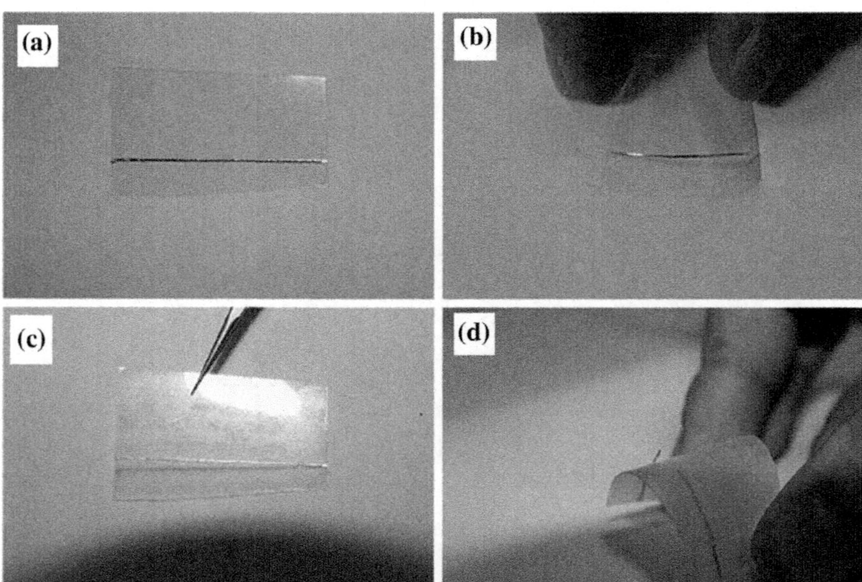

Fig. 13.26 The adhesion between the printed liquid metal and PVC substrate without the PDMS [38]. **a** The liquid metal line is printed on the PVC substrate at room temperature. **b** The liquid metal line bends with the PVC substrate at room temperature. **c** The metal line still adheres to the PVC surface when frozen. **d** The frozen metal line separates from the PVC easily when the PVC substrate is bent. These phenomena suggest that volumetric changes in the alloy due to phase transition do not cause spontaneous separation. All pictures reproduced with permission

the thermal tension at the interface between the PDMS and the metal becomes stronger, which would hold the metal tightly. Meanwhile, the PDMS tends to transform along the vectors to the center and move up. While the metal-PVC interface is flat and smooth, the adhesion force is not strong enough to drag the frozen metal out of the PDMS channels. All the above effects lead to the consequence that the PDMS substrate and the liquid metal circuit separate from the PVC substrate successfully.

13.12.2 Liquid Metal Flexible Circuits for Wireless Communication with Mobile Phone

To demonstrate the good performance of the flexible consumer electronics, a transparent band has been particularly implemented by using the above fabrication strategy [38] (see more details in Figs. 13.27 and 13.28). As shown in Fig. 13.29a, the band is 20 cm long and 2 cm wide. Eight LEDs are connected to an MCU chip and can light up according to the downloaded program. Owing to its fluidity and

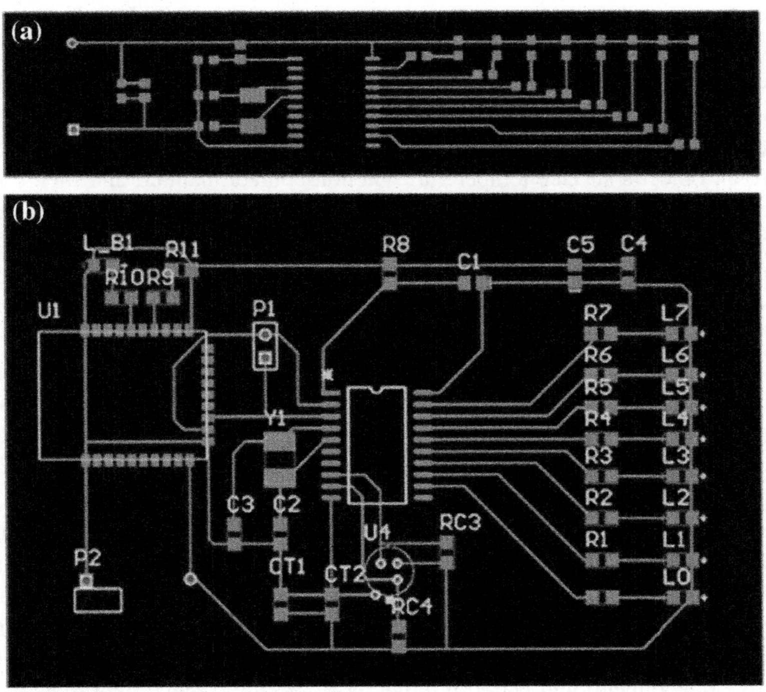

Fig. 13.27 Layouts of the functional flexible circuits printed with the liquid metal [38]. **a** Circuit layout of the programmable band. **b** Circuit layout of the wireless temperature sensor module. Picture reproduced with permission

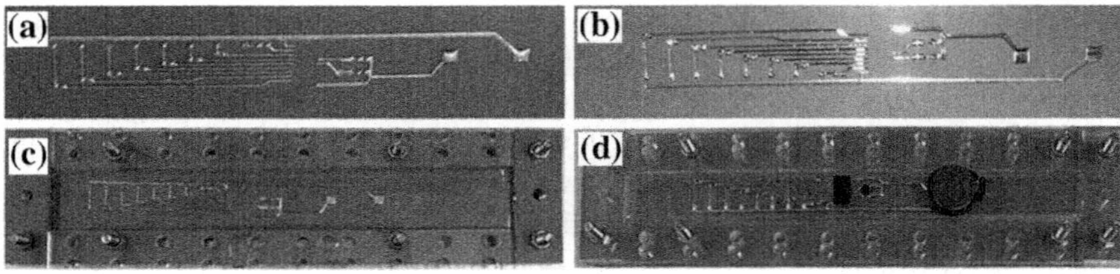

Fig. 13.28 Fabrication procedures of the band [38]. **a** Mirrored circuit layout printed on the top of the PVC film in the "after peeling" approach. **b** Circuit pattern printed on the top of the PVC substrate in the "before peeling" approach. **c** Covered with liquid PDMS solution after printing the circuit in the "after peeling" approach. **d** Covered with liquid PDMS solution after placing the electronic components in the "before peeling" approach. All pictures reproduced with permission

conductivity, the liquid metal offers more conveniences for the flexible circuit board fabrication. The role of the liquid metal is not only serving as the interconnections among the functional components, but also the binder bonding these components. The fine connection between liquid metal and the components has been proven in Fig. 13.29b, which is an SEM image of a resistor in the circuit. Since the liquid metal is deformable and PDMS is flexible, such transparent band is able to be rolled and twisted arbitrarily while working (Fig. 13.29c).

The dual-trans fabrication strategy opens a wide variety for multiple applications of the liquid metal soft circuits, especially for biomedical use purpose [38]. Figure 13.29d shows the optical images of a soft sensor module with the functions of temperature measurement and wireless communication with a mobile phone. As displayed in Fig. 13.29e, controlled by the mobile phone app, the module is able to acquire an object's surface temperature via non-contact manner, and then transmit wirelessly the data to the mobile phone via Bluetooth. Whenever the app sends a requirement, the Bluetooth transfers it to the MCU via the RS232 protocol. Once receiving the code, the MCU reads out the temperature from the sensor via another two-wired digital communication protocol immediately and returns the data. After receiving the Bluetooth-transmitted data packages, the app interprets the temperature value and the real-time curve is drawn on the screen. Owing to the flexibility of the PDMS films and the strechability of the liquid metal lines, the wireless temperature measurement circuit ensures such capabilities such as bending, stretching and twisting, and no noticeable failure of the functionality appears. The test result as depicted in the curve indicates fast response and stability of the measurement. Furthermore, Fig. 13.29f shows a smaller PDMS module with the similar function as that in Fig. 13.29d. Here, the film is capable to match and stick to the skin compliantly for continuous temperature monitoring. Figure 13.30 displays the temperature measurement curves when putting the circuit on the hand, joint and chest, respectively (Fig. 13.31).

Unlike the conventional patterning methods, the liquid metal dual-trans printing is a substrate-transferred strategy with high efficiency, precision and robustness. It is material-saving, and also ensures "what you see is what you get", which makes a

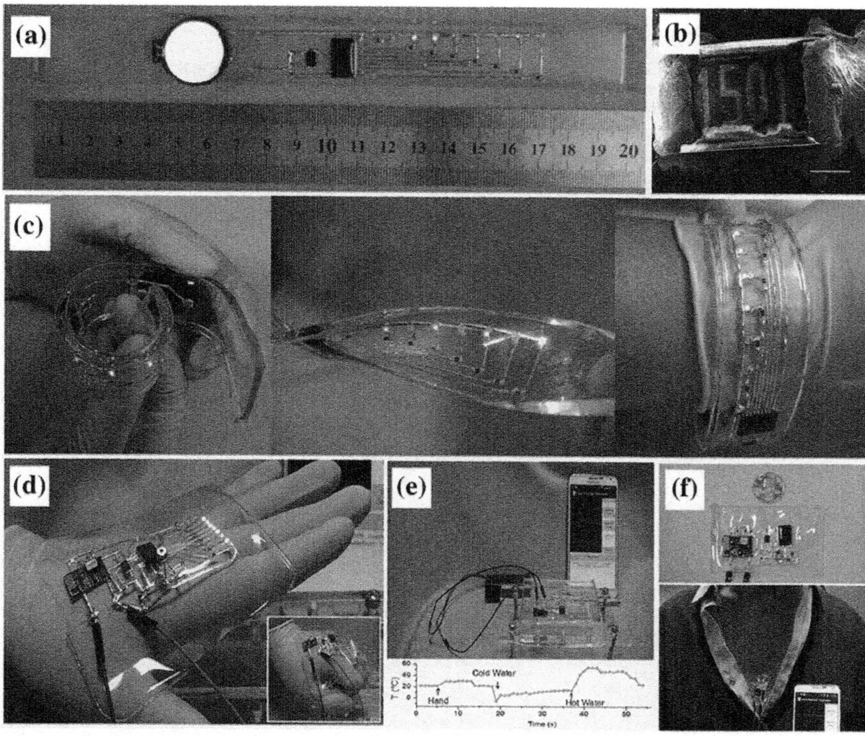

Fig. 13.29 Programmable flexible printing circuits fabricated by the dual-trans method [38]. **a** The top view of the transparent band with programmed lighting. **b** SEM image of the connection between a resistor and the liquid metal circuit wire. Scale bar, 500 μm. **c** The good performance of the band when rolled, twisted, and even formed as a wristband. **d** Flexible temperature measurement circuit with MCU, infrared temperature sensor and Bluetooth module. **e** Real-time and wireless temperature measurement system containing mobile phone and flexible liquid metal circuit, and the curve of temperature measured with the flexible wireless sensor module. **f** Packaged and integrated flex temperature measurement circuit which can stick to the skin compliantly. All pictures reproduced with permission

customized electrical design much easier. Yet the key lies in the temperature-controlled freeze phase transition of the alloy and the subsequent adhesion change. The simple manipulation successfully solves the problem of the low wetting ability of the alloy to the elastic substrates. And the transfer procedure naturally leads to channels that firmly hold the alloy inside without needing to make any extra efforts. The unique method has been proven quite suitable for manufacturing flexible electronics and totally compatible with current IC techniques. For instance, the naturally formed channels just fit for fixing IC pins, while the fluidity of the alloy warrants the robustness of the circuits under arbitrary deformations.

With these fundamental advantages, the present fabrication is capable of branching with various substrate materials and manipulations. For instance, in addition to PDMS, other elastic materials such as RTV (Room Temperature

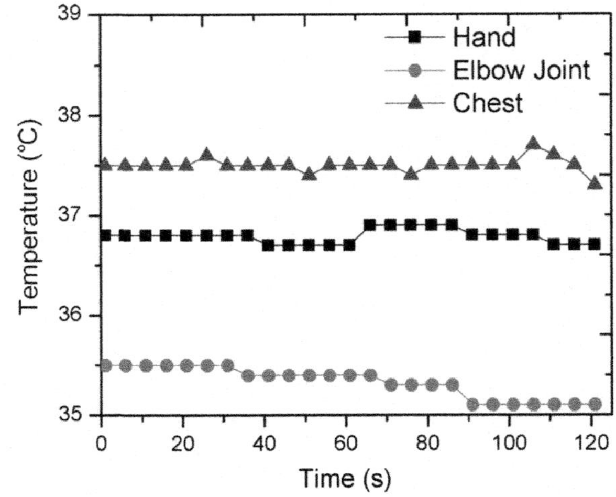

Fig. 13.30 Temperature transient results obtained by the flexible wireless temperature measurement module and mobile phone [38]. Picture reproduced with permission

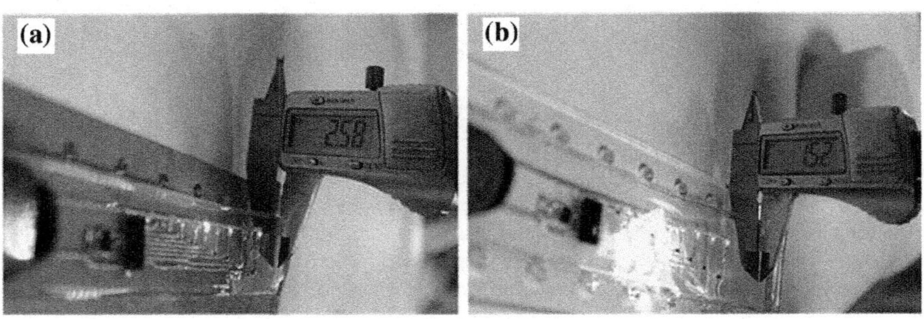

Fig. 13.31 The adjustable substrate thickness of the encased bands [38]. **a** The thickness of the band in Fig. 13.29 is measured as 2.58 mm. **b** The thickness of another band with identical structure and function, which is measured as 1.52 mm. All pictures reproduced with permission

Vulcanized) silicone rubber could also be exploited as the flexible substrate for more variations in stretchability and other characteristics. What's more, some of the existing techniques could also be compatible and complementary with the dual-trans printing method. For example, the deposition of the liquid metal circuit layout can be done through adopting screen spraying or painting. Other than that, by drilling holes through the substrate, it is possible to quickly make double-side or multi-layer structures as well. Of course, there also exist certain limitations that should be noticed. The resolution of the dual-trans printing is mainly determined by the direct printing device (50 μm). And if the pins are aligned with the component's bottom, additional efforts might be spared to ensure a good connection with the liquid metal wires.

Overall, the value of the new fabrication technique looks profound. Regardless of the time and cost reduction, it is more worthy of mentioning that with this pervasive method, everyone is able to make, design and create flexible electronic gadgets in diverse shapes at home. With a pre-designed layout document downloaded from website in advance, all needed stuffs for making a user end electronic circuit are just the easily available materials, oven, refrigerator and other common household goods. Thus it provides a rather convenient style for electronic innovation and individual implementation, which will become much more accessible than ever before.

13.13 Conclusion

In summary, a series of biomedical sensor systems, particularly for quantitative measurement of various physiological signals, through combining the directly printed alloy electrode and the mobile phone were illustrated. By virtue of the low melting point, the introduced liquid metal ink makes it possible for the direct writing or printing of the biomedical circuits in a moment. Unlike the prior art, the current fabrication process appears rather straightforward, labor-saving and cost-effective. This is expected to fulfill certain increasing needs in the coming home or society health care. In some cases, the developed sensors have already displayed rather beneficial properties. For example, according to the measurements, the sensors have large stretchability (up to 250%), high repeatability (>500 stretches), stable electrical properties (0.077–0.23 pF/mm^2), and a fast response time (<10 ms). Meanwhile, with the developed mobile phone platform, the present system enables diagnosis at the point of care. Whenever needed, liquid metal electronics can be conveniently developed into various biomedical sensors including those closely contacting with the skin or even implanted into the human body [42]. In the near future, people can even possibly make their own sensors, record the test results for late check or just transmit them to the doctors via mobile phones. Overall, according to the progresses ever made so far, the alloy senor and mobile phone system have shown high reliability for the biomedical detection. Nevertheless, there still exist certain limitations which need to be fully addressed. Such problem can be fixed by improved engineering to ensure the standardization of liquid metal biomedical sensors in the coming time.

References

1. Yi L, Li J, Guo C, Li L, Liu J (2015) Liquid metal ink enabled rapid prototyping of electrochemical sensor for wireless glucose detection on the platform of mobile phone. ASME J Med Dev 9(4):044507
2. Martinez AW, Phillips ST, Whitesides GM (2010) Diagnostics for the developing world: microfluidic paper-based analytical devices. Anal Chem 82:3–10

3. Bruzewicz DA, Reches M, Whitesides GM (2008) Low-cost printing of PDMS barriers to define microchannels in paper. Anal Chem 80:3387–3392
4. Martinez AW, Phillips ST, Carrilho E, Thomas SW, Sindi H, Whitesides GM (2008) Simple telemedicine for developing regions: camera phones and paper-based microfluidic devices for real-time, off-site diagnosis. Anal Chem 80:3699–3707
5. Ellerbee AK, Phillips ST, Siegel AC et al (2009) Quantifying colorimetric assays in paper-based microfluidic devices by measuring the transmission of light through paper. Anal Chem 81:8447–8452
6. Lee DS, Jeon BG, Ihm C, Park JK, Jung MY (2010) A simple and smart telemedicine device for developing regions: a pocket-sized colorimetric reader. Lab Chip 11(1):120–126
7. Dantu V, Vempati J, Srivilliputhur S (2014) Non-invasive blood glucose monitor based on spectroscopy using a smartphone. Eng Med Biol Soc 3695–3698
8. Chun HJ, Park YM, Yong DH, Jang YH, Yoon HC (2014) Paper-based glucose biosensing system utilizing a smartphone as a signal reader. Biochip J 8(3):218–226
9. Fujimoto T, Kawahara S, Fuchigami Y et al (2017) Portable electrochemical sensing system attached to smartphones and its incorporation with paper-based electrochemical glucose sensor. Int J Electr Comput Eng 7(3):1423–1429
10. Huang YW, Ugaz VM (2013) Smartphone-based detection of unlabeled DNA via electrochemical dissolution. Analyst 138(9):2522–2526
11. Wang J (2006) Electrochemical biosensors: towards point-of-care cancer diagnostics. Biosens Bioelectron 21:1887–1892
12. Dungchai W, Chailapakul O, Henry CS (2009) Electrochemical detection for paper-based microfluidics. Anal Chem 81:5821–5826
13. Nie Z, Nijhuis CA, Gong J et al (2010) Electrochemical sensing in paper-based microfluidic devices. Lab Chip 10:477–483
14. Ahn CH, Choi JW, Beaucage G, Nevin JH, Lee JB, Puntambekar A, Lee JY (2004) Disposable smart lab on a chip for point-of-care clinical diagnostics. Proc IEEE 92:154–173
15. Sia SK, Linder V, Parviz BA, Siegel A, Whitesides GM (2004) An integrated approach to a portable and low-cost immunoassay for resource-poor settings. Angew Chem Int Ed 43:498–502
16. Soper SA, Brown K, Ellington A et al (2006) Point-of-care biosensor systems for cancer diagnostics/prognostics. Biosens Bioelectron 21:1932–1942
17. Dittrich PS, Tachikawa K, Manz A (2006) Micro total analysis systems: latest advancements and trends. Anal Chem 78:3887–3907
18. Cho YK, Lee JG, Park JM, Lee BS, Lee Y, Ko C (2007) One-step pathogen specific DNA extraction from whole blood on a centrifugal microfluidic device. Lab Chip 7:565–573
19. Haun JB, Castro CM, Wang R, Peterson VM, Marinelli BS, Lee H, Weissleder R (2011) Micro-NMR for rapid molecular analysis of human tumor samples. Sci Transl Med 3:1–13
20. Liu J, Yu Y, Liu L (2011) Biomedical engineering on a mobile phone (in Chinese). Science Press, Beijing, pp 1–30
21. Lillehoj PB, Huang MC, Ho CM (2013) A handheld, cell phone-based electrochemical biodetector. In: IEEE, international conference on MICRO electro mechanical systems, pp 53–56
22. Lillehoj PB, Huang MC, Truong N, Ho CM (2013) Rapid electrochemical detection on a mobile phone. Lab Chip 13(15):2950–2955
23. Sun A, Wambach T, Venkatesh AG, Hall W (2016) A low-cost smartphone-based electrochemical biosensor for point-of-care diagnostics. In: Biomedical circuits & systems conference, pp 190–190
24. Gao Y, Li H, Liu J (2012) Direct writing of flexible electronics through room temperature liquid metal ink. PLoS ONE 7:e45485
25. Wang L, Liu J (2014) Liquid phase 3D printing for quickly manufacturing conductive metal objects with low melting point alloy ink. Sci China Technol Sci 57(9):1721–1728
26. Zhou J, Sun Y, Xue F (2005) Properties of low melting point Sn-Zn-Bi solders. J Alloy Compd 397:260–264

27. Whitesides GM (2004) Whitesides' group: writing a paper. Adv Mater 16:1375–1377
28. Russo A, Ahn BY, Adams JJ, Duoss EB, Bernhard JT, Lewis JA (2011) Pen-on-paper flexible electronics. Adv Mater 23:3426–3430
29. Martinez AW, Phillips ST, Wiley BJ, Gupta M, Whitesides GM (2008) FLASH: a rapid method for prototyping paper-based microfluidic devices. Lab Chip 8:2146–2150
30. Apilux A, Dungchai W, Siangproh W, Praphairaksit N, Henry CS, Chailapakul O (2010) Lab-on-paper with dual electrochemical/colorimetric detection for simultaneous determination of gold and iron. Anal Chem 82:1727–1732
31. Yeh JTC (1982) Characterization of in-based eutectic alloys used in Josephson packaging. Metall Trans A 13A:1547–1562
32. Nie Z, Deiss F, Liu X, Akbulut O, Whitesides GM (2010) Integration of paper-based microfluidic devices with commercial electrochemical readers. Lab Chip 10:3163–3169
33. Sheng L, Teo S, Liu J (2016) Liquid metal painted stretchable capacitor sensor devices for wearable healthcare electronics. J Med Biol Eng 36(2):265–272
34. Carcia PF, McLean RS, Reilly MH (2003) Transparent ZnO thin-film transistor fabricated by rf magnetron sputtering. Appl Phys Lett 82:1117–1119
35. Li HY, Yang Y, Liu J (2012) Printable tiny thermocouple by liquid metal gallium and its matching metal. Appl Phys Lett 101:073511
36. Gregory OJ, Busch E, Fralick GC, Chen XM (2010) Preparation and characterization of ceramic thin film thermocouples. Thin Solid Films 518:6093–6098
37. Bradley CC (1962) The experimental determination of the thermoelectric power in liquid metals and alloys. Phil Mag 7:1337–1347
38. Wang Q, Yang Y, Yang J, Liu J (2015) Fast fabrication of flexible functional circuits based on liquid metal dual-trans printing. Adv Mater 27:7109–7116
39. Khang DY, Jiang HQ, Huang Y, Rogers JA (2006) A stretchable form of single-crystal silicon for high-performance electronics on rubber substrates. Science 311:208–212
40. Zheng Y, He Z, Yang J, Liu J (2014) Personal electronics printing via tapping mode composite liquid metal ink delivery and adhesion mechanism. Sci Rep 4:4588
41. Boley JW, White EL, Chiu GTC, Kramer R (2014) Direct writing of gallium-indium alloy for stretchable electronics. Adv Funct Mater 24:3501–3507
42. Zhao ZN, Lin J, Zhang J, Yu Y, Yuan B, Fan C, Wang L, Liu J (2018) Liquid metal enabled flexible electronic system for eye movement tracking. IEEE Sens J 18(6):2592–2598

Chapter 14
Liquid Metal Enabled Wearable Electronics

Abstract This chapter summarizes recent developments in the field of wearable devices where liquid metal technologies may find important contributions. Particular focus was put on potential use of liquid metal electronics in monitoring and therapy for chronic diseases including diabetes, heart disease, Parkinson's disease, chronic kidney disease and movement disability after neurologic injuries. Meanwhile, typical wearable liquid metal electronics in the emerging applications will be briefly explained. Some key enabling technologies allowing for the implementation of liquid metal enabled wearable monitoring and therapy devices is given, such as miniaturization of electronic circuits, data analysis techniques, telecommunication strategy and physical therapy etc. For the illustration of future developments, research directions worth of pursuing are outlined.

Keywords Wearable electronics · Health care · Liquid metal

14.1 Wearable Systems for Managing Chronic Diseases

Chronic disease is a long-lasting physiological status that can be controlled but not cured. Owing to the portability and continuous action, wearable devices are regarded as promising ways for management and rehabilitation of patients with chronic diseases. Along with the development of mobile health care, the wearable therapy on some specific diseases especially chronic ones is receiving increasing attentions in recent years. Among the many potential ways to realize such target, wearable soft electronics are especially promising due to their easy going styles. Clearly, liquid metal electronics will play unique role for such endeavors. This chapter is to summarize recent developments in the field of wearable devices where liquid metal technologies may find important contributions. Particular focus was put on potential use of liquid metal electronics in monitoring and therapy for chronic diseases including diabetes, heart disease, Parkinson's disease, chronic kidney disease and movement disability after neurologic injuries [1]. Meanwhile, typical

J. Liu and L. Yi, *Liquid Metal Biomaterials*,
Springer Series in Biomaterials Science and Engineering10,
https://doi.org/10.1007/978-981-10-5607-9_14

wearable liquid metal electronics in the emerging applications will be briefly explained. Some key enabling technologies allowing for the implementation of liquid metal enabled wearable monitoring and therapy devices is given, such as miniaturization of electronic circuits, data analysis techniques, telecommunication strategy and physical therapy etc. For the illustration of future developments, research directions worth of pursuing are outlined.

14.2 Challenges in Current Health Care

With the progresses in science and technology, residents in industrialized cities are now living longer, but with multiple complicated health conditions [2]. Clinical operations are also increasingly accurate. However, prevalence of chronic disease and aging population begin to trouble the healthcare system accompanying rising costs [3]. Chronic diseases like diabetes, high blood pressure, Parkinson's disease and so forth have limited treatment methods due to complicated and confused causes while narrow part of pathologic phenomenon and biological mechanisms have been approved in current biological sciences [4–6]. Surgery might be a solution to certain chronic diseases, for example, implanting electrodes in the brain of Parkinson's disease patient to control tremble and dyskinesia [7]. However, the high cost of surgical operations and large risk of postoperative infection overwhelm the elderly patients who are the main group of chronic diseases. The most frequent therapies are regular drug and healthy behaviors of diet and exercise which contribute to relieving the incurable burden and improving health outcome and quality of life [8, 9]. Clearly, the optimal therapy for chronic diseases will be complex and require upgrading the health care system. However, part of the solutions may lie in how we take advantage of current technological advances to develop efficient system that is required to cope with the increased life expectancy. Along this direction, liquid metal enabled soft electronics as addressed in this book will serve well for such purposes.

The conception of mobile health appears on the scene to relieve the pressure of clinic management and to intervene the reinforcement of preventive medicine [10]. There have been many breakthroughs in monitoring system using mobile electronic devices like mobile phone and personal digital assistant, which could implement electrocardiogram monitoring, diabetes control and dermatosis care and more [11–13]. On this sound foundation, an emerging research trend of mobile health places more importance on developing therapy technique which is perhaps an ultimate goal of wearable electronics. As the developments of wireless communication and data analysis technologies, continuous transmission of patients' health status information to remote center can receive intervention from physicians and acquire complete self-management to chronic diseases [14, 15]. Also, the approach of physical therapy including electrical stimulation, phototherapy, ultrasound and so on can be used to intervene the body, focus on musculoskeletal, neuromuscular, cardiovascular, pulmonary and integumentary disorders [16]. Besides, the miniaturization of equipment and the development of circulation system based on existing heavy therapeutic devices open a door to wearable therapy devices. Figure 14.1 showed the wearable monitoring and therapy devices throughout the body via the methods mentioned above, which feature long-term functional treatment to one or more kinds of chronic diseases, exploding into a prominence in the field of health care over the last few decades. As can be anticipated, liquid metal can be found important in such newly emerging field of biomedicine.

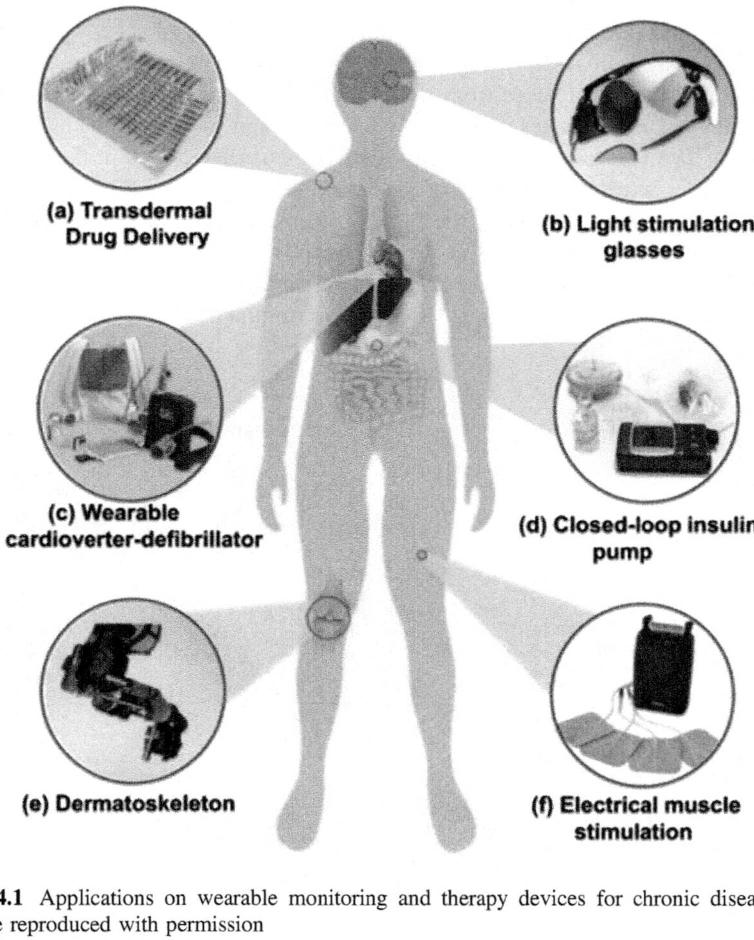

Fig. 14.1 Applications on wearable monitoring and therapy devices for chronic diseases [1]. Picture reproduced with permission

14.3 Conventional Key Enabling Wearable Electronics

Wearable devices for patients' monitoring and therapy means applying the portable and wearable systems to the medical field, including physiological and biochemical monitoring out of hospital, movement assistance, precise drug delivery, physical therapy and more. Recent advances in sensor technology, microelectronics, microelectromechanical system (MEMS), data analysis technology, telecommunication and physical therapy have led to the progress of wearable systems for patients' monitoring and therapy, although many of them are based on conventional rigid electronics but not liquid metal soft technologies.

The miniaturization of electronic circuits rooted in the microelectronics has played an important role on the wearable devices. Looking back to history, it is not surprised to find how to downsize and realize flexible the medical equipment via a gradual process. Using electrocardiogram (ECG) as an example, Fig. 14.2 illustrates the evolution of devices from water buckets, bench-top and portable sizes to the recent wearable devices like belt, wrist strap and clothing [17], which may evolve into flexible and stretchable film with organic electronics in the next stage [18]. One conception closely relevant to wearable devices is the continuous monitoring and therapy. In the past, the large sized sensors and front-end electronics made the hardware too obtrusive to be suitable for long-term monitoring of physiological and biochemical data. Now developments in the field of microelectronics have allowed researchers to develop miniaturized circuits possessing

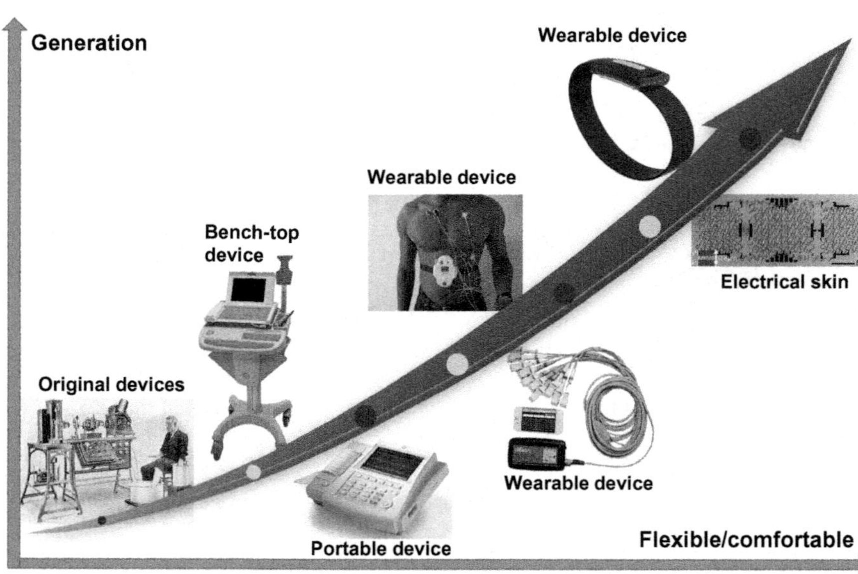

Fig. 14.2 Evolution of ECG devices with the miniaturization of electronic circuits [17, 18]. All pictures reproduced with permission

sensing capability, microcontroller functions and radio transmission. MEMS has also enabled the development of miniaturization, which can realize batch fabrication reducing the cost of electronic components significantly. In addition, MEMS is the foundation of microneedle for transcutaneous detection and drug delivery. The painless and precise characteristics promise microneedle large prospects in the application of wearable monitoring and therapy devices. To focus our attention on the medical aspects, we do not particular explain how to innovate liquid metal into such needs but rather leave typical examples in late sections of this chapter.

Wearable systems for monitoring and therapy often integrate multiple sensors into a network which is coordinated with other actuator and processor units by wireless communication. Conducting this kind of short-range information transmission inside the wearable device, Bluetooth is a preferable choice. As for the long-range data transmission to remote severs, an information gateway, which is a personal device such as smart phone or personal computer with powerful processors and large memory capacity, is needed to gather the physiological signals from the sensor network, preprocess the received data and retransmit them to a central server. Advances in wireless communication have enabled the remote transmission of data in a short time. There are many different wireless technologies that can serve this goal. Such technologies including WLAN, WiMAX as well as mobile phone communication standards like 4G can offer wide coverage and pervasive network access.

Data management is the bridge connecting complex human bodies' parameters and specific healthcare services. Automatic integration of collected data or manual input into research database offers the opportunity for the medical community or the caregiver to predict personal health trends, make early detection of disorders, get insight into illness evolution, improve medicine therapy and rehabilitation process. This would help patients suffering chronic disease more likely to feel in control of their health as well. System may not rely on the active participation and intervention of the user when the closed loop between sensor network and actuators like pump and electrode carry out the therapy function directly. One of the major obstacles to the adoption of wearable device is to develop soft and comfortable technologies. Besides, effective algorithm to control the dynamic physiological parameters and deal with emergencies are also important issues. For example, smart algorithms for the closed loop insulin pump are urgently needed to accomplish the proper medicine titration in various occasions including exercise, diet and overnight avoiding time lags in subcutaneous glucose sensing and insulin action [19].

Here, physical therapy for wearable device mainly refers to two aspects: functional trainings and physical agent therapies including electrotherapy, phototherapy, ultrasound therapy, magnetotherapy, compression therapy and so on. Functional trainings combined with wearable devices could provide physically disabled individuals due to neurological disorders with high intensity and repetitive training and augmented feedback to improve performance [20]. It is now widely accepted that the brain has the potential for neural repair following stroke and other injuries through neural plasticity [21]. Positive rehabilitation through neuroplasticity depends on the functional tasks and the number of repetitions both of which the wearable therapy systems can meet in our review. With regard to physical agent therapies, the most comprehensive applied approach is electrotherapy. Direct current therapy is also called transdermal iontophoresis, which uses an electric field to move both charged and uncharged drugs across the skin [22]. Also, reverse iontophoresis extracting glucose from the skin is applied in the continuous glucose monitoring and provide a foothold for artificial pancreas. Another electrotherapy is functional electrical stimulation (FES) that stimulates the patient's muscles through configured electrical impulses to generate joint movement as a way of gait compensation. In general, although there is not thorough and systematic cognition on the therapeutic mechanism of wearable devices, liquid metal remains a potentially useful remedy to seek for rehabilitation scheme from the basic physical methods and biochemical effects following up the current technologies.

14.4 Wearable Sensors for Physiological Parameters Monitoring

Physiological measures for health monitoring include body temperature, respiration rate, heart rate, electrocardiogram (ECG), electroencephalogram (EEG), blood pressure (BP), blood glucose, blood oxygen saturation (SpO_2), electromyography (EMG) and muscle activity. Until recently, continuous monitoring of physiological parameters can only be realized in the hospital setting. However, the possibility of accurate, continuous and long-term monitoring of physiological parameters out of hospital is a reality with developments in the field of wearable technology. Clearly, the liquid metal materials can be applied to develop various wearable sensors for different types of physiological parameters monitoring. Such unconventional soft electronics would offer innovative ways to realize important soft devices which will be very beneficial for use in health care situations.

14.4.1 Bioelectrical Signal Monitoring

The activities of human organs, such as heart, muscle, brain and so on, can generate bioelectric signals which are defined as electric potentials between points in living cells and can be measured with a group of different techniques.

ECG is one of the most widely used bioelectrical signal and many wearable ECG systems have been available in the market to date. A wearable system named "Life Guard" to monitor the physiological status of astronauts in space was developed by Stanford University and NASA [17], where ECG signals and heart rate were acquired with traditional button electrodes providing ECG Lead II and V5. Thereafter the spread of mobile phone and the GSM (global system for mobile communication) mobile telephony network pushed the wearable ECG device with

Table 14.1 Non-adherent capacitive ECG sensing devices that liquid metal may contribute

Devices	Location of ECG electrodes	Measured signals	Refs.	Year
ECG monitoring system	Attached on T-shirts	ECG	[28]	2006
ECG of neonates and infants	Attached on underwear	ECG	[38]	2006
Wearable smart shirt	Attached on shirt with wireless network	ECG, heart rate, physical activity	[39]	2009
Wearable ECG sensor	Integrated into a cotton T-shirt	ECG	[40]	2012
Ambulatory ECG monitoring	Integrated on underwear	ECG	[41]	2007
Non-contact ECG/ EEG electrodes	Integrated into fabric and clothing	ECG, EEG	[42]	2010
ECG measurement in clinical practice	Integrated into a pillow of a pre-ambulance bed	ECG	[43]	2009
Sleeping bed	Between the mattress and bed sheet	ECG, heart rate, blood pressure	[44]	2009
Aachen smart-chair	Integrated into the backrest and pad of a chair	ECG	[45]	2007
Non-contact chair based system	Integrated into the backrest of a chair	ECG, BCG, heart rate, blood pressure	[46]	2012
Non-contacting ECG measurement	Attached on toilet seat	ECG	[47]	2004
Wireless steering wheel	Integrated into steering wheel	ECG, heart rate	[48]	2012

real-time telemonitoring to a new stage [23], which could help out-patients record their conditions for clinical analysis, emergency detection and effective rescue [11, 24, 25]. To get broader wearable application and better user experience, the electrode of ECG may deserve a discussion. Conventional wet ECG sensor always accounted for the complete market for medical use [26] but the drawbacks were also obvious that the pastes or gels to keep the electrical contact could cause skin irritation and discomfort. Especially when sweating in rigorous physical exercise, the electrodes might become loose and break electrical contact. Therefore, new dry-contact and noncontact electrodes through biopotential sensor technologies, using the skin and the electrode as the two layers of a capacitor, were researched to address these problems. Gruetzmann et al. [27] demonstrated a foam electrode which displayed outstanding stability with increased resistance to motion artifact versus the wet electrode. Park et al. [28] developed a wearable capacitive ECG monitoring system that did not require direct contact to the skin but possessed comparable performance to gold standard conventional electrodes. More typical nonadherent capacitive ECG sensing devices are summarized in Table 14.1. They could not only be worn by the subjects in the form of clothing, belts, watches and shoes, but also be embedded into ambient environment such as mattress or back of chair, bed, steering wheel of car and more. The major challenges of wearable ECG devices with non-adherent are the capacitive mismatch due to motion artifacts and the high contact impedance due to the indirect contact [29].

EMG is a good measure of the strength of contraction of the muscle, which can be used as a diagnostics tool for identifying neuromuscular diseases, or as a control signal for prosthetic devices. For the two typical EMG: surface EMG and intra-muscular EMG, the former is more commonly used for wearable monitoring. Though there is some variation in surface EMG compared with original EMG, it can response the pattern of muscle contraction to a certain extent and provided a lot of information for action recognition [30]. As EMG signals contain some undesired sources like ECG artifacts, filtering techniques is suggested to eliminate all the noises. For real-time monitoring, the classification of EMG signals is an important issue [31]. Accurate hand gesture classification including the position and pressure of finger presses, as well as the tapping and lifting gestures across has been realized by using forearm electromyography [32, 33]. Gruebler and Suzuki [34] presented the design of a wearable device for reading positive expressions from facial EMG signals. Applications of this wearable sensor can be extended to the medical support by long-term facial expression recognition during therapeutic interventions. Besides, the combination of SEMG and ACC signals was demonstrated to have the superiority both fine subtle actions and large-scale movements [35]. Further, the identification of highly discriminative features has been realized by extracting information from the EMG signals for the automatic assistance of people instability, which could be applied in continuous daily activity monitoring and fall detection [36, 37].

EEG is a non-invasive method for measuring brain activity. Compared with EMG control for body limbs, EEG-based brain-computer interfaces (BCI) translate brain activity into control signals without physical movement, which can aid communication for individuals with severe disabilities [49]. Though the clinical potential of enabling communication through an EEG BCI remains unclear, many key issues including the classification algorithms [50], the acquisition of BCI control [51], psychological principles of BCI use [52], and wireless and wearable EEG system design [53] have been discussed. Besides BCI communication, EEG monitoring can be applied to automated diagnosis of epilepsy [54–56], Alzheimer's disease [57], and even sleep disordered breathing [58]. Many time-domain [59, 60], frequency-domain [61–66], time-frequency analysis [67], energy distribution in the time-frequency plane [68, 69], wavelet features [62, 70] and chaotic features such as entropies [60, 71] are used for seizure detection. At the lab level, liquid metal electronics has already been able to be used for making soft ECG or EEG circuits.

14.4.2 Acoustic Sensor Monitoring

Physiological acoustic signals from the human body include heart sounds, respiratory sounds, gastrointestinal sounds, limb joint sounds and more. Their continuous monitoring and quantitative analysis are expected to play important role in the emerging wearable and mobile healthcare field. Here, two kinds of acoustic sensors where liquid metal may have potential value were discussed.

The first introduced sensor was microphone, which can be subdivided into electret, MEMS and piezoelectric film microphones. Corbishley and Rodríguez-Villegas [72] demonstrated a miniaturized and wearable system for respiratory rate monitoring. By developing techniques to filter the noise sources and interference artifacts, the average success in the measurement of breathing rate had achieved 91.3%. On the basis of breathing rate monitoring technology, heart rate could also be extracted by placing a small sensor at the neck [73]. Moreover, the sensing methods of joint acoustical emissions from the knee were also proposed in many researches [74–76]. Friction between the structures and articulating components of the knee joint gives rise to various kinds of vibrations, which can be continuously monitored by miniature microphones places on the knee for wearable rehabilitation assessment. Changes in joint sounds during recovery from musculoskeletal injury could be quantified by analyzing the consistency of the knee acoustical emission during different activities [75].

Another kind of acoustic senor was accelerometer, which could detect the vibration of the skin due to sounds generated inside human body [77]. Typical applications of acoustic accelerometer sensors covered vocal behavior monitoring [78], heart sound monitoring [79], respiratory sound monitoring [80], fetal monitoring [81], and even gastrointestinal sound monitoring [82]. Compared to microphones, accelerometers appear more sensitive to motion noise. Some algorithms have been developed to remove motion artifacts. Pandia et al. [83] provided a method to effectively extract heart sound signals from accelerometer data. Besides, friction noise generated between the sensor and the skin or clothes is also a big challenge. There are a lot of methods to reduce or prevent such noise.

14.4.3 Optical Signal Monitoring

Due to that there is not light source in human body, photoplethysmographic (PPG) sensing can be applied which involves a light-emitting diode to emit light into tissue and a photodiode to measure the amount of light reflected from or transmitted through the tissue. Since blood flow to the skin can be modulated via multiple physiological systems, the PPG can be adopted to monitor SpO_2 [84], heart rate [85], respiration rate [86] and BP [87].

In recent researches, the PPG sensors have been explored to design compact and lightweight for wearable measurement, which can be placed in different sites including the finger, wrist, brachia, earlobe, external ear cartilage, and the superior auricular region. Commercial clinical PPG sensors commonly use the finger, earlobe and forehead [88]. Earlobe sensors have become popular as pulse rate monitors because the transmitted PPG signal amplitude from the earlobe provides the largest perfusion value. Patterson et al. [89] introduced an ear-worn and flexible PPG sensor for heart rate monitoring, which is suitable for long-term and continuous monitoring due to its location and unobtrusive design. To minimize motion artifacts, researchers performed a double ring design to reduce influences from the external forces, acceleration and ambient light [90, 91]. Xu et al. [92] developed a near-infrared phototransistor with high sensitivity based on organic bulk heterojunction. This phototransistor can be used as the detection unit in a PPG sensor for continuous finger pulse wave monitoring. Besides, novel PPG sensors with the wristwatch-type design have also been developed. Unlike previous methods that obtained signals from the capillaries in the skin, this method measures the signal from the radial artery and the ulnar artery of the wrist. Nemati et al. [93] proposed a promising wrist watch with PPG sensors for atrial fibrillation monitoring, which is the first study of enough high accuracy for general population without an ambulatory Holter electrocardiographic monitor. Lastly, compared with other peripheral body locations, forehead sensors appear more sensitive to pulsatile signal changes under low perfusion conditions [94]. The forehead structure including the thin-skin layer and the prominent bone helps to direct light back to the photo detector, showing the result of decreased motion artifacts during different physical activities.

The present lab had ever developed an ear wearable liquid metal soft device for blood oxygen monitoring. Elderly people, intensive care patients, extreme athletes are demanding the continuous monitoring of blood oxygen, heart rate, temperature and other physiological parameters. But most of the currently available wearable physiological monitoring equipments are non-flexible, difficult to fix and affecting appearance. Therefore, they are generally not applicable for long-term monitoring of physiological parameters. In addition, the ear canals as natural body cavities which are near the brain tissue, can shield external signals and be used as perfect sites for physiological signal acquisition and non-invasive deep brain stimulation.

Liquid metal itself has good conductivity and fluidity. With the development of advanced additive manufacturing technology, it now became possible to produce more complex flexible wearable equipment with liquid metal. This lab proposed a flexible wearable sensing system using gallium-indium-based liquid metal alloy as circuit wires, pads and electrodes, and PDMS as packaging material (Fig. 14.3). The sensing and stimulating effects of the ear wearable device were tested and demonstrated.

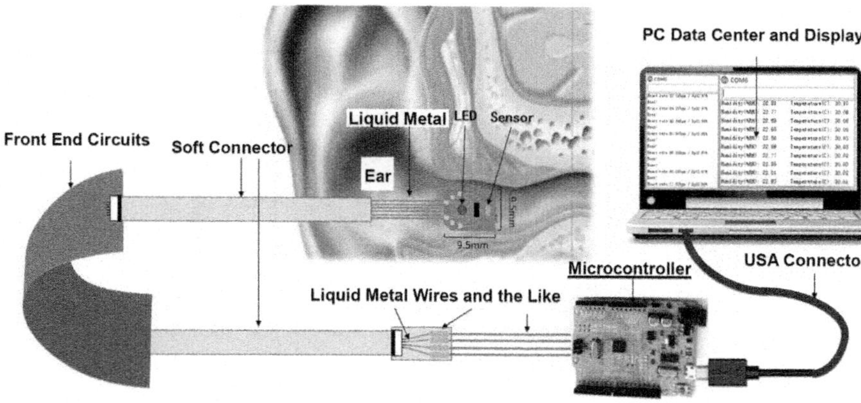

Fig. 14.3 Ear canals wearable liquid metal soft electronics for physiological signals monitoring and stimulation (*Note* Q. J. Zou, Design of Ear Canal Physiological Sensing System based on Liquid Metal Soft Electronics, B.S. Thesis, Department of Biomedical Engineering, Tsinghua University, Beijing, China, 2017). All pictures reproduced with permission

14.4.4 Biochemistry Index Monitoring

Biochemical index monitoring has recently gained a lot of interest among researches in the field of wearable technology. The former chapter has presented an example of using liquid metal to directly print out and coat glucose sensor. But potential innovations are many. Within the category of chronic disease management, continuous glucose monitoring (CGM), has more potential benefits than capillary blood glucose in the management of patients with type 1 diabetes [95].

The technology of CGM was introduced 15 years ago when some devices were approved by the U.S. Food and Drug Administration (FDA) and CE in Europe [96] for use, based on invasive subcutaneous sensor, minimally invasive microneedle and noninvasive methods mainly including transdermal and optical measurement [97]. The MiniMed (Medtronic Diabetes, Northridge, California) Continuous Glucose Monitoring was an invasive device using a subcutaneous needle-type amperometric enzyme electrode based on GO_x [98, 99], which was attached on the abdomen of patient with a fixed belt. It acquired signal every 10 s and saved an average of the signal in memory every 5 min. Potts et al. [100] combined reverse iontophoresis extracting glucose from intact skin with an in situ glucose sensor in a device called the GlucoWatch G2 Biographer (GW2B, Cygnus, Redwood City, California) just like an electronic watch that was convenient for children to wear. Clinical researches including controlled clinical environment and the home environment had suggested the accuracy was relatively constant but not reliably in large blood glucose variation such as hypoglycemia [101, 102]. More current representative commercial CGM devices are provided in Table 14.2, with noninvasive

Table 14.2 Main reported commercial CGM devices that liquid metal may innovate

Brand name	Symphony	HG1-c	GlucoTrack	FreeStyle navigator
Method	Ultrasound-based transdermal permeation	Raman spectroscopy	Ultrasonic, thermal and electromagnetic sensing	Enzyme-tipped catheter
Country	USA	USA	Israel	USA
Company	Echo Therapeutics	C8 MediSensors	Integrity Applications	Abbott
Website	http://echotx.com/	http://www.c8medisensors.com/	https://www.integrity-apps.com/	http://www.abbott.com/
Display	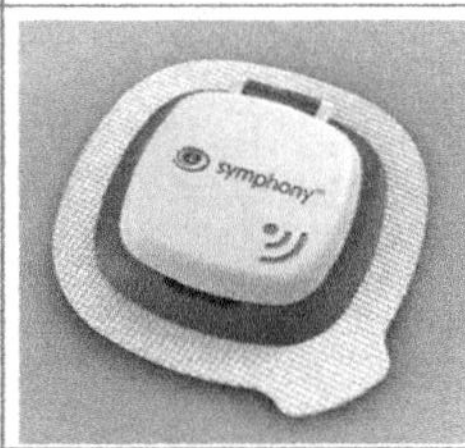	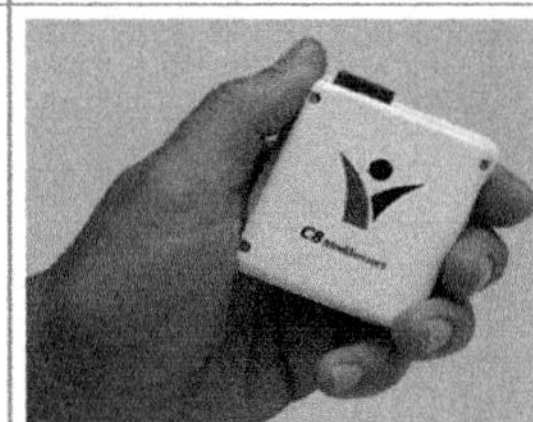	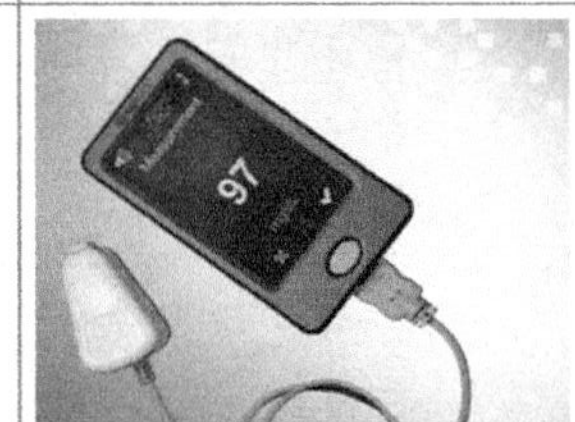	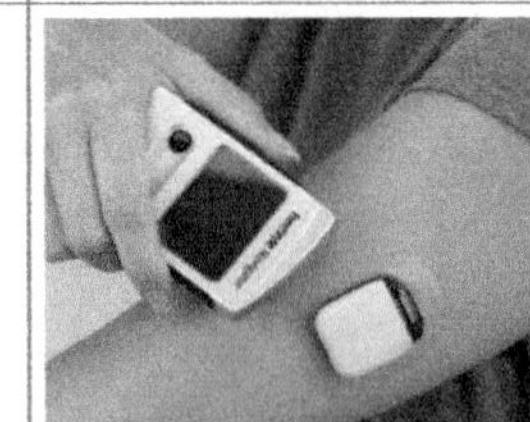
Characteri-stics	Permeated skin measurement with some irritation [110, 111], needing fast warm-up [112, 113]	Scanning the skin with monochromatic source [114] and returning spectroscopy having high discrimination for glucose [115, 116]	Attaching clip on the earlobe with abundant blood supply and not affected by activities [117, 118]	Minimally invasive [119], needing warm-up about one hour and providing early-warning about high or low glucose [120]

All pictures reproduced with permission

method including ultrasonic, optical, electromagnetic, thermal and enzymatic sensing. It is observed that these devices are all small size, light weight and easy to wear. Further applications of the CGM devices may become a critical component of the closed loop insulin delivery system [97–99]. However, three main accuracy limitations of CGM technology must be improved, including the calibration in rapidly changing condition [103, 104], the time lag due to blood-to-interstitial glucose transport and sensor processing [105, 106], as well as the error from random noise confound CGM data [107–109].

14.4.5 Pressure Signal Monitoring

Human body's pressure monitoring is an extensive concept, ranged from the obvious daily activity like the foot plantar pressure [121] to the subtle signal like the vibration of pulse [122].

In terms of daily activities monitoring, extensive research efforts have been made to access the accuracy of wearable sensors. Sazonov et al. [123] developed an in-shoe pressure and acceleration sensor system for automatic recognition of postures and activities in patients with stroke, which could classify activities including sitting, standing and walking and detecting whether subjects were simultaneously performing arm reaching movements. Besides, combined wireless communication, the work undertaken by Bamberg et al. [124] had received much attention.

On the other hand, with the development of flexible electronics, pressure sensors have emerged as a highly active field. The mimicry of human skin to sense pressure is a topic of innovative research. Many physiological monitoring studies in this field have been made as shown in Fig. 14.4. Bao's team [125] developed a flexible pressure sensor based on organic thin film transistors and used it to monitor continuous radial artery pulse wave with no invasion and high fidelity. Pang et al. [126] showed a flexible sensor that was based on two interlocked arrays of high-aspect-ratio Pt-coated polymeric nanofibres. Gong et al. [127] used ultrathin gold nanowires to develop wearable sensor for real-time monitoring of blood pulses. Other flexible systems were concentrated on human motion monitoring, such as the silk-molded pressure sensor for speaking recognition [128], the carbon nanotube strain sensor for movement and breathing [129], as well as the system including sensor, memory and actuator for diagnosis of movement disorders [130]. Among these endeavors, the electrodes are generally made via conventional manufacture ways. As an alternative, liquid metal can be adopted in a large extent to replace the functional units in the coming time.

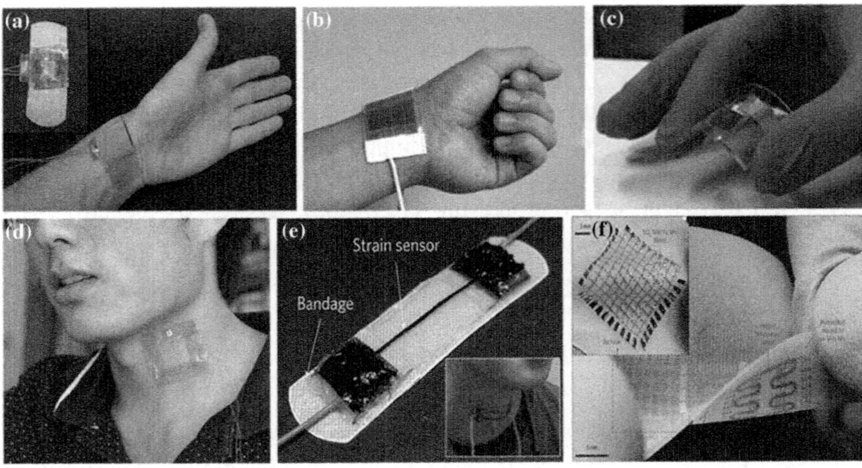

Fig. 14.4 Flexible electronics for various physiological measurements: **a** A flexible pressure sensor for continuous radial artery pulse wave [125]. **b** A flexible sensor for physical force of heart beat measurement [126]. **c** A flexible sensor for real-time monitoring of blood pulses [127]. **d** A silk-molded pressure sensor for speaking recognition [128]. **e** A strain sensor for movement and breathing monitoring [129]. **f** A system for movement disorder diagnosis [130]. All pictures reproduced with permission

14.5 Typical Applications of Wearable Electronics for Chronic Disease Therapy

Based on the rapid development in monitoring systems for various physiological parameters, an emerging research trend of wearable system is to put more importance on developing therapy technique [1]. Applications about wearable therapy devices with long-term monitoring can be divided into two systems, namely remote medical treatment and direct remedial treatment, while physiological parameters extracted from sensors can provide indicators of health status and have tremendous diagnostic value as well as therapeutic evaluations. Figure 14.5 demonstrates a whole framework of remote medical treatment based on the monitoring of wearable sensors. These wearable sensors deployed according to the clinical application of interest are connected to mobile devices to gather different physiological information regarding the status of the individual. Such measurements can be wirelessly forwarded to a medical center via a mobile phone. The professional physicians in medical center will give intervention to patients' behaviors based on the transmitted data, which can also be shared with families to keep acquaintance and deal with emergency situations whenever necessary. Systems for direct remedial treatment also rely on the wearable monitoring, but they take therapeutic measures directly like drug injection, defibrillation, auditory signal stimulation and more rather than relay suggestion from physician and behavior feedbacks remotely. To focus on the chronic disease therapy, the following sections illustrate several typical wearable

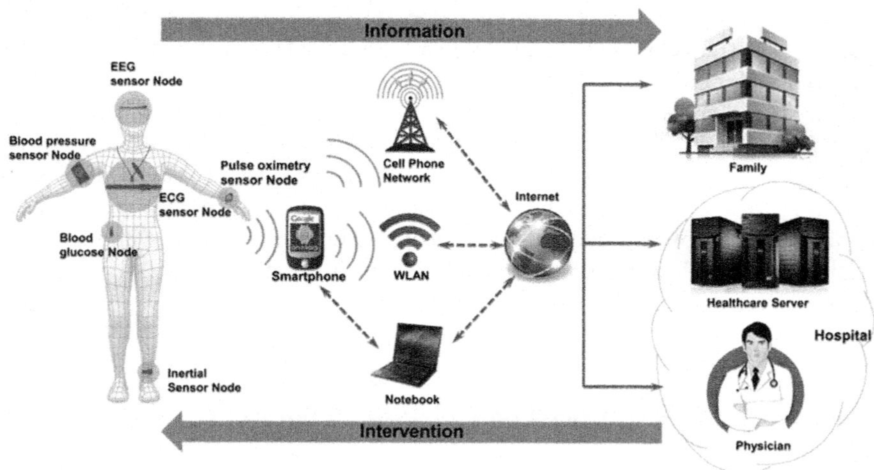

Fig. 14.5 Framework of telemedicine based on the monitoring of wearable sensors [1]. Picture reproduced with permission

applications by dividing them into different functional assistance including organ, limb as well as daily habit management, and then explain their respective developments and existing problems.

14.6 Organ Function Assistance

The major hazard of chronic disease lies in the damage of vital organs like heart, pancreas and kidney. For patients with severe symptoms, the immediate and continuous function assistance of organ is very necessary when organs exhibit hormone imbalance or rhythm disorder. Wearable therapy devices for organ function assistance, which are also called as artificial organs, are aimed to timely respond to one or more abnormal conditions and maintain the homeostasis.

14.6.1 Wearable Cardioverter-Defibrillator for Heart Disease

Sudden cardiac death that mainly resulting from tachyarrhythmia is a major cause of mortality in industrialize populations, the rate of which in the United States, Netherlands, Ireland and China range from 50 to 100 cases per 100,000 in the general population annually [131]. After a few years of clinical investigation [132, 133], the wearable cardioverter-defibrillator (WCD) that could provide an effective technology to improve survival rate of patients with a previous episode of sudden death, left ventricular dysfunction or ventricular tachyarrhythmias [134] was approved and introduced into practice until two years ago.

Currently, there are two WCD models available, the older LifeVest3100 and the new LifeVest 4000 [ZOLL Lifecor Corporation (ZOOL), Pittsburgh, PA, USA] [135]. However, the application of WCD useful for acute phase care is still limited according to the clinical practice [136] because it can only be a bridge to ICD (implantable cardioverter-defibrillator) or help avoid unnecessary ICD implantation. As also partially addressed in former chapters, it is no doubt liquid metal electronics will play ever important role in this area.

14.6.2 Wearable Closed-Loop Insulin Pump for Diabetes

Diabetes, with approximately 220 million diagnosed people in the worldwide [1], presents an indispensable problem to the health and social care systems. It is a chronic illness that requires continuing medical treatment and ongoing self-management to control the progression due to lack of permanent cure. In terms of continuing medical treatment for diabetes, insulin control of high blood glucose is the most effective means and the artificial pancreas that deliver extrinsic insulin automatically [137] has been proven a promising method.

The artificial pancreas (AP) is made up of CGM device and insulin pump while insulin delivery is modulated subcutaneously according to real-time interstitial glucose levels [138]. The major challenge in AP closed-loop system is refining the phase processes including overnight control, meals control and exercise control to avoid hypoglycemia. Now the simplest form of a closed-loop is to suspend insulin delivery at low glucose levels. Buckingham et al. [139] used five predictive algorithms to realize overnight control avoiding hypoglycemia in children and young adults with type 1 diabetes mellitus. In the clinical trial, insulin suspension was initiated at normoglycemia when the glucose trend was decreasing, and this measure prevented hypoglycemia on 75% of nights without a rebound to hyperglycemia. Del et al. [140] developed a new modular MPC algorithm focusing on meal control as the rapid rise of post-meal glucose is difficult to avert due to the inherent delays in subcutaneous insulin absorption and action, which showed satisfactory dinner control versus open-loop. This system running on a smart-phone in outpatient conditions reduced hypoglycemia but accompanied with marginal increase in average glycemia resulting from a possible overemphasis on hypoglycemia safety [141]. Co-administration of insulin and glucagon was investigated by El-Khatib et al. [142] to control the blood glucose at normal range. The MiniMed Paradigm® REAL-Time system was launched as early as 2006, which integrated real-time CGM with an insulin deliver device [143]. It was small in size so patients could wear it almost anywhere such as under the clothing in a leg pouch or on the belt like a mobile. Insulin delivery and CGM were made possible through tiny components patients wear for up to six days at a time [1]. Clearly, liquid metal can be applied in a group of technologies to tackle diabetes diseases including sensor as well as insulin pump etc.

14.6.3 Wearable Artificial Kidney for Chronic Kidney Disease

A wearable artificial kidney (WAK) is a long-held aim in the treatment of patients with chronic kidney disease [144, 145]. Though the WAK is not commercialized owing to some technical problems, numerous efforts has been carried out for decades and the breakthroughs and the issues are summarized in Table 14.3. Treatment modalities of dialysis includes hemodialysis (HD), hemofiltration (HF) and peritoneal dialysis (PD), while all three need to minimize the huge dialysate supply system to realize wearability and portability [146]. Pioneers proposed the concept that continuous regeneration and reuse of a small amount of dialysate in a closed-loop system instead of using large volumes of dialysate in a single pass configuration as done in conventional dialysis. Kolff et al. [147, 148] provided a portable WAK system consisted of pumps, batteries, dialyzers and a charcoal regeneration cartridge. Due to large dialysate volume for electrolyte balance, it was portable rather than wearable. Murisasco et al. [149, 150] developed a more advanced regeneration module based on the combination of sorbents and enzyme which was called recirculating dialysis (REDY) system. This cartridge used for purifying the dialysate included urease for removal of urea, charcoal for absorption of non-urea organic toxins, zirconium phosphate for removal of potassium and ammonium, and zirconium oxide for removal of phosohate. However, a large amount of zirconium phosphate required to remove the generated ammonium limits further miniaturization. After that, more different approaches were tried. Gura et al. [151, 152] developed a belt-type wearable HD machine that can accomplish dialysate regeneration with 375 ml of dialysate volume and got acceptable clinical results. Roberts et al. [153] proposed a concept of tidal PD using a hemofilter and REDY sorbent cartridge for WAK. Ronco and Fecondini [154] showed the concept of a wearable device called ViWAK based on sorbent cartridge technology and double-lumen PD catheter. In the coming time, developing soft electronics via liquid metal is a good way for future innovation in the area.

Table 14.3 Wearable artificial kidney that liquid metal may contribute

Name	TM	Technology breakthrough	Issues	Clinical experiment	Years	Refs.
Portable WAK	HD	A charcoal regeneration cartridge	Large dialysate volume	5 patients, 3 h, 6 times per week	1976	[147, 148]
Continuous Hemofiltratiom	HF	Sorbent and enzyme technology (REDY)	Large amount of zirconium phosphate	2 patients, one for 1 month and another for 1 month	1986	[149, 150]
Flow-thru PD	PD	Concept of tidal PD, REDY sorbent cartridge	Additional injection system for glucose and bicarbonate	Before clinical	1999	[151]
The WAK	HD	Pulsatile pump, REDY sorbent cartridge	Variation of composition and PH in dialysate	8 patients for 4–8 h	2007	[152]
ViWAK	PD	Remote control, double lumen PD catheter	Variation of composition and PH in dialysate, glucose injection	Before clinical	2007	[153]
The WHF	HF	Pulsatile pump, improved middle molecule clearance	Low small solute clearance	6 patients for 6 h	2008	[155]

14.7 Limb Function Assistance

The aim of wearable therapy devices applied on limb function assistance is to facilitate the patient's task performance after a neurological injury. Without these wearable devices, training based on manual assistance is exhausting for the staff, and the duration of training is thus limited by the fatigue of the therapist. Besides, the manual assistance is lack of the repeatability of training and quantitative evaluation of curative effect. These disadvantages can be relieved or even overcome with the use of wearable therapy devices.

14.7.1 Therapy of Parkinson's Disease Based on Symptoms Monitoring

Parkinson's disease is a common neurodegenerative disorder caused by a deficiency of dopamine due to the severe neuronal dysfunction in the substantia nigra pars compacta [156], which affects about 3% of the population over the age of 65 years and more than 500,000 U.S. residents [157]. Current therapy is mainly based on pharmacotherapy, which just maintains effective for a while but eventually develop complications like motor fluctuations and psychiatric disturbances.

Another key factor reducing the patients' quality of life is motion problems such as tremor, freezing of gait, postural instability. Bächlin et al. [158] developed a wearable system with acceleration sensors to detect freezing of gait (FOG) and provided a rhythmic auditory signal to stimulate the patients to resume walking. Ferrarin et al. [159] demonstrated a pair of optical stimulating glasses that provided different types of continuous optic flow and intermittent stimuli synchronous with external events. After prolonged testing, the device showed a remarkable increase in stride length for all subjects. Espay et al. [160] examined the efficacy of a closed-loop wearable visual-auditory curing device in 13 patients with Parkinson's disease with off-state gait impairment. From the physiological aspect, electronic stimulation based on liquid metal soft circuit has important potential for developing wearable technologies.

14.7.2 Wearable Rehabilitation Robots in Neurologic Injuries

This area belongs to the one that liquid metal can play diverse roles. Wearable robots known as robotic exoskeleton and powered orthoses are being developed for movement disabilities caused by neurologic injuries like stroke, traumatic brain and spinal cord injuries [161, 162]. Positive outcome of physical rehabilitation depends heavily on functional task-oriented training that can be realized by mechanical and electrical devices with high-intensity and repetitive training.

Traditionally, actuators of the devices are provided in three forms: electric current, hydraulic fluid or pneumatic pressure. The electrical actuators are most common because of their ease to use. Hasegawa et al. [163] introduced an exoskeleton assistive hand. Rocon et al. [164] proposed an exoskeleton for tremor assessment and suppression with DC motors actuator. Powered orthosiswith electric motors controlled by joint angle were also developed to assist elbow rehabilitation or foot drop gait [165, 166]. Pneumatic artificial muscle was used in upper extremity therapy robot [167] and soft robotic device for ankle foot rehabilitation [168], while its weight was generally light compared to other actuators but also have slow and non-linear dynamic response.

Pylatiuk et al. [169] proposed to apply the miniaturized and flexible fluidic actuators in the elbow orthosis. Moreover, another specific electrical stimulation known as functional electrical stimulation (FES) is the natural actuator of body muscles instead of traditional external actuators. FES allows patients to exercise muscle and prevent muscular atrophy [170]. However, disadvantages also lie in the appearance of muscle fatigue and control of joint trajectories [171]. Freeman et al.

[172] and Li et al. [173] proposed two systems combining FES with assistive force. In the coming time, liquid metal electronics can be fully explored to develop soft stimulator or control system for various rehabilitation needs.

14.8 Daily Habit Management Assistance

The diabetes' self-management tasks such as blood glucose monitoring, physical exercise and diet are inherently data intensive, which requires acquisition, storage and analysis of large amounts of data on a regular basis [174]. One way that has been proposed to help individuals better manage their diabetes is to make full use of smart-phone technology. El-Gayar et al. [175] reviewed 16 articles and 71 applications and divided the features of app functions into two classes. The primary features included blood glucose monitoring, medication, diet management and physical exercise. To form a long-term record and get professional analysis from health care provider, some apps needed patients enter manually into the mobile phone and others realized data entry automation just for blood glucose through blue-tooth [176]. The second features included weight, blood pressure, education, alert, decision support and social networking. It was important to note that decision support which mainly referred to automated analysis and ruled-based interpretation of data on an individual basis was a comprehensive but crucial part of diabetes management. WellDoc published some clinical results that documented the positive impact of their multipronged approach to patient and physician satisfaction [177, 178]. New paid application system called BlueStar was launched which is showing increasing value for large scale health care [179].

14.9 Printing Liquid Metal on Clothes to Compose Wearable Electronic Device

As explained before, wearable liquid metal electronics can be many in its working styles. For illustration purpose, this section illustrates the basics of liquid metal spraying printing which has generalized purpose on developing wearable electronic textile [180].

14.9.1 About Smart Textiles

Smart textiles represent an attractive direction in wearable health care ranging from physiological signals monitoring [181] to emergency assistance [182], which are also expected to have a place in continuous therapy [183]. An important process for smart textiles is the realization of stretchable or flexible circuits to meet comfortable wearing and free movement. Up to now, conductive yarns, stainless steel wires and copper wires are all common materials as interconnection lines in textile's circuits. Possible methods to integrate these filaments into textiles include weaving [184], knitting [185], embroidery [186], lamination [187] and stitching [188]. However, the trade-off of mechanical and electrical characteristics is an important bottleneck for textiles with conductive filaments. Increasing the conductive filaments for higher conductivity diminishes the flexibility. In turn, the necessary conductivity cannot be ensured when the metal layers are too thin to form the final product [189, 190].

Electronic functional inks, ranging from semiconductors and conductors with organic and inorganic materials, are alternatives for circuit fabrication in specific areas of a fabric or garment. Sirringhaus et al. developed inject printing of all-polymer transistor circuits with water-based ink of the conducting polymer [191]. Petukhov et al. presented nickel and copper conductive patterns by reactive inkjet printing avoiding common electroplating method [192]. Jeong et al. provided a method to minimize the surface oxidation of Cu nanoparticles and fabricated highly conductive Cu patterns in a plastic substrate [193]. Someya et al. demonstrated a stretchable organic transistor matrix and a wearable electromyogram sensor printed with Ag-based conductive ink [194]. Hu et al. used single-walled carbon nanotube ink to form capacitors on textiles as wearable power devices [195].

Room temperature liquid metal consisting of the gallium and its alloys is a rising hotspot research subject as electronic functional ink. It is rather convenient to fabricate flexible electronics such as conductive interconnects [196], electrodes [197], capacitors [198], inductors [199], stretchable antennas [200], strain sensor [201, 202], pressure sensor [203] and more. Meanwhile, various printing technologies including direct writing [204–207], spraying printing [208–210] and 3D printing [211] have been put forward for liquid metal patterning.

14.9.2 Spraying Printing of Liquid Metal on Cloth

The present lab disclosed for the first time that [208], liquid metal can be printed on nearly all desired substrates subject to an atomizing process. As Fig. 14.6a indicated [180], liquid metal in the airbrush broke up into droplets resulting from the high pressure nitrogen gas. Mixing with nitrogen gas, these droplets were exposed to the air and formed thin oxidation film on the surface. Excellent adhesion and special morphological structures were observed when these oxidized droplets struck the substrate. Figure 14.6b demonstrated a stereo light microscope image of oxidized liquid metal droplets after impacting transparent glass substrate. As was seen, these liquid metal droplets on the substrate presented irregular shapes with spin margins. Gently dropping a small amount of 0.5 mol/L NaOH on substrate, the droplets immersed in solution restored original shine and shrank into spheres in situ due to elimination of the oxide films on their surfaces. In order to make a

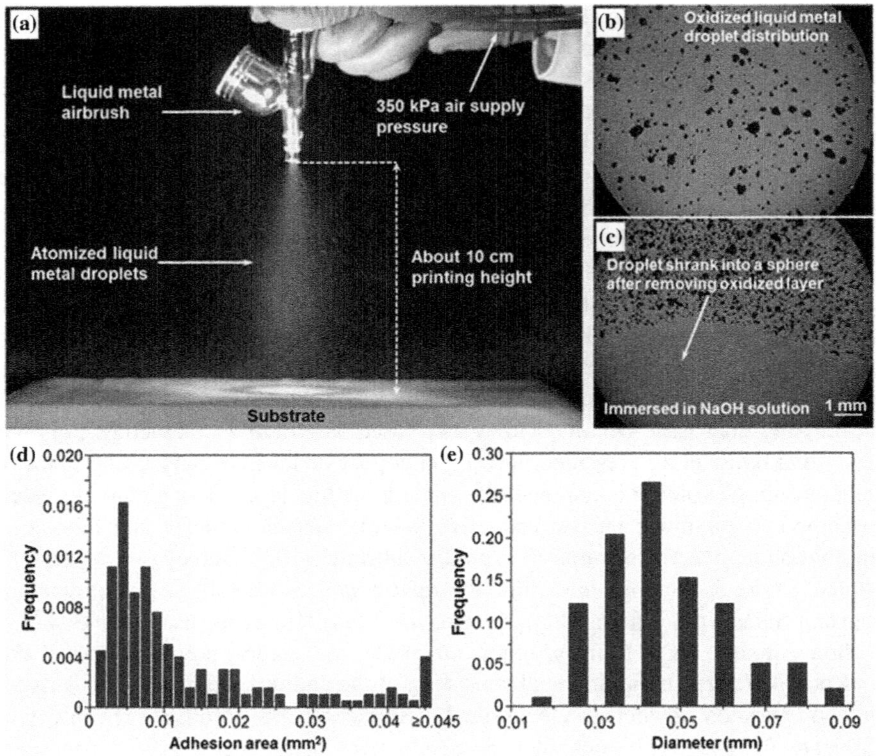

Fig. 14.6 Basic definition of atomized liquid metal droplets based on spraying printing [180]. **a** The droplets generated by the airbrush. **b** The stereo light microscope image of oxidized liquid metal droplets on transparent glass substrate via spraying printing. **c** The stereo light microscope image of liquid metal droplets immersed in NaOH solution to remove the oxidized layer. **d** The statistic graph of the size distribution of oxidized droplets after impacting the substrate. **e** The statistic graph of the size distribution of the droplets after being removed the oxidized layer and shrinking into spheres. All pictures reproduced with permission

quantitative analysis on the liquid metal droplets on substrate, we selected the droplets in dense area as statistic samples which were shown in Fig. 14.6c. Based on the microscope image in vertical view, the size of these samples was counted and got the results of Fig. 14.6d, e. As shown, the area of liquid metal droplets unrolling on the upper part distributed between 0.015 and 0.112 mm^2, while the diameter of liquid metal droplets shrinking into spheres on the lower part ranged from 0.017 to 0.086 mm. Because the unrolling area of droplets was proportional to the shrinking spherical volume which was related to the third power of its diameter, the distribution tendency of statistical data in Fig. 14.6d was consistent with the result in Fig. 14.6e. Besides, the result in Fig. 14.6e which was approximately normal distribution with the mean of 0.043 mm also confirmed that the liquid metal droplets generated by this method were atomized homogeneously.

Because gallium can be easily oxidized, the surface of liquid metal droplet will form a dense oxide film which predominately contains oxides of gallium to protect the bulk material from further oxidation [212]. On the one hand, from the view of droplets' morphology, a yield stress directly attributable to the solid-like oxide film obscures the intrinsic behavior of the liquid metal [213], leading these liquid metal droplets randomly form into shapes such as cones rather than tend to be spherical as Newtonian fluid. Therefore, these liquid metal droplets sputtered like mud and presented irregular shapes with spin margins when bumping into the substrate. After eliminating their surface oxide films, they could shrink into spheres like normal fluid to minimize their surface area and surface free energy. On the other hand, oxidation of liquid metal will lead to the decrease of contact angle and the increase of surface tension. Also, the smaller the volume of the liquid metal droplet, the higher the ratio of oxides accounts for. Generally, the Young-Dupre equation [214] determines the adhesion work of a liquid drop on a solid surface.

To explore whether oxide film is the only determining factor that ensures liquid metal to adhere to the cloth in spraying printing technology, Gui et al. conducted several control experiments as shown in Fig. 14.7 [180]. First of all, two kinds of liquid metals including the unoxidized liquid metal before filling into the airbrush container and the oxidized liquid metal collected from airbrush nozzle were chosen. Then, two kinds of liquid metals were painted with a brush or made to strike clothes substrate from a height respectively. In every experiment 0.1 mL of liquid metal was used. For a full oxidative process of liquid metal in air, the time of painting was

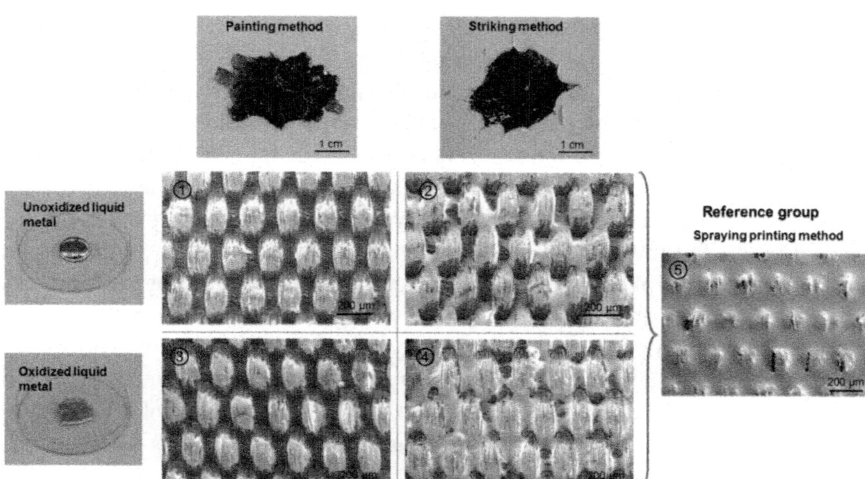

Fig. 14.7 Adhesive effect of liquid metal on the cloth with different oxidation degrees and different handling methods [180]. The environmental scanning electron microscope images of five groups' samples were displayed, which in order were as: ① The group of painting unoxidized liquid metal; ② The group of striking unoxidized liquid metal; ③ The group of painting oxidized liquid metal; ④ The group of striking oxidized liquid metal and ⑤ The reference group of spraying printing unoxidized liquid metal. All pictures reproduced with permission

set to 100 s and the height of free fall striking was selected at 1.5 m. Next, every experimental sample would be gently wiped to move the liquid metal not adhering to the cloth, which then was observed to analyze the adhesion of remaining liquid metal on cloth via field emission environmental scanning electron microscope. For comparison, an experimental sample that spraying printing liquid metal on cloth was also wiped and observed via the same way as above. General experimental process and detailed microscope results were demonstrated in Fig. 14.7.

By observing the phenomena in five groups of experiments, Gui et al. found the following facts [180]. Firstly, when using painting method with a brush, liquid metal just adhered to the upper woof yarns instead of the lower warp yarns whether unoxidized or oxidized. As the scanning electron microscope results of group ① and group ③ shown in Fig. 14.7, there were liquid metal arrays distributing on the raised part of all woof yarns, but there was hardly any liquid metal on warp yarns and the concave part of woof yarns. The adhesive effect of liquid metal in the two groups was different from that of spraying printing in reference group, which indicates that oxide film is not the only determining factor to ensure liquid metal to adhere to the cloth in spraying printing technology. Secondly, both two kinds of liquid metal could adhere to the upper woof yarns and the lower warp yarns if using striking method from 1.5 m height. However, the oxidized one worked better with regard to the lower yarns' adhesive result. The areas not covered by liquid metal in group ④ were less than those in group ②, all of which were on the warp yarns or the concave part of woof yarns. It should be pointed out that, in these two groups, the fine adhesive area of liquid metal as shown in Fig. 14.7 was only a small round area which meant the impact center on cloth. Except for the impact center, other areas with liquid metal spreading had the same microscope results as painting groups, existing only liquid metal arrays on the raised part of all woof yarns. These experimental phenomena prove that oxide film provides the foundation for liquid metal to adhere to cloth and the adhesive effect improves with the oxidative degree increases. Also, the pressure force generated by impacting enables liquid metal to drill into the lower yarns of cloth and brings a qualitative leap in adhesive effect compared with the painting method. Thirdly, relative to striking groups, the reference group with spraying printing method had a further improvement in adhesive effect. As the sample of reference group illustrated, liquid metal completely covered the lower warp yarns and the concave part of woof yarns, integrating interconnected lines and surrounding the liquid metal arrays on the raised part of woof yarns. Neglecting air resistance, the terminal velocity of the falling liquid metal droplet in striking groups can be calculated according to the formula of uniformly accelerating rectilinear motion $v = \sqrt{2gh}$, where acceleration of gravity g is 9.8 m/s^2, the free fall height h is 1.5 m and the calculation result of terminal velocity v is 5.42 m/s. In contrast, the initial impact velocities of tiny liquid metal droplets range from 10.3 to 12.8 m/s when using spraying printing method. Because the initial impact velocity in spraying printing group is larger than that in striking groups and the pressure force generated by impacting is positively related to the impact velocity [215], the pressure force on cloth of spraying printing group is also greater. This interprets the reason why the adhesive effect of lower yarns in reference group was better than those in group ② and group ④. Generally, by comparing these five groups of experiments, it can be found that the pressure force of liquid metal generated by impacting is the determining factor that ensures its fine adhesion on cloth, and the adhesive effect improves as the pressure increases.

14.9.3 Performance Analysis of Liquid Metal Conductors Printed on Clothes

In order to explore the printing results of liquid metal on clothes, selected six kinds of clothes whose characteristics were listed in Table 14.4 can be used [180]. The separation points of clothes were mainly concentrated on the pore size and the surface feature because they had greater impact than the material type on spraying printing of liquid metal.

Through printing a flexible conductor of liquid metal on these six kinds of clothes, Gui et al. made evaluation via three ways including stereo light microscope, 3D shape measuring microscope, field emission environmental scanning electron microscope [180]. Top views of liquid metal conductors were presented in Fig. 14.8a, b, and a cross-section view of these conductors along the transverse symmetry axis was exhibited in Fig. 14.8c. Though all conductors were verified to work properly, in terms of conductor evenness, they showed different print qualities which mainly depended on the pore size and surface feature of cloth. The highest print quality existed in sample ①, which was directly attributable to the compact and smooth cloth. Similar conductor evenness was shown in sample ②, sample ③ and sample ④ since there were pores in the former two and there was little fluff in the latter. In contrast to sample ④, sample ⑤ had coarser conductor because there was more and longer fluff in the surface of cloth. The worst print quality was presented in sample ⑥ when there were not only large pores but also lots of long fluff in the surface of cloth. Compared with sample ⑤, the cloth used in sample ⑥ had more fluff which was obliquely upward in different angles on the loose cloth. From the cross section view of Fig. 14.8c, it was found that liquid metal droplets stacked relatively flat on the base of the cloth in sample ⑤, but a large number of

Table 14.4 Characteristics of different clothes for liquid metal spraying printing [180]

Cloth number	Color	Material	Pore size	Surface feature
1	Yellow	Terylene	Compact	Smooth
2	Red	Chinlon	Small pore	Smooth
3	Deep blue	Linen	Large pore	Rare fluff
4	Deep pink	Terylene	Compact	Little fluff
5	Brown	Acrylon	Compact	Some fluff
6	Light blue	Terylene mainly	Large pore	Lots of fluff

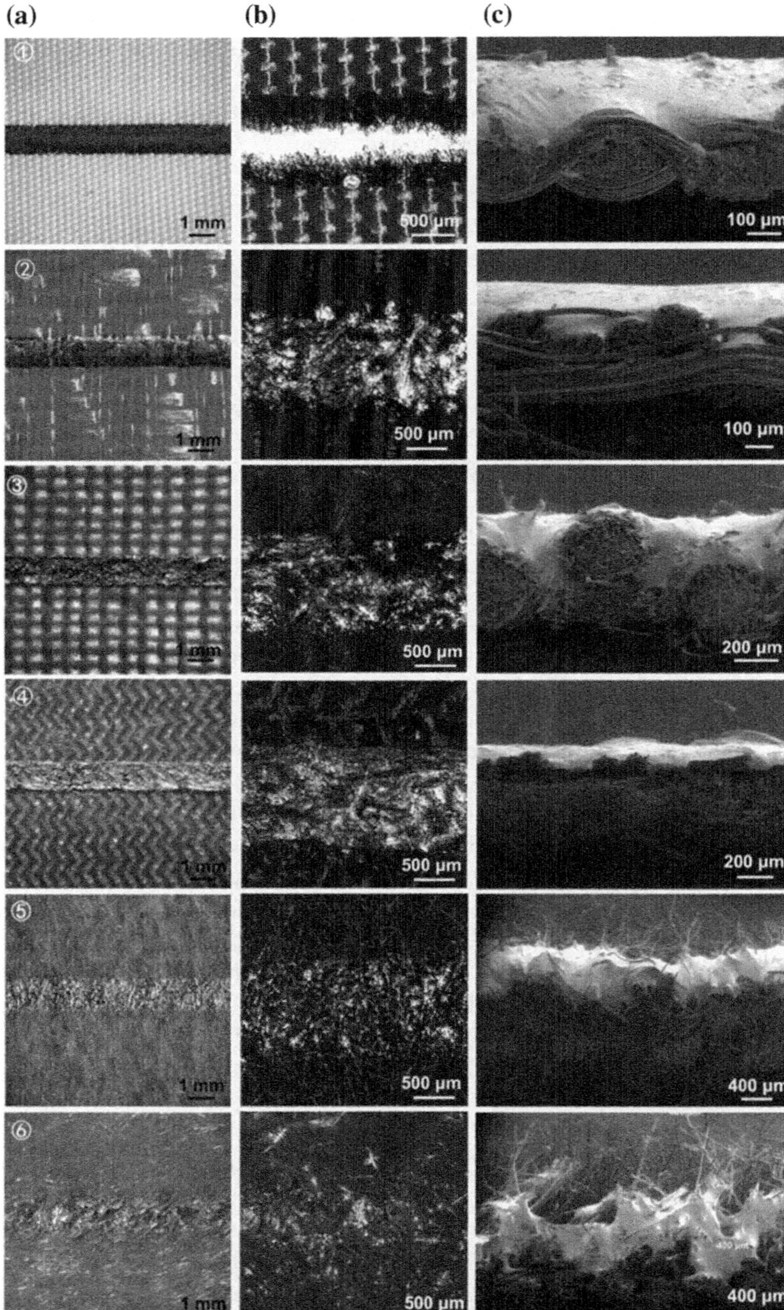
(a)
(b)
(c)
①
②
③
④
⑤
⑥
1 mm
500 μm
100 μm
200 μm
400 μm

◄**Fig. 14.8** Liquid metal conductors on different kinds of clothes [180]. **a** The stereo light microscope images of liquid metal conductors from an overlooking perspective. **b** The 3D shape measuring microscope images of liquid metal conductors from an overlooking perspective. **c** The environmental scanning electron microscope images of liquid metal conductors' section from a front perspective. All pictures reproduced with permission

droplets unevenly accumulated on the fluff rather than on the base of cloth in sample ⑥. Clearly, liquid metal droplets would stick to the fluff in both two cases due to the excellent adhesion. However, the long and decumbent fluff in sample ⑤ has small resistance against liquid metal droplets which allowed them to get to the base of cloth smoothly, while the forked fluff in sample ⑥ hindered liquid metal droplets from approaching to the base to some extent and led a large number of droplets to accumulate on the fluff unevenly.

Additionally, to quantitatively study the printing quality and explore spraying printing precision, four masks of different widths including 0.3, 0.5, 0.8 and 1.0 mm were used to print conductors on six kinds of clothes. In the printing process, other variables including the length of these masks, air supply pressure, printing time, airbrush height and its movement speed all remained constant. Then, the resistances of these conductors were measured for 6 times and took the average values. The results were shown in Table 14.5. Here, the cloth number was consistent with that in Fig. 14.8. As can be seen, these resistance results were also generally in accordance with the above microscope analysis. Conductors on cloth ① showed the smallest resistance whatever the width was. Conductors on cloth ② and cloth ③ had similar resistances in 0.8 and 1.0 mm but differed in narrower widths. Conductors on cloth ④ had slightly bigger resistances than those on cloth ② and cloth ③. Conductors on cloth ⑤ and cloth ⑥ increased significantly in resistance compared with formers. As the used mask was narrower, the difficulty of forming working conductor that needed connecting these liquid metal droplets into a continuous line increased. When using the mask of 0.3 mm width, the first five

Table 14.5 Resistances of liquid metal conductors with different widths on various clothes

Cloth number	0.3 mm	0.5 mm	0.8 mm	1.0 mm
1	0.48 Ω	0.28 Ω	0.22 Ω	0.18 Ω
2	1.47 Ω	0.77 Ω	0.55 Ω	0.48 Ω
3	2.20 Ω	1.08 Ω	0.53 Ω	0.41 Ω
4	3.46 Ω	1.98 Ω	1.41 Ω	1.03 Ω
5	26.80 Ω	15.91 Ω	7.26 Ω	6.69 Ω
6	Broken circuit	0.25×10^6 Ω	1.44×10^3 Ω	9.03 Ω

clothes could easily print out interconnected conductors but the last one appeared broken circuit.

14.10 Fabrication of Flexible Circuits on Clothes and Washing Resistance Testing

As investigated by Gui et al. [180], the process steps to fabricate flexible circuits of liquid metal on clothes can be spilt into two parts, including the printing part and the encapsulation part as shown in Fig. 14.9. First, a designed mask can be pressed on the flat cloth to conduct spraying printing with a liquid metal airbrush roughly 5–10 cm above the substrate. After this process finishes, the mask should be removed carefully to avoid smudging the liquid metal circuit. Then, the electronic components such as micro control units, resistors, capacitors, Bluetooth module and sensors can be put into the circuits according to layout design. The printing part is done when proper work of circuit is tested and verified. Next follows the encapsulation part. Firstly, a 2-mm-thickness hollow flat plate assorted with the designed mask is positioned on the cloth to determine the external contour of circuit encapsulation. Then plenty of PDMS is perfused into hollow areas of the flat plate to completely cover these liquid metal lines and electronic components on cloth, which will immediately be put into constant temperature box at 90 °C for 1.5 h to accelerate curing of PDMS. The liquid metal circuit thus is encapsulated to fix electronic components to resist destroying. After cooling down, one needs to cut the cured PDMS along the plate edge to take out the circuit on cloth. Lastly, the back of

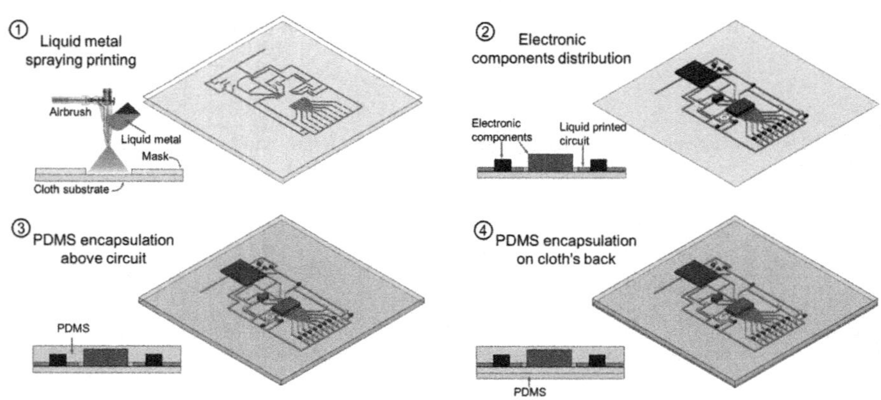

Fig. 14.9 Schematic illustrations of the fabrication process of flexible liquid metal circuit on cloth [180]. ① The step of spraying printing liquid metal circuits on cloth with a designed mask. ② The step of putting electronic components into circuit according to layout design. ③ The step of encapsulating liquid metal lines and electronic components with PDMS. ④ The step of encapsulating the cloth's back with PDMS. All pictures reproduced with permission

the cloth should also be encapsulated with PDMS to keep liquid metal from oozing out of the cloth pore, by following the same steps mention above.

In the process of encapsulation part, heavy permeation on cloth, which is related to the viscosity of encapsulation material, will occur and lead to an ambiguous contour of circuit encapsulation if using the freshly prepared PDMS. The viscosity of PDMS will increase during the curing procedure where temperature and time are major control variables. Because the viscosity of PDMS is hard to control at relatively high temperature, for example, PDMS will lose its liquidity in less than an hour if the temperature is set to 50 °C, one could rest PDMS at room temperature (27 °C) to ensure a wide time range (about 7 h) to choose suitable viscosity for encapsulation. In order to quantitatively study the permeation of PDMS with different viscosity on cloth, we conducted permeability testing on cloth with PDMS that was rested for 0–6 h at room temperature, in which the cloth was that provided the best spraying printing quality above, the hollow part of flat plate was 47 mm × 47 mm × 2 mm, and the condition of accelerating curing was 90 °C for 1.5 h. As shown in Fig. 14.10a, PDMS respectively rested for 1, 3 and 5 h congruously presented different permeation widths in transverse and longitudinal directions. The transverse permeation width was greater than the longitudinal permeation width as woven texture in the two directions was discrepant. Average value of the permeation width in two directions was taken as general permeation

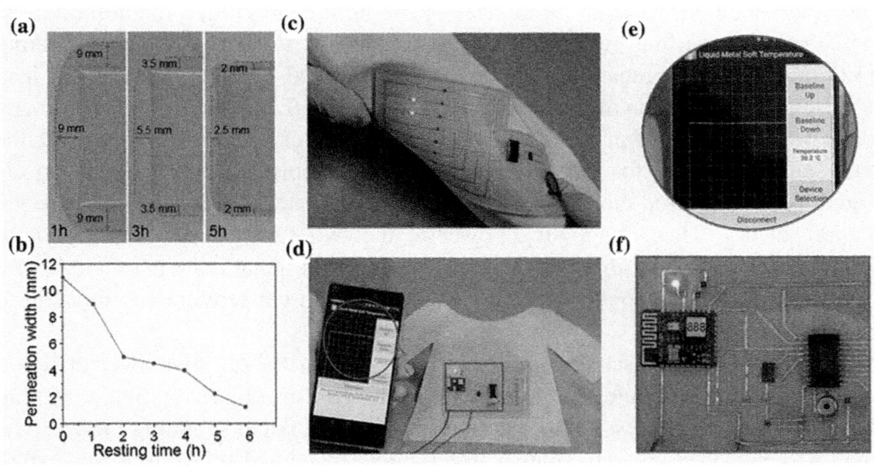

Fig. 14.10 Practical demonstration of the printing and encapsulation of flexible liquid metal circuits [180]. **a** The different permeation widths of PDMS that rested for different hours along the transverse and longitudinal directions of cloth. **b** The general permeation width of PDMS on cloth as a function of resting time. **c** The flexible blinking LED module with programmable function. **d** The infrared temperature measurement module with wireless communication to mobile phone. **e** Real-time temperature measurement displayed and stored on the physiological monitoring platform of mobile phone app. **f** The flexible temperature measurement circuit with liquid metal lines, MCU chip, infrared temperature sensor and Bluetooth. All pictures reproduced with permission

width on cloth, and its relationship with the resting time of PDMS were analyzed in Fig. 14.10b. In terms of the penetration width on cloth, PDMS rested for 6 h with 1.25 mm penetration width on cloth is a fine choice to control the external contour of circuit encapsulation efficiently.

Further, to demonstrate the fine property of smart textile combined with liquid metal, two flexible circuits on cloth were designed through the above fabrication method of printing and encapsulation. Figure 14.10c worked as a blinking LED module with programmable function in which eight LEDs were connected with a MCU chip and could blink according to the downloaded program. Besides, eight resistors, two capacitors and one crystal oscillator were used to perform the blinking. Outside the circuit, the encapsulation contour had distinct boundary whose penetration width was about 1.25 mm. Due to the deformable ability of liquid metal and the flexibility of PDMS, the whole circuit still worked properly while deforming as shown here. Figure 14.10d was an infrared temperature measurement module owning wireless communication function with mobile phone. It could realize non-contact continuous body temperature monitoring by directly printing liquid metal circuits on the textile. Measurement results were displayed and stored as shown in Fig. 14.10e when the Bluetooth transmitted data to the physiological monitoring platform in mobile phone app. Figure 14.10f presented specific details of the liquid metal spraying printing circuit in which liquid metal lines were all 0.5 mm width. It should be noted that the liquid metal was not only the wiring on cloth but also the interconnection with electronic components, protecting these electronic components from disconnecting during the circuit deformation process.

To conduct washing resistance testing, two samples of programmable blinking LED module were prepared. Sample 1 was immersed in soapy water for 3 h in which the concentration of domestic detergent was 1 g/L and the pH value of soapy water was about 8.5. Sample 2 was placed in the water bath cauldron keeping the temperature at 50 °C for 3 h. After 3 h, the two samples were removed from the liquid and were rinsed thoroughly with running tap water. Drying method used the natural air-dry. Then, reapplying power to the two samples, all LEDs on both samples were still working, which verified that liquid metal circuits on cloth with PDMS encapsulation could withstand alkaline or high temperature environment to some extent.

Overall, with the discovery of determining factors to adhesive effect of liquid metal on cloth, one could try more ways to improve the current spraying printing technology, such as pressurized printing liquid metal circuits, adding electrostatic charge to enhance the interactions between liquid metal and substrate. After testing the printing results of various clothes, more choices would be presented for the materials of electronic textiles with different functions. For instance, smooth cloth is capable of printing liquid metal as conducting line and rough cloth with fluff might be used for fabricating resistive heater of high resistance. The resistance difference between the liquid metal lines on two kinds of cloth can be over thousand-fold. Clearly, as the realization of various wearable functional modules via liquid metal, it can be expected that quickly fabricating flexible electronics on cloth would welcome a bright future in the coming time.

14.11 Liquid Metal Based Stretchable Radiation-Shielding Film

14.11.1 About Flexible Liquid Metal Radiation-Shielding Film

Liquid metal itself can even serve as health care shelter. In this respect, Deng et al. [216] reported a stretchable and flexible radiation-shielding film based on room-temperature liquid metal. Conceptual experiments showed that the liquid metal based printing technology can achieve an ultrathin flexible radiation-shielding film with a thickness of 0.3 mm. Moreover, the yield strength and ultimate strength of the liquid metal film appear much better than those of a conventional lead-particle-containing radiation-shielding material. In order to evaluate the radiation-shielding performance of the liquid metal material, X-ray radiation experiments to compare the liquid metal film and conventional lead-particle-based shielding material under different stretching conditions were performed. The results indicate that the liquid metal shielding film could achieve a certain radiation-shielding performance. Furthermore, because of the screen-printing properties of liquid metal, a low-cost X-ray mask method using a liquid metal selective radiation-shielding film was also studied, which could serve as a highly efficient and practical method for the medical X-ray shielding applications or semiconductor lithography industry.

Until now, various types of radioactive rays have been extensively applied in the development of radioactive medicine and nuclear technology applications. Concurrently, the harmful effects of X-rays on the human body, e.g., skin burns, hair loss, leucopenia, and even myeloma, have gradually been recognized [217–220]. Hence, the research on radiation-shielding materials has become a significant and urgent subject. Currently, low energy X-ray shielding is usually made of lead glass or lead rubber. However, lead glass, which is a rigid material, is not suitable for flexible shielding applications. Although lead rubber possesses certain flexibility, due to the dispersed structures, a lead rubber shielding material is usually thick, with limited tensile deformation and a small ultimate tensile stress [221–223]. Therefore, the current flexible medical radiation shielding, including shielding gloves, shielding clothes, and local shielding, is inconvenient to use. Moreover, there is a risk of toxicity from the lead-containing materials [224–227].

Unlike the existing ones, the stretchable radiation-shielding material based on liquid metal can be quite thin, which is therefore highly flexible [216]. Figure 14.11a illustrates the conventional lead rubber used in Shuang Ying PC14 radiation-shielding gloves, which have a thickness of 2 mm and the density of 1.6 g/cm^3. Figure 14.11 Billustrates the liquid metal based stretchable radiation-shielding film, which has a thickness of only 0.3 mm. The liquid metal is the alloy $Ga_{61}In_{25}Sn_{13}Zn_1$ (the subscript represents the mass ratio), which has a melting point of 8 °C and the density of 6.2 g/cm^3. Based on the screen printing process, the liquid metal was evenly coated on the silicon film. The smaller film

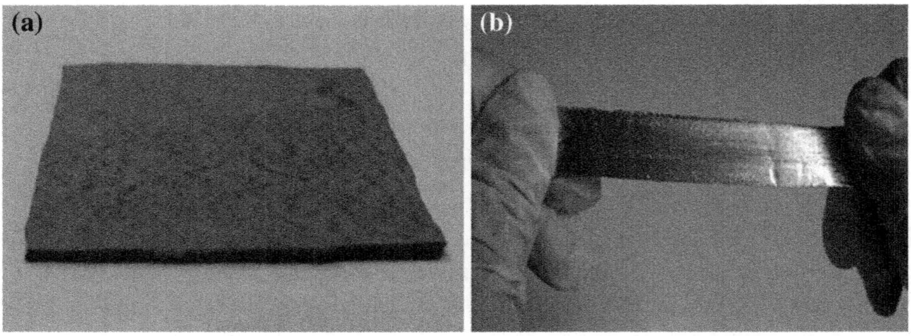

Fig. 14.11 **a** Conventional lead-rubber flexible radiation-shielding material. **b** Liquid metal based ultrathin radiation-shielding material [216]. All pictures reproduced with permission

thickness can produce a more comfortable experience for users, which is of great importance in the field of radiation-shielding clothes.

In order to comparatively evaluate the radiation-shielding performance of the liquid metal radiation-shielding material, 20 mm × 30 mm × 2 mm samples of both the lead rubber and liquid metal shielding film were employed in a radiation-shielding experiment. The liquid metal radiation-shielding material was fabricated by coating liquid metal onto a 2-mm-thick silicon film using a screen-printing method. Figure 14.12 shows the testing platform that was used to study the shielding performances of materials with different lengths: 30, 35, 40, 45, and 50 mm, respectively. A GE Optima X-ray machine was employed for the experiments, with an X-ray tube voltage of 55 kV and a tube current of 6.3 mAs.

Fig. 14.12 Platform for radiation-shielding experiments [216]. Picture reproduced with permission

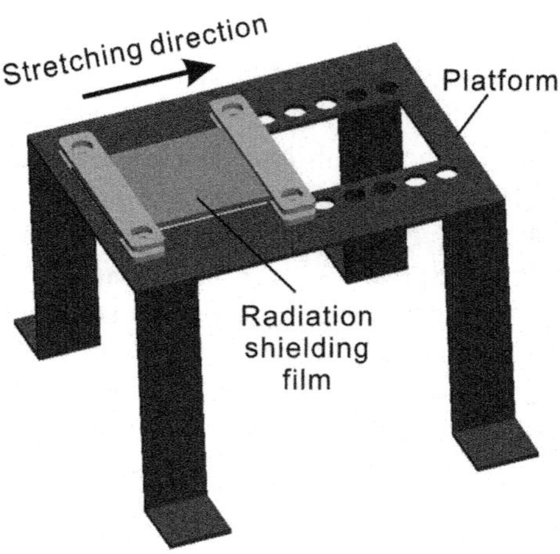

14.11.2 *Mechanical Properties of Liquid Metal Stretchable Shielding Material*

One of the greatest advantages of the liquid metal radiation-shielding material lies in its high flexibility. Figure 14.13 illustrates the stretching elongation percentages of the traditional lead rubber and liquid metal shielding materials under different stretching forces, respectively [216]. The materials for this experiment were 100 mm × 5 mm × 2 mm strips, and each material was stretched in the 100 mm direction. Figure 14.13 shows that when the stretching force is 12.5 N, the traditional lead rubber has obviously reached its yield limit. However, when the stretching force is 15 N, the liquid metal shielding material still has good flexibility and does not reach its yield limit. This is mainly because the even dispersion of lead particles in the conventional lead rubber weakens its tensile strength. In contrast, the liquid metal of the liquid-metal radiation-shielding material is only coated on the rubber surface, which maintains the high flexibility of the rubber base.

The liquid metal radiation-shielding material possesses not only a higher yield strength, but also a higher ultimate strength. Figure 14.14 shows a comparison of the tension limits of the lead-rubber shielding material and liquid metal shielding

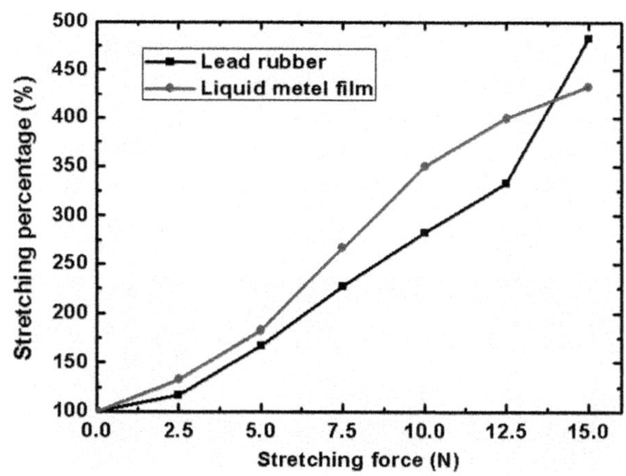

Fig. 14.13 Stretching elongation percentages of conventional lead rubber and liquid metal shielding material under different stretching forces [216]. Picture reproduced with permission

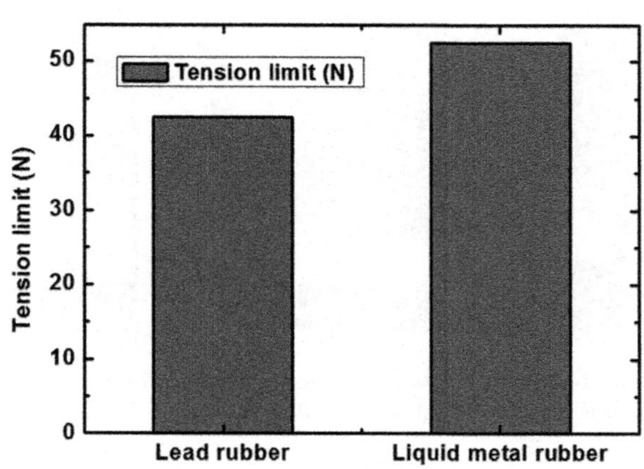

Fig. 14.14 Comparison of tension limits of lead-rubber and liquid metal shielding materials [216]. Picture reproduced with permission

material [216]. It can be seen that the liquid metal radiation-shielding material possesses a higher tension limit. This is mainly because the lead particles contained in the lead-rubber shielding material lower the tensile strength of the rubber base. In contrast, the shielding metal of the liquid metal shielding material is mainly distributed on the flexible rubber surface, which does not affect the mechanical strength of the rubber, and thus allows a higher tension limit.

14.11.3 Radiation-Shielding Performance of Liquid Metal Material

Figure 14.15a, b shows X-ray photographs of the silicon film uncoated and coated with the liquid metal, respectively [216]. It can be seen from Fig. 14.15 that the uncoated silicon film can hardly block X-rays, whereas when it is coated with the liquid metal, it can obviously block X-rays. Since it was difficult to evenly coat it with liquid metal using a screen in the lab, and the liquid metal coating was thin, dark spots show up in Fig. 14.15b, indicating a slightly inferior shielding effect.

Figure 14.16 shows the radiation-shielding abilities of the conventional lead-rubber and liquid metal shielding materials under different stretching conditions [216]. The original length of 30 mm was stretched to lengths of 35, 40, 45, and 50 mm, respectively. In the radiation photograph data processing, the mean gray-scale of the shielded area was employed as the evaluation criterion. In the case of complete shielding, the photograph was pure white, with a gray value of 255. Therefore, the radiation-shielding capability could be defined as $\eta = G/G_0$, where

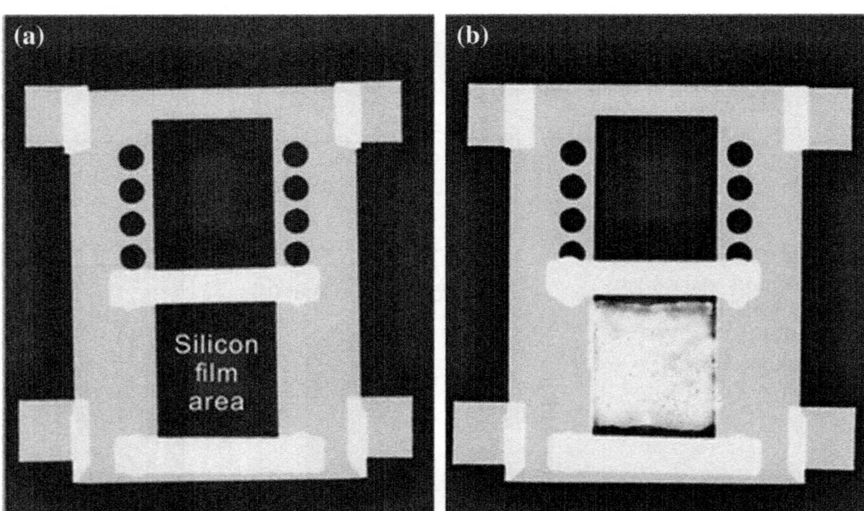

Fig. 14.15 Comparison of X-ray photographs of silicon film [216]. **a** uncoated with liquid metal and **b** coated with liquid metal. All pictures reproduced with permission

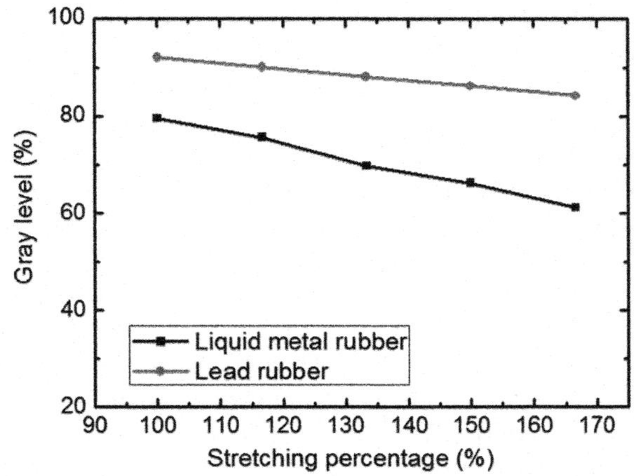

Fig. 14.16 Comparison of radiation-shielding performances of lead-rubber and liquid metal materials under different stretching conditions [216]. Picture reproduced with permission

G is the gray-scale value of the shielded area, G_0 is 255 (complete shielding), and η is the gray level.

It can be seen from Fig. 14.16 that the radiation-shielding ability gradually weakens with an increase in the stretching elongation for either material. This is mainly because the thickness of the shielding metal decreases with stretching. Hence, there is a stretching limit for the liquid metal radiation-shielding material. Once this stretching limit is reached, its radiation-shielding effect weakens. Furthermore, Fig. 14.16 shows that the performance of the current liquid metal radiation-shielding material cannot yet reach the performance of the conventional lead-particle-containing radiation-shielding material. This is mainly because the liquid metal coating is relatively thin. In addition, the current liquid metal material is mainly a gallium-based alloy, which has a radiation-shielding ability that is inferior to lead. From the practical aspect, the best solution is applying multilayer structure for liquid metal shielding film, which can effectively improve the radiation shielding capability, while retained the tensile strength of liquid metal shielding film. Besides, the greatest advantages of liquid metal shielding film lie in its high flexibility, biological safety, and higher adaptability, which is of great importance for applications to medical gloves, body coating, etc.

Generally, the attenuation of X-rays in a solid follows the simple exponential attenuation law. The linear attenuation coefficient of X-rays for a certain substance is related to the incident photon energy and shielding material atomic number. The total mass attenuation coefficient of the composite shielding material should be the summation of the mass attenuation coefficients of each element in the compound multiplied by its mass fraction in the shielding material. Thus, in the case of the liquid metal radiation-shielding film, the radiating shielding effect is mainly produced by the properties and thickness of the coated liquid metal. Although the lead particles in conventional lead rubber are evenly dispersed in the rubber, while the liquid metal in a liquid metal shielding material is coated on the surface of the rubber film, their radiation-shielding capabilities are both subject to the metal mass per unit area. Based on this theory, one can assume that multilayer liquid metal shielding film could offer much better shielding performance since the stacked liquid metal enhances the shielding capability.

Liquid metal possesses an outstanding radiation-shielding ability. Because of its adjustable viscosity, selective surface printing can be conveniently achieved using some conventional approaches like cold spraying and screen printing. Hence, liquid metal can be used not only to produce full-shielding medical materials, but also to efficiently produce a selective X-ray film using screen-printing technology. Figure 14.17 shows a selective X-ray shielding film fabricated using a liquid metal screen printing method, along with its X-ray radiation photograph [216]. It can be seen that liquid metal can be conveniently printed onto any rigid or flexible base. The coated liquid metal can produce an outstanding radiation-shielding effect and high resolution. Therefore, the liquid metal selective radiation-shielding method can achieve an extremely low-cost and highly efficient X-ray lithography mask, which is of great value in the X-ray lithography field. Moreover, in medical applications, selective local shielding can also be rapidly achieved using a liquid metal printing, without molding. Thus, it will cost less.

Overall, because of its excellent flexibility and good shielding capacity, liquid metal based radiation-shielding technology offers a promising solution for dealing with medical X-ray shielding applications. In addition, liquid metal based selective radiation shielding can be used to fabricate an extremely low-cost and highly efficient X-ray lithography mask. Overall, such a liquid metal based stretchable radiation-shielding film represents a feasible and cost-effective technology for the coming medical X-ray shielding applications.

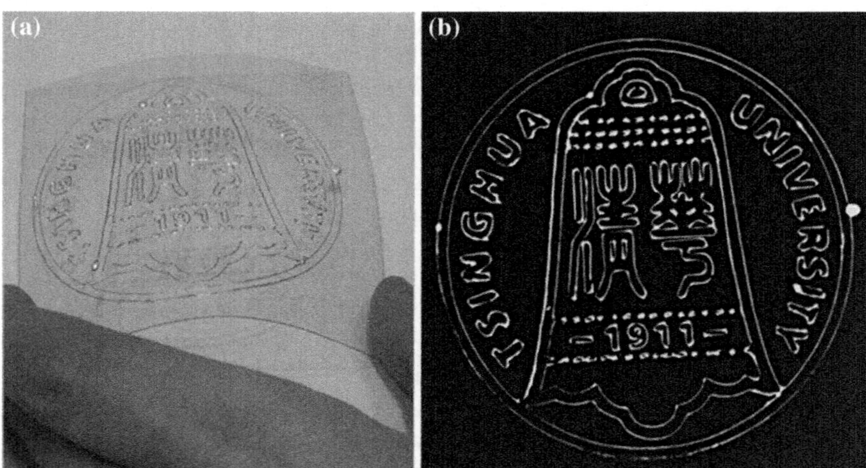

Fig. 14.17 **a** Liquid metal based screen-printed selective X-ray shielding film and **b** related X-ray radiation photograph [216]. All pictures reproduced with permission

14.12 Conclusion

This chapter provides an overview on current status and future prospects about the liquid metal wearable devices related to health care. Long-term or continuous wearable monitoring systems with unobtrusive sensors took in many advanced technologies like the electronic circuit, MEMS and nanotechnology, as well as novel approaches like noncontact ECG and glucose monitoring through blood substitutes. On this basis, information technology expedited the treatment with pharmaceutical products becoming more accurate with continuous automatic processes to dispense an effective dose of drug to treat disease. Besides, the scope of chronic disease treatment through wearable devices is broadened as the miniaturization of therapy equipment and clinical rehabilitation evidences with attempting various remedy methods.

So far, most systems are still in their prototype stages and there remain many problems to be solved. Some emerging directions for wearable monitoring and therapy devices are especially worthy of being emphasized in the near future. For example, flexible electronics, where electronic circuits are manufactured on flexible substrates such as paper, cloth fabrics and directly on human body to provide sensing, powering and interconnecting functions, have a broad range application like smart textile and transcutaneous film as new wearable monitoring systems. It is worth mentioning that, rapid advances in this field promise to allow one to print a full circuit on fabric or skin and new materials like liquid metal have the potential to directly print on skin to take effect. In the end, business models of liquid metal enabled flexible wearable monitoring and therapy devices need to be established. Only such wearable devices are used and accepted by patients as a reliable, multifunctional and easy-to-use technology, can they relieve the severe burdens of medical system and go farther in the avenue of improving quality of life.

References

1. Gui H, Liu J (2018) Latest progresses in developing wearable monitoring and therapy systems for managing chronic diseases. arXiv:1802.01747
2. Gulley SP, Rasch EK, Chan L (2011) If we build it, who will come? Working-age adults with chronic health care needs and the medical home. Med Care 49(2):149–155
3. Hung WW, Ross JS, Boockvar KS, Siu AL (2011) Recent trends in chronic disease, impairment and disability among older adults in the United States. BMC Geriatr 11(1):47–59
4. World Health Organization (2005) Preventing chronic diseases: a vital investment: WHO Global Report
5. Yach D, Hawkes C, Gould CL, Hofman KJ (2004) The global burden of chronic diseases: overcoming impediments to prevention and control. JAMA 291:2616–2622
6. Chodosh J, Morton SC, Mojica W, Maglione M, Suttorp MJ, Hilton L, Rhodes S, Shekelle P (2005) Meta-analysis: chronic disease self-management programs for older adults. Ann Intern Med 143(6):427–438
7. Starr PA, Vitek JL, Bakay RA (1998) Ablative surgery and deep brain stimulation for Parkinson's disease. Neurosurgery 43(5):989–1013

8. Who J, Diet FE (2003) Consultation, nutrition and the prevention of chronic diseases. World Health Organ Tech Rep Ser 916(i–viii)
9. Holman H, Lorig K (2004) Patient self-management: a key to effectiveness and efficiency in care of chronic disease. Public Health Rep 119(3):239–243
10. Wootton R (2012) Twenty years of telemedicine in chronic disease management-an evidence synthesis. J Telemedicine Telecare 18(4):211–220
11. Liu L, Liu J (2011) Mobile phone-enabled control of medical care and handicapped assistance. Expert Rev Med Devices 8(6):757–768
12. Morón MJ, Luque R, Casilari E (2014) On the capability of smartphones to perform as communication gateways in medical wireless personal area networks. Sensors 14(1):575–594
13. Jurik AD, Weaver AC (2008) Remote medical monitoring. Computer 41(4):96–99
14. Carson ER, Cramp DG, Morgan A, Roudsari AV (1998) Clinical decision support, systems methodology, and telemedicine: their role in the management of chronic disease. IEEE Trans Inf Technol Biomed 2(2):80–88
15. Celler BG, Lovell NH, Basilakis J (2003) Using information technology to improve the management of chronic disease. Med J Aust 179(5):242–246
16. Pagliarulo MA (2013) Introduction to physical therapy. Elsevier Health Sciences, Amsterdam
17. Montgomery K, Mundt C, Thonier G, et al (2004) Lifeguard-a personal physiological monitor for extreme environments. In: 26th annual international conference of the IEEE. Vol 1, pp 2192–2195
18. Yeo WH, Kim YS, Lee J et al (2013) Multifunctional epidermal electronics printed directly onto the skin. Adv Mater 25(20):2773–2778
19. Dudde R, Vering T, Piechotta G, Hintsche R (2006) Computer-aided continuous drug infusion: setup and test of a mobile closed-loop system for the continuous automated infusion of insulin. IEEE Trans Inf Technol Biomed 10(2):395–402
20. Graham J (2014) Technology for rehabilitating the upper limb after stroke: the hand. Br J Neurosci Nursing 10:19–24
21. Senelick RC (2010) Technological advances in stroke rehabilitation-high tech marries high touch. US Neurol 6(2):102–104
22. Prausnitz MR, Mitragotri S, Langer R (2004) Current status and future potential of transdermal drug delivery. Nat Rev Drug Discovery 3(2):115–124
23. Wen C, Yeh MF, Chang KC, Lee RG (2008) Real-time ECG telemonitoring system design with mobile phone platform. Measurement 41(4):463–470
24. Chen X, Ho CT, Lim T, Kyaw TZ (2007) Cellular phone based online ECG processing for ambulatory and continuous detection. Comput Cardiol, 653–656
25. Jin Z, Sun Y, Cheng AC (2009) Predicting cardiovascular disease from real-time electrocardiographic monitoring: an adaptive machine learning approach on a cell phone. In: 2009 annual international conference of the IEEE, pp 6889–6892
26. Chi YM, Jung TP, Cauwenberghs G (2010) Dry-contact and noncontact biopotential electrodes: methodological review. IEEE Rev Biomed Eng 3:106–119
27. Gruetzmann A, Hansen S, Müller J (2007) Novel dry electrodes for ECG monitoring. Physiol Meas 28(11):1375–1390
28. Park C, Chou PH, Bai Y, Matthews R, Hibbs A (2006) An ultra-wearable, wireless, low power ECG monitoring system. In: Biomedical circuits and systems conference. BioCAS IEEE, pp 241–244
29. Chi YM, Deiss SR, Cauwenberghs G (2009) Non-contact low power EEG/ECG electrode for high density wearable biopotential sensor networks. In: 6th international workshop on IEEE, pp 246–250
30. Costanza E, Inverso SA, Allen R, Maes P (2007) Intimate interfaces in action: assessing the usability and subtlety of EMG-based motionless gestures. In: Conference on human factors in computing systems. ACM, pp 819–828

31. Nazmi N, Abdul RMA, Yamamoto SI, Ahmad SA, Zamzuri H, Mazlan SA (2016) A review of classification techniques of EMG signals during isotonic and isometric contractions. Sensors 16(8):1304
32. Saponas TS, Tan DS, Morris D, Balakrishnan R (2008) Demonstrating the feasibility of using forearm electromyography for muscle-computer interfaces. In: Proceedings of the SIGCHI conference on human factors in computing systems, ACM, pp 515–524
33. Chavan VB, Mhala NN (2015) Development of hand gesture recognition framework using surface EMG and accelerometer sensor for mobile devices. Int Res J Eng Technol 2(5):232–238
34. Gruebler A, Suzuki K (2014) Design of a wearable device for reading positive expressions from facial EMG signals. IEEE Trans Affect Comput 5(3):227–237
35. Zhang X, Chen X, Li Y, Lantz V, Wang K, Yang J (2011) A framework for hand gesture recognition based on accelerometer and EMG sensors. IEEE Trans Syst Man Cybern Part A Syst Hum 41(6):1064–1076
36. Leone A, Rescio G, Caroppo A, Siciliano P (2015) A wearable EMG-based system pre-fall detector. Procedia Eng 120:455–458
37. Cheng J, Chen X, Shen M (2013) A framework for daily activity monitoring and fall detection based on surface electromyography and accelerometer signals. IEEE J Biomed Health Informatics 17(1):38–45
38. Kato T, Ueno A, Kataoka S, Hoshino H, Ishiyama Y (2006) An application of capacitive electrode for detecting electrocardiogram of neonates and infants. In: 28th annual international conference of the IEEE engineering in Medicine and Biology Society, pp 916–919
39. Lee YD, Chung WY (2009) Wireless sensor network based wearable smart shirt for ubiquitous health and activity monitoring. Sens Actuators B Chem 140(2):390–395
40. Nemati E, Deen MJ, Mondal T (2012) A wireless wearable ECG sensor for long-term applications. IEEE Commun Mag 50(1):36–43
41. Yama Y, Ueno A, Uchikawa Y (2007) Development of a wireless capacitive sensor for ambulatory ECG monitoring over clothes. In: 29th annual international conference of the IEEE, pp 5727–5730
42. Chi YM, Cauwenberghs G (2010) Wireless non-contact EEG/ECG electrodes for body sensor networks. In: International conference on IEEE body sensor networks (BSN), pp 297–301
43. Eilebrecht B, Czaplik M, Walter M, Wartzek T, Rossaint R, Leonhardt S (2009) Implementation of a capacitive ECG measurement system in clinical practice: an interim report. In: World congress on medical physics and biomedical engineering, Munich, Germany, pp 370–372
44. Gu WB, Poon CCY, Leung HK, Sy MY, Wong MYM, Zhang YT (2009) A novel method for the contactless and continuous measurement of arterial blood pressure on a sleeping bed. In: Annual international conference of the IEEE, pp 6084–6086
45. Aleksandrowicz A, Leonhardt S (2007) Wireless and non-contact ECG measurement system-the "Aachen SmartChair". Int VLSI J 47(4):4–5
46. Baek HJ, Chung GS, Kim KK, Park KS (2012) A smart health monitoring chair for nonintrusive measurement of biological signals. IEEE Trans Inf Technol Biomed 16(1):150–158
47. Kim KK, Lim YK, Park KS (2004) The electrically noncontacting ECG measurement on the toilet seat using the capacitively-coupled insulated electrodes. In: 26th annual international conference of the IEEE, vol 1, pp 2375–2378
48. Gómez-Clapers J, Casanella R (2012) A fast and easy-to-use ECG acquisition and heart rate monitoring system using a wireless steering wheel. IEEE Sens J 12(3):610–616
49. Moghimi S, Kushki A, Marie GA, Chau T (2013) A review of EEG-based brain-computer interfaces as access pathways for individuals with severe disabilities. Assistive Technol 25 (2):99–110

50. Lotte F, Congedo M, Lécuyer A, Lamarche F, Arnaldi B (2007) A review of classification algorithms for EEG-based brain-computer interfaces. J Neural Eng 4(2):R1
51. Curran EA, Stokes MJ (2003) Learning to control brain activity: a review of the production and control of EEG components for driving brain-computer interface (BCI) systems. Brain Cogn 51(3):326–336
52. Kübler A, Neumann N, Kaiser J, Kotchoubey B, Hinterberger T, Birbaumer NP (2001) Brain-computer communication: self-regulation of slow cortical potentials for verbal communication. Arch Phys Med Rehabil 82(11):1533–1539
53. Lin CT, Ko LW, Chang MH, Duann JR, Chen JY, Su TP, Jung TP (2010) Review of wireless and wearable electroencephalogram systems and brain-computer interfaces-a mini-review. Gerontology 56(1):112–119
54. Acharya UR, Fujita H, Sudarshan VK, Bhat S, Koh JE (2015) Application of entropies for automated diagnosis of epilepsy using EEG signals: a review. Knowl-Based Syst 88:85–96
55. Kondziella D, Friberg CK, Wellwood I, Reiffurth C, Fabricius M, Dreier JP (2015) Continuous EEG monitoring in aneurysmal subarachnoid hemorrhage: a systematic review. Neurocrit Care 22(3):450–461
56. Acharya UR, Sree SV, Swapna G, Martis RJ, Suri JS (2013) Automated EEG analysis of epilepsy: a review. Knowl Based Syst 45(3):147–165
57. Bhat S, Acharya UR, Dadmehr N, Adeli H (2015) Clinical neurophysiological and automated EEG-based diagnosis of the Alzheimer's disease. Eur Neurol 74(3–4):202–210
58. Motamedi-Fakhr S, Moshrefi-Torbati M, Hill M, Hill CM, White PR (2014) Signal processing techniques applied to human sleep EEG signals-a review. Biomed Signal Process Control 10(2):21–33
59. Meier R, Dittrich H, Schulze-Bonhage A, Aertsen A (2008) Detecting epileptic seizures in long-term human EEG: a new approach to automatic online and real-time detection and classification of polymorphic seizure patterns. J Clin Neurophysiol 25(3):119–131
60. Minasyan GR, Chatten JB, Chatten MJ, Harner RN (2010) Patient-specific early seizure detection from scalp EEG. J Clin Neurophysiol 27(3):163–178
61. Correa AG, Laciar E, Patiño H, Valentinuzzi ME (2007) Artifact removal from EEG signals using adaptive filters in cascade. J Phys Conf 2007, 012081 (IOP Publishing)
62. Güler I, Übeyli ED (2005) Adaptive neuro-fuzzy inference system for classification of EEG signals using wavelet coefficients. J Neurosci Methods 148(2):113–121
63. Subasi A (2007) EEG signal classification using wavelet feature extraction and a mixture of expert model. Expert Syst Appl 32(4):1084–1093
64. Aarabi A, Fazel-Rezai R, Aghakhani Y (2009) A fuzzy rule-based system for epileptic seizure detection in intracranial EEG. Clin Neurophysiol 120(9):1648–1657
65. Polat K, Güneş S (2007) Classification of epileptiform EEG using a hybrid system based on decision tree classifier and fast Fourier transform. Appl Math Comput 187(2):1017–1026
66. Chan AM, Sun FT, Boto EH, Wingeier BM (2008) Automated seizure onset detection for accurate onset time determination in intracranial EEG. Clin Neurophysiol 119(12):2687–2696
67. Niederhauser JJ, Esteller R, Echauz J, Vachtsevanos G, Litt B (2003) Detection of seizure precursors from depth-EEG using a sign periodogram transform. IEEE Trans Bio-med Eng 50(4):449–458
68. Gabor AJ (1998) Seizure detection using a self-organizing neural network: validation and comparison with other detection strategies. Electroencephalogr Clin Neurophysiol 107 (1):27–32
69. Tzallas AT, Tsipouras MG, Fotiadis DI (2007) Automatic seizure detection based on time-frequency analysis and artificial neural networks. Comput Intell Neurosci 4:80510
70. Abibullaev B, Seo HD, Kim MS (2010) Epileptic spike detection using continuous wavelet transforms and artificial neural networks. Int J Wavelets Multiresolut Inf Process 8:33–48
71. Yuan Q, Zhou W, Li S, Cai D (2011) Epileptic EEG classification based on extreme learning machine and nonlinear features. Epilepsy Res 96(1–2):29–38

72. Corbishley P, Rodríguez-Villegas E (2008) Breathing detection: towards a miniaturized, wearable, battery-operated monitoring system. IEEE Trans Biomed Eng 55(1):196–204
73. Chen G, Imtiaz SA, Aguilar-Pelaez E, Rodriguez-Villegas E (2015) Algorithm for heart rate extraction in a novel wearable acoustic sensor. Healthcare Technol Lett 2(1):28
74. Teague CN, Hersek S, Toreyin H et al (2016) Novel methods for sensing acoustical emissions from the knee for wearable joint health assessment. IEEE Trans Biomed Eng 63 (8):1581–1590
75. Inan OT, Hersek S, Teague CN et al (2016) A stethoscope for the knee: investigating joint acoustical emissions as novel biomarkers for wearable joint health assessment. J Acoust Soc Am 139(4):2175–2176
76. Teague C, Hersek S, Töreyin H et al (2015) Novel approaches to measure acoustic emissions as biomarkers for joint health assessment. In: IEEE 12th international conference on wearable and implantable body sensor networks (BSN), pp 1–6
77. Hu Y, Kim EG, Cao G, Liu S, Xu Y (2014) Physiological acoustic sensing based on accelerometers: a survey for mobile healthcare. Ann Biomed Eng 42(11):2264–2277
78. Mehta DD, Zañartu M, Feng SW, Cheyne II HA, Hillman RE (2012) Mobile voice health monitoring using a wearable accelerometer sensor and a smartphone platform. IEEE Trans Biomed Eng 59(11):3090–3096
79. Bombardini T, Sicari R, Bianchini E, Picano E (2011) Abnormal shortened diastolic time length at increasing heart rates in patients with abnormal exercise-induced increase in pulmonary artery pressure. Cardiovasc Ultrasound 9(1):1–9
80. Bucklin CL, Das M, Luo SL (2010) An inexpensive accelerometer-based sleep-apnea screening technique. Proc IEEE Int Aerospace Electron Conf 7675(1):396–399
81. Khlif MS, Boashash B, Layeghy S, Ben-Jabeur T, Mesbah M, East C, Colditz P (2011) Time-frequency characterization of tri-axial accelerometer data for fetal movement detection. In: IEEE international symposium on signal processing and information technology, pp 466–471
82. Li B, Wang JR, Ma YL (2012) Bowel sounds and monitoring gastrointestinal motility in critically ill patients. Clin Nurse Specialist 26(1):29–34
83. Pandia K, Ravindran S, Cole R, Kovacs GT, Giovangrandi L (2010) Motion artifact cancellation to obtain heart sounds from a single chest-worn accelerometer. In: ICASSP, pp 590–593
84. Mendelson Y, Duckworth RJ, Comtois G (2006) A wearable reflectance pulse oximeter for remote physiological monitoring. In: 28th annual international conference of the IEEE engineering in Medicine and Biology Society, EMBS'06, pp 912–915
85. Celka P, Verjus C, Vetter R, Renevey P, Neuman V (2004) Motion resistant earphone located infrared based heart rate measurement device. Biomed Eng
86. Shaltis PA, Reisner A, Asada HH (2006) Wearable, cuff-less PPG-based blood pressure monitor with novel height sensor. Engineering in Medicine and Biology Society, 2006. In: EMBS'06. 28th annual international conference of the IEEE, pp 908–911
87. Leonard PA, Clifton D, Addison PS, Watson JN, Beattie T (2006) An automated algorithm for determining respiratory rate by photoplethysmogram in children. Acta Paediatr 95 (9):1124–1128
88. Tamura T, Maeda Y, Sekine M, Yoshida M (2014) Wearable photoplethysmographic sensors-past and present. Electronics 3(2):282–302
89. Patterson JAC, McIlwraith DC, Yang GZ (2009) A flexible, low noise reflective PPG sensor platform for ear-worn heart rate monitoring. In: Sixth International Workshop on Wearable and Implantable Body Sensor Networks. IEEE, pp 286–291
90. Rhee S, Yang BH, Asada HH (2001) Artifact-resistant power-efficient design of finger-ring plethysmographic sensors. IEEE Trans Biomed Eng 48(7):795–805
91. Asada HH, Shaltis P, Reisner A, Rhee S, Hutchinson RC (2003) Mobile monitoring with wearable photoplethysmographic biosensors. IEEE Eng Med Biol Mag 22(3):28–40

92. Xu H, Li J, Leung BHK, Poon CC, Ong BS, Zhang Y, Zhao N (2013) A high-sensitivity near-infrared phototransistor based on an organic bulk heterojunction. Nanoscale 5 (23):11850–11855
93. Nemati S, Ghassemi MM, Ambai V, Isakadze N, Levantsevych O, Shah A, Clifford GD (2016) Monitoring and detecting atrial fibrillation using wearable technology. In: 38th annual international conference of the IEEE engineering in Medicine and Biology Society (EMBC), pp 3394–3397
94. Grubb MR, Carpenter J, Crowe JA, Teoh J, Marlow N, Ward C, Mann C, Sharkey D, Hayes-Gill BR (2014) Forehead reflectance photoplethysmography to monitor heart rate: preliminary results from neonatal patients. Physiol Meas 35(5):881
95. Juvenile Diabetes Research Foundation Continuous Glucose Monitoring Study Group (2008) Continuous glucose monitoring and intensive treatment of type 1 diabetes. New England J Med 359(14):1464–1476
96. Klonoff DC (2005) Continuous glucose monitoring roadmap for 21st century diabetes therapy. Diabetes Care 28(5):1231–1239
97. Oliver NS, Toumazou C, Cass AEG, Johnston DG (2009) Glucose sensors: a review of current and emerging technology. Diabet Med 26(3):197–210
98. Hovorka R, Allen JM, Elleri D et al (2010) Manual closed-loop insulin delivery in children and adolescents with type 1 diabetes: a phase 2 randomised crossover trial. Lancet 375 (9716):743–751
99. Clarke WL, Anderson S, Breton M, Patek S, Kashmer L, Kovatchev B (2009) Closed-loop artificial pancreas using subcutaneous glucose sensing and insulin delivery and a model predictive control algorithm: the Virginia experience. J Diabetes Sci Technol 3(5):1031–1038
100. Potts RO, Tamada J, Tierney MJ (2002) Glucose monitoring by reverse iontophoresis. Diabetes/metab Res Rev 18(S1):S49–S53
101. Tierney MJ, Tamada JA, Potts RO, Jovanovic L, Garg S (2001) Clinical evaluation of the GlucoWatch® biographer: a continual, non-invasive glucose monitor for patients with diabetes. Biosens Bioelectron 16:621–629
102. Diabetes Research in Children Network (DirecNet) Study Group (2004) Accuracy of the glucowatch g2 biographer and the continuous glucose monitoring system during hypoglycemia. experience of the diabetes research in children network (direcnet. Diabetes Care 27:722
103. Rebrin K, Steil GM, Antwerp WP, Mastrototaro JJ (1999) Subcutaneous glucose predicts plasma glucose independent of insulin: implications for continuous monitoring. Am J Physiol 277(1):E561–E571
104. Steil GM, Rebrin K, Hariri F, Jinagonda S, Tadros S, Darwin C, Saad MF (2005) Interstitial fluid glucose dynamics during insulin-induced hypoglycaemia. Diabetologia 48(9):1833–1840
105. Aussedat B, Dupire-Angel M, Gifford R, Klein JC, Wilson GS, Reach G (2000) Interstitial glucose concentration and glycemia: implications for continuous subcutaneous glucose monitoring. Am J Physiol Endocrinol Metab 278(4):E716–E728
106. Kovatchev B, Clarke W (2008) Peculiarities of the continuous glucose monitoring data stream and their impact on developing closed-loop control technology. J Diab Sci Technol 2 (1):158–163
107. Clarke WL, Kovatchev B (2007) Continuous glucose sensors: continuing questions about clinical accuracy. J Diab Sci Technol 1(5):669–675
108. Diabetes Research in Children Network (DirecNet) Study Group (2008) The accuracy of the Guardian® RT continuous glucose monitor in children with type 1 diabetes. Diab Technol Ther 10(4):266–272
109. Garg SK, Smith J, Beatson C, Lopez-Baca B, Voelmle M, Gottlieb PA (2009) Comparison of accuracy and safety of the SEVEN and the Navigator continuous glucose monitoring systems. Diab Technol Ther 11(2):65–72

110. Chuang H, Trieu MQ, Hurley J, Taylor EJ, England MR, Nasraway SA (2008) Pilot studies of transdermal continuous glucose measurement in outpatient diabetic patients and in patients during and after cardiac surgery. J Diab Sci Technol 2(4):595–602
111. Keenan DB, Mastrototaro JJ, Voskanyan G, Steil GM (2009) Delays in minimally invasive continuous glucose monitoring devices: a review of current technology. J Diab Sci Technol 3(5):1207–1214
112. Saur NM, England MR, Menzie W et al (2014) Accuracy of a novel noninvasive transdermal continuous glucose monitor in critically ill patients. J Diab Sci Technol 8(5):945–950
113. Vashist SK (2012) Non-invasive glucose monitoring technology in diabetes management: a review. Anal Chim Acta 750(11):16–27
114. Lipson J, Bernhardt J, Block U et al (2009) Requirements for calibration in noninvasive glucose monitoring by Raman spectroscopy. J Diab Sci Technol 3(2):233–241
115. Caduff A, Dewarrat F, Talary M, Stalder G, Heinemann L, Feldman Y (2006) Non-invasive glucose monitoring in patients with diabetes: a novel system based on impedance spectroscopy. Biosens Bioelectron 22(5):598–604
116. Caduff A, Talary MS, Mueller M, Dewarrat F, Klisic J, Donath M, Heinemann L, Stahel WA (2009) Non-invasive glucose monitoring in patients with Type 1 diabetes: a multisensor system combining sensors for dielectric and optical characterisation of skin. Biosens Bioelectron 24:2778–2784
117. Harman-Boehm I, Gal A, Raykhman AM, Zahn JD, Naidis E, Mayzel Y (2009) Noninvasive glucose monitoring: a novel approach. J Diab Sci Technol 3(2):253–260
118. Harman-Boehm I, Gal A, Raykhman AM, Naidis E, Mayzel Y (2010) Noninvasive glucose monitoring: increasing accuracy by combination of multi-technology and multi-sensors. J Diab Sci Technol 4(3):583–595
119. Feldman B, Brazg R, Schwartz S, Weinstein R (2003) A continuous glucose sensor based on Wired Enzyme™ technology-results from a 3-day trial in patients with type 1 diabetes. Diabs Technol Ther 5(5):769–779
120. Vashist SK (2013) Continuous glucose monitoring systems: a review. Diagnostics 3(4):385–412
121. Abdul RAH, Zayegh A, Begg RK, Wahab Y (2012) Foot plantar pressure measurement system: a review. Sensors 12(7):9884–9912
122. Zang Y, Zhang F, Di C, Zhu D (2015) Advances of flexible pressure sensors toward artificial intelligence and health care applications. Mater Horiz 2(2):140–156
123. Sazonov ES, Fulk G, Sazonova N, Schuckers S (2009) Automatic recognition of postures and activities in stroke patients. In: Annual international conference of the IEEE engineering in Medicine and Biology Society, pp 2200–2203
124. Bamberg SJM, Benbasat AY, Scarborough DM, Krebs DE, Paradiso JA (2008) Gait analysis using a shoe-integrated wireless sensor system. IEEE Trans Inf Technol Biomed 12(4):413–423
125. Schwartz G, Tee BCK, Mei J, Appleton AL, Kim D, Wang H, Bao Z (2013) Flexible polymer transistors with high pressure sensitivity for application in electronic skin and health monitoring. Nat Commun 4(5):1859
126. Pang C, Lee GY, Kim T, Kim SM, Kim HN, Ahn SH, Suh KY (2012) A flexible and highly sensitive strain-gauge sensor using reversible interlocking of nanofibres. Nat Mater 11 (9):795–801
127. Gong S, Schwalb W, Wang Y, Tang Y, Si J, Shirinzadeh B, Cheng W (2014) A wearable and highly sensitive pressure sensor with ultrathin gold nanowires. Nat Commun 5(2):3132
128. Wang X, Gu Y, Xiong Z, Zhang T (2014) Silk-molded flexible, ultrasensitive, and highly stable electronic skin for monitoring human physiological signals. Adv Mater 26(9):1336–1342
129. Yamada T, Hayamizu Y, Yamamoto Y, Yomogida Y, Izadi-Najafabadi A, Futaba DN, Hata K (2011) A stretchable carbon nanotube strain sensor for human-motion detection. Nat Nanotechnol 6(5):296–301

130. Son D, Lee J, Qiao S, Ghaffari R et al (2014) Multifunctional wearable devices for diagnosis and therapy of movement disorders. Nat Nanotechnol 9(5):397–404
131. Deo R, Albert CM (2012) Epidemiology and genetics of sudden cardiac death. Circulation 125(4):620–637
132. Auricchio A, Klein H, Geller CJ, Reek S, Heilman MS, Szymkiewicz SJ (1998) Clinical efficacy of the wearable cardioverter-defibrillator in acutely terminating episodes of ventricular fibrillation. Am J Cardiol 81(10):1253–1256
133. Reek S, Geller JC, Meltendorf U, Wollbrueck A, Szymkiewicz SJ, Klein HU (2003) Clinical efficacy of a wearable defibrillator in acutely terminating episodes of ventricular fibrillation using biphasic shocks. Pacing Clin Electrophysiol Pace 26(10):2016–2022
134. Feldman AM, Klein H, Tchou P et al (2004) Use of a wearable defibrillator in terminating tachyarrhythmias in patients at high risk for sudden death. Pacing Clin Electrophysiol Pace 27(1):4–9
135. Klein HU, Goldenberg I, Moss AJ (2013) Risk stratification for implantable cardioverter defibrillator therapy: the role of the wearable cardioverter-defibrillator. Eur Heart J 34 (29):2230–2242
136. Sasaki S, Tomita H, Shibutani S et al (2014) Usefulness of the wearable cardioverter-defibrillator in patients at high risk for sudden cardiac death. Circ J 78 (12):2987–2989
137. Hovorka R (2011) Closed-loop insulin delivery: from bench to clinical practice. Nat Rev Endocrinol 7(7):385–395
138. Cobelli C, Renard E, Kovatchev B (2011) Artificial pancreas: past, present, future. Diabetes 60(11):2672–2682
139. Buckingham B, Chase HP, Dassau E et al (2010) Prevention of nocturnal hypoglycemia using predictive alarm algorithms and insulin pump suspension. Diab Care 33(5):1013–1017
140. Del Favero S, Bruttomesso D, Palma F et al (2014) First use of model predictive control in outpatient wearable artificial pancreas. Diab Care 37(5):1212–1215
141. Kovatchev BP, Renard E, Cobelli C et al (2014) Safety of outpatient closed-loop control: first randomized crossover trials of a wearable artificial pancreas. Diab Care 37(7):1789–1796
142. El-Khatib FH, Russell SJ, Nathan DM, Sutherlin RG, Damiano ER (2010) A bihormonal closed-loop artificial pancreas for type 1 diabetes. Sci Transl Med 2(27):27ra27–27ra27
143. Mastrototaro J, Lee S (2009) The integrated miniMed paradigm REAL-Time insulin pump and glucose monitoring system: implications for improved patient outcomes. Diab Technol Ther 11(S1):S37–S43
144. Kjellstrand CM, Rosa AA, Shideman JR, Rodrigo F, Davin T, Lynch RE (1978) Optimal dialysis frequency and duration: the "unphysiology hypothesis". Kidney Int Suppl 8(8): S120–S124
145. Kooman JP, Joles JA, Gerritsen KGF (2015) Creating a wearable artificial kidney: where are we now? Expert Rev Med Devices 12(4):373–376
146. Kim JC, Garzotto F, Nalesso F, Cruz D, Kim JH, Kang E, Kim HC, Ronco C (2011) A wearable artificial kidney: technical requirements and potential solutions. Expert Rev Med Devices 8(5):567–579
147. Jacobsen SC, Stephen RL, Bulloch EC, Luntz RD, Kolff WJ (1975) A wearable artificial kidney: functional description of hardware and clinical results. Proc Clin Dialysis Transplant Forum 5(5):65–71
148. Stephens RL, Jacobsen SC, Atkin-Thor E, Kolff W (1975) Portable/wearable artificial kidney (WAK)-initial evaluation. In: Proceedings of the European Dialysis and Transplant Association. European Dialysis and Transplant Association vol 12, issue 2, pp 511–518
149. Reynier JP, Ragon A (1985) A continuous hemofiltration system using sorbents for hemofiltrate regeneration. Clin Nephrol 26:S53–S57
150. Roberts M (1993) Wearable artificial kidneys for continuous dialysis: a personal view. ASAIO J 39(1):19–23

151. Gura V, Beizai M, Ezon C, Polaschegg H (2005) Continuous renal replacement therapy for end-stage renal disease. In: 14th international course on hemodialysis. Vicenza, vol 149, issue 2, pp 325–333
152. Davenport A, Gura V, Ronco C, Beizai M, Ezon C, Rambod E (2007) A wearable haemodialysis device for patients with end-stage renal failure: a pilot study. Lancet 370 (9604):2005–2010
153. Roberts M, Ash SR, Lee DBN (1999) Innovative peritoneal dialysis: flow-thru and dialysate regeneration. ASAIO J 45(5):372–378
154. Ronco C, Fecondini L (2007) The Vicenza wearable artificial kidney for peritoneal dialysis (ViWAK PD). Blood Purif 25(4):383–388
155. Gura V, Ronco C, Nalesso F et al (2008) A wearable hemofilter for continuous ambulatory ultrafiltration. Kidney Int 74(4):537–538
156. Lang AE, Lozano AM (1998) Parkinson's disease. N Engl J Med 339:1044–1053
157. Patel S, Lorincz K, Hughes R et al (2009) Monitoring motor fluctuations in patients with Parkinson's disease using wearable sensors. IEEE Trans Inf Technol Biomed 13(6):864–873
158. Bächlin M, Plotnik M, Roggen D, Maidan I, Hausdorff JM, Giladi N, Troster G (2010) Wearable assistant for parkinson's disease patients with the freezing of gait symptom. IEEE Trans Inf Technol Biomed 14(2):436–446
159. Ferrarin M, Brambilla M, Garavello L, Di CA, Pedotti A, Rabuffetti M (2004) Microprocessor-controlled optical stimulating device to improve the gait of patients with Parkinson's disease. Med Biol Eng Comput 42(3):328–332
160. Espay AJ, Baram Y, Dwivedi AK et al (2010) At-home training with closed-loop augmented-reality cueing device for improving gait in patients with Parkinson disease. J Rehabil Res Dev 47(6):573–581
161. Maciejasz P, Eschweiler J, Gerlach-Hahn K, Jansen-Troy A, Leonhardt S (2014) A survey on robotic devices for upper limb rehabilitation. J Neuroeng Rehabil 11(1):3
162. Zhang M, Davies TC, Xie S (2013) Effectiveness of robot-assisted therapy on ankle rehabilitation-a systematic review. J Neuroeng Rehabil 10(1):30
163. Hasegawa Y, Mikami Y, Watanabe K, Sankai Y (2008) Five-fingered assistive hand with mechanical compliance of human finger. In: International conference on IEEE, pp 718–724
164. Rocon E, Belda-Lois JM, Ruiz AF, Manto M, Moreno JC, Pons JL (2007) Design and validation of a rehabilitation robotic exoskeleton for tremor assessment and suppression. IEEE Trans Neural Syst Rehabil Eng 15(3):367–378
165. Vanderniepen I, Van HR, Van DM, Sankai Y (2009) Orthopaedic rehabilitation: a powered elbow orthosis using compliant actuation. In: International conference on IEEE rehabilitation robotics, pp 172–177
166. Blaya J, Herr H (2004) Adaptive control of a variable-impedance ankle-foot orthosis to assist drop-foot gait. IEEE Trans Neural Syst Rehabil Eng 12(1):24–31
167. Balasubramanian S, Wei R, Perez M, Shepard B, Koeneman E, Koeneman J, He JR (2008) An exoskeleton robot for assisting rehabilitation of arm functions. Virtual Rehabilitation, pp 163–167
168. Park YL, Chen B, Pérez-Arancibia NO, Stirling L, Wood RJ, Goldfield EC, Nagpal R (2014) Design and control of a bio-inspired soft wearable robotic device for ankle-foot rehabilitation. Bioinspiration Biomimetics 9(1):016007
169. Pylatiuk C, Kargov A, Gaiser I, Werner T, Schulz S, Bretthauer G (2009) Design of a flexible fluidic actuation system for a hybrid elbow orthosis. In: International conference on IEEE rehabilitation robotics, pp 167–171
170. Hamid S, Hayek R (2008) Role of electrical stimulation for rehabilitation and regeneration after spinal cord injury: an overview. Eur Spine J 17(9):1256–1269
171. Del-Ama AJ, Koutsou AD, Moreno JC, De-Los-Reyes A, Gil-Agudo Á, Pons JL (2012) Review of hybrid exoskeletons to restore gait following spinal cord injury. J Rehabil Res Dev 49(4):497–514

172. Freeman CT, Hughes AM, Burridge JH, Chappell PH, Lewin PL, Rogers E (2009) A robotic workstation for stroke rehabilitation of the upper extremity using FES. Med Eng Phys 31 (3):364–373
173. Li R, Hu XL, Tong KY (2008) Combined electromyography (EMG)-driven system with functional electrical stimulation (FES) for poststroke rehabilitation. In: 2nd IEEE RAS & EMBS international conference on IEEE biomedical robotics and biomechatronics, pp 642–646
174. Holtz B, Lauckner C (2012) Diabetes management via mobile phones: a systematic review. Telemedicine J Ez-Health 18(3):175–184
175. El-Gayar O, Timsina P, Nawar N, Eid W (2013) Mobile applications for diabetes self-management: status and potential. J Diab Sci Technol 7(1):247–262
176. Årsand E, Tatara N, Hartvigsen G (2010) Mobile phone-based self-management tools for type 2 diabetes: the few touch application. J Diab Sci Technol 4(2):328–336
177. Quinn CC, Clough SS, Minor JM, Lender D, Okafor MC, Gruber-Baldini A (2008) WellDoc™ mobile diabetes management randomized controlled trial: change in clinical and behavioral outcomes and patient and physician satisfaction. Diab Technol Ther 10(3):160–168
178. Katz R, Mesfin T, Barr K (2012) Lessons from a community-based mHealth diabetes self-management program: "it's not just about the cell phone". J Health Commun 17:67–72
179. Salber P, Niksch A (2015) Digital health tools for diabetes. J Ambulatory care Manage 38 (2):196–199
180. Gui H, Tan S, Wang Q, Yu Y, Liu F, Liu J (2017) Spraying printing of liquid metal electronics on various clothes to compose wearable functional device. Sci China Technol Sci 60(2):306–316
181. Axisa F, Schmitt PM, Gehin C, Delhomme G, McAdams E, Dittmar A (2005) Flexible technologies and smart clothing for citizen medicine, home healthcare, and disease prevention. IEEE Trans Inf Technol Biomed 9(3):325–936
182. Patel S, Park H, Bonato P, Chan L, Rodgers M (2012) A review of wearable sensors and systems with application in rehabilitation. J Neuroeng Rehabil 9(1):1–17
183. Cherenack K, Pieterson LV (2012) Smart textiles: challenges and opportunities. J Appl Phys 112:091301–091314
184. Cottet D, Grzyb J, Kirstein T, Troster G (2003) Electrical characterization of textile transmission lines. IEEE Trans Adv Packag 26(2):182–190
185. Huang CT, Shen CL, Tang CF, Chang SH (2008) A wearable yarn-based piezo-resistive sensor. Sens Actuators, A 141(2):396–403
186. Roh JS, Chi YS, Lee JH, Tak Y, Nam S, Kang TJ (2010) Embroidered wearable multiresonant folded dipole antenna for FM reception. IEEE Antennas Wireless Propag Lett 9(1):803–806
187. Ouyang Y, Chappell WJ (2008) High frequency properties of electro-textiles for wearable antenna applications. IEEE Trans Antennas Propag 56(2):381–389
188. Berzowska J, Coelho MK, and vilkas: Kinetic electronic garments. IEEE International Symposium on Wearable Computers, 2005, 82–85
189. Gimpel S, Mohring U, Muller H, Neudeck A (2004) Textile-based electronic substrate technology. J Ind Text 33(33):179–189
190. Vervust T, Buyle G, Bossuyt F, Vanfleteren J (2012) Integration of stretchable and washable electronic modules for smart textile applications. J Textile Inst Proc Abstr 103(10):1127–1138
191. Sirringhaus H, Kawase T, Friend RH, Shimoda T, Inbasekaran M, Wu W, Woo EP (2000) High-resolution inkjet printing of all-polymer transistor circuits. Science 290(5499):2123–2126
192. Petukhov DI, Kirikova MN, Bessonov AA, Bailey MJ (2014) Nickel and copper conductive patterns fabricated by reactive inkjet printing combined with electroless plating. Mater Lett 132(132):302–306

193. Jeong S, Woo K, Kim D et al (2008) Controlling the thickness of the surface oxide layer on Cu nanoparticles for the fabrication of conductive structures by ink-jet printing. Adv Func Mater 18(5):679–686
194. Matsuhisa N, Kaltenbrunner M, Yokota T, Jinno H, Kuribara K, Sekitani T, Someya T (2015) Printable elastic conductors with a high conductivity for electronic textile applications. Nat Commun 6:7461
195. Hu L, Pasta M, Mantia FL et al (2010) Stretchable, porous, and conductive energy textiles. Nano Lett 10(2):708–714
196. Wang Q, Yu Y, Yang J, Liu J (2015) Fast fabrication of flexible functional circuits based on liquid metal dual-trans printing. Adv Mater 27(44):7109–7116
197. Liu Y, Gao M, Mei S, Han Y, Liu J (2013) Ultra-compliant liquid metal electrodes with in-plane self-healing capability for dielectric elastomer actuators. Appl Phys Lett 103(6):242
198. Gao Y, Li H, Liu J (2013) Directly writing resistor, inductor and capacitor to composite functional circuits: a super-simple way for alternative electronics. PLoS ONE 8(8):e69761–e69768
199. Lazarus N, Meyer CD, Bedair SS, Nochetto H, Kierzewski IM (2014) Multilayer liquid metal stretchable inductors. Smart Mater Struct 23(23):085036-10
200. Cheng S, Rydberg A, Hjort K, Wu ZG (2009) Liquid metal stretchable unbalanced loop antenna. Appl Phys Lett 94(14):5524
201. Cheng S, Wu Z (2011) A microfluidic, reversibly stretchable, large-area wireless strain sensor. Adv Func Mater 21(12):2282–2290
202. Fassler A, Majidi C (2013) Soft-matter capacitors and inductors for hyperelastic strain sensing and stretchable electronics. Smart Mater Struct 22(5):055023–055028
203. Park YL, Majidi C, Kramer R, Berard P, Wood RJ (2010) Hyperelastic pressure sensing with a liquid-embedded elastomer. J Micromech Microeng 20(12):125029–125034
204. Zheng Y, Zhang Q, Liu J (2013) Pervasive liquid metal based direct writing electronics with roller-ball pen. AIP Adv 3(11):2123
205. Zheng Y, He ZZ, Yang J, Liu J (2014) Personal electronics printing via tapping mode composite liquid metal ink delivery and adhesion mechanism. Sci Rep 4(6179):4588
206. Gao Y, Li H, Liu J (2012) Direct writing of flexible electronics through room temperature liquid metal ink. PLoS One 7(9): e45485-10
207. Boley JW, White EL, Chiu GTC, Kramer RK (2014) Direct writing of gallium-indium alloy for stretchable electronics. Adv Func Mater 24(23):3501–3507
208. Zhang Q, Gao Y, Liu J (2014) Atomized spraying of liquid metal droplets on desired substrate surfaces as a generalized way for ubiquitous printed electronics. Appl Phys A 116 (3):1091–1097
209. Wang L, Liu J (2015) Ink spraying based liquid metal printed electronics for directly making smart home appliances. ECS J Solid State Sci Technol 4(4):3057–3062
210. Guo C, Yu Y, Liu J (2014) Rapidly patterning conductive components on skin substrates as physiological testing devices via liquid metal spraying and pre-designed mask. J Mater Chem B 2(35):5739–5745
211. Wang L, Liu J (2014) Liquid phase 3D printing for quickly manufacturing conductive metal objects with low melting point alloy ink. Sci China Technol Sci 57(9):1721–1728
212. Regan MJ, Tostmann H, Pershan PS, Magnussen OM, Dimasi E, Ocko BM, Deutsch M (1997) X-ray study of the oxidation of liquid-gallium surfaces. Phys Rev B 55(16):10786–10790
213. Xu Q, Oudalov N, Guo Q, Jarger HM, Brown E (2012) Effect of oxidation on the mechanical properties of liquid gallium and eutectic gallium-indium. Phys Fluids 24 (6):063101–063113
214. Schrader ME (1995) Young-Dupre revisited. Langmuir 11(9):3585–3589
215. Engel OG (1955) Waterdrop collisions with solid surfaces. J Res Nat Bureau Standards 54 (5):281–298
216. Deng YG, Liu J (2015) Liquid metal based stretchable radiation-shielding film. ASME J Med Devices 9(1):014502–014502-4

217. Antic V, Stankovic K, Vujisic M, Osmokrovic P (2013) Comparison of various methods for designing the shielding from ionising radiation at PET-CT installations. Radiat Prot Dosimetry 154(2):245–249
218. Li QF, Xing QZ, Kong CC (2009) Physical analysis of the radiation shielding for the medical accelerators. J Appl Phys 105(3):1–4
219. McCaffrey JP, Tessier F, Shen H (2012) Radiation shielding materials and radiation scatter effects for interventional radiology (IR) physicians. Med Phys 39(7):4537–4546
220. Romanets Y, Bernardes AP, Dorsival A et al (2013) Radiation protection, radiation safety and radiation shielding assessment of HIE-ISOLDE. Radiat Prot Dosimetry 155(3):351–363
221. Arranz-Andres J, Perez E, Cerrada ML (2014) Lightweight nanocomposites based on polypropylene and aluminum nanoparticles and their shielding capability to ionizing radiation. IEEE Trans Nanotechnol 13(3):502–509
222. Li Z, Nambiar S, Zheng W, Yeow JTW (2013) PDMS/single-walled carbon nanotube composite for proton radiation shielding in space applications. Mater Lett 108(10):79–83
223. Shin JW, Lee JW, Yu S et al (2014) Polyethylene/boron-containing composites for radiation shielding. Thermochim Acta 585(2):5–9
224. McCaffrey JP, Mainegra-Hing E, Shen H (2009) Optimizing non-Pb radiation shielding materials using bilayers. Med Phys 36(12):5586–5594
225. Schlattl H, Zankl M, Eder H, Hoeschen C (2007) Shielding properties of lead-free protective clothing and their impact on radiation doses. Med Phys 34(11):4270–4280
226. Yue K, Luo WY, Dong XQ, Wang CS, Wu GH, Jiang MW, Zha YZ (2009) A new lead-free radiation shielding material for radiotherapy. Radiat Prot Dosimetry 133(4):256–260
227. Zia N, Fakhar-E-Alam M, Atif M et al (2014) Designing of sophisticated automatic lead shielding to reduce radiation dose of Tc-99m. J Optoelectronics Adv Mater 16(3–4):443–450

Chapter 15
Liquid Alkali Alloy for Chemothermal Therapy of Tumor

Abstract This chapter illustrated the role of alkali liquid metal in developing new generation tumor hyperthermia-chemothermal therapy. The unique merits as offered by the method were outlined. It can be found that the chemothermal therapy based on liquid alkali alloy materials owns a clinical potential to contribute to low cost, safe and effective ablation of tumors, as it can provide truly localized heating through exothermic chemical reactions, possibly even on an outpatient basis.

Keywords Liquid alkali alloy · Chemothermal tumor therapy · Liquid metal

15.1 Introduction

Liquid metals have many different forms. Some of them can be very active when exposed to air or just contact with water. A critical issue for developing liquid metal biotechnologies is to fully explore its capabilities to quickly tackle major disease such as tumor. Endeavors on such metal material have led to unconventional biomedical technology. One of such trials is on developing new generation chemothermal therapy. As gradually realized in recent years, chemothermal therapy is serving as a new hyperthermia treatment modality on tumor based on the heat released from exothermic chemical reaction between the injected reactants and the target diseased tissues. With the highly minimally invasive feature and localized heating performance, such method is expected to overcome the ubiquitous shortcomings encountered by many existing hyperthermia approaches in ablating irregular tumor. This chapter illustrates the concept and application of chemothermal therapy enabled from alkali metal, a form of liquid alloy [1]. The basic principles and unique features of alkali-metal-enabled thermal/chemical ablation are introduced. The prospects and possible challenges facing chemothermal ablation are discussed. Such liquid alkali alloy and its enabled tumor therapy are expected to open clinical possibilities for precise tumor treatment via a minimally invasive way.

J. Liu and L. Yi, *Liquid Metal Biomaterials*,
Springer Series in Biomaterials Science and Engineering10,
https://doi.org/10.1007/978-981-10-5607-9_15

In clinics, hyperthermia has long been an important tumor treatment modality, besides the classical radiotherapy and chemotherapy [2]. Different from the routinely adopted radiotherapy and chemotherapy, such method only changes the temperature of diseased tissues and induces minor side effect which wins its fame as a "Green Therapy" [3]. Up to now, a wide variety of hyperthermia approaches based on different heat generation principles have been established, such as microwave [4, 5], high intensity focused ultrasound [6, 7], radiofrequency [8, 9], magnetic fluids [10–13], laser [14–16], and hot medium [17], etc. However, the major drawbacks in these approaches lie in the cost and inevitable thermal damage to the surrounding healthy tissues along the path that heat energy is transmitted from outside to the target tumor embedded inside the human body. For a widespread clinical application of hyperthermia, two important but extremely difficult issues are (a) generation of a high enough temperature increase should be confined only within the target region (tumors) and leaving all the surrounding healthy tissues intact, and (b) temperature detection and control within as well as outside the target region should be easily available [18, 19]. Due to the irregular shapes of tumors, there is still a long way for the current hyperthermia techniques to satisfactorily address the above two issues. So for many years, there is a great need to establish a highly localized, economic, safe, efficient and powerful heating strategy for thermal ablation of tumor.

In view of these important goals, efforts were made by the present lab in recent years in exploratory researches on methodology of hyperthermia, particularly a method which can generate high enough heat energy only in the target tissue. Clearly, a promising solution to targeted heating on tumor is by exothermic chemical reaction [20]. It is well known that many chemical reactions release heat. Therefore, through choosing appropriate exothermic chemical reactants and injecting them into the target tumor, the corresponding exothermic chemical reaction could release enough heat to thermally ablate the tumor tissue [21, 22]. In such modality, only the reactant such as liquid NaK is to be injected into the tumor tissue, which would result in exothermic reaction when reacting with water in the tissue, and would thermally ablate the tumor [23]. Here, the ingredient in tumor tissue such as water also serves as the reactant for such purpose. It should be pointed out that the reaction simultaneously generates a caustic environment with a higher pH than normal tissue. However, due to the fact that only extremely small amount of liquid NaK is needed for this case, the pH value in the tissues surrounding the injection site will be not too high after treatment. Based on the above consideration, we proposed a series of exothermic-reaction-based hyperthermia methods with high intensity heat release effect on the target tissue, in which the residual reactants and resultants can be easily absorbed by human body [21–23]. Among them, the method of alkali-metal thermal/chemical ablation [23] is especially typical examples. It can ensure that high intensity heat is only released at the target tissue site but not the surrounding healthy tissues.

15.2 Basic Principle of Alkali-Metal Enabled Thermal/ Chemical Ablation

The exothermic-reaction-based hyperthermia can be defined as chemothermal therapy or ablation. This concept was first proposed by the authors' group [21–24], and subsequently, similar works were reported by other researchers [25–28]. Compared with most of the existing hyperthermia strategies, the heating involved in chemothermal therapy is highly localized which will remarkably reduce the thermal damage and mechanical trauma to the surrounding healthy tissues. This method opens the clinical possibilities for a low cost but highly efficient tumor treatment that is minimally invasive by using surgical syringes with diameter smaller than 1 mm.

A basic alkali metal ablation uses the exothermic chemical reaction between ingredient in tissue (water) and alkali metal (Na, K, or NaK) [23]. After injection or transplantation of only an extremely small amount of such metals into the target tissue, a significant temperature increase or even combustion at the target site can occur, which results in thermal ablation of the tumor. The heat generation rate of such reaction is very high. For example, mixing alkali metal of sodium with a matched amount of water would release 281.778 kJ/mol of heat, as shown by Eq. (15.1). Similar research occurs on another alkali metal: potassium (Eq. 15.2). Besides, an immediate product of the reaction, such as NaOH, KOH further contributes to the heating if dissolved in water, and further raises the temperature of the targeted tissue.

$$2\text{Na} + 2\text{H}_2\text{O} = 2\text{NaOH} + \text{H}_2 \uparrow \; + 281.778 \text{ kJ/mol} \quad (15.1)$$

$$\text{K} + \text{H}_2\text{O} = \text{KOH} + 1/2\text{H}_2 \uparrow \; + 140.008 \text{ kJ/mol} \quad (15.2)$$

As illustrated in Fig. 15.1, the above event has multi-mode therapeutic effects. Extraction of water from cells due to the hygroscopic nature of alkalis may cause damage to the tissue [29]. Alkalis also dissolve proteins of the tissues to form alkaline proteinate which is soluble and contains hydroxyl ions. These ions cause further chemical reaction and magnify injury to the diseased tissues [30]. One merit of the present method is that the remaining reactant such as Na^+ is friendly and absorbable by the living tissues, since it is a basic element of the physiological fluid. Therefore, after the thermal ablation therapy, the alkalis are expected not to cause any significant adverse effect when appropriately administered.

Figure 15.2 shows the temperature variation of an in vitro test of fresh beef using heating generated by alkali metal, in which 0.3 g of sodium was introduced into the beef. A temperature increase of about 90 °C was recorded at site A which is at the center of the reaction region. The highest temperature level during the reaction can be quickly elevated to 90 °C and then kept at above 60 °C, far higher than that required to thermally kill tumor tissue. At point B, the temperature is still kept above 40 °C during the reaction process. At points C and D, temperature elevation

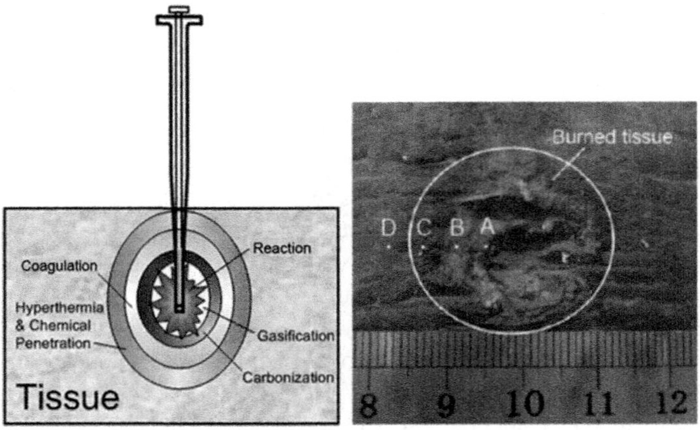

Fig. 15.1 Thermal and chemical effects on the target tissue due to exothermic chemical reaction between alkali metal and the water in the biological tissue [23]. All pictures reproduced with permission

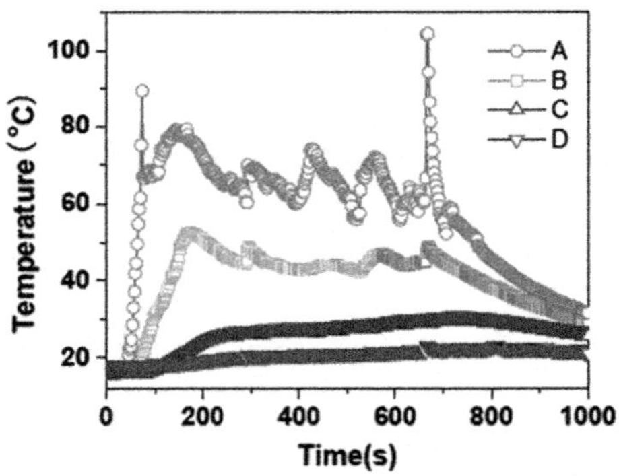

Fig. 15.2 Tissue temperature variation during reaction process [23].
Picture reproduced with permission

is however not significant. Inspection of the target tissues showed that, a nearly round area with radius of 2.5 cm had been burned. All these results were achieved through injecting only a small amount of sodium into the target site.

Considering that infrared thermometer was quite useful for monitoring the temperature field of viable tumor during the treating process, Rao et al. introduced this method to quantify the heating issues of the alkali metal ablation of tumor [31]. The colorful image allows for a clear display of the damage zone as sodium reacting with water during the treatment process. Figure 15.3 showed thermal maps of tumor surface in a BALB/c mouse before and after injection of two sodium capsules. The maps were pseudo-color images, where the respective bar gives information about color-temperature relation. Prior to sodium injection, the tumor region can be clearly differentiated from normal tissue due to lower temperature displaying

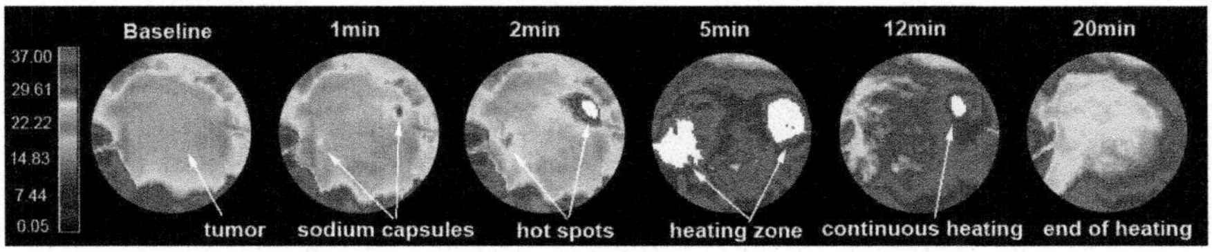

Fig. 15.3 Infrared maps on the tumor surface prior to and after sodium capsules injection over time [31] (the six cases include: prior to, 1, 2, 5, 12 and 20 min after sodium injection, respectively). The maps are pseudo-color images, the color bar at the left hand side gives information regarding the color-temperature relation. Picture reproduced with permission

in green color. Hot spots appeared when two sodium capsules were delivered into tumor. Gradually, heating zone around the sodium capsules increased with development of exothermic reaction. Heating continues for several minutes until reaction ended.

Infrared images also showed that the body temperature increase in tested mice during sodium treatment process (left vs. middle in Fig. 15.4). During this sodium exothermic reaction, the average surface temperature of tumor was raised to 34.2 ± 6.5 °C from its original 24.9 ± 1.1 °C. In addition, following a computer processing on the digital temperature data, the tumor volume was found to decrease after treatment, which can be clearly disclosed from the outer contour. The average temperature sampled over tumor masses before treatment within a 132 × 132 pixel region was significantly higher than those over the same tumor position 1 day after treatment (24.91 ± 1.14 vs. 23.48 ± 0.82).

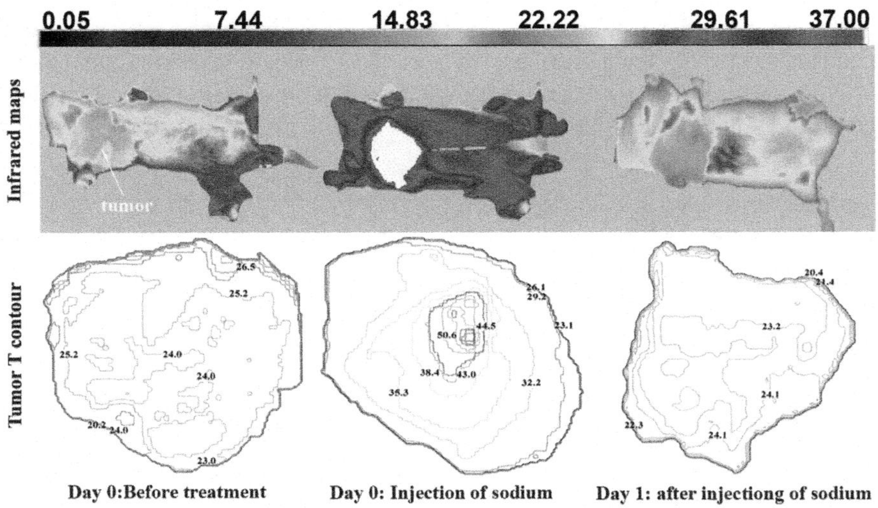

Fig. 15.4 Infrared imaging before and after sodium capsule injection, illustrating the thermal zone during treatment, and the difference of temperature distribution in tumor between before and after sodium treatment [31]. Picture reproduced with permission

15.3 Anti-tumor Effect of Alkali-Metal-Enabled Thermal/Chemical Ablation

To disclose the fundamental mechanisms of tumor treatment by the alkali-metal-enabled thermal ablation, Rao et al. conducted a series of experiment using EMT6 tumor-bearing animal model [24]. Eight mice with tumors ranging from 1.0 to 1.5 cm were randomized into four groups. Two mice in the control group were given no therapy. In the second group, two mice received intratumoral injection of 1.5 ml of NaOH solution (1 mol/l, pH = 14) at a rate of about 0.03 ml/s into the center of the tumor. In the third group, another two mice underwent sodium treatment, with 0.03 ± 0.005 g of encapsulated sodium inserted into the tumor center along the horizontal direction. In the fourth group, hyperthermia was induced by electrical heating using a needle of 2.5 mm diameter with the same thermal dosage as that in sodium treatment group (the third group). Tumor dimensions in each group were measured daily after the treatment, and the tumor volume was determined according to Carlsson formula [32]:

$$V = \frac{1}{2} a \times b^2 \tag{15.3}$$

where a is the longest diameter (mm) and b is the shortest diameter (mm). Tumor tissues at treatment site of 4 mice, one from each of the 4 groups, were resected and histologically examined by light microscopy immediately after treatment. Tumors were cut into 5 μm frozen sections and prepared for histological assessment with hematoxylin and eosin staining.

Tumor volume for each group was recorded daily after the treatment, and the results are exhibited in Fig. 15.5. Strong necrosis of tumor occurred in sodium treatment group. No significant necrosis occurred in electric heating group. On the sixth day and the tenth day, the tumor disappeared in the sodium group. Therefore, the results suggest that the chemical effect of the sodium treatment is more

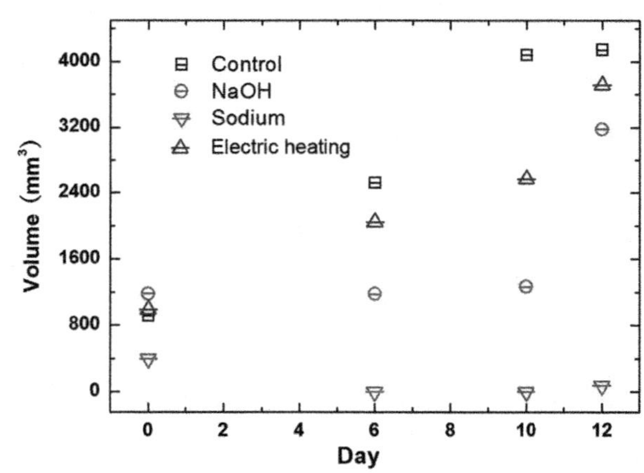

Fig. 15.5 Tumor volumes change in four groups during the 12 days after treatment. Mice in control group, NaOH group, sodium group and electric heating group underwent no treatment, intratumoral injection of NaOH solution, sodium capsule therapy and heating needle therapy, respectively [24]. Picture reproduced with permission

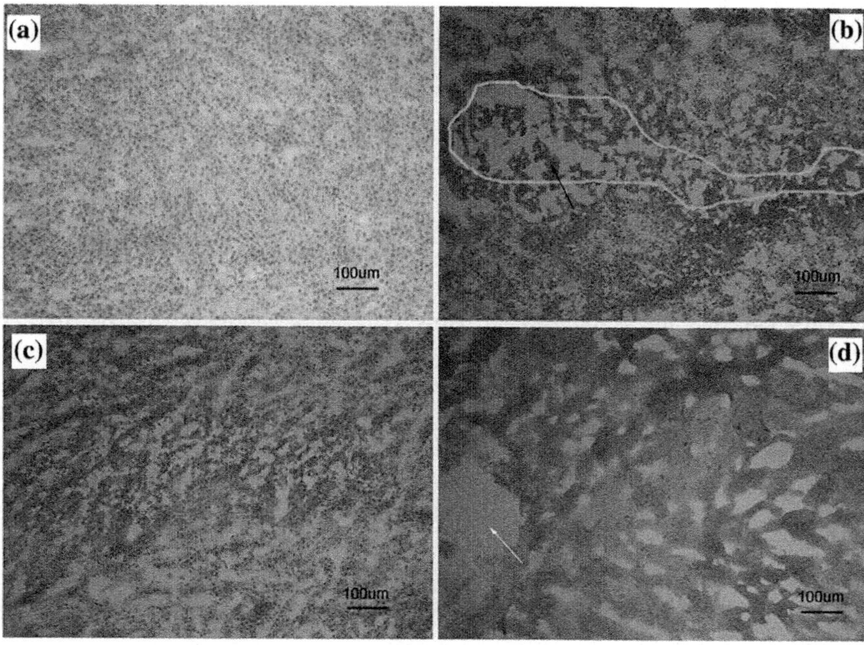

Fig. 15.6 Hematoxylin/eosin staining of EMT6 tumor immediately after treatment for the four groups. **a** The control group showed infiltrating growth trend. **b** The NaOH group showed necrotic tumor cells (marked by black arrow) and a region of necrotic tumor cells indicated by the grey line. **c** The electric heating group showed no significant change. **d** The sodium group showed cell necrosis around the injection zone indicated by the white arrow [24]. Picture reproduced with permission (Color figure online)

important than the thermal ablation effect. Figure 15.6 shows the histological images for the above four groups, respectively. Untreated tumors showed infiltrating growth trend in the control group, as shown in Fig. 15.6a. There is a partial destruction area in the group treated with NaOH solution injection, with the grey line indicating the region of necrotic tumor cells, as shown in Fig. 15.6b. In the hyperthermia group, tumors surrounding the heating site showed no evidence of cell death, as shown in Fig. 15.6c. In the sodium-treated group, the tumor cell structure completely disappeared and its nucleus was dissolved around the injection zone, as shown in Fig. 15.6d. In summary, the alkali-metal-enabled thermal ablation has a better inhibitory effect on tumor growth compared to the thermal or chemical treatment alone. Histological examination revealed complete destruction of tumor tissues, suggesting that sodium could be employed as a therapeutic agent to destroy malignant tumors.

15.4 Development Trends of Alkali Metal Enabled Thermal/Chemical Ablation

The alkali-metal-based ablation provides both thermal and chemical effects during treatment and could result in significant tumor necrosis. The heat released from the chemical reaction between alkali metal and water provides thermal ablation treatment that could be confined within the target tissues. Such heating performance, almost impossible by many advanced thermal ablation applicators, may be developed into an effective and minimally invasive tumor treatment through injecting only a small amount of alkali metal. However, safety should always be the first priority for patients and clinicians when performing such treatment. Administrating a completely safe tumor treatment puts high demand for designing such as practical device (Fig. 15.7). While reaction between bare alkali metal and tissue is rather strong and rapid, encapsulated alkali metal may provide a heat release process that can be more easily controlled, safer, and more feasible for clinical application.

Although previous results indicated that the alkali-metal-enabled thermal ablation can produce a complete necrosis around the tissues where the reactant is introduced, incomplete destruction of the malignant cells is possible due to the fact that tumor shape is usually irregular. Therefore, appropriate dosage and conformal

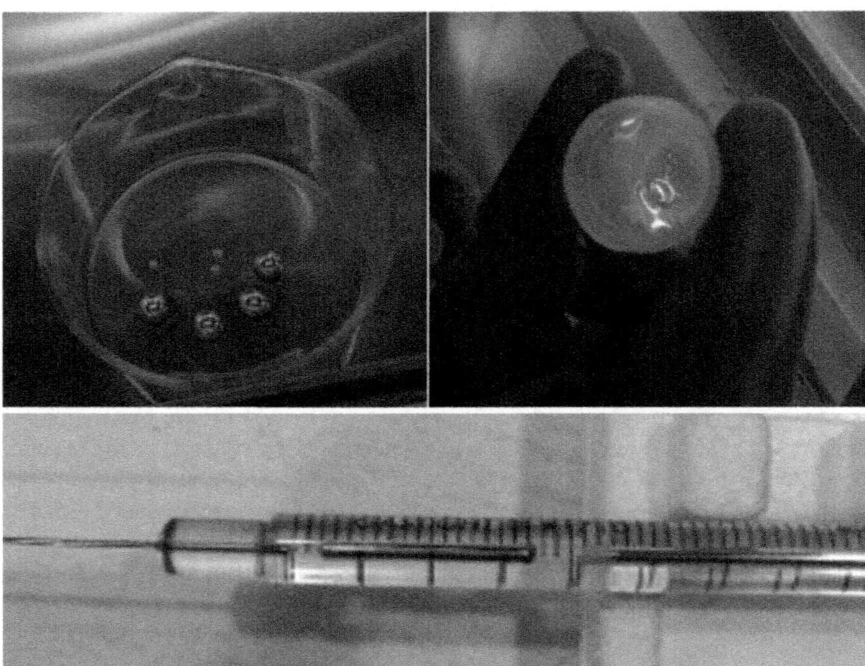

Fig. 15.7 Safe restoration of liquid NaK alloy in silicon oil (above) and a well packaged syringe with liquid alloy inside (below)

treatment is important in minimizing damage to normal tissue while maximizing tumor cell necrosis. This can be conveniently achieved by injecting reactants of alkali metal fluid such as NaK alloy into multiple regions under the guidance of a medical imaging system [33]. In addition, some commonly used temperature sensors such as thermocouples or infrared thermometer can be employed to monitor in situ the temperature hike due to heat generation by reaction between alkali metal and water in tissue.

Clearly, localized ablation using alkali metal is potentially an effective, safe and low cost way to treat malignant tumors. However, using alkali metal as chemothermal ablation agent is still at its incubating stage. Research efforts are needed both in device improvement and thermal dosage investigation in the near future.

15.5 Dosage Issue of Alkali Alloy Therapy

Although thermal ablation to kill tumor with high temperature is playing an increasingly important role in oncological clinics, hyperthermia in conjunction with other therapy usually can produce superior results compared with that of a single treatment. In many existing studies, better outcomes have been achieved with combinations of hyperthermia and radiotherapy, chemotherapy [34] or radiochemotherapy [3]. In clinical practice, hyperthermia and chemical ablation alone have been widely adopted. Attempts were also made on combining these two therapies for a better output. The exothermic-chemical-reaction-based ablation therapy could result in more significant tumor necrosis through both thermal and chemical effects. Previous results on the chemothermal therapy have demonstrated better effectiveness in tumor cell necrosis than thermal or chemical ablation alone. The fact that the heated tumor cells in alkaline environment can generate significant damage [24] also proves the chemothermal effect is not just a simple superposition of thermal effect and chemical effect; i.e., it is a synergistic effect. The underlying mechanism of the chemothermal ablation needs to be investigated. For the new chemothermal method, the emphasis still lies in that no additional surgical equipment but injection of only an extremely small amount of matched reactants is needed to achieve effective destruction of tumor.

Theoretically speaking, the kinetics of the destruction process of living tumor tissue can be described as the first-order chemical reaction process dependent on activation energy, temperature and frequency factor [34]. A generalized expression for the damage rate is given by the Arrhenius formulation:

$$\frac{d\Omega}{dt} = K = P \cdot \exp(-\frac{E_a}{RT}) \tag{15.4}$$

where Ω represents damage, t is time, K is the damage rate, P is a constant corresponding to chemical reaction frequency (1/s), E_a is the activation energy (J/mol), R is universal gas constant (J/mol K), and T is the absolute temperature (K). P and

E_a are normally determined by curve-fitting the experimental data. Since chemothermal ablation combines both effects of hyperthermia and chemical ablation, the activation energy for chemothermal ablation should be expressed as:

$$E_a = E_t + E_c \tag{15.5}$$

where E_t is activation energy reflecting thermal effect, E_c is activation energy characterizing the chemical contribution. In Eq. (15.4), P increases with E_a and is exponentially dependent on the entropy of activation [35]. As a result, the injury rate still increases with E_a, although Eq. (15.4) seemingly indicates that the injury rate decreases with E_a. The above equations explain why the anti-tumor effect of chemothermal ablation is not a linear superposition of thermal and chemical effects, but a synergy with a combined effect greater than each of the two.

The exothermic chemical reaction between acid and base (or between alkali metal and water) suggests a viable protocol for the combined thermal ablation and chemical therapy. Using the heat released from the exothermic chemical reaction, safe thermal ablation may be achieved and confined within only the target. In addition, the alkaline environment further induce a swelling of tissues with liquefied and coagulation necrosis, and hence cell death. Such performance suggests an effective and minimally invasive thermal/chemical ablation for tumor treatment. The reactants used in the chemothermal ablation during injection are at room temperature which is safe for the tissues surrounding the injection needle. Therefore, unnecessary burning injury to the healthy tissues can be avoided. The chemothermal method also allows therapeutic monitoring and guidance. Since the injected amount of the matched reactants is rather small and with no anti-electromagnetic effect, the chemothermal ablation is compatible with most routinely used clinical image devices such as MRI, ultrasound and X-CT. Injection of chemical substances may also possibly be adopted as an imaging enhancer. In future clinics, to detect in situ the heat dosage during chemothermal therapy, some common temperature sensors such as thermal couples can also be adopted for monitoring and administrating the ablation procedure.

15.6 Conclusion

This chapter illustrated the use of alkali liquid metal to develop new generation tumor hyperthermia—chemothermal therapy. It can be found that the chemothermal therapy based on such special materials has a clinical potential to contribute to low cost, safe and effective ablation of tumors, as it can provide highly localized heating through exothermic chemical reactions, possibly even on an outpatient basis. The thermal dosage of chemothermal therapy (including acid-base neutralization-reaction-enabled thermal ablation, alkali-metal-enabled thermal ablation, and possible other candidates) can easily be controllable by adjusting the amount of the alkali liquid metal and the related reactant(s). The temperature achieved by the chemothermal procedures can be monitored by common temperature sensors such as thermocouples. Different from the conventional hyperthermia strategies, the new method can combine thermal and chemical ablation via controlling the dosage of reactant. In addition, new modality of hybrid cryosurgery and hyperthermia can be developed through combining chemothermal method and any cryosurgical applicator. Moreover, it is worth exploring chemothermal procedures for treating cardiac and vascular diseases.

It should be emphasized that the newly developed chemothermal therapy is overall still at its stage of incubation and proof of clinical concept. Much research is needed (such as animal and clinical tests for safety and efficacy, development of the corresponding medical devices, and thermal dosage investigation) before possible clinical implementation.

References

1. Deng ZS, Liu J (2013) Chemothermal therapy for localized heating and ablation of tumor. J Healthc Eng 4(3):409–425
2. Liu J, Deng ZS (2008) Physics of tumor hyperthermia (in Chinese). Science Press, Beijing
3. Falk MH, Issels RD (2001) Hyperthermia in oncology. Int J Hyperth 17:1–18
4. Samaras GM, Cheung AY (1981) Microwave hyperthermia for cancer therapy. CRC Criti Rev Bioeng 5:123–184
5. Dong BW, Zhang J, Liang P et al (2003) Sequential pathological and immunologic analysis of percutaneous microwave coagulation therapy of hepatocellular carcinoma. Int J Hyperth 19:119–133
6. Madersbacher S, Pedevilla M, Vingers L, Susani M, Marberger M (1995) Effect of high-intensity focused ultrasound on human prostate cancer in vivo. Can Res 55:3346–3351
7. Cordeiro ER, Cathelineau X, Thüroff S, Marberger M, Crouzet S, Rosette J (2012) High-intensity focused ultrasound (HIFU) for definitive treatment of prostate cancer. BJU Int. https://doi.org/10.1111/j.1464-410X.2012.11262.x
8. Wood BJ, Ramkaransingh JR, Fojo T, Walther MM, Libutti SK (2002) Percutaneous tumor ablation with radio frequency. Cancer 94:443–451
9. Rossi S, Garbagnati F, Lencioni R et al (2000) Percutaneous radio-frequency thermal ablation of nonresectable hepatocellular carcinoma after occlusion of tumor blood supply. Radiology 217:119–126
10. Jordan A, Wust P, Fahling H, John W, Hinz A, Felix R (1993) Inductive heating of ferrimagnetic particles and magnetic fluids-physical evaluation of their potential for hyperthermia. Int J Hyperth 9:51–68
11. Jordan A, Scholz R, Maier-Hauff K et al (2006) The effect of thermotherapy using magnetic nanoparticles on rat malignant glioma. J Neurooncol 78:7–14
12. Moroz P, Jones SK, Gray BN (2002) The effect of tumour size on ferromagnetic embolization hyperthermia in a rabbit liver tumour model. Int J Hyperth 18:129–140
13. Haase C, Nowak U (2012) Role of dipole-dipole interactions for hyperthermia heating of magnetic nanoparticle ensembles. Phys Rev B 85:045435
14. Dai LJ, Hua GR, Qian AP, Qian ZY (2012) Investigation on local optical parameters of liver tumors in laser-induced thermotherapy. Appl Mech Mater 121–126:3998–4002
15. Vogl TJ, Straub R, Zangos S, Mack MG, Eichler K (2004) MR-guided laser-induced thermotherapy (LITT) of liver tumours: experimental and clinical data. Int J Hyperth 20:713–724

16. Lindner U, Trachtenberg J, Lawrentschuk N (2010) Focal therapy in prostate cancer: modalities, findings and future considerations. Nat Rev Urol 7:562–571
17. Honda N, Guo Q, Uchida H, Ohishi H, Hiasa Y (1994) Percutaneous hot saline injection therapy for hepatic tumors: an alternative to percutaneous ethanol injection therapy. Radiology 190:53–57
18. Roemer RB (1999) Engineering aspects of hyperthermia therapy. Annu Rev Biomed Eng 1:347–376
19. Soares PI, Ferreira IM, Igreja RA, Novo CM, Borges JP (2012) Application of hyperthermia for cancer treatment: recent patents review. Recent Pat Anti-Cancer Drug Discov 7:64–73
20. Liu J, Deng ZS, Rao W (2008) Way to ultra low cost tumor hyperthermia treatment: targeted high intensity thermochemical ablation therapy (in Chinese). Sci Technol Rev 26(2):78–84
21. Deng ZS, Liu J, Zhou YX (2006) Tumor hyperthermia method based on exothermic chemical reaction. China Patent No. 200610083646.6
22. Deng ZS, Liu J (2007) Minimally invasive thermotherapy method for tumor treatment based on an exothermic chemical reaction. Minim Invasive Ther Allied Technol 16:341–346
23. Rao W, Liu J (2008) Tumor thermal ablation therapy using alkali metals as powerful self heating seeds. Minim Invasive Ther Allied Technol 17(1):43–49
24. Rao W, Liu J, Zhou YX, Yang Y, Zhang H (2008) Anti-tumor effect of sodium-induced thermochemical ablation therapy. Int J Hyperth 24:675–681
25. Misselt AJ, Edelman TL, Choi JH, Bischof JC, Cressman EN (2009) A hydrophobic gel phantom for study of thermochemical ablation: initial results using a weak acid and weak base. J Vasc Interv Radiol 20:1352–1358
26. Cressman EN, Tseng HJ, Talaie R, Henderson BM (2010) A new heat source for thermochemical ablation based on redox chemistry: initial studies using permanganate. Int J Hyperth 26:327–337
27. Freeman LA, Anwer B, Brady RP, Smith BC, Edelman TL, Misselt AJ, Cressman EN (2010) In vitro thermal profile suitability assessment of acids and bases for thermochemical ablation: underlying principles. J Vasc Interv Radiol 21:381–385
28. Farnam JL, Smith BC, Johnson BR, Estrada R, Edelman TL, Farah R, Cressman EN (2010) Thermochemical ablation in an ex-vivo porcine liver model using acetic acid and sodium hydroxide: proof of concept. J Vasc Interv Radiol 21:1573–1578
29. Acikel C, Ulkur E, Guler MM (2001) Prolonged intermittent hydrotherapy and early tangential excision in the treatment of an extensive strong alkali burn. Burns 27:293–296
30. Mozingo DW, Smith AA, McManus WF, Pruitt BA, Mason AD (1988) Chemical burns. J Trauma 28:642–647
31. Rao W, Liu J (2008) Tumor thermal ablation therapy using alkali metals as powerful self heating seeds, unpublished report
32. Carlsson G, Gullberg B, Hafström L (1983) Estimation of liver tumor volume using different formulas—an experimental study in rats. J Cancer Res Clin Oncol 105:20–23
33. Rao W, Liu J (2009) Injectable liquid alkali alloy based tumor thermal ablation therapy. Minim Invasive Ther Allied Technol 18:30–35
34. Haaga JR, Exner AA, Wang YD, Stowe NT, Tarcha PJ (2006) Combined tumor therapy by using radiofrequency ablation and 5-FU-laden polymer implants: evaluation in rats and rabbits. Radiology 238:911–918
35. He X (2011) Thermostability of biological systems: fundamentals, challenges, and quantification. Open Biomed Eng J 5:47–73

Printed by Printforce, the Netherlands